Primary and M

Kenneth Cardona • Shishir K. Maithel
Editors

Primary and Metastatic Liver Tumors

Treatment Strategy and Evolving Therapies

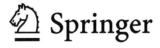
Springer

Editors
Kenneth Cardona
Division of Surgical Oncology
Winship Cancer Institute
Emory University Hospital Midtown
Atlanta, GA
USA

Shishir K. Maithel
Division of Surgical Oncology
Winship Cancer Institute
Emory University Hospital
Atlanta, GA
USA

ISBN 978-3-030-06339-9   ISBN 978-3-319-91977-5   (eBook)
https://doi.org/10.1007/978-3-319-91977-5

© Springer Nature Switzerland AG 2018
Softcover re-print of the Hardcover 1st edition 2018
This work is subject to copyright. All rights are reserved by the Publisher, whether the whole or part of the material is concerned, specifically the rights of translation, reprinting, reuse of illustrations, recitation, broadcasting, reproduction on microfilms or in any other physical way, and transmission or information storage and retrieval, electronic adaptation, computer software, or by similar or dissimilar methodology now known or hereafter developed.
The use of general descriptive names, registered names, trademarks, service marks, etc. in this publication does not imply, even in the absence of a specific statement, that such names are exempt from the relevant protective laws and regulations and therefore free for general use.
The publisher, the authors and the editors are safe to assume that the advice and information in this book are believed to be true and accurate at the date of publication. Neither the publisher nor the authors or the editors give a warranty, express or implied, with respect to the material contained herein or for any errors or omissions that may have been made. The publisher remains neutral with regard to jurisdictional claims in published maps and institutional affiliations.

Printed on acid-free paper

This Springer imprint is published by the registered company Springer Nature Switzerland AG
The registered company address is: Gewerbestrasse 11, 6330 Cham, Switzerland

Foreword

It gives me great pleasure to write a brief foreword for this book edited by two outstanding young surgical oncologists both graduates of the surgical oncology fellowship at Memorial Sloan Kettering Cancer Center. The editors set out to describe treatment modalities and strategies in the management of primary and metastatic liver tumors. They and a team of expert contributors have succeeded admirably.

There is a full consideration of anatomy, surgical and ablative therapy, regionally applied treatment, and of course radiation and medical therapy, with guidance as to the strategies of using these modalities in combination. In addition, there is extensive discussion of the place of liver transplantation in the management of liver tumors.

New and evolving approaches in diagnosis and treatment are described and lend insight into contemporary knowledge. This is no small achievement if one recognizes the many major developments that have taken place in recent years.

This volume deserves a prominent place on the bookshelves of all interested in the management of liver tumors.

L.H. Blumgart, MD, DSc(H), FRCS, FACS
Memorial Sloan-Kettering Cancer Center,
New York, NY, USA

Preface

Primary and metastatic liver tumors mandate a multidisciplinary approach to optimize patient care, requiring input from surgical, medical, radiation, and interventional specialties. Experts from each of these disciplines must work in harmony to deliver the best treatment plan, often individualized to each patient. A mastery and thorough understanding of what each specialty contributes and has to offer to each case is paramount.

To this end, *Primary and Metastatic Liver Tumors: Treatment Strategy and Evolving Therapies* brings together the expertise of the various disciplines involved in the care of patients with this disease and provides a comprehensive multidisciplinary overview and approach to patients with liver tumors. This textbook offers clinicians evidence-based, high-yield, and cutting-edge information related to the treatment of primary and metastatic liver tumors from a 360° perspective. Additionally, the text provides insight into evolving therapies and future directions within the field.

We are personally grateful and indebted to all the contributing authors. They represent a group of nationally and internationally renowned physicians within their respective fields and are the current and future leaders in their discipline. We hope that this textbook serves as a valuable resource to the practicing clinician when treating patients afflicted with liver tumors.

Atlanta, GA, USA   Kenneth Cardona
                                                                                                      Shishir K. Maithel

Contents

Part I Introduction

1. **Patient Selection and Technical Considerations**............   3
   Vasilena Zheleva, Cecilia G. Ethun, and Yuman Fong

2. **Radiographic Assessment for Liver Tumors** 15
   Daniel Fouladi, Nannan Shao, Manijeh Zarghampour,
   Ankur Pandey, Pallavi Pandey, and Ihab R. Kamel

Part II Primary Liver Tumors

3. **Liver Transplantation for Hepatocellular Carcinoma:
   The Challenge of Organ Availability**.................... 37
   Christopher Sonnenday

4. **Surgical Approach in Hepatocellular Carcinoma:
   Resection Versus Transplantation** 45
   Vikrom K. Dhar and Shimul A. Shah

5. **Locoregional Therapies in the Management
   of Hepatocellular Carcinoma**........................... 57
   Alexa O. Levey, R. Mitch Ermentrout, Zachary L. Bercu,
   and Darren D. Kies

6. **Role of Radiation Therapy in Hepatocellular Carcinoma** 73
   Emma B. Holliday, Eugene J. Koay, and Christopher H. Crane

7. **Medical Therapy Options for Advanced Disease
   in Hepatocellular Carcinoma**........................... 91
   Imane El Dika and Ghassan K. Abou-Alfa

8. **Guidelines for Resection of Intrahepatic
   Cholangiocarcinoma**.................................. 99
   Richard Tang, Nicholas Latchana, Amir A. Rahnemai-Azar,
   and Timothy M. Pawlik

9. **Regional Liver-Directed Therapies for Intrahepatic
   Cholangiocarcinoma**.................................. 111
   Nikitha Murali, Lynn Jeanette Savic, Nariman Nezami,
   Julius Chapiro, and Jean-François Geschwind

10 **Role of Radiation Therapy for Intrahepatic Cholangiocarcinoma**............................. 125
Sagar A. Patel, Florence K. Keane, and Theodore S. Hong

11 **Current and Emerging Medical Therapies for Advanced Disease in Intrahepatic Cholangiocarcinoma**... 137
Aileen Deng and Steven Cohen

12 **Pathological Classification and Surgical Approach to Hepatocellular Adenomas**............................. 153
Safi Dokmak

13 **Regional Therapies for Hepatic Adenoma**............. 169
Jack P. Silva and T. Clark Gamblin

14 **Pathologic Classification of Preinvasive Cystic Neoplasms of the Intra- and Extrahepatic Bile Ducts**.................. 177
Brian Quigley, Burcin Pehlivanoglu, and Volkan Adsay

15 **Indications for Resection of Preinvasive Cystic Neoplasms of the Intra- and Extrahepatic Bile Ducts**.................. 187
Jad Abou-Khalil and Flavio G. Rocha

Part III Metastatic Liver Tumors

16 **Patient Selection and Surgical Approach to Colorectal Cancer Liver Metastases**..................... 197
Jordan M. Cloyd and Thomas A. Aloia

17 **Ablative Techniques for Colorectal Cancer Liver Metastases** . 207
Camilo Correa-Gallego and T. Peter Kingham

18 **Hepatic Arterial Therapy for Colorectal Cancer Liver Metastases**....................................... 217
Neal Bhutiani and Robert C. G. Martin II

19 **Hepatic Artery Infusion Therapy for Colorectal Cancer Liver Metastases**............................... 233
Camilo Correa-Gallego and Michael I. D'Angelica

20 **Patient Selection and Surgical Approach to Neuroendocrine Tumor Liver Metastases**............... 243
Kendall J. Keck and James R. Howe

21 **Liver-Directed Therapies for Neuroendocrine Metastases**.... 255
Erica S. Alexander and Michael C. Soulen

22 **Systemic Therapy for the Management of Neuroendocrine Tumor Liver Metastases**............................... 267
Stephanie M. Kim and Jennifer R. Eads

23 **Patient Selection and Guidelines for Resection and Liver-Directed Therapies: Non-colorectal, Non-neuroendocrine Liver Metastases** 279
Zhi Ven Fong, George A. Poultsides, and Motaz Qadan

Part IV Evolving Therapies

24 **Liver Transplantation for Other Cancers**................. 291
Sandra Garcia-Aroz, Min Xu, and William C. Chapman

25 **Radiation Therapy for Liver Metastases** 311
Arya Amini and Karyn A. Goodman

26 **MRI-Guided Laser Ablation of Liver Tumors**.............. 323
Sherif G. Nour

27 **Hepatic Artery Infusion Therapy for Primary Liver Tumors** . 333
Matthew S. Strand and Ryan C. Fields

28 **Two-Stage Approach to Liver Resection**.................. 373
Kerollos Nashat Wanis and Roberto Hernandez-Alejandro

Index 387

Contributors

Ghassan K. Abou-Alfa, MD Memorial Sloan Kettering Cancer Center, New York, NY, USA

Weil Cornel Medical College, New York, NY, USA

Jad Abou-Khalil, MD, MSc, FRCSC Department of Surgery, The Ottawa Hospital, Ottawa, ON, Canada

Volkan Adsay, MD Department of Pathology, Koç University Hospital, Istanbul, Turkey

Erica S. Alexander, MD Department of Diagnostic Radiology, Hospital of the University of Pennsylvania, Philadelphia, PA, USA

Thomas A. Aloia, MD Department of Surgical Oncology, University of Texas MD Anderson Cancer Center, Houston, TX, USA

Arya Amini, MD Department of Radiation Oncology, University of Colorado Cancer Center, Aurora, CO, USA

Zachary L. Bercu, MD, RPVI Department of Radiology, Division of Interventional Radiology and Image-Guided Medicine, Emory University School of Medicine, Atlanta, GA, USA

Neal Bhutiani, MD Department of Surgery, Division of Surgical Oncology, University of Louisville, Louisville, KY, USA

Department of Microbiology and Immunology, University of Louisville, Louisville, KY, USA

Julius Chapiro, MD Department of Diagnostic Radiology, Yale University School of Medicine, New Haven, CT, USA

Department of Radiology and Biomedical Imaging, Yale New Haven Hospital, Yale School of Medicine, New Haven, CT, USA

William C. Chapman, MD Section of Transplantation, Division of General Surgery, Transplant Center, Department of Surgery, Washington University School of Medicine Saint Louis, Saint Louis, MO, USA

Jordan M. Cloyd, MD Division of Surgical Oncology, The Ohio State University Wexner Medical Center, Columbus, OH, USA

Steven Cohen, MD Rosenfeld Cancer Center at Abington Jefferson Health, Abington, PA, USA

Department of Medical Oncology, Sidney Kimmel Cancer Center, Thomas Jefferson University Hospital, Philadelphia, PA, USA

Camilo Correa-Gallego, MD Department of Surgery, Memorial Sloan Kettering Cancer Center, New York, NY, USA

Christopher H. Crane, MD Department of Radiation Oncology, Memorial Sloan-Kettering Cancer Center, New York, NY, USA

Michael I. D'Angelica, MD Division of Hepatopancreatobiliary Surgery, Department of Surgery, Memorial Sloan Kettering Cancer Center, New York, NY, USA

Aileen Deng, MD Sidney Kimmel Cancer Center, Thomas Jefferson University Hospital, Philadelphia, PA, USA

Vikrom K. Dhar, MD Department of Surgery, University of Cincinnati College of Medicine, Cincinnati Research in Outcomes and Safety in Surgery (CROSS), Cincinnati, OH, USA

Safi Dokmak, MD Department of HBP Surgery and Liver Transplantation, Beaujon Hospital, Clichy, France

Assistance Publique Hôpitaux de Paris, Paris, France

Jennifer R. Eads, MD Division of Hematology and Oncology, Perelman Center for Advanced Medicine, University of Pennsylvania, Philadelphia, PA, USA

Imane El Dika, MD Memorial Sloan Kettering Cancer Center, New York, NY, USA

R. Mitch Ermentrout, MD Department of Radiology, Division of Interventional Radiology and Image-Guided Medicine, Emory University School of Medicine, Atlanta, GA, USA

Cecilia G. Ethun, MD, MS Division of Surgical Oncology, Department of Surgery, Emory University School of Medicine, Atlanta, GA, USA

Ryan C. Fields, MD Department of Surgery, Alvin J. Siteman Cancer Center, Barnes-Jewish Hospital, Washington University School of Medicine, St. Louis, MO, USA

Yuman Fong, MD Department of Surgery, City of Hope National Medical Center, Duarte, CA, USA

Zhi Ven Fong, MD Codman Center for Clinical Effectiveness in Surgery, Massachusetts General Hospital and Harvard Medical School, Boston, MA, USA

Daniel Fouladi, MD Department of Radiology, Johns Hopkins, Baltimore, MD, USA

T. Clark Gamblin, MD, MBA Division of Surgical Oncology, Department of Surgery, Medical College of Wisconsin, Milwaukee, WI, USA

Sandra Garcia-Aroz, MD Section of Transplantation, Division of General Surgery, Transplant Center, Department of Surgery, Washington University School of Medicine Saint Louis, Saint Louis, MO, USA

Jean-François Geschwind, MD PreScience Labs LLC, Westport, CT, USA

Karyn A. Goodman, MD, MS Department of Radiation Oncology, University of Colorado Cancer Center, Aurora, CO, USA

Roberto Hernandez-Alejandro, MD Division of Transplantation, HPB Surgery, Department of Surgery, University of Rochester, Rochester, NY, USA

Emma B. Holliday, MD Department of Radiation Oncology, The University of Texas MD Anderson Cancer Center, Houston, TX, USA

Theodore S. Hong, MD Department of Radiation Oncology, Massachusetts General Hospital, Boston, MA, USA

James R. Howe, MD Department of General Surgery, University of Iowa Hospitals and Clinics, Iowa City, IA, USA

University of Iowa College of Medicine, Iowa City, IA, USA

Ihab R. Kamel, MD, PhD Russell H. Morgan Department of Radiology and Radiological Science, Johns Hopkins University, Baltimore, MD, USA

Florence K. Keane, MD Department of Radiation Oncology, Massachusetts General Hospital, Boston, MA, USA

Kendall J. Keck, BSE, MD Department of General Surgery, University of Iowa Hospitals and Clinics, Iowa City, IA, USA

Darren D. Kies, MD Piedmont South Imaging, Newnan, GA, USA

Stephanie M. Kim, MD Division of Hematology and Oncology, University Hospitals Seidman Cancer Center, Case Comprehensive Cancer Center, Cleveland, OH, USA

T. Peter Kingham, MD Division of Hepatopancreatobiliary Surgery, Memorial Sloan Kettering Cancer Center, New York, NY, USA

Eugene J. Koay, MD, PhD Department of Radiation Oncology, The University of Texas MD Anderson Cancer Center, Houston, TX, USA

Nicholas Latchana, MS, MD Department of Surgery, The Ohio State University Wexner Medical Center, Columbus, OH, USA

Alexa O. Levey, MD Department of Radiology, Division of Interventional Radiology and Image-Guided Medicine, Emory University School of Medicine, Atlanta, GA, USA

Robert C.G. Martin II, MD, PhD Division of Surgical Oncology, Upper Gastrointestinal and Hepato-Pancreatico-Biliary Clinic, Louisville, KY, USA

Nikitha Murali, BA Department of Diagnostic Radiology, Yale University School of Medicine, New Haven, CT, USA

Nariman Nezami, MD Department of Diagnostic Radiology, Yale University School of Medicine, New Haven, CT, USA

Department of Radiology and Biomedical Imaging, Yale New Haven Hospital, Yale School of Medicine, New Haven, CT, USA

Sherif G. Nour, MD, FRCR Interventional MRI Program, Department of Radiology and Imaging Sciences, Emory University Hospitals and School of Medicine, Atlanta, GA, USA

Divisions of Abdominal Imaging, Interventional Radiology and Image-Guided Medicine, Department of Radiology and Imaging Sciences, Emory University Hospitals and School of Medicine, Atlanta, GA, USA

Ankur Pandey, MD Russell H. Morgan Department of Radiology and Radiological Science, Johns Hopkins University, Baltimore, MD, USA

Pallavi Pandey, MD Russell H. Morgan Department of Radiology and Radiological Science, Johns Hopkins University, Baltimore, MD, USA

Sagar A. Patel, MD Harvard Radiation Oncology Program, Harvard Medical School, Boston, MA, USA

Timothy M. Pawlik, MD, MPH, PhD Department of Surgery, The Ohio State University Wexner Medical Center, Columbus, OH, USA

Burcin Pehlivanoglu, MD Department of Pathology and Laboratory Medicine, Emory University School of Medicine, Atlanta, GA, USA

George A. Poultsides, MD, MS Division of Surgical Oncology, Department of Surgery, Stanford University Medical Center, Stanford University School of Medicine, Stanford University Hospital, Stanford, CA, USA

Motaz Qadan, MD, PhD Codman Center for Clinical Effectiveness in Surgery, Massachusetts General Hospital and Harvard Medical School, Boston, MA, USA

Division of Surgical Oncology, Department of Surgery, Massachusetts General Hospital, Boston, MA, USA

Brian Quigley, MD Department of Pathology and Laboratory Medicine, Emory University School of Medicine, Atlanta, GA, USA

Amir A. Rahnemai-Azar, MD Department of Surgery, University of Washington Medical Center, Seattle, WA, USA

Flavio G. Rocha, MD Section of General, Thoracic and Vascular Surgery, Virginia Mason Medical Center, Seattle, WA, USA

Lynn Jeanette Savic, MD Department of Diagnostic Radiology, Yale University School of Medicine, New Haven, CT, USA

Department of Radiology and Biomedical Imaging, Yale School of Medicine, New Haven, CT, USA

Shimul A. Shah, MD, MHCM Division of Transplantation, Department of Surgery, University of Cincinnati College of Medicine, Cincinnati Research in Outcomes and Safety in Surgery (CROSS), Cincinnati, OH, USA

Nannan Shao, MD Russell H. Morgan Department of Radiology and Radiological Science, Johns Hopkins University, Baltimore, MD, USA

Jack P. Silva Division of Surgical Oncology, Department of Surgery, Medical College of Wisconsin, Milwaukee, WI, USA

Christopher Sonnenday, MD, MHS Department of Surgery, University of Michigan, Ann Arbor, MI, USA

Michael C. Soulen, MD Department of Radiology, Abramson Cancer Center, University of Pennsylvania, Philadelphia, PA, USA

Matthew S. Strand, MD Department of Surgery, Alvin J. Siteman Cancer Center, Barnes-Jewish Hospital, Washington University School of Medicine, St. Louis, MO, USA

Richard Tang, MD Department of Surgery, The Ohio State University Wexner Medical Center, Columbus, OH, USA

Kerollos Nashat Wanis, MD Department of Surgery, London Health Sciences Centre, Western University, London, ON, Canada

Min Xu, MD Section of Transplantation, Division of General Surgery, Transplant Center Department of Surgery, Washington University School of Medicine Saint Louis, Saint Louis, MO, USA

Manijeh Zarghampour, MD Department of Radiology, Johns Hopkins, Baltimore, MD, USA

Vasilena Zheleva, MD Department of Surgery, City of Hope National Medical Center, Duarte, CA, USA

Part I
Introduction

Patient Selection and Technical Considerations

Vasilena Zheleva, Cecilia G. Ethun, and Yuman Fong

Introduction

Hepatic resection plays a critical role in the multimodality management of various primary and secondary liver malignancies and in many cases represents the only potentially curative intervention for such diseases. Over the past few decades, we have seen considerable advancements in our locoregional and systemic therapeutic options for the treatment of hepatic malignancies, which has paralleled a breadth of technical improvements in liver surgery and which in turn has increased the number of patients who could be candidates for hepatic resection. Hence each patient with a hepatic malignancy, primary or secondary, should be carefully assessed and evaluated by a surgeon with expertise in treating hepatic tumors and discussed in a multidisciplinary care setting. When considering a patient for hepatic resection, three factors must be carefully assessed by the treating surgeon: (1) surgical fitness of the patient, (2) oncologic appropriateness, and (3) technical resectability.

V. Zheleva · Y. Fong (✉)
Department of Surgery, City of Hope National Medical Center, Duarte, CA, USA
e-mail: vzheleva@coh.org; yfong@coh.org

C. G. Ethun
Division of Surgical Oncology, Department of Surgery, Emory University School of Medicine, Atlanta, GA, USA
e-mail: cethun@emory.edu

If the patient is considered to be an appropriate surgical candidate, the hepatic resection will provide an oncological benefit, and the extent of planned resection leaves an adequate future liver remnant (FLR), practically all patients should be candidates for hepatic resection. This chapter will focus on and discuss these three factors within the context of patients with primary and secondary hepatic malignancies being considered for hepatic resection.

Surgical Fitness of Patient

Patient selection plays a crucial role in minimizing morbidity and mortality following hepatic resection. Thus, the general health status of the surgical patient and determining their ability to tolerate surgery (i.e., determine surgical fitness) are critical when assessing a patient for hepatic resection. A thorough clinical assessment of the patient consisting, but not limited to, a detailed history and physical examination, as well as any ancillary tests required to evaluate the patient's performance status, should be performed preoperatively on all patients. Pre-existing comorbidities can contribute substantially to surgical morbidity and mortality; therefore, the aim of a thorough preoperative clinical assessment should be to identify patients with prohibitive operative risks and those with manageable conditions that can be medically optimized prior to surgical resection. It is important to note that advanced age should not be considered as an absolute contraindication to surgery as hepatic resections are now routinely performed in the elderly patient.

Determining a patient's surgical fitness can be quite subjective; thus several risk indices have been developed to assist the clinician in appropriately risk-stratifying patients for surgery. Those commonly used in the perioperative setting include the American Society of Anesthesiologists (ASA) scale, the Acute Physiology and Chronic Health Evaluation (APACHE) score, the Eastern Cooperative Oncology Group (ECOG) Performance Status, the Charlson Comorbidity Index (CCI), and the Revised Cardiac Risk Index (RCRI) [1–4]. More recently, the concept of *frailty* has been introduced as an important surgical risk assessment tool, and numerous frailty scores are available to help guide the clinician in patient selection [5, 6].

Oncologic Appropriateness

What is paramount for the clinician treating patients with primary or secondary hepatic malignancies is to understand that tumor biology will ultimately dictate and determine the outcome of the patient; therefore, having an in-depth understanding of the natural history, treatment options, and oncological outcome of such tumors is crucial. The value of hepatic resection is ultimately measured by its impact on oncological outcome (i.e., survival). As part of the oncological assessment for hepatic resection, a comprehensive preoperative evaluation should be performed to assess and determine the extent of disease and ultimate tumor burden. The presence of extrahepatic disease (especially oligometastatic disease) while not an absolute contraindication to surgery must be taken into consideration and weighed against the risks and benefits of hepatic resection as part of the treatment plan—thus emphasizing the importance of discussing these cases, regardless of the extent of the disease, in a multidisciplinary setting where all therapeutic options, including surgical resection, are considered [7].

Preoperative Evaluation

A comprehensive preoperative evaluation, including but not limited to endoscopic, cross-sectional, and functional imaging, and in certain cases laparoscopy, should be performed to assess the extent of disease. More specifically, a computerized tomography (CT) scan of the chest in conjunction with either a triphasic CT scan or magnetic resonance imaging (MRI) of the abdomen and pelvis should be obtained. In certain cases, additional investigation of extrahepatic disease is warranted, and this can be ascertained with a positron emission tomography (PET) scan [8–11]. Finally, despite considerable advances in cross-sectional and functional imaging, approximately 9–36% of patients with hepatic malignancies can have occult, subradiographic metastatic disease at the time of surgery [12–16]. Thus, in order to avoid an unnecessary laparotomy, staging laparoscopy can be considered in certain, select cases [15–19].

Tumor-Related Factors

Hepatocellular Carcinoma

Hepatocellular carcinoma (HCC) is the most common primary liver tumor and the third most common cause of cancer-related death worldwide [20]. To date, surgery, either in the form of liver transplantation or hepatic resection, is considered the primary curative treatment modality for HCC—with tumor burden and degree of underlying liver dysfunction predominantly dictating which surgical intervention to pursue [21, 22]. From an oncologic standpoint, four major clinical prognostic indicators (tumor size, multifocality, vascular invasion, and extrahepatic spread) have been identified and serve as the basis for various clinical staging systems and prognostic models currently available for HCC [23, 24]. While implementation of such models (i.e., Milan Criteria, University of California Expanded Criteria) in patients undergoing liver transplantation has resulted in reproducible, favorable outcomes, these models or staging systems have not been able to predict similar, consistent outcomes in patients undergoing hepatic resection [25, 26]. Thus, translating these clinical indicators into oncologic criteria for hepatic resection has proven to be problematic.

Traditionally, tumor size has been an important predictor of outcome for patients with HCC. However, while implementation of size restrictions (i.e., Milan criteria) has been shown to be associated with improvements in outcomes in patients undergoing liver transplantation for HCC, the same cannot be said when considering patients for hepatic resection where several groups have demonstrated favorable, long-term survival following resection of large (>10 cm) HCC, thus questioning the prognostic significance of tumor size alone [27–31]. More recently, studies have demonstrated a link between tumor size and vascular invasion with increasing tumor size being associated with increasing rates of vascular invasion [29, 32, 33]. Thus, while tumor size in itself may not be a strong independent predictor and should not by itself guide surgical treatment, it is important to note that increasing tumor size may be associated with more aggressive tumor biology (i.e., vascular invasion) and should be taken into account when considering hepatic resection.

Multifocal HCC is routinely encountered in clinical practice and has independently been shown to be a strong prognostic indicator. However, the ability to determine whether the presence of multiple tumors is representative of multicentric hepatocarcinogenesis versus intrahepatic metastasis remains unclear to date [34–36]. Regardless of the underlying pathogenesis of multifocality, the presence of multiple tumors is associated with a worse prognosis when compared to similar solitary HCC tumors [24, 37, 38].

Vascular invasion, either microvascular or macrovascular, is another well-established independent prognostic factor in patients with HCC and when present has been associated with increased frequency of intrahepatic and systemic metastasis and consequently worse outcomes [23, 37–41]. Clearly, our ability to ascertain microvascular invasion in the preoperative setting is limited, and thus its importance is primarily discussed in the postoperative setting. However, the value of hepatic resection in patients with major vascular invasion identified on staging imaging remains debatable and should be considered in select cases only.

Intrahepatic Cholangiocarcinoma

Intrahepatic cholangiocarcinoma (ICC) is the second most common primary liver tumor encountered, with a rising incidence across both hemispheres [42, 43]. To date, surgical resection is the only curative treatment option for patients with ICC [44]. Similar to HCC, numerous prognostic indicators (tumor size, multifocality, vascular invasion, and extrahepatic disease) have been identified and incorporated into various clinical staging systems and nomograms in an attempt to improve upon the risk stratification and estimation of survival of patients with ICC [45–50].

The applicability of tumor size as a prognostic indicator to stratify patients with ICC remains controversial. On one hand, numerous reports have found no independent association between tumor size and survival in patients with ICC, to the point that the prognostic value of tumor size was refuted in one of the earliest proposed staging systems for ICC [45, 46, 51–53]. On the other hand, several groups have found that, while not an independent predictor of outcome, increasing tumor size is associated with an increased incidence of adverse pathological features (nodal involvement, multiple tumors, vascular invasion, and poorly differentiated tumors) [54, 55], suggesting that larger tumor size may be indicative of more aggressive tumor biology. Nonetheless, tumor size has been incorporated into the recent eighth edition of the AJCC staging system, which similar to the staging system proposed by the Liver Cancer Study Group of Japan, when stratified by size, a worse survival was associated with an increasing tumor size (T stage) [48].

Similarly, the presence of multiple tumors is a significant prognostic factor for survival in patients with ICC. Multifocal intrahepatic disease, similar to HCC, may be secondary to multicentric hepatocarcinogenesis or intrahepatic metastases, both of which have been associated with poor survival outcomes in patients with ICC

[47, 50, 52, 54, 56–58]. Thus, in patients with multifocal ICC, hepatic resection should be reserved for only select cases of patients, and alternative therapies, such as systemic chemotherapy and/or arterial-based locoregional therapies, should be considered as first-line therapy.

Colorectal Cancer Liver Metastases

With approximately 25% of patients with colorectal cancer presenting with metastatic disease and another 50% eventually developing metastases (the majority being in the liver), colorectal cancer liver metastasis (CRLM) represents the most common secondary liver malignancy encountered in clinical practice for which hepatic resection is performed [59, 60]. In patients with CRLM, hepatic resection has become the standard of care, with a 5-year survival rate exceeding 50% in recent series [61, 62].

It is important to note that only 20–25% of patients with CRLM present with *resectable* disease, and the challenge is identifying which of these patients would benefit from hepatic resection. To this end, similar to other hepatic malignancies, various prognostic factors (synchronous liver disease, primary tumor node status and histology, number and size of liver tumors, CEA level, disease-free interval, and the presence of extrahepatic disease) have been identified and incorporated into numerous clinical risk scores and nomograms in an attempt to help guide the clinician in appropriately selecting patients that would benefit from surgery for CRLM. While most studies are in agreement as to the significance of these factors and their effect on survival, no one factor has unequivocally been shown to affect outcomes [63–67].

Certainly, there is little question that patients with many risk factors do worse than patients with few. However, the line that separates the biologically resectable from the biologically unresectable patients is yet to be defined.

Technical Resectability

In regard to hepatic resection, technical resectability is primarily defined by the quantity and quality of hepatic parenchyma that will remain after resection. This is critical because the risk of major morbidity and mortality from hepatic resection is directly related to the relative volume of hepatic parenchyma preserved—the FLR. An adequate FLR is defined as two adjacent liver segments with appropriate hepatic arterial and portal venous inflow, venous outflow, and biliary drainage, which is sufficient to allow for liver regeneration and preservation of liver function in the postoperative period. Thus, hepatic tumors are considered technically resectable when a negative resection margin can be achieved via resection of all hepatic disease, and an adequate FLR will remain.

Assessment of Liver Function

Preoperative assessment of baseline liver function is a critical first step in determining whether a patient will be an appropriate candidate for hepatic resection. Hence, all patients being considered for resection should be assessed for preoperative liver dysfunction. The risk of postoperative morbidity and mortality has been shown to proportionally increase with worsening degree of hepatocellular compromise in patients with underlying liver dysfunction who are undergoing hepatic resection [68–71]. Unfortunately, assessment of liver function is not simple and can be perplexing. To date, a plethora of imaging modalities, functional studies, serum-based analyses, and predictive models exist to assess a patient's baseline hepatic function; however, no single study has been undoubtedly proven to be superior to another in terms of estimating baseline preoperative liver function or predicting postoperative hepatic insufficiency.

The Child-Turcotte-Pugh (CTP) score is a common and frequently used clinical scoring system to predict liver-related mortality in cirrhotic patients and takes into account both clinical measures and laboratory values, including presence of ascites, encephalopathy, total serum bilirubin, INR, and serum albumin [72]. Although initially developed to assess risk of death following portacaval shunt procedures, the CTP score has subsequently been studied in patients undergoing elective hepatic resection, and an elevated CTP score has been associated with increased morbidity and mortality [69, 71, 73]. Hepatic resection is thus routinely performed with acceptable morbidity and mortality in patients with a class A CTP score, but normally considered prohibitive in class B and C patients.

The model for end-stage liver disease (MELD) is another principal clinical scoring system frequently used to evaluate preoperative hepatic function and is based on a patient's bilirubin, international normalized ratio (INR), and creatinine [74]. Traditionally used to predict survival in cirrhotic patients awaiting liver transplantation, the MELD score is nowadays commonly used in assessing perioperative risk in patients undergoing major abdominal procedures, including hepatic resections [74–77]. A conservative, yet routinely referenced, MELD score of <9 is used as a cutoff score for considering a patient for hepatic resection as this score has been associated with acceptable postoperative risk in cirrhotic patients [76, 77].

An additional method of assessment of hepatic function is to assess for portal hypertension which is an indirect measurement of advanced cirrhosis. Severe portal hypertension can be characterized by the presence of splenomegaly, gastroesophageal varices, and/or thrombocytopenia (<100,000/μL). Patients with significant portal hypertension have an increased risk of mortality associated with hepatic resection and when present should be considered a contraindication to hepatic resection [33]. If the presence of portal hypertension is unclear, portal pressures can be investigated by determining transjugular hepatic vein wedge pressures—with a wedge pressure >10 mmHg defining portal hypertension and a high-risk patient [34].

Indocyanine green (ICG) clearance is an alternative assessment tool used to evaluate hepatic function in patients with chronic liver disease being considered for hepatic resection. ICG is an anionic organic dye that is selectively taken up by hepatocytes and excreted in bile and indirectly reflects hepatocyte blood flow and functional capacity. It is typically measured as a percent serum clearance at 15 min [78]. An ICG cutoff of <10% at 15 min has been reported to be safe for extended resection, a cutoff of 10–20% for hemihepatectomy, 20–30% for segmentectomy, and enucleation for those with >40% ICG clearance [79]. It is important to note that this test although widely used in Asia is only rarely performed in the United States.

Biliary Anatomy and Vascular Inflow/Outflow

Considerable improvements in our currently available cross-sectional imaging armamentarium allow for in-depth characterization of the relationship between the hepatic tumors and the hepatic vasculature (portal vein branches and hepatic veins). This characterization is critical for determination of resectability and for surgical planning. Additionally, mapping of the biliary anatomy in regard to its relationship to the hepatic tumor(s) is paramount and is also provided by current, high-quality cross-sectional imaging. Thin-cut, triphasic computed tomography and Eovist-enhanced magnetic resonance imaging (MRI) of the liver provide the clinician with such detailed characterization. When biliary obstruction is present, cholangiography may additionally help delineate extent of biliary involvement and can be obtained endoscopically, percutaneously, or with MRI.

Previously, major vascular involvement (portal vein or inferior vena cava) by the tumor was considered a contraindication to surgery, as resection of these tumors incurred significant perioperative morbidity and was associated with a worse prognosis. However, improvements in our systemic and locoregional therapeutic options for hepatic malignancies as well as our surgical technique and perioperative management of such patients have expanded our definition of resectability, and major vascular invasion is no longer seen as an absolute contraindication in select patients [80–86].

Assessment of Future Liver Remnant (FLR)

The unique ability of the liver to functionally compensate and regenerate allows for hepatic resections to be undertaken; however, the extent of resection (minor versus major) will depend heavily on the presence of underlying chronic liver disease (cirrhosis, steatosis, steatohepatitis, etc.), such that, in an otherwise healthy liver with no history or evidence of chronic liver disease, approximately 80% of the parenchymal liver volume can be removed safely with a low risk of postoperative hepatic dysfunction. Nonetheless, the segmental distribution of the liver's functional capacity is variable and not uniform from person to person [87]. Thus, appropriate of assessment of the FLR by preoperative volumetric analysis is critical, especially when considering major or extended hepatic resections. Various assessment tools and formulas are available for such situations.

Usually, the FLR is standardized to total liver volume (TLV) and is expressed as the percentage of the TLV that will remain after hepatic resection. Various methods for measuring such liver volume have been reported. One such method is using cross-sectional imaging (CT or MRI) and three-dimensional volumetry to calculate FLR volume [88–90]. However, calculation of TLV on cross-sectional imaging is not without limitations, as tumor size and number, biliary obstruction, and presence of chronic liver disease may affect true estimate of TLV.

Another method of determining TLV is to estimate the TLV using a mathematical formula based on body surface area (TLV [cm^3] = −794.41 + 1267.28 × body surface area [m^2]). A recent meta-analysis validated this method and found it to be superior to other similar formulas [91, 92].

The challenge, however, is determining if the estimated FLR is appropriate enough to maintain adequate hepatic function in a patient with underlying chronic liver disease or in someone who has had *acute* liver injury from recent systemic therapy. To date, many of the chemotherapeutic options available have been linked to some form of direct liver injury and dysfunction. Although the exact pathogenesis is not entirely understood, chemotherapy-related liver injury is a well-known entity, and increasing duration of preoperative chemotherapy (>12 weeks) has been shown to increase the risk of postoperative complications and, more specifically, hepatic dysfunction [93–100]. Thus, in patients with fibrosis or cirrhosis, the FLR volume is recommended to be at least 40–50% of TLV [101, 102]. In patients who receive short-duration preoperative chemotherapy, a FLR of at least 20–30% is adequate to undergo hepatic resection [100, 103]. However, for those receiving a prolonged course (>12 weeks) of preoperative chemotherapy, a FLR volume of at least 30% (if not 40%) is recommended in this cohort of patients [100, 104, 105].

A FLR volume ≤20% has been found to be the strongest independent predictor of postoperative liver insufficiency and a significant risk factor for postoperative hepatic dysfunction and failure [106–108]. To this end, various techniques and approaches are available to the clinician to manage the patient with an inadequate FLR with the goal of not only proceeding to hepatic resection but also minimizing postoperative hepatic dysfunction. Such techniques include portal vein embolization/ligation, two-stage hepatectomy, and associating liver partition with portal vein ligation for staged hepatectomy. These will be discussed further in detail in subsequent chapters.

Conclusion

Hepatic resection plays a critical role in the multimodality management of various primary and secondary liver malignancies and in many cases represents the only potentially curative intervention. When considering a patient for hepatic resection, three key factors must be carefully assessed by the treating surgeon: (1) surgical fitness of the patient, (2) oncologic appropriateness, and (3) technical resectability. However, as our understanding of tumor biology evolves, as operative techniques improve, as locoregional and systemic therapies grow, and as selection of patients for resection expand, the interplay between these three key factors in considering a patient for hepatic resection will be difficult to navigate, and thus one must continuously strive to improve and refine one's understanding of this complex clinical scenario.

References

1. Saklad M. Grading of patients for surgical procedures. Anesthesiology. 1941;2:281–4.
2. Oken MM, Creech RH, Tormey DC, Horton J, Davis TE, McFadden ET, Carbone PP. Toxicity and response criteria of the Eastern Cooperative Oncology Group. Am J Clin Oncol. 1982;5(6):649–55.
3. Charlson ME, Pompei P, Ales KL, MacKenzie CR. A new method of classifying prognostic comorbidity in longitudinal studies: development and validation. J Chronic Dis. 1987;40(5):373–83.
4. Goldman L, Caldera DL, Nussbaum SR, Southwick FS, Krogstad D, Murray B, Burke DS, O'Malley TA, Goroll AH, Caplan CH, et al. Multifactorial index of cardiac risk in noncardiac surgical procedures. N Engl J Med. 1977;297(16):845–50.
5. Makary MA, Segev DL, Pronovost PJ, Syin D, Bandeen-Roche K, Patel P, Takenaga R, Devgan L, Holzmueller CG, Tian J, et al. Frailty as a predictor of surgical outcomes in older patients. J Am Coll Surg. 2010;210(6):901–8.
6. Revenig LM, Canter DJ, Taylor MD, Tai C, Sweeney JF, Sarmiento JM, Kooby DA, Maithel SK, Master VA, Ogan K. Too frail for surgery? Initial results of a large multidisciplinary prospective study examining preoperative variables predictive of poor surgical outcomes. J Am Coll Surg. 2013;217(4):665–70 e661.
7. Maithel SK, Ginsberg MS, D'Amico F, DeMatteo RP, Allen PJ, Fong Y, Blumgart LH, Jarnagin WR, D'Angelica MI. Natural history of patients with subcentimeter pulmonary nodules undergoing hepatic resection for metastatic colorectal cancer. J Am Coll Surg. 2010;210(1):31–8.
8. Ramos E, Valls C, Martinez L, Llado L, Torras J, Ruiz S, Gamez C, Serrano T, Fabregat J, Rafecas A. Preoperative staging of patients with liver metastases of colorectal carcinoma. Does PET/CT really add something to multidetector CT? Ann Surg Oncol. 2011;18(9):2654–61.
9. Petrowsky H, Wildbrett P, Husarik DB, Hany TF, Tam S, Jochum W, Clavien PA. Impact of integrated positron emission tomography and computed tomography on staging and management of gallbladder cancer and cholangiocarcinoma. J Hepatol. 2006;45(1):43–50.
10. Selzner M, Hany TF, Wildbrett P, McCormack L, Kadry Z, Clavien PA. Does the novel PET/CT imaging modality impact on the treatment of patients with metastatic colorectal cancer of the liver? Ann Surg. 2004;240(6):1027–34; discussion 1026–1035.
11. Wiering B, Krabbe PF, Jager GJ, Oyen WJ, Ruers TJ. The impact of fluor-18-deoxyglucose-positron emission tomography in the management of colorectal liver metastases. Cancer. 2005;104(12):2658–70.
12. Figueras J, Valls C, Rafecas A, Fabregat J, Ramos E, Jaurrieta E. Resection rate and effect of postoperative chemotherapy on survival after surgery for colorectal liver metastases. Br J Surg. 2001;88(7):980–5.
13. Jarnagin WR, Conlon K, Bodniewicz J, Dougherty E, DeMatteo RP, Blumgart LH, Fong Y. A clinical scoring system predicts the yield of diagnostic laparoscopy in patients with potentially resectable hepatic colorectal metastases. Cancer. 2001;91(6):1121–8.
14. Jarnagin WR, Fong Y, Ky A, Schwartz LH, Paty PB, Cohen AM, Blumgart LH. Liver resection for metastatic colorectal cancer: assessing the risk of occult irresectable disease. J Am Coll Surg. 1999;188(1):33–42.
15. Rahusen FD, Cuesta MA, Borgstein PJ, Bleichrodt RP, Barkhof F, Doesburg T, Meijer S. Selection of patients for resection of colorectal metastases to the liver using diagnostic laparoscopy and laparoscopic ultrasonography. Ann Surg. 1999;230(1):31–7.
16. Goere D, Wagholikar GD, Pessaux P, Carrere N, Sibert A, Vilgrain V, Sauvanet A, Belghiti J. Utility of staging laparoscopy in subsets of biliary cancers: laparoscopy is a powerful diagnostic tool in patients with intrahepatic and gallbladder carcinoma. Surg Endosc. 2006;20(5):721–5.
17. Biondi A, Tropea A, Basile F. Clinical rescue evaluation in laparoscopic surgery for hepatic metastases by colorectal cancer. Surg Laparosc Endosc Percutan Tech. 2010;20(2):69–72.
18. Gholghesaei M, van Muiswinkel JM, Kuiper JW, Kazemier G, Tilanus HW, Ijzermans JN. Value of laparoscopy and laparoscopic ultrasonography in determining resectability of colorectal hepatic metastases. HPB (Oxford). 2003;5(2):100–4.
19. Jarnagin WR, Bodniewicz J, Dougherty E, Conlon K, Blumgart LH, Fong Y. A prospective analysis of staging laparoscopy in patients with primary and secondary hepatobiliary malignancies. J Gastrointest Surg. 2000;4(1):34–43.
20. Jemal A, Bray F, Center MM, Ferlay J, Ward E, Forman D. Global cancer statistics. CA Cancer J Clin. 2011;61(2):69–90.
21. Forner A, Llovet JM, Bruix J. Hepatocellular carcinoma. Lancet. 2012;379(9822):1245–55.
22. Jarnagin W, Chapman WC, Curley S, D'Angelica M, Rosen C, Dixon E, Nagorney D, American Hepato-Pancreato-Biliary Association, Society of Surgical Oncology, Society for Surgery of the Alimentary Tract. Surgical treatment of hepatocellular carcinoma: expert consensus statement. HPB (Oxford). 2010;12(5):302–10.
23. Vauthey JN, Lauwers GY, Esnaola NF, Do KA, Belghiti J, Mirza N, Curley SA, Ellis LM, Regimbeau JM, Rashid A, et al. Simplified staging for hepatocellular carcinoma. J Clin Oncol. 2002;20(6):1527–36.
24. Edge SB, Byrd DR, Compton CC, Fritz AG, Greene FL, Trotti A III. Liver. In: Edge SB, Byrd DR, Compton CC, Fritz AG, Greene FL, Trotti III A, editors. AJCC cancer staging manual. 7th ed. New York, NY: Springer; 2010.
25. Mazzaferro V, Regalia E, Doci R, Andreola S, Pulvirenti A, Bozzetti F, Montalto F, Ammatuna

M, Morabito A, Gennari L. Liver transplantation for the treatment of small hepatocellular carcinomas in patients with cirrhosis. N Engl J Med. 1996;334(11):693–9.
26. Mazzaferro V, Bhoori S, Sposito C, Bongini M, Langer M, Miceli R, Mariani L. Milan criteria in liver transplantation for hepatocellular carcinoma: an evidence-based analysis of 15 years of experience. Liver Transpl. 2011;17(Suppl 2):S44–57.
27. Lee NH, Chau GY, Lui WY, King KL, Tsay SH, Wu CW. Surgical treatment and outcome in patients with a hepatocellular carcinoma greater than 10 cm in diameter. Br J Surg. 1998;85(12):1654–7.
28. Ng KK, Vauthey JN, Pawlik TM, Lauwers GY, Regimbeau JM, Belghiti J, Ikai I, Yamaoka Y, Curley SA, Nagorney DM, et al. Is hepatic resection for large or multinodular hepatocellular carcinoma justified? Results from a multi-institutional database. Ann Surg Oncol. 2005;12(5):364–73.
29. Pawlik TM, Poon RT, Abdalla EK, Zorzi D, Ikai I, Curley SA, Nagorney DM, Belghiti J, Ng IO, Yamaoka Y, et al. Critical appraisal of the clinical and pathologic predictors of survival after resection of large hepatocellular carcinoma. Arch Surg. 2005;140(5):450–7; discussion 457–458.
30. Poon RT, Fan ST, Wong J. Selection criteria for hepatic resection in patients with large hepatocellular carcinoma larger than 10 cm in diameter. J Am Coll Surg. 2002;194(5):592–602.
31. Zhou XD, Tang ZY, Ma ZC, Wu ZQ, Fan J, Qin LX, Zhang BH. Surgery for large primary liver cancer more than 10 cm in diameter. J Cancer Res Clin Oncol. 2003;129(9):543–8.
32. Pawlik TM, Delman KA, Vauthey JN, Nagorney DM, Ng IO, Ikai I, Yamaoka Y, Belghiti J, Lauwers GY, Poon RT, et al. Tumor size predicts vascular invasion and histologic grade: implications for selection of surgical treatment for hepatocellular carcinoma. Liver Transpl. 2005;11(9):1086–92.
33. Tsai TJ, Chau GY, Lui WY, Tsay SH, King KL, Loong CC, Hsia CY, Wu CW. Clinical significance of microscopic tumor venous invasion in patients with resectable hepatocellular carcinoma. Surgery. 2000;127(6):603–8.
34. Li Q, Wang J, Juzi JT, Sun Y, Zheng H, Cui Y, Li H, Hao X. Clonality analysis for multicentric origin and intrahepatic metastasis in recurrent and primary hepatocellular carcinoma. J Gastrointest Surg. 2008;12(9):1540–7.
35. Morimoto O, Nagano H, Sakon M, Fujiwara Y, Yamada T, Nakagawa H, Miyamoto A, Kondo M, Arai I, Yamamoto T, et al. Diagnosis of intrahepatic metastasis and multicentric carcinogenesis by microsatellite loss of heterozygosity in patients with multiple and recurrent hepatocellular carcinomas. J Hepatol. 2003;39(2):215–21.
36. Yamamoto T, Kajino K, Kudo M, Sasaki Y, Arakawa Y, Hino O. Determination of the clonal origin of multiple human hepatocellular carcinomas by cloning and polymerase chain reaction of the integrated hepatitis B virus DNA. Hepatology. 1999;29(5):1446–52.
37. Lei HJ, Chau GY, Lui WY, Tsay SH, King KL, Loong CC, Wu CW. Prognostic value and clinical relevance of the 6th edition 2002 American Joint Committee on cancer staging system in patients with resectable hepatocellular carcinoma. J Am Coll Surg. 2006;203(4):426–35.
38. Poon RT, Fan ST. Evaluation of the new AJCC/UICC staging system for hepatocellular carcinoma after hepatic resection in Chinese patients. Surg Oncol Clin N Am. 2003;12(1):35–50, viii.
39. Llovet JM, Bustamante J, Castells A, Vilana R, Ayuso Mdel C, Sala M, Bru C, Rodes J, Bruix J. Natural history of untreated nonsurgical hepatocellular carcinoma: rationale for the design and evaluation of therapeutic trials. Hepatology. 1999;29(1):62–7.
40. Pawarode A, Voravud N, Sriuranpong V, Kullavanijaya P, Patt YZ. Natural history of untreated primary hepatocellular carcinoma: a retrospective study of 157 patients. Am J Clin Oncol. 1998;21(4):386–91.
41. Vauthey JN, Klimstra D, Franceschi D, Tao Y, Fortner J, Blumgart L, Brennan M. Factors affecting long-term outcome after hepatic resection for hepatocellular carcinoma. Am J Surg. 1995;169(1):28–34; discussion 25–34.
42. McGlynn KA, Tarone RE, El-Serag HB. A comparison of trends in the incidence of hepatocellular carcinoma and intrahepatic cholangiocarcinoma in the United States. Cancer Epidemiol Biomark Prev. 2006;15(6):1198–203.
43. Shaib YH, Davila JA, McGlynn K, El-Serag HB. Rising incidence of intrahepatic cholangiocarcinoma in the United States: a true increase? J Hepatol. 2004;40(3):472–7.
44. Dodson RM, Weiss MJ, Cosgrove D, Herman JM, Kamel I, Anders R, Geschwind JF, Pawlik TM. Intrahepatic cholangiocarcinoma: management options and emerging therapies. J Am Coll Surg. 2013;217(4):736–50 e734.
45. Nathan H, Aloia TA, Vauthey JN, Abdalla EK, Zhu AX, Schulick RD, Choti MA, Pawlik TM. A proposed staging system for intrahepatic cholangiocarcinoma. Ann Surg Oncol. 2009;16(1):14–22.
46. Okabayashi T, Yamamoto J, Kosuge T, Shimada K, Yamasaki S, Takayama T, Makuuchi M. A new staging system for mass-forming intrahepatic cholangiocarcinoma: analysis of preoperative and postoperative variables. Cancer. 2001;92(9):2374–83.
47. Wang Y, Li J, Xia Y, Gong R, Wang K, Yan Z, Wan X, Liu G, Wu D, Shi L, et al. Prognostic nomogram for intrahepatic cholangiocarcinoma after partial hepatectomy. J Clin Oncol. 2013;31(9):1188–95.
48. Yamasaki S. Intrahepatic cholangiocarcinoma: macroscopic type and stage classification. J Hepato-Biliary-Pancreat Surg. 2003;10(4):288–91.
49. Edge SB, Byrd DR, Compton CC, Fritz AG, Greene FL, Trotti A III. Intrahepatic bile ducts. In: Edge SB,

Byrd DR, Compton CC, Fritz AG, Greene FL, Trotti III A, editors. AJCC cancer staging manual. 7th ed. New York, NY: Springer; 2010.
50. Hyder O, Marques H, Pulitano C, Marsh JW, Alexandrescu S, Bauer TW, Gamblin TC, Sotiropoulos GC, Paul A, Barroso E, et al. A nomogram to predict long-term survival after resection for intrahepatic cholangiocarcinoma: an Eastern and Western experience. JAMA Surg. 2014;149(5):432–8.
51. Choi SB, Kim KS, Choi JY, Park SW, Choi JS, Lee WJ, Chung JB. The prognosis and survival outcome of intrahepatic cholangiocarcinoma following surgical resection: association of lymph node metastasis and lymph node dissection with survival. Ann Surg Oncol. 2009;16(11):3048–56.
52. de Jong MC, Nathan H, Sotiropoulos GC, Paul A, Alexandrescu S, Marques H, Pulitano C, Barroso E, Clary BM, Aldrighetti L, et al. Intrahepatic cholangiocarcinoma: an international multi-institutional analysis of prognostic factors and lymph node assessment. J Clin Oncol. 2011;29(23):3140–5.
53. Inoue K, Makuuchi M, Takayama T, Torzilli G, Yamamoto J, Shimada K, Kosuge T, Yamasaki S, Konishi M, Kinoshita T, et al. Long-term survival and prognostic factors in the surgical treatment of mass-forming type cholangiocarcinoma. Surgery. 2000;127(5):498–505.
54. Ribero D, Pinna AD, Guglielmi A, Ponti A, Nuzzo G, Giulini SM, Aldrighetti L, Calise F, Gerunda GE, Tomatis M, et al. Surgical approach for long-term survival of patients with intrahepatic cholangiocarcinoma: a multi-institutional analysis of 434 patients. Arch Surg. 2012;147(12):1107–13.
55. Spolverato G, Ejaz A, Kim Y, Sotiropoulos GC, Pau A, Alexandrescu S, Marques H, Pulitano C, Barroso E, Clary BM, et al. Tumor size predicts vascular invasion and histologic grade among patients undergoing resection of intrahepatic cholangiocarcinoma. J Gastrointest Surg. 2014;18(7):1284–91.
56. Endo I, Gonen M, Yopp AC, Dalal KM, Zhou Q, Klimstra D, D'Angelica M, DeMatteo RP, Fong Y, Schwartz L, et al. Intrahepatic cholangiocarcinoma: rising frequency, improved survival, and determinants of outcome after resection. Ann Surg. 2008;248(1):84–96.
57. Spolverato G, Kim Y, Alexandrescu S, Popescu I, Marques HP, Aldrighetti L, Clark Gamblin T, Miura J, Maithel SK, Squires MH, et al. Is hepatic resection for large or multifocal intrahepatic cholangiocarcinoma justified? Results from a multi-institutional collaboration. Ann Surg Oncol. 2015;22(7):2218–25.
58. Weber SM, Jarnagin WR, Klimstra D, DeMatteo RP, Fong Y, Blumgart LH. Intrahepatic cholangiocarcinoma: resectability, recurrence pattern, and outcomes. J Am Coll Surg. 2001;193(4):384–91.
59. Manfredi S, Lepage C, Hatem C, Coatmeur O, Faivre J, Bouvier AM. Epidemiology and management of liver metastases from colorectal cancer. Ann Surg. 2006;244(2):254–9.
60. Weiss L, Grundmann E, Torhorst J, Hartveit F, Moberg I, Eder M, Fenoglio-Preiser CM, Napier J, Horne CH, Lopez MJ, et al. Haematogenous metastatic patterns in colonic carcinoma: an analysis of 1541 necropsies. J Pathol. 1986;150(3):195–203.
61. House MG, Ito H, Gönen M, Fong Y, Allen PJ, DeMatteo RP, Brennan MF, Blumgart LH, Jarnagin WR, D'Angelica MI. Survival after hepatic resection for metastatic colorectal cancer: trends in outcomes for 1,600 patients during two decades at a single institution. J Am Coll Surg. 2010;210(5):744–52, 745–752.
62. Tomlinson JS, Jarnagin WR, DeMatteo RP, Fong Y, Kornprat P, Gonen M, Kemeny N, Brennan MF, Blumgart LH, D'Angelica M. Actual 10-year survival after resection of colorectal liver metastases defines cure. J Clin Oncol. 2007;25(29):4575–80.
63. Fong Y, Fortner J, Sun RL, Brennan MF, Blumgart LH. Clinical score for predicting recurrence after hepatic resection for metastatic colorectal cancer: analysis of 1001 consecutive cases. Ann Surg. 1999;230(3):309–18; discussion 318–321.
64. Kato T, Yasui K, Hirai T, Kanemitsu Y, Mori T, Sugihara K, Mochizuki H, Yamamoto J. Therapeutic results for hepatic metastasis of colorectal cancer with special reference to effectiveness of hepatectomy: analysis of prognostic factors for 763 cases recorded at 18 institutions. Dis Colon Rectum. 2003;46(10 Suppl):S22–31.
65. Nordlinger B, Guiguet M, Vaillant JC, Balladur P, Boudjema K, Bachellier P, Jaeck D. Surgical resection of colorectal carcinoma metastases to the liver. A prognostic scoring system to improve case selection, based on 1568 patients. Association Francaise de Chirurgie. Cancer. 1996;77(7):1254–62.
66. Rees M, Tekkis PP, Welsh FK, O'Rourke T, John TG. Evaluation of long-term survival after hepatic resection for metastatic colorectal cancer: a multifactorial model of 929 patients. Ann Surg. 2008;247(1):125–35.
67. Wei AC, Greig PD, Grant D, Taylor B, Langer B, Gallinger S. Survival after hepatic resection for colorectal metastases: a 10-year experience. Ann Surg Oncol. 2006;13(5):668–76.
68. Bruix J, Castells A, Bosch J, Feu F, Fuster J, Garcia-Pagan JC, Visa J, Bru C, Rodes J. Surgical resection of hepatocellular carcinoma in cirrhotic patients: prognostic value of preoperative portal pressure. Gastroenterology. 1996;111(4):1018–22.
69. Franco D, Capussotti L, Smadja C, Bouzari H, Meakins J, Kemeny F, Grange D, Dellepiane M. Resection of hepatocellular carcinomas. Results in 72 European patients with cirrhosis. Gastroenterology. 1990;98(3):733–8.
70. Teh SH, Nagorney DM, Stevens SR, Offord KP, Therneau TM, Plevak DJ, Talwalkar JA, Kim WR, Kamath PS. Risk factors for mortality after surgery in patients with cirrhosis. Gastroenterology. 2007;132(4):1261–9.

71. Schroeder RA, Marroquin CE, Bute BP, Khuri S, Henderson WG, Kuo PC. Predictive indices of morbidity and mortality after liver resection. Ann Surg. 2006;243(3):373–9.
72. Pugh RN, Murray-Lyon IM, Dawson JL, Pietroni MC, Williams R. Transection of the oesophagus for bleeding oesophageal varices. Br J Surg. 1973;60(8):646–9.
73. Maithel SK, Kneuertz PJ, Kooby DA, Scoggins CR, Weber SM, Martin RC 2nd, McMasters KM, Cho CS, Winslow ER, Wood WC, et al. Importance of low preoperative platelet count in selecting patients for resection of hepatocellular carcinoma: a multi-institutional analysis. J Am Coll Surg. 2011;212(4):638–48; discussion 648–650.
74. Kamath PS, Wiesner RH, Malinchoc M, Kremers W, Therneau TM, Kosberg CL, D'Amico G, Dickson ER, Kim WR. A model to predict survival in patients with end-stage liver disease. Hepatology. 2001;33(2):464–70.
75. Wiesner RH, McDiarmid SV, Kamath PS, Edwards EB, Malinchoc M, Kremers WK, Krom RA, Kim WR. MELD and PELD: application of survival models to liver allocation. Liver Transpl. 2001;7(7):567–80.
76. Teh SH, Christein J, Donohue J, Que F, Kendrick M, Farnell M, Cha S, Kamath P, Kim R, Nagorney DM. Hepatic resection of hepatocellular carcinoma in patients with cirrhosis: model of end-stage liver disease (MELD) score predicts perioperative mortality. J Gastrointest Surg. 2005;9(9):1207–15; discussion 1215.
77. Cucchetti A, Ercolani G, Vivarelli M, Cescon M, Ravaioli M, La Barba G, Zanello M, Grazi GL, Pinna AD. Impact of model for end-stage liver disease (MELD) score on prognosis after hepatectomy for hepatocellular carcinoma on cirrhosis. Liver Transpl. 2006;12(6):966–71.
78. Caesar J, Shaldon S, Chiandussi L, Guevara L, Sherlock S. The use of indocyanine green in the measurement of hepatic blood flow and as a test of hepatic function. Clin Sci. 1961;21:43–57.
79. Imamura H, Seyama Y, Kokudo N, Maema A, Sugawara Y, Sano K, Takayama T, Makuuchi M. One thousand fifty-six hepatectomies without mortality in 8 years. Arch Surg. 2003;138(11):1198–206; discussion 1206.
80. Nuzzo G, Giordano M, Giuliante F, Lopez-Ben S, Albiol M, Figueras J. Complex liver resection for hepatic tumours involving the inferior vena cava. Eur J Surg Oncol. 2011;37(11):921–7.
81. Hemming AW, Reed AI, Langham MR Jr, Fujita S, Howard RJ. Combined resection of the liver and inferior vena cava for hepatic malignancy. Ann Surg. 2004;239(5):712–9; discussion 719–721.
82. Ali SM, Clark CJ, Zaydfudim VM, Que FG, Nagorney DM. Role of major vascular resection in patients with intrahepatic cholangiocarcinoma. Ann Surg Oncol. 2013;20(6):2023–8.
83. Shi J, Lai EC, Li N, Guo WX, Xue J, Lau WY, Wu MC, Cheng SQ. Surgical treatment of hepatocellular carcinoma with portal vein tumor thrombus. Ann Surg Oncol. 2010;17(8):2073–80.
84. Wu CC, Hsieh SR, Chen JT, Ho WL, Lin MC, Yeh DC, Liu TJ, P'Eng FK. An appraisal of liver and portal vein resection for hepatocellular carcinoma with tumor thrombi extending to portal bifurcation. Arch Surg. 2000;135(11):1273–9.
85. Pesi B, Ferrero A, Grazi GL, Cescon M, Russolillo N, Leo F, Boni L, Pinna AD, Capussotti L, Batignani G. Liver resection with thrombectomy as a treatment of hepatocellular carcinoma with major vascular invasion: results from a retrospective multicentric study. Am J Surg. 2015;210(1):35–44.
86. Pawlik TM, Poon RT, Abdalla EK, Ikai I, Nagorney DM, Belghiti J, Kianmanesh R, Ng IO, Curley SA, Yamaoka Y, et al. Hepatectomy for hepatocellular carcinoma with major portal or hepatic vein invasion: results of a multicenter study. Surgery. 2005;137(4):403–10.
87. Abdalla EK, Denys A, Chevalier P, Nemr RA, Vauthey JN. Total and segmental liver volume variations: implications for liver surgery. Surgery. 2004;135(4):404–10.
88. Heymsfield SB, Fulenwider T, Nordlinger B, Barlow R, Sones P, Kutner M. Accurate measurement of liver, kidney, and spleen volume and mass by computerized axial tomography. Ann Intern Med. 1979;90(2):185–7.
89. Saito S, Yamanaka J, Miura K, Nakao N, Nagao T, Sugimoto T, Hirano T, Kuroda N, Iimuro Y, Fujimoto J. A novel 3D hepatectomy simulation based on liver circulation: application to liver resection and transplantation. Hepatology. 2005;41(6):1297–304.
90. Yamanaka J, Saito S, Fujimoto J. Impact of preoperative planning using virtual segmental volumetry on liver resection for hepatocellular carcinoma. World J Surg. 2007;31(6):1249–55.
91. Vauthey JN, Abdalla EK, Doherty DA, Gertsch P, Fenstermacher MJ, Loyer EM, Lerut J, Materne R, Wang X, Encarnacion A, et al. Body surface area and body weight predict total liver volume in western adults. Liver Transpl. 2002;8(3):233–40.
92. Johnson TN, Tucker GT, Tanner MS, Rostami-Hodjegan A. Changes in liver volume from birth to adulthood: a meta-analysis. Liver Transpl. 2005;11(12):1481–93.
93. Karoui M, Penna C, Amin-Hashem M, Mitry E, Benoist S, Franc B, Rougier P, Nordlinger B. Influence of preoperative chemotherapy on the risk of major hepatectomy for colorectal liver metastases. Ann Surg. 2006;243(1):1–7.
94. Nakano H, Oussoultzoglou E, Rosso E, Casnedi S, Chenard-Neu MP, Dufour P, Bachellier P, Jaeck D. Sinusoidal injury increases morbidity after major hepatectomy in patients with colorectal liver metastases receiving preoperative chemotherapy. Ann Surg. 2008;247(1):118–24.

95. Pawlik TM, Olino K, Gleisner AL, Torbenson M, Schulick R, Choti MA. Preoperative chemotherapy for colorectal liver metastases: impact on hepatic histology and postoperative outcome. J Gastrointest Surg. 2007;11(7):860–8.
96. Vauthey JN, Pawlik TM, Ribero D, Wu TT, Zorzi D, Hoff PM, Xiong HQ, Eng C, Lauwers GY, Mino-Kenudson M, et al. Chemotherapy regimen predicts steatohepatitis and an increase in 90-day mortality after surgery for hepatic colorectal metastases. J Clin Oncol. 2006;24(13):2065–72.
97. Kishi Y, Zorzi D, Contreras CM, Maru DM, Kopetz S, Ribero D, Motta M, Ravarino N, Risio M, Curley SA, et al. Extended preoperative chemotherapy does not improve pathologic response and increases postoperative liver insufficiency after hepatic resection for colorectal liver metastases. Ann Surg Oncol. 2010;17(11):2870–6.
98. Nordlinger B, Sorbye H, Glimelius B, Poston GJ, Schlag PM, Rougier P, Bechstein WO, Primrose JN, Walpole ET, Finch-Jones M, et al. Perioperative chemotherapy with FOLFOX4 and surgery versus surgery alone for resectable liver metastases from colorectal cancer (EORTC intergroup trial 40983): a randomised controlled trial. Lancet. 2008;371(9617):1007–16.
99. Cleary JM, Tanabe KT, Lauwers GY, Zhu AX. Hepatic toxicities associated with the use of preoperative systemic therapy in patients with metastatic colorectal adenocarcinoma to the liver. Oncologist. 2009;14(11):1095–105.
100. Shindoh J, Tzeng CW, Aloia TA, Curley SA, Zimmitti G, Wei SH, Huang SY, Mahvash A, Gupta S, Wallace MJ, et al. Optimal future liver remnant in patients treated with extensive preoperative chemotherapy for colorectal liver metastases. Ann Surg Oncol. 2013;20(8):2493–500.
101. Shirabe K, Shimada M, Gion T, Hasegawa H, Takenaka K, Utsunomiya T, Sugimachi K. Postoperative liver failure after major hepatic resection for hepatocellular carcinoma in the modern era with special reference to remnant liver volume. J Am Coll Surg. 1999;188(3):304–9.
102. Clavien PA, Petrowsky H, DeOliveira ML, Graf R. Strategies for safer liver surgery and partial liver transplantation. N Engl J Med. 2007;356(15):1545–59.
103. Kishi Y, Abdalla EK, Chun YS, Zorzi D, Madoff DC, Wallace MJ, Curley SA, Vauthey JN. Three hundred and one consecutive extended right hepatectomies: evaluation of outcome based on systematic liver volumetry. Ann Surg. 2009;250(4):540–8.
104. Azoulay D, Castaing D, Krissat J, Smail A, Hargreaves GM, Lemoine A, Emile JF, Bismuth H. Percutaneous portal vein embolization increases the feasibility and safety of major liver resection for hepatocellular carcinoma in injured liver. Ann Surg. 2000;232(5):665–72.
105. Narita M, Oussoultzoglou E, Fuchshuber P, Pessaux P, Chenard MP, Rosso E, Nobili C, Jaeck D, Bachellier P. What is a safe future liver remnant size in patients undergoing major hepatectomy for colorectal liver metastases and treated by intensive preoperative chemotherapy? Ann Surg Oncol. 2012;19(8):2526–38.
106. Abdalla EK, Barnett CC, Doherty D, Curley SA, Vauthey JN. Extended hepatectomy in patients with hepatobiliary malignancies with and without preoperative portal vein embolization. Arch Surg. 2002;137(6):675–80; discussion 671–680.
107. Ribero D, Abdalla EK, Madoff DC, Donadon M, Loyer EM, Vauthey JN. Portal vein embolization before major hepatectomy and its effects on regeneration, resectability and outcome. Br J Surg. 2007;94(11):1386–94.
108. Vauthey JN, Pawlik TM, Abdalla EK, Arens JF, Nemr RA, Wei SH, Kennamer DL, Ellis LM, Curley SA. Is extended hepatectomy for hepatobiliary malignancy justified? Ann Surg. 2004;239(5):722–30; discussion 722–730.

Radiographic Assessment for Liver Tumors

2

Daniel Fouladi, Nannan Shao, Manijeh Zarghampour, Ankur Pandey, Pallavi Pandey, and Ihab R. Kamel

Liver tumors comprising both benign and malignant entities are relatively common, sometimes difficult to diagnose, and maybe associated with significant morbidity and mortality [1]. Imaging studies play a substantial role in the management of hepatic tumors, because accurate and rapid diagnosis could lead to better outcome with less complications and improvement of patients' quality of life and overall survival [2].

Benign Hepatic Tumors

Benign hepatic tumors constitute a variety of neoplasms with different histopathological and imaging characteristics. Hepatic cyst, hepatic hemangioma, focal nodular hyperplasia (FNH), and hepatocellular adenoma are the four most common benign hepatic neoplasms. Intrahepatic biliary cystadenoma and bile duct hamartoma are less frequently seen benign hepatic tumors [3, 4].

Hepatic Cyst

There is no communication between these benign developmental lesions and the biliary tree [5]. A simple hepatic cyst appears as a homogeneous and hypoattenuating lesion on computed tomography (CT) images (Fig. 2.1a), with no enhancement after administration of intravenous (IV) contrast material [6]. Hepatic cyst can be easily diagnosed on magnetic resonance imaging (MRI), and the lesion is homogenously hyperintense on T2-weighted images (Fig. 2.1b) and hypointense on T1-weighted images. No enhancement develops after IV contrast administration (Fig. 2.1c). With intracystic bleeding, a high signal intensity with a fluid-fluid level may be seen on both T1- and T2-weighted images [6].

Hepatic Hemangioma

Hemangiomas are the most common non-cystic benign hepatic neoplasms. Depending on the imaging findings, they are categorized as typical and atypical. Typical hemangiomas comprise three distinct histological subtypes, including cavernous hemangioma, capillary hemangioma,

D. Fouladi · M. Zarghampour
Department of Radiology, Johns Hopkins,
Baltimore, MD, USA
e-mail: dfoulad1@jhmi.edu; mzargha1@jhmi.edu

N. Shao · A. Pandey · P. Pandey · I. R. Kamel (✉)
Russell H. Morgan Department of Radiology and Radiological Science, Johns Hopkins University, Baltimore, MD, USA
e-mail: nshao1@jhmi.edu; Apandey9@jhmi.edu; ppandey1@jhmi.edu; ikamel@jhmi.edu

© Springer Nature Switzerland AG 2018
K. Cardona, S. K. Maithel (eds.), *Primary and Metastatic Liver Tumors*,
https://doi.org/10.1007/978-3-319-91977-5_2

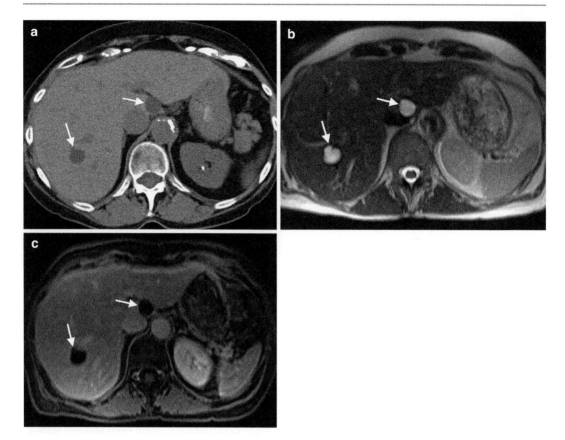

Fig. 2.1 Hepatic cysts. These are well-defined hypoattenuating lesions (arrows) on un-enhanced CT (**a**). On MRI the lesions are homogenously very hyperintense on T2-weighted image (**b**) and hypointense with no enhancement in the portal venous phase (**c**)

and sclerosed hemangioma [7]. Heterogeneously large, giant, and rapidly filling hemangiomas are three major examples in the atypical group [8, 9].

Generally, typical hemangiomas are homogeneous hyperechoic masses with well-defined margins and posterior acoustic enhancement on ultrasound (US) [7, 10]. Color Doppler US may not detect intralesional slow blood flow in a hemangioma. However, some authors have found that this modality can be useful in evaluating hepatic hemangiomas by detecting intratumoral venous signals and revealing peripheral feeding vessels, large penetrating arteries, and portal venous flow within and around hemangiomas [11–17].

The lesion is usually well defined and hypoattenuating compared to the surrounding tissue on un-enhanced CT. After administration of IV contrast material, a discontinuous, nodular, peripheral enhancement develops in the hepatic arterial phase (HAP), which progresses to more centripetal fill-in during the portal venous phase (PVP) and results in irregular fill-in and an isoattenuating or hyperattenuating appearance in the delayed phase [14]. The density of a cavernous hemangioma is the same as that of a blood vessel [7]. Capillary hemangiomas, like other typical hepatic hemangiomas, appear mildly hypodense, but sometimes they may appear isodense on noncontrast CT [18]. The kinetics of enhancement is rapid and very similar to that of the aorta, i.e., an early, homogenous intense enhancement in the HAP is usually seen [19]. The presence of hypodense focal nodular patches that correspond to sclerotic zones is the main CT feature of sclerosed hemangiomas [20].

On T2-weighted images, hepatic hemangiomas are hyperintense with a well-defined margin, but the intensity is less than that of the

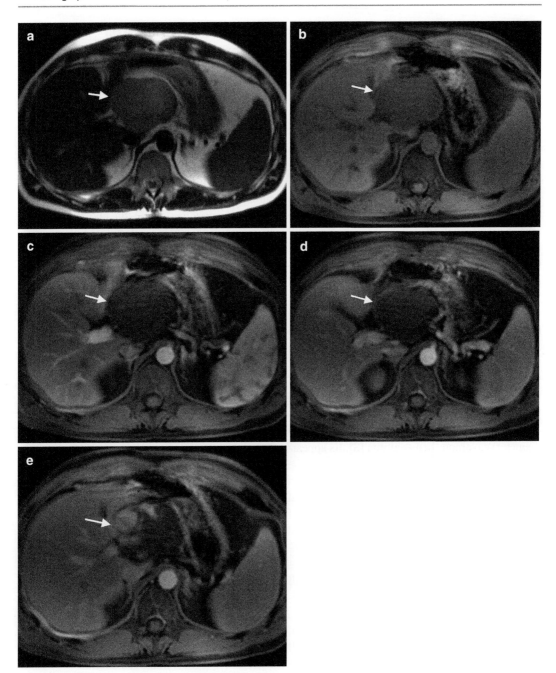

Fig. 2.2 Hepatic hemangiomas. These have a well-defined margin (arrow) and are mildly hyperintense on T2-weighted image (**a**). The lesions are hypointense on un-enhanced T1-weighted image (**b**), with gradual peripheral nodular enhancement that begins in the hepatic arterial phase (**c**) and progresses through the portal venous (**d**) and delayed (**e**) phases

cerebrospinal fluid (CSF) or a hepatic cyst (Fig. 2.2a). The lesion is generally hypointense on T1-weighted images (Fig. 2.2b). After administration of IV gadolinium, the lesion shows peripheral nodular discontinuous enhancement that progresses centripetally in the delayed phase (Fig. 2.2b–e). The contrast kinetics in capillary hemangiomas is similar to that with CT, i.e., a uniform and rapid enhancement often develops [21]. In sclerosed hemangiomas the zones of central sclerosis appear hypointense, and the overall signal of the lesion is heterogeneous on T2-weighted images. After administration of IV contrast material, a peripheral nodular enhancement develops and progresses very slowly. An early transient perilesional enhancement is a classical finding. Sometimes sclerosed hemangiomas do not enhance at all.

Large hemangiomas appear heterogeneous in US. On un-enhanced CT the lesion may be seen hypoattenuating and heterogeneous with low attenuated central areas. After administration of IV contrast material, filling is incomplete during the PVP and delayed phase. On T1-weighted images, the lesion is observed as a marginated hypointense mass containing hypointense septa and a hypointense cleft. On T2-weighted images, the internal septa remain hypointense, but the cleft is hyperintense. Enhancement is similar to that described with CT, and the internal septa and cleft remain hypointense [22, 23].

A giant hemangioma is a large (over 4 cm in diameter) cavernous hemangioma [8]. Its appearance is heterogeneous on US, with a hypodense central zone on CT. On T2-weighted images, a hyperintense lesion with a hypointense central scar is a typical finding. After administration of IV contrast material, a nodular peripheral enhancement is seen and followed by an incomplete centripetal filling [8].

Rapidly filling hemangiomas are usually small in size. Differentiating rapidly filling hemangiomas from hypervascular tumors is difficult. Although T2-weighted images may be helpful, some hypervascular tumors such as islet cell metastases also show a similar intensity on such images. The best diagnostic imaging finding is using delayed-phase CT or MR images, in which hemangiomas, unlike hypervascular metastases, remain hyperattenuating or hyperintense. Attenuation identical to that of the aorta during all phases of enhancement is another differentiating clue [8].

Focal Nodular Hyperplasia

FNH, defined as a nodule composed of normal-appearing hepatocytes in an otherwise normal liver [24], is the second most common benign hepatic tumor after hemangioma. Histopathologically, FNH is categorized into two major groups, classic (80%) and nonclassic (20%). Three key elements are present in classic FNH lesions including an abnormal nodular architecture, cholangiolar proliferation, and malformed vessels. In nonclassic type, the cholangiolar proliferation is always present, but one of the other two elements may be missing [25].

US is often not contributory for evaluating classic FNH since the lesion may be hypoechoic, isoechoic, or hyperechoic to surrounding liver parenchyma (Fig. 2.3a). When the central scar is large, the conspicuity of the lesion increases [26]. A hypoattenuated or isoattenuated lobulated homogeneous lesion is the typical finding on un-enhanced CT [26]. A hyperattenuating lesion may be seen if the background liver is fatty. After administration of IV contrast material, the entire lesion except for the central scar immediately becomes hyperattenuating in the HAP owing to the hypervascularity of the tumor. In the PVP and delayed phase, the lesion becomes more hypo-/isoattenuating compared to the liver, and the central scar may become slightly enhanced in up to 80% of cases because of the presence of abundant myxomatous stroma (Fig. 2.3b) [9, 27]. MRI is the modality of choice for detecting FNH (sensitivity, 70%; specificity, 98%) [28]. FNH lesions are slightly hyperintense or isointense on T2-weighted images (94–100%) (Fig. 2.3c), and a hyperintense central scar is evident in 84% of cases because of the presence of vascular channels, bile ductules, and edema. On T1-weighted images, FNH lesions are usually isointense or hypointense (94–100%). The central scar is also hypointense on T1-weighted images (Fig. 2.3d) [28]. With the use of gadolinium chelates, enhancement is homogenous and intense in the HAP (Fig. 2.3e), and the central scar enhances in the later phases [29]. Lesions are isointense to the liver during the PVP and delayed phases (Fig. 2.3f–g) [30–32]. The central scar demonstrates high signal intensity on delayed-phase imaging because of the accumulation of the contrast material [28].

Hepatocellular Adenoma

Using pathological and genetic features, hepatocellular adenomas (liver cell adenoma) can be classified into four distinct categories including inflammatory, hepatocyte nuclear factor 1 alpha (HNF-1a)-mutated, b-catenin-mutated, and unclassified subtypes [33, 34]. Inflammatory hepatocellular adenoma (IHA) is the most common subtype and shows the highest risk of intratumoral hemorrhage (30%) [35]. HNF-1a-mutated hepatocellular adenoma is the second most common subtype and is the most benign type of hepatocellular adenoma [36]. The b-catenin-mutated hepatocellular adenoma bears the highest risk of malignancy [37].

Grayscale US is not an accurate imaging modality for diagnosing hepatocellular adenomas, because it is neither adequately sensitive nor specific in determining the nature of liver lesions, particularly when they are small or an abnormal

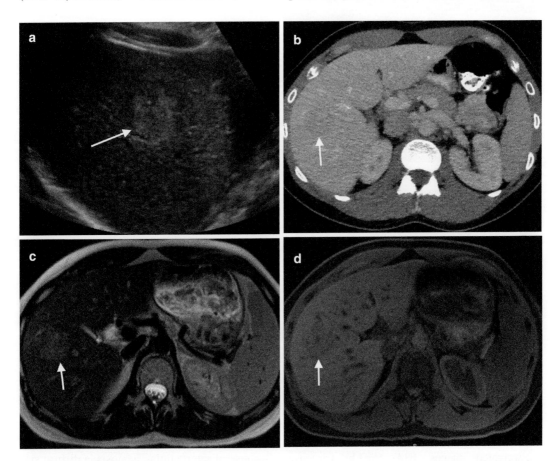

Fig. 2.3 Hepatic focal nodular hyperplasia. The lesion (arrow) is hyperechoic on grayscale ultrasonography (**a**) and is iso- to slightly hypoattenuating on delayed-phase CT (**b**). On MRI the lesion is a slightly hyperintense lesion on T2-weighted image (**c**) and slightly hypointense lesion on un-enhanced T1-weighted image (**d**) and becomes significantly hyperintense in the hepatic arterial phase (**e**). The lesion is iso- to slightly hypointense during the portal venous (**f**) and delayed (**g**) phases

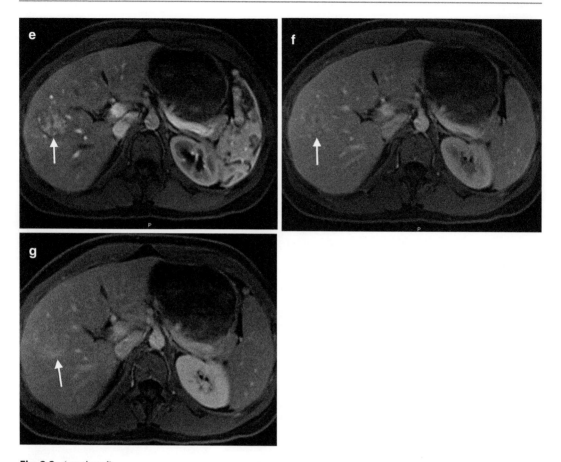

Fig. 2.3 (continued)

hepatic background further deteriorates their typical echoic or vascular profile [38].

IHAs are generally observed as nonhomogeneous hyperattenuating masses on un-enhanced CT and show enhancement similar to that in MRI when IV contrast material is administered [36]. CT is capable of depicting intracellular and intercellular lipid deposits in HNF-1a-mutated hepatocellular adenomas [39].

Multiphase dynamic contrast-enhanced MRI is the method of choice in diagnosing and subtyping hepatocellular adenomas [40]. On T2-weighted images, IHAs are hyperintense (Fig. 2.4a) with a peripheral region of hyperintensity that correlates with areas of sinusoidal dilatation (atoll sign). On T1-weighted images, IHAs are found as isointense to hyperintense hypervascular lesions with negligible heterogeneous or signal drop-off on chemical shift sequences [41, 42]. When a gadolinium-based contrast material is administered, an intense enhancement is usually present during the HAP (Fig. 2.4b) that persists in the PVP (Fig. 2.4c) and delayed phase [41, 43]. A combination of marked T2 hyperintensity and persistently delayed enhancement has been found highly sensitive (85%) and specific (87%) for the diagnosis of IHAs [41].

On T2-weighted images, HNF-1a-mutated hepatocellular adenomas show isointensity to mild hyperintensity (Fig. 2.5a) [41, 43]. Because of intercellular steatosis, a diffuse signal drop-off occurs on T1-weighted out-of-phase sequences (sensitivity, 86%; specificity, 100%) (Fig. 2.5b, c). On T1-weighted images, the lesion is isointense or hyperintense depending on the presence of fat, glycogen, or bleeding (Fig. 2.5d) [41].

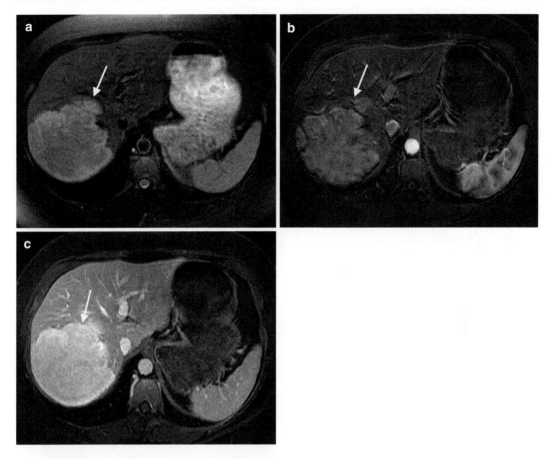

Fig. 2.4 Hepatic inflammatory adenoma. The lesion (arrow) demonstrates hyperintensity on T2-weighted image (**a**), with enhancement during the hepatic arterial (**b**) and portal venous (**c**) phases

In 35–77% of cases of HNF-1a-mutated hepatocellular adenomas, microscopic intratumoral fat deposits can be detected at MRI [44]. With using a gadolinium-based contrast material, a moderate enhancement is observed in the HAP (Fig. 2.5e) but in contrast to that in IHAs does not persist on to the PVP and delayed phase (Fig. 2.5f, g) [41].

Unclassified and b-catenin-mutated subtypes demonstrate no specific imaging feature [36, 41, 45].

Intrahepatic Biliary Cystadenoma

This cystic neoplasm can be either unilocular or multilocular. It appears as a cyst containing anechoic or hypoechoic content at US imaging. Mural nodules, papillary projections, and septal or wall calcification may be seen. The content could be hypoattenuating to hyperattenuating. Calcification of septa or cyst wall is also possible. Septal enhancement may be also present. Depending on the content of the cyst fluid, the signal intensity of intrahepatic biliary cystadenoma is variable on MR images [30, 46, 47].

Bile Duct Hamartoma

Bile duct hamartomas or von Meyenburg complexes originate from abnormally developed embryonic bile ducts [48]. In non-contrast CT, there are multiple hypoattenuating cysts distributed throughout the liver and usually are less than 1.5 cm in diameter [49, 50]. In contrast to simple

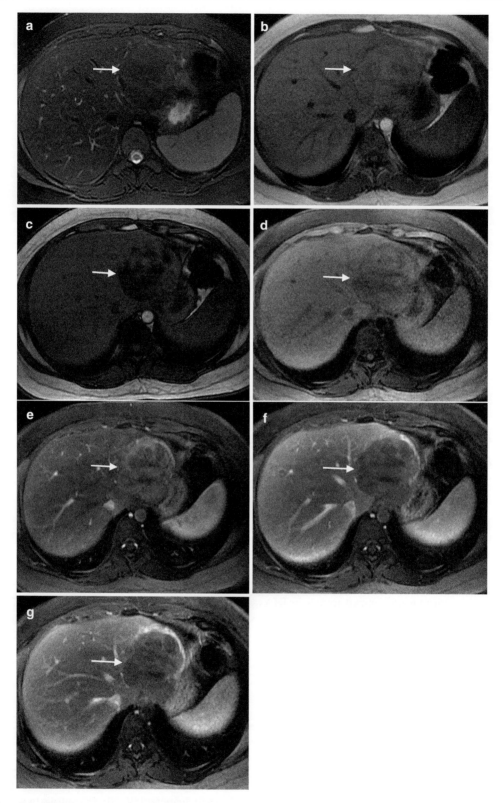

Fig. 2.5 HNF-1a-mutated hepatocellular adenoma (arrow). The lesion is isointense on T2-weighted image (**a**), with signal drop from in-phase (**b**) to out-of-phase (**c**). The lesion is iso- to hypointense on un-enhanced T1-weighted image (**d**) and shows variable enhancement in the hepatic arterial (**e**), portal venous (**f**), and delayed (**g**) phases

hepatic cysts, bile duct hamartomas show an irregular outline. No enhancement is usually seen after administration of IV contrast material [51, 52]. These cysts are hypointense on T1-weighted images and hyperintense on T2-weighted images. After administration of gadolinium, there might be homogenous enhancement or no enhancement at all. Some authors have reported a thin rim of enhancement in certain cases [5, 52].

Malignant Hepatic Tumors

Hepatic malignancies can be classified as primary and secondary (metastatic). In the primary group, tumors are pathologically of epithelial or nonepithelial origin. Major primary malignant hepatic tumors with epithelial origin in adults are hepatocellular carcinoma (HCC), intrahepatic cholangiocarcinoma (ICC), and cholangiocellular cystadenocarcinoma. The major nonepithelial tumors are lymphoma and carcinoid tumors [53]. Liver metastases are the most common hepatic malignancies [54].

Primary Malignant Hepatic Tumors

Hepatocellular Carcinoma

HCC is the most common primary hepatic cancer [55] and the third most common cause of malignancy-related death [56]. Unlike most malignancies, HCC can be diagnosed on the basis of imaging findings only because the blood supply of advanced HCC is exclusively provided by abnormal hepatic arteries, resulting in characteristic patterns after enhancement [57]. CT and MRI are very sensitive and specific modalities in detecting HCC. Generally, a diagnostic problem emerges when the lesion is small (<2 cm) [58, 59].

A small focal lesion is usually hypoechoic on US (Fig. 2.6a), whereas large lesions could be heterogeneous in echogenicity depending on the presence of fat, fibrosis, necrosis, or calcification [60]. Since the majority of cases with HCC occur in the setting of a cirrhotic liver, the diagnosis of diffuse HCCs may be difficult (cirrhotomimetic-type HCC).

A significant enhancement during the late HAP followed by a rapid washout in the PVP is the characteristic feature of HCCs on CT (Fig. 2.6b, c). Other supporting findings are internal mosaic patterns, vascular invasions, presence of fat, and documentation of a continuous lesion growth in serial images [61].

Findings are variable on T2-weighted (Fig. 2.6d) and T1-weighted (Fig. 2.6e) images depending on the presence of intratumoral fat and the intensity of the surrounding liver [62]. With the administration of gadolinium, a late arterial enhancement followed by a rapid washout is generally seen, but a persistent rim enhancement (capsule) may be observed (Fig. 2.6f–h). Since many patients with HCC are also cirrhotic, differentiating small lesions from regenerative liver nodules may be difficult. Sometimes small foci of arterial enhancement may be detected within a nodule (nodule-in-nodule appearance) [63].

Differentiating between regenerative/dysplastic nodules and early/late HCC in cirrhotic patients is difficult at un-enhanced CT or MRI. Regenerative nodules are usually isointense on un-enhanced CT and T1-weighted images, whereas dysplastic nodules and HCC lesions may be isointense, hyperintense, or hypointense. On unenhanced T1-weighted out-of-phase images, nodules except for cirrhotic ones may show signal loss, particularly if they are fatty. On unenhanced T2-weighted and diffusion-weighted (DW) images, lesion intensity is variable, but dysplastic nodules never become hyperintense. When using contrast agents in the arterial and venous phases, regenerative nodules are isointense and/or hypointense, respectively. Dysplastic lesions are often isointense or hypointense in both phases. Early HCC lesions are also predominantly isointense or hypointense, but progressed lesions are typically hyperintense and hypointense in the arterial and venous phases, respectively [56].

Fibrolamellar hepatocellular carcinoma is a clinicopathologically distinct tumor from HCCs [64]. This tumor is usually a well-circumscribed mass with mixed echogenicity and a hyperechoic center at US examination. On non-contrast CT, fibrolamellar hepatocellular carcinomas are generally large, heterogeneous, lobulated lesions with hypoattenuation [65]. In over 65% of cases, a central scar with radiating septa and bands, calcification foci (35–68%), and necrosis is present [65, 66]. The scar can be stellate or amorphous in shape [67]. After administration of IV contrast material, heterogeneous hyperattenuation in the HAP with variable patterns of enhancement during the remaining phases is a typical finding [65]. The enhancement of central scars is also variable. In over half of the cases, a significant lymphadenopathy exists predominantly in the hilum or in the hepaticoduodenal ligament [67]. Fibrolamellar hepatocellular carcinoma is usually hypointense on T1-weighted images and hyperintense on T2-weighted images [65]. The central scar is typically hypointense on both T1- and T2-weighted images. Features after administration of IV contrast material are similar to those described on CT [64].

Intrahepatic Cholangiocarcinoma

ICC or peripheral bile duct carcinoma is the second most common primary hepatic malignancy. There are several subtypes of ICCs. Intrahepatic exophytic nodular tumors (mass-forming) are often located at the periphery and have a fibrotic central portion that may lead to a capsular retraction. Periductal infiltrating intrahepatic tumors, on the other hand, are most common at the hilum

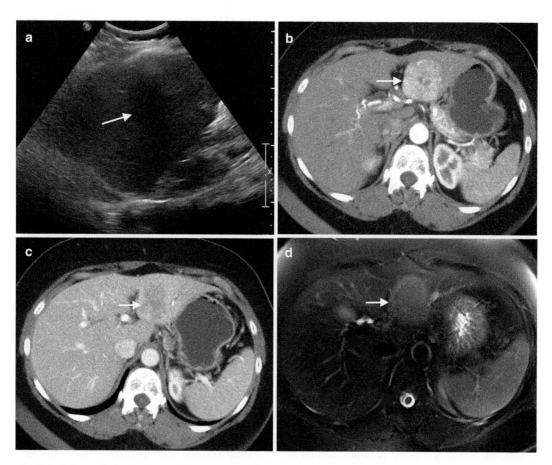

Fig. 2.6 Hepatocellular carcinoma (thick arrow). The lesion appears hypoechoic on grayscale ultrasonography (**a**). CT shows significant enhancement in the arterial phase (**b**) followed by washout in the venous phase (**c**). On MRI the lesion is slightly hyperintense on T2-weighted image (**d**), hypointense on un-enhanced T1-weighted image (**e**), with intense enhancement and central necrosis (thin arrow) in the hepatic arterial phase (**f**) followed by rapid washout during the portal venous (**g**) and delayed (**h**) phases. A capsule is visible on T1-weighted images in both the portal venous and delayed phases (dotted arrows)

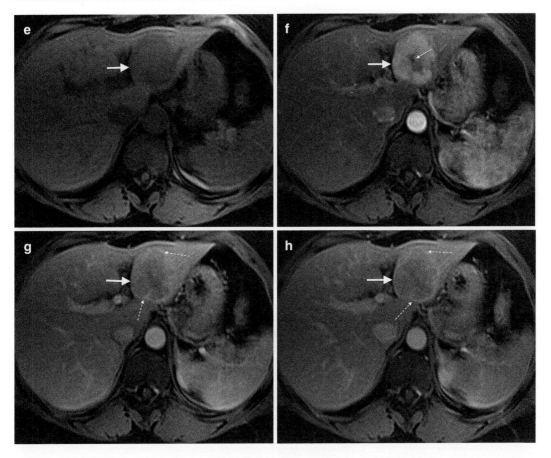

Fig. 2.6 (continued)

(Klatskin tumors) but can be found in the combination of mass-forming tumors [68]. Intraductal tumors are less frequent and are usually detected because of changes in duct caliber with or without a conspicuous mural or polypoid mass [69].

Mass-forming tumors are homogeneous lesions with intermediate echogenicity and irregular but well-defined margin, a peripheral hypoechoic rim, and capsular retractions at US [69]. Satellite (daughter) nodules are frequently seen [70]. Periductal infiltrating intrahepatic tumors are associated with narrowed/dilated bile ducts without a recognizable mass. Sometimes a diffuse bile duct thickening may be the predominant feature [69]. Intraductal tumors can be seen as diffuse duct ectasia with or without a visible papillary mass, a polypoid mass within a localized ductal dilatation, cast-like lesions within a mild ductal dilatation, or a focal stricture with mild proximal ductal dilatation. In the case of an existing polypoid mass, it is usually hyperechoic [69].

On CT, mass-forming tumors are typically homogeneous and hypoattenuating with irregular, mild heterogeneous enhancement in the periphery and gradual centripetal enhancement (Fig. 2.7a, b) [68, 69], reflecting the presence of abundant fibrotic stroma within the tumor [69]. Other features include capsular retractions, satellite nodules, distal bile duct dilation, narrowed portal veins, and regional hepatic atrophy in case of vascular invasion(s) [68–71]. The presence of periductal infiltrating tumors can be suspected when narrowed/dilated duct(s) and diffuse periductal thickening are evident, particularly at the hilum. In the peripheral liver, a combination of the periductal and mass-forming types is more frequent than a pure periductal infiltrating tumor. Detection of duct ectasia with or without

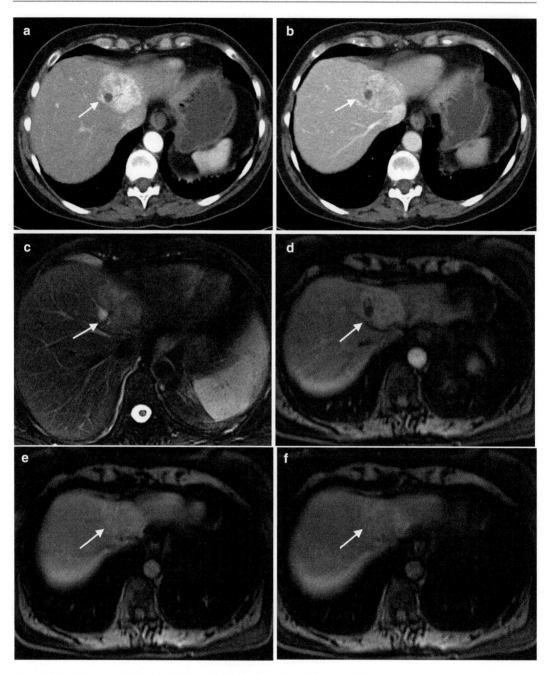

Fig. 2.7 Intrahepatic cholangiocarcinoma (arrow). CT shows heterogeneous enhancement in the hepatic arterial (**a**) and portal venous (**b**) phases. On MRI the lesion is hyperintense on T2-weighted image (**c**), with progressive enhancement in the hepatic arterial (**d**), portal venous (**e**), and delayed (**f**) phases

a polypoid mass is a sign of intraductal tumors. The wall generally appears intact. Sometimes because of copious mucin production, only a marked intrahepatic bile duct dilatation is present. The mass is hypoattenuating with enhancement after gadolinium administration [69]. Un-enhanced CT is useful for discrimination between stones and ICCs [72, 73].

MR findings are identical to those described with CT [68]. The T2-weighted images and the contrast-enhanced T1-weighted images are of particular importance in the diagnosis of ICCs [74]. Typically, lesions are hyperintense on T2-weighted images (Fig. 2.7c) and hypointense on T1-weighted images, but the latter may vary significantly on the basis of the histopathological content of the tumor, i.e., the amount of intratumoral fibrosis, necrosis, and mucin, as well as the tumor subtype. Because of hypovascularity, enhancement after administration of gadolinium may be heterogeneous or slow but progressive (Fig. 2.7d–f) [75].

Cholangiocellular (Biliary) Cystadenocarcinoma

On imaging, these rare malignant tumors are similar to their benign counterparts, i.e., biliary cystadenomas. A solitary, capsulated cystic mass with internal septa, mural nodules, polypoid projections, and capsular calcification is the most typical finding on CT [48]. The signal intensity on MR images varies depending on the presence of hemorrhage, protein content, and solid components [76, 77].

Secondary (Metastatic) Malignant Hepatic Tumors

Liver metastases are up to 40 times more common than primary hepatic tumors [78]. The most common primary malignant tumors that cause metastases to the liver are lung, breast, colon, pancreas, and melanoma [79]. Generally, metastatic lesions are multiple in number with poorly defined borders [80].

The most common features of hepatic metastases on US are hypoechogenicity (65% of cases), round well-circumscribed contours, tumor mass effect on adjacent tissue/structures, hypoechoic halo, and variable appearances such as cystic necrosis, calcification, and infiltration [81]. Calcifications are usually present in metastases from ovarian, breast, renal, lung, thyroid, and mucinous gastrointestinal tumors [80]. Cystic liver metastases are from either cystic malignancies, such as pancreatic mucinous cystadenocarcinoma and ovarian carcinoma, or solid primary lesions such as leiomyosarcoma, melanoma, carcinoid tumors, pheochromocytoma, neuroblastoma, pancreatic neuroendocrine tumor, and gastrointestinal stromal tumor [82, 83].

Hypoattenuation is the most common finding related to liver metastases on un-enhanced CT (Fig. 2.8a), reflecting glycogen scarcity or increased tumor water content. Hypodense liver metastases with intralesional amorphous calcified areas usually are primary gastric or colonic mucinous cancers [84]. After administration of contrast material, documentation of a lesser degree of enhancement compared to the surrounding tissue is a key finding, unless in fatty livers that may cause the lesions to appear iso- or even hyperattenuating compared to background liver. The pattern of enhancement is not uniform, including a dominant peripheral enhancement, central filling during the PVP, or washout in the delayed phase [85]. "Peripheral washout sign" or "peripheral low-density area sign" refers to the presence of low-density bands in the periphery of liver metastases originating from the stomach, colon, pancreas, gallbladder, and breast during the PVP or delayed phase and reflects the existence of abundant tumor cells in the peripheral areas versus coagulative necrosis and desmoplastic reactions in the central area [86]. In contrast, newer histopathological data suggest that the peripheral rim enhancement is actually related to extralesional areas with desmoplastic reactions, vascular proliferation, and inflammation [87]. Manifestations of liver metastases are variable at MRI. Generally, the lesions are hypo- to isointense on T1-weighted images (Fig. 2.8b) and iso- to hyperintense on T2-weighted images without using IV contrast material [88]. Mixed signal intensity on T1-weighted images may be present when there is intratumoral hemorrhage, necrosis, or mucin production. Rarely metastatic tumors are hyperintense on T1-weighted images, as is seen with those from pancreatic insulinoma. This rare finding has been attributed to the effects of insulin, leading to triglyceride accumulation in hepatocytes [89]. High T1 signals have also been reported with liver metastasis from colonic ade-

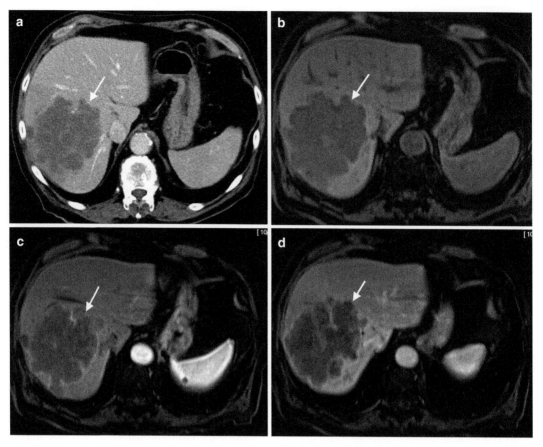

Fig. 2.8 Colorectal metastasis (arrows). These are hypodense with irregular borders on CT in the portal venous phase (**a**). On MRI these are hypointense on T1-weighted image (**b**), with rim enhancement in the hepatic arterial (**c**) and portal venous (**d**) phases

nocarcinoma, melanoma, ovarian adenocarcinoma, myeloma, and pancreatic mucinous cystadenocarcinoma because of intratumoral hemorrhage, melanin, extracellular methemoglobin, and protein content [90]. In case of intratumoral fibrosis and necrosis, the lesion may appear hypointense on T2-weighted images [84].

After IV administration of gadolinium, enhancements could be lesional or perilesional on T1-weighed images [91]. Colorectal cancer metastases may show a hyperintense peripheral halo or rim on T2-weighted images because of central necrosis, fibrin, or mucin [92–94]. The "doughnut sign" and the "target sign" are also common in metastatic lesions, generally seen on T1- and T2-weighted images, respectively. The former represents a hypointense rim surrounding an irregular or ovoid central region with lower signal intensity. The latter is composed of a rim surrounding a central area with higher signal intensity [92].

The pattern of enhancement in metastatic liver tumors also varies by the size of the lesion. In small lesions, enhancement is usually uniform, whereas in larger lesions, a transient rim enhancement tends to appear (Fig. 2.8c, d). Most liver metastases are hypovascular and hence they are best visualized during the PVP. Such tumors may show an enhancing ring during the HAP [80]. The primary malignancies with hypervascular liver metastases such as thyroid and renal cell carcinomas, pheochromocytoma, pancreatic neuroendocrine tumors, melanoma (Fig. 2.9), sarcoma, and carcinoid tumors show moderate to full enhancement during the HAP [95]. An early enhancement usually occurs in the form of a con-

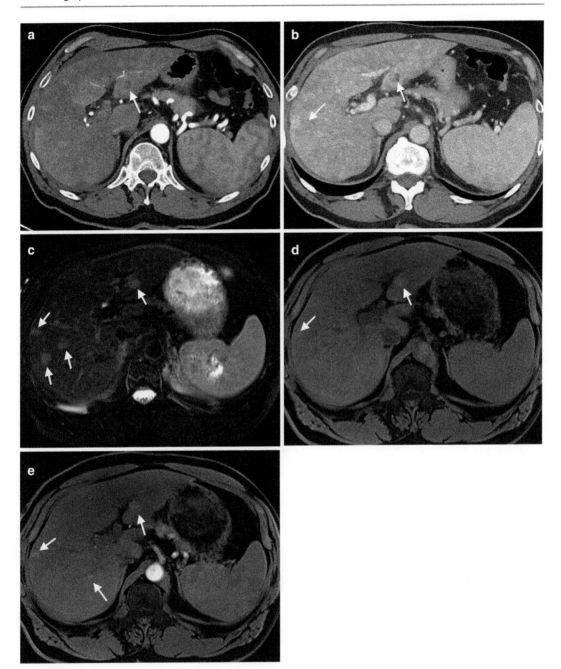

Fig. 2.9 Melanoma metastasis (arrows). These are hypointense on CT images in the arterial (**a**) and portal venous (**b**) phases. On MRI the lesions are hyperintense on T2-weighted image (**c**) and mildly hyperintense on unenhanced T1-weighted image due to the presence of melanin (**d**). The lesion demonstrates hypervascularity in the hepatic arterial phase (**e**)

tinuous rim with progressive centripetal fill-in [80]. These hypervascular metastatic lesions become iso- or hypointense during the PVP, and a peripheral washout sign (development of a hypointense peripheral rim compared to the center of the lesion) can be seen during the delayed phase [96]. Breast-liver metastases are usually hypovascular, but occasionally hypervascular cases may be encountered, as well. Of note, metastases from papillary cystic ovarian tumors do not show enhancement [78].

Hepatic metastases do not contain functioning hepatocytes. So, their intensity remains constant after using hepatobiliary contrast agents, whereas the normal liver shows a marked reduction in signal intensity, resulting in a dramatic increase in liver-to-lesion contrast [97].

References

1. Edrei Y, Gross E, Corchia N, Tsarfaty G, Galun E, Pappo O, et al. Vascular profile characterization of liver tumors by magnetic resonance imaging using hemodynamic response imaging in mice. Neoplasia. 2011;13(3):244–53.
2. Llovet JM, Bruix J. Novel advancements in the management of hepatocellular carcinoma in 2008. J Hepatol. 2008;48(Suppl 1):S20–37. https://doi.org/10.1016/j.jhep.2008.01.022.
3. Choi BY, Nguyen MH. The diagnosis and management of benign hepatic tumors. J Clin Gastroenterol. 2005;39(5):401–12.
4. Margonis GA, Ejaz A, Spolverato G, Rastegar N, Anders R, Kamel IR, et al. Benign solid tumors of the liver: management in the modern era. J Gastrointest Surg. 2015;19(6):1157–68. https://doi.org/10.1007/s11605-014-2723-x.
5. van Sonnenberg E, Wroblicka JT, D'Agostino HB, Mathieson JR, Casola G, O'Laoide R, et al. Symptomatic hepatic cysts: percutaneous drainage and sclerosis. Radiology. 1994;190(2):387–92. https://doi.org/10.1148/radiology.190.2.8284385.
6. Mathieu D, Vilgrain V, Mahfouz AE, Anglade MC, Vullierme MP, Denys A. Benign liver tumors. Magn Reson Imaging Clin N Am. 1997;5(2):255–88.
7. Klotz T, Montoriol PF, Da Ines D, Petitcolin V, Joubert-Zakeyh J, Garcier JM. Hepatic haemangioma: common and uncommon imaging features. Diagn Interv Imaging. 2013;94(9):849–59. https://doi.org/10.1016/j.diii.2013.04.008.
8. Vilgrain V, Boulos L, Vullierme MP, Denys A, Terris B, Menu Y. Imaging of atypical hemangiomas of the liver with pathologic correlation. Radiographics. 2000;20(2):379–97. https://doi.org/10.1148/radiographics.20.2.g00mc01379.
9. Lencioni R, Cioni D, Bartolozzi C, Baert AL. Focal liver lesions: detection, characterization, ablation. Milan: Springer; 2005.
10. Yu JS, Kim MJ, Kim KW, Chang JC, Jo BJ, Kim TH, et al. Hepatic cavernous hemangioma: sonographic patterns and speed of contrast enhancement on multiphase dynamic MR imaging. AJR Am J Roentgenol. 1998;171(4):1021–5. https://doi.org/10.2214/ajr.171.4.9762989.
11. Tanaka S, Kitamura T, Fujita M, Nakanishi K, Okuda S. Color Doppler flow imaging of liver tumors. AJR Am J Roentgenol. 1990;154(3):509–14. https://doi.org/10.2214/ajr.154.3.2154912.
12. Perkins AB, Imam K, Smith WJ, Cronan JJ. Color and power Doppler sonography of liver hemangiomas: a dream unfulfilled? J Clin Ultrasound. 2000;28(4):159–65.
13. Nino-Murcia M, Ralls PW, Jeffrey RB Jr, Johnson M. Color flow Doppler characterization of focal hepatic lesions. AJR Am J Roentgenol. 1992;159(6):1195–7. https://doi.org/10.2214/ajr.159.6.1332456.
14. Yamashita Y, Ogata I, Urata J, Takahashi M. Cavernous hemangioma of the liver: pathologic correlation with dynamic CT findings. Radiology. 1997;203(1):121–5. https://doi.org/10.1148/radiology.203.1.9122378.
15. Hanafusa K, Ohashi I, Himeno Y, Suzuki S, Shibuya H. Hepatic hemangioma: findings with two-phase CT. Radiology. 1995;196(2):465–9. https://doi.org/10.1148/radiology.196.2.7617862.
16. Kim KW, Kim TK, Han JK, Kim AY, Lee HJ, Choi BI. Hepatic hemangiomas with arterioportal shunt: findings at two-phase CT. Radiology. 2001;219(3):707–11. https://doi.org/10.1148/radiology.219.3.r01ma05707.
17. Naganuma H, Ishida H, Konno K, Hamashima Y, Komatsuda T, Ishida J, et al. Hepatic hemangioma with arterioportal shunts. Abdom Imaging. 1999;24(1):42–6.
18. Kim T, Federle MP, Baron RL, Peterson MS, Kawamori Y. Discrimination of small hepatic hemangiomas from hypervascular malignant tumors smaller than 3 cm with three-phase helical CT. Radiology. 2001;219(3):699–706. https://doi.org/10.1148/radiology.219.3.r01jn45699.
19. Caseiro-Alves F, Brito J, Araujo AE, Belo-Soares P, Rodrigues H, Cipriano A, et al. Liver haemangioma: common and uncommon findings and how to improve the differential diagnosis. Eur Radiol. 2007;17(6):1544–54. https://doi.org/10.1007/s00330-006-0503-z.
20. Shim KS, Suh JM, Yang YS, Kim JG, Kang SJ, Jeon JS, et al. Sclerosis of hepatic cavernous hemangioma: CT findings and pathologic correlation. J Korean Med Sci. 1995;10(4):294–7. https://doi.org/10.3346/jkms.1995.10.4.294.
21. Semelka RC, Brown ED, Ascher SM, Patt RH, Bagley AS, Li W, et al. Hepatic hemangiomas: a multi-institutional study of appearance on T2-weighted and serial gadolinium-enhanced gradient-echo MR images. Radiology. 1994;192(2):401–6. https://doi.org/10.1148/radiology.192.2.8029404.
22. Soyer P, Dufresne AC, Somveille E, Scherrer A. Hepatic cavernous hemangioma: appearance on T2-weighted fast spin-echo MR imaging with and without fat suppression. AJR Am J Roentgenol. 1997;168(2):461–5. https://doi.org/10.2214/ajr.168.2.9016227.
23. Choi BI, Han MC, Park JH, Kim SH, Han MH, Kim CW. Giant cavernous hemangioma of the liver: CT and MR imaging in 10 cases. AJR Am J Roentgenol. 1989;152(6):1221–6. https://doi.org/10.2214/ajr.152.6.1221.

24. International Working Party. Terminology of nodular hepatocellular lesions. Hepatology. 1995;22(3):983–93.
25. Nguyen BN, Flejou JF, Terris B, Belghiti J, Degott C. Focal nodular hyperplasia of the liver: a comprehensive pathologic study of 305 lesions and recognition of new histologic forms. Am J Surg Pathol. 1999;23(12):1441–54.
26. Shirkhoda A, Farah MC, Bernacki E, Madrazo B, Roberts J. Hepatic focal nodular hyperplasia: CT and sonographic spectrum. Abdom Imaging. 1994;19(1):34–8.
27. Shamsi K, De Schepper A, Degryse H, Deckers F. Focal nodular hyperplasia of the liver: radiologic findings. Abdom Imaging. 1993;18(1):32–8.
28. Mortele KJ, Praet M, Van Vlierberghe H, Kunnen M, Ros PR. CT and MR imaging findings in focal nodular hyperplasia of the liver: radiologic-pathologic correlation. AJR Am J Roentgenol. 2000;175(3):687–92. https://doi.org/10.2214/ajr.175.3.1750687.
29. Hussain SM, Terkivatan T, Zondervan PE, Lanjouw E, de Rave S, Ijzermans JN, et al. Focal nodular hyperplasia: findings at state-of-the-art MR imaging, US, CT, and pathologic analysis. Radiographics. 2004;24(1):3–17. ; discussion 8–9. https://doi.org/10.1148/rg.241035050.
30. Horton KM, Bluemke DA, Hruban RH, Soyer P, Fishman EK. CT and MR imaging of benign hepatic and biliary tumors. Radiographics. 1999;19(2):431–51. https://doi.org/10.1148/radiographics.19.2.g99mr04431.
31. Seale MK, Catalano OA, Saini S, Hahn PF, Sahani DV. Hepatobiliary-specific MR contrast agents: role in imaging the liver and biliary tree. Radiographics. 2009;29(6):1725–48. https://doi.org/10.1148/rg.296095515.
32. Mortele KJ, Praet M, Van Vlierberghe H, de Hemptinne B, Zou K, Ros PR. Focal nodular hyperplasia of the liver: detection and characterization with plain and dynamic-enhanced MRI. Abdom Imaging. 2002;27(6):700–7. https://doi.org/10.1007/s00261-001-0140-6.
33. Bioulac-Sage P, Rebouissou S, Thomas C, Blanc JF, Saric J, Sa Cunha A, et al. Hepatocellular adenoma subtype classification using molecular markers and immunohistochemistry. Hepatology. 2007;46(3):740–8. https://doi.org/10.1002/hep.21743.
34. Thomeer MG, ME EB, de Lussanet Q, Biermann K, Dwarkasing RS, de Man R, et al. Genotype-phenotype correlations in hepatocellular adenoma: an update of MRI findings. Diagn Interv Radiol. 2014;20(3):193–9. https://doi.org/10.5152/dir.2013.13315.
35. Bioulac-Sage P, Balabaud C, Zucman-Rossi J. Subtype classification of hepatocellular adenoma. Dig Surg. 2010;27(1):39–45. https://doi.org/10.1159/000268406.
36. Katabathina VS, Menias CO, Shanbhogue AK, Jagirdar J, Paspulati RM, Prasad SR. Genetics and imaging of hepatocellular adenomas: 2011 update. Radiographics. 2011;31(6):1529–43. https://doi.org/10.1148/rg.316115527.
37. Farges O, Dokmak S. Malignant transformation of liver adenoma: an analysis of the literature. Dig Surg. 2010;27(1):32–8. https://doi.org/10.1159/000268405.
38. Xu HX, Liu GJ, Lu MD, Xie XY, Xu ZF, Zheng YL, et al. Characterization of small focal liver lesions using real-time contrast-enhanced sonography: diagnostic performance analysis in 200 patients. J Ultrasound Med. 2006;25(3):349–61.
39. Prasad SR, Wang H, Rosas H, Menias CO, Narra VR, Middleton WD, et al. Fat-containing lesions of the liver: radiologic-pathologic correlation. Radiographics. 2005;25(2):321–31. https://doi.org/10.1148/rg.252045083.
40. Agrawal S, Agarwal S, Arnason T, Saini S, Belghiti J. Management of hepatocellular adenoma: recent advances. Clin Gastroenterol Hepatol. 2015;13(7):1221–30. https://doi.org/10.1016/j.cgh.2014.05.023.
41. Laumonier H, Bioulac-Sage P, Laurent C, Zucman-Rossi J, Balabaud C, Trillaud H. Hepatocellular adenomas: magnetic resonance imaging features as a function of molecular pathological classification. Hepatology. 2008;48(3):808–18. https://doi.org/10.1002/hep.22417.
42. van Aalten SM, Thomeer MG, Terkivatan T, Dwarkasing RS, Verheij J, de Man RA, et al. Hepatocellular adenomas: correlation of MR imaging findings with pathologic subtype classification. Radiology. 2011;261(1):172–81. https://doi.org/10.1148/radiol.11110023.
43. Lewin M, Handra-Luca A, Arrive L, Wendum D, Paradis V, Bridel E, et al. Liver adenomatosis: classification of MR imaging features and comparison with pathologic findings. Radiology. 2006;241(2):433–40. https://doi.org/10.1148/radiol.2412051243.
44. Grazioli L, Federle MP, Brancatelli G, Ichikawa T, Olivetti L, Blachar A. Hepatic adenomas: imaging and pathologic findings. Radiographics. 2001;21(4):877–92. https://doi.org/10.1148/radiographics.21.4.g01jl04877; discussion 92–4.
45. Thompson MD, Monga SP. WNT/beta-catenin signaling in liver health and disease. Hepatology. 2007;45(5):1298–305. https://doi.org/10.1002/hep.21651.
46. Levy AD, Murakata LA, Abbott RM, Rohrmann CA Jr. From the archives of the AFIP. Benign tumors and tumorlike lesions of the gallbladder and extrahepatic bile ducts: radiologic-pathologic correlation. Armed Forces Institute of Pathology. Radiographics. 2002;22(2):387–413. https://doi.org/10.1148/radiographics.22.2.g02mr08387.
47. Lewin M, Mourra N, Honigman I, Flejou JF, Parc R, Arrive L, et al. Assessment of MRI and MRCP in diagnosis of biliary cystadenoma and cystadenocarcinoma. Eur Radiol. 2006;16(2):407–13. https://doi.org/10.1007/s00330-005-2822-x.
48. Mortele KJ, Ros PR. Cystic focal liver lesions in the adult: differential CT and MR imaging features.

Radiographics. 2001;21(4):895–910. https://doi.org/10.1148/radiographics.21.4.g01jl16895.
49. Martinoli C, Cittadini G Jr, Rollandi GA, Conzi R. Case report: imaging of bile duct hamartomas. Clin Radiol. 1992;45(3):203–5.
50. Wohlgemuth WA, Bottger J, Bohndorf K. MRI, CT, US and ERCP in the evaluation of bile duct hamartomas (von Meyenburg complex): a case report. Eur Radiol. 1998;8(9):1623–6. https://doi.org/10.1007/s003300050599.
51. Slone HW, Bennett WF, Bova JG. MR findings of multiple biliary hamartomas. AJR Am J Roentgenol. 1993;161(3):581–3. https://doi.org/10.2214/ajr.161.3.8352110.
52. Semelka RC, Hussain SM, Marcos HB, Woosley JT. Biliary hamartomas: solitary and multiple lesions shown on current MR techniques including gadolinium enhancement. J Magn Reson Imaging. 1999;10(2):196–201.
53. Bosman FT, World Health Organization, International Agency for Research on Cancer. WHO classification of tumours of the digestive system, vol. 3. 4th ed. Lyon: International Agency for Research on Cancer; 2010.
54. Shamsi K, de Schepper AMA. Medical imaging of focal liver lesions : a clinico-radiologic approach. Amsterdam: Elsevier; 1994.
55. Robbins SL, Kumar V, Cotran RS. Robbins and cotran pathologic basis of disease. 8th ed. Philadelphia: Saunders/Elsevier; 2010.
56. Choi JY, Lee JM, Sirlin CB. CT and MR imaging diagnosis and staging of hepatocellular carcinoma: part I. Development, growth, and spread: key pathologic and imaging aspects. Radiology. 2014;272(3):635–54. https://doi.org/10.1148/radiol.14132361.
57. McEvoy SH, McCarthy CJ, Lavelle LP, Moran DE, Cantwell CP, Skehan SJ, et al. Hepatocellular carcinoma: illustrated guide to systematic radiologic diagnosis and staging according to guidelines of the American Association for the Study of Liver Diseases. Radiographics. 2013;33(6):1653–68. https://doi.org/10.1148/rg.336125104.
58. Digumarthy SR, Sahani DV, Saini S. MRI in detection of hepatocellular carcinoma (HCC). Cancer Imaging. 2005;5:20–4. https://doi.org/10.1102/1470-7330.2005.0005.
59. Chou R, Cuevas C, Fu R, Devine B, Wasson N, Ginsburg A, et al. Imaging techniques for the diagnosis of hepatocellular carcinoma: a systematic review and meta-analysis. Ann Inter Med. 2015;162(10):697–711. https://doi.org/10.7326/M14-2509.
60. Lau WY. Hepatocellular carcinoma. World Scientific Publication: Hackensack; 2008.
61. Choi BI, Lee JM. Advancement in HCC imaging: diagnosis, staging and treatment efficacy assessments: imaging diagnosis and staging of hepatocellular carcinoma. J Hepatobiliary Pancreat Sci. 2010;17(4):369–73. https://doi.org/10.1007/s00534-009-0227-y.
62. Willatt JM, Hussain HK, Adusumilli S, Marrero JA. MR imaging of hepatocellular carcinoma in the cirrhotic liver: challenges and controversies. Radiology. 2008;247(2):311–30. https://doi.org/10.1148/radiol.2472061331.
63. Parente DB, Perez RM, Eiras-Araujo A, Oliveira Neto JA, Marchiori E, Constantino CP, et al. MR imaging of hypervascular lesions in the cirrhotic liver: a diagnostic dilemma. Radiographics. 2012;32(3):767–87. https://doi.org/10.1148/rg.323115131.
64. Ganeshan D, Szklaruk J, Kundra V, Kaseb A, Rashid A, Elsayes KM. Imaging features of fibrolamellar hepatocellular carcinoma. AJR Am J Roentgenol. 2014;202(3):544–52. https://doi.org/10.2214/AJR.13.11117.
65. Ichikawa T, Federle MP, Grazioli L, Madariaga J, Nalesnik M, Marsh W. Fibrolamellar hepatocellular carcinoma: imaging and pathologic findings in 31 recent cases. Radiology. 1999;213(2):352–61. https://doi.org/10.1148/radiology.213.2.r99nv31352.
66. Blachar A, Federle MP, Ferris JV, Lacomis JM, Waltz JS, Armfield DR, et al. Radiologists' performance in the diagnosis of liver tumors with central scars by using specific CT criteria. Radiology. 2002;223(2):532–9. https://doi.org/10.1148/radiol.2232010801.
67. Smith MT, Blatt ER, Jedlicka P, Strain JD, Fenton LZ. Best cases from the AFIP: fibrolamellar hepatocellular carcinoma. Radiographics. 2008;28(2):609–13. https://doi.org/10.1148/rg.282075153.
68. Han JK, Choi BI, Kim AY, An SK, Lee JW, Kim TK, et al. Cholangiocarcinoma: pictorial essay of CT and cholangiographic findings. Radiographics. 2002;22(1):173–87. https://doi.org/10.1148/radiographics.22.1.g02ja15173.
69. Chung YE, Kim MJ, Park YN, Choi JY, Pyo JY, Kim YC, et al. Varying appearances of cholangiocarcinoma: radiologic-pathologic correlation. Radiographics. 2009;29(3):683–700. https://doi.org/10.1148/rg.293085729.
70. Lim JH. Cholangiocarcinoma: morphologic classification according to growth pattern and imaging findings. AJR Am J Roentgenol. 2003;181(3):819–27. https://doi.org/10.2214/ajr.181.3.1810819.
71. Vilgrain V. Staging cholangiocarcinoma by imaging studies. HPB. 2008;10(2):106–9. https://doi.org/10.1080/13651820801992617.
72. Jung AY, Lee JM, Choi SH, Kim SH, Lee JY, Kim SW, et al. CT features of an intraductal polypoid mass: differentiation between hepatocellular carcinoma with bile duct tumor invasion and intraductal papillary cholangiocarcinoma. J Comput Assist Tomogr. 2006;30(2):173–81.
73. Neitlich JD, Topazian M, Smith RC, Gupta A, Burrell MI, Rosenfield AT. Detection of choledocholithiasis: comparison of unenhanced helical CT and endoscopic retrograde cholangiopancreatography. Radiology. 1997;203(3):753–7. https://doi.org/10.1148/radiology.203.3.9169700.
74. Maetani Y, Itoh K, Watanabe C, Shibata T, Ametani F, Yamabe H, et al. MR imaging of intrahepatic cholangiocarcinoma with pathologic correlation. AJR Am

J Roentgenol. 2001;176(6):1499–507. https://doi.org/10.2214/ajr.176.6.1761499.
75. Vanderveen KA, Hussain HK. Magnetic resonance imaging of cholangiocarcinoma. Cancer Imaging. 2004;4(2):104–15. https://doi.org/10.1102/1470-7330.2004.0018.
76. Palacios E, Shannon M, Solomon C, Guzman M. Biliary cystadenoma: ultrasound, CT, and MRI. Gastrointest Radiol. 1990;15(4):313–6.
77. Buetow PC, Midkiff RB. MR imaging of the liver. Primary malignant neoplasms in the adult. Magn Reson Imaging Clin N Am. 1997;5(2):289–318.
78. Namasivayam S, Martin DR, Saini S. Imaging of liver metastases: MRI. Cancer Imaging. 2007;7:2–9. https://doi.org/10.1102/1470-7330.2007.0002.
79. Kamel IR, Bluemke DA. MR imaging of liver tumors. Radiol Clin N Am. 2003;41(1):51–65.
80. Sica GT, Ji H, Ros PR. CT and MR imaging of hepatic metastases. AJR Am J Roentgenol. 2000;174(3):691–8. https://doi.org/10.2214/ajr.174.3.1740691.
81. Wernecke K, Vassallo P, Bick U, Diederich S, Peters PE. The distinction between benign and malignant liver tumors on sonography: value of a hypoechoic halo. AJR Am J Roentgenol. 1992;159(5):1005–9. https://doi.org/10.2214/ajr.159.5.1329454.
82. Chen MY, Bechtold RE, Savage PD. Cystic changes in hepatic metastases from gastrointestinal stromal tumors (GISTs) treated with Gleevec (imatinib mesylate). AJR Am J Roentgenol. 2002;179(4):1059–62. https://doi.org/10.2214/ajr.179.4.1791059.
83. Lee SY, Chuang JH, Huang CB, Hsiao CC, Wan YL, Ng SH, et al. Congenital bilateral cystic neuroblastoma with liver metastases and massive intracystic haemorrhage. Br J Radiol. 1998;71(851):1205–7. https://doi.org/10.1259/bjr.71.851.10434918.
84. Kanematsu M, Kondo H, Goshima S, Kato H, Tsuge U, Hirose Y, et al. Imaging liver metastases: review and update. Eur J Radiol. 2006;58(2):217–28. https://doi.org/10.1016/j.ejrad.2005.11.041.
85. Bartolozzi C. Magnetic resonance imaging in liver disease : technical approach, diagnostic imaging of liver neoplasms, focus on a new superparamagnetic contrast agent. Stuttgart: George Thieme Verlag; 2003.
86. Muramatsu Y, Takayasu K, Moriyama N, Shima Y, Goto H, Ushio K, et al. Peripheral low-density area of hepatic tumors: CT-pathologic correlation. Radiology. 1986;160(1):49–52. https://doi.org/10.1148/radiology.160.1.3012632.
87. Semelka RC, Hussain SM, Marcos HB, Woosley JT. Perilesional enhancement of hepatic metastases: correlation between MR imaging and histopathologic findings-initial observations. Radiology. 2000;215(1):89–94. https://doi.org/10.1148/radiology.215.1.r00mr2989.
88. Saini S, Nelson RC. Technique for MR imaging of the liver. Radiology. 1995;197(3):575–7. https://doi.org/10.1148/radiology.197.3.7480718.
89. Silva AC, Evans JM, McCullough AE, Jatoi MA, Vargas HE, Hara AK. MR imaging of hypervascular liver masses: a review of current techniques. Radiographics. 2009;29(2):385–402. https://doi.org/10.1148/rg.292085123.
90. Kelekis NL, Semelka RC, Woosley JT. Malignant lesions of the liver with high signal intensity on T1-weighted MR images. J Magn Reson Imaging. 1996;6(2):291–4.
91. Danet IM, Semelka RC, Leonardou P, Braga L, Vaidean G, Woosley JT, et al. Spectrum of MRI appearances of untreated metastases of the liver. AJR Am J Roentgenol. 2003;181(3):809–17. https://doi.org/10.2214/ajr.181.3.1810809.
92. Wittenberg J, Stark DD, Forman BH, Hahn PF, Saini S, Weissleder R, et al. Differentiation of hepatic metastases from hepatic hemangiomas and cysts by using MR imaging. AJR Am J Roentgenol. 1988;151(1):79–84. https://doi.org/10.2214/ajr.151.1.79.
93. Outwater E, Tomaszewski JE, Daly JM, Kressel HY. Hepatic colorectal metastases: correlation of MR imaging and pathologic appearance. Radiology. 1991;180(2):327–32. https://doi.org/10.1148/radiology.180.2.2068294.
94. Sica GT, Ji H, Ros PR. Computed tomography and magnetic resonance imaging of hepatic metastases. Clin Liver Dis. 2002;6(1):165–79, vii.
95. Bressler EL, Alpern MB, Glazer GM, Francis IR, Ensminger WD. Hypervascular hepatic metastases: CT evaluation. Radiology. 1987;162(1 Pt 1):49–51. https://doi.org/10.1148/radiology.162.1.3024210.
96. Mahfouz AE, Hamm B, Wolf KJ. Peripheral washout: a sign of malignancy on dynamic gadolinium-enhanced MR images of focal liver lesions. Radiology. 1994;190(1):49–52. https://doi.org/10.1148/radiology.190.1.8259426.
97. Low RN. Contrast agents for MR imaging of the liver. J Magn Reson Imaging. 1997;7(1):56–67.

Part II

Primary Liver Tumors

Liver Transplantation for Hepatocellular Carcinoma: The Challenge of Organ Availability

Christopher Sonnenday

Introduction

In patients with end-stage liver disease and early-stage hepatocellular carcinoma (HCC), liver transplantation provides the most definitive therapy option, addressing both the patient's chronic liver disease and their malignancy. While appropriate debate continues about the extent of tumor burden able to be addressed by transplantation, patients with advanced liver disease who are not candidates for resection have transplantation as their only potentially curative treatment option. In the modern era, liver transplant outcomes are excellent, with short-term survival outcomes rivaling that of hepatic resection (4–8% 90-day mortality) and long-term recurrence rates that are lower than 10% in most centers [1]. Even with extended selection criteria, long-term transplant outcomes among patients with HCC are equivalent to patients undergoing liver transplantation for other indications.

However, liver transplantation remains a therapy with inherently limited application due to the profound mismatch between organ availability and demand. While much debate has occurred about which patients with HCC are best served with transplantation, the reality remains that liver transplantation is not an "off-the-shelf" therapy, with inherent challenges in patient selection and obligate delays in offering definitive therapy, while a donor organ is identified. Furthermore, access to transplantation varies significantly among both individuals and populations, subject to multiple factors including availability of living donor liver transplantation (LDLT), supply of deceased donor organs relative to local waitlist volume, policy measures that control access of HCC patients to deceased donor organs, and transplant center donor and recipient selection criteria. To add complexity to the decision-making about the use of transplantation for patients with HCC, the amount of time an individual patient waits for transplant appears to have significant impact on outcome, emphasizing the always central importance of tumor biology and the uncertain influence of "bridging therapies" (liver-directed therapies applied while patients are waiting for transplant). Counter to initial intuition, more immediate access to transplant (as in the case of LDLT, or in areas with shorter waiting times for a deceased donor organ) does not always provide better long-term survival outcomes, especially in patients with more advanced tumors. It is therefore imperative that providers treating patients with HCC understand the access of their individual patient to liver transplantation, as it has direct impact on clinical decision-making and selection of therapies.

C. Sonnenday
Department of Surgery, University of Michigan, Ann Arbor, MI, USA
e-mail: csonnend@umich.edu

In the following chapter, the issues of organ supply and allocation will be addressed as it relates to liver transplantation for HCC. The indications for transplantation for HCC, particularly relative to other therapies, are discussed elsewhere in this text and will not be specifically addressed.

History of Liver Transplantation for HCC

Many of the initial cases of liver transplantation were performed in patients with advanced malignancy [2]. In many ways, liver transplantation seems the ideal therapy for hepatic malignancy, with total hepatectomy extending limits of hepatic resection. As many of the earliest cases of liver transplantation ended in early mortality due to technical and immunologic failures, the risk of recurrent disease was not initially realized. However, early series of HCC patients documented excessively high recurrence rates (75%+) with expedited cancer-related mortality [3]. It was not until Mazzaferro's seminal series of patients with early-stage HCC undergoing successful liver transplantation that the primacy of patient selection and tumor burden was established [4]. The Milan criteria established in this study have been stretched and challenged since that time, but they remain the standard for low recurrence risk in this patient population.

MELD-Based Allocation and HCC Exception Policy

In the United States, recognition of the Milan criteria corresponded temporally with the adoption of the model for end-stage liver disease (MELD) as the scoring system for liver transplant allocation. MELD, a multivariate model including serum bilirubin, serum creatinine, and international normalized ratio (INR) for prothrombin time that is transformed to an integer from 6 to 40, was initially designed to predict mortality after transjugular intrahepatic portosystemic shunt (TIPS) but was also shown to predict waitlist mortality for liver transplantation [5, 6]. MELD was instituted as the metric for waitlist prioritization in 2002 and was immediately associated with a decrease in waitlist mortality and waiting time. At the time of the adoption of MELD-based allocation, it was recognized that patients with HCC would require MELD "exception" points proportionate to their priority for transplantation, as the majority of patients with HCC listed for transplant did not have end-stage disease associated with elevated MELD scores. Patient selection for liver transplantation is driven by modified TNM staging for HCC (Table 3.1). Initial MELD exception scores granted by the Organ Procurement and Transplantation Network (OPTN) included 29 points for patients with T2 tumors and 24 points for patients with T1 tumors.

Since the adoption of MELD-based allocation, the amount of priority given to HCC patients via MELD exception has evolved continuously in response to waitlist and transplant outcomes of HCC patients relative to other populations (Table 3.2) [7]. Initial policy changes aimed to decrease MELD exception points given to patients with T2 lesions to 22 points in 2003 and then 22 points in 2005. As it became clear that patients with small, solitary lesions had good outcomes with liver-directed therapy (e.g., ablation) alone, the MELD exception given to patients with T1 tumors was eliminated in 2004. Thus, the United Network for Organ Sharing (UNOS)/OPTN criteria for transplant came to differ from the original Milan criteria with the exclusion of patients with T1 tumors.

Table 3.1 UNOS modified TNM staging for hepatocellular carcinoma

T stage	T1	Solitary tumor <2 cm
	T2	Solitary tumor 2–5 cm; 2–3 nodules all less than 3 cm
	T3	Solitary tumor >5 cm; 2–3 nodules with at least one >3 cm
	T4a	Four or more tumors
	T4b	T2, T3, or T4b tumor with gross vascular involvement
N stage	N1	Regional lymph node involvement
M stage	M1	Any extrahepatic metastatic disease beyond regional nodes

Table 3.2 UNOS/OPTN exception policy for HCC (Adapted from Rich NE et al.) [7]

Year of policy change	MELD exception points and policy details
2002	29 exception points for T2 lesions 24 exception points for T1 lesions
2003	24 exception points for T2 lesions 20 exception points for T1 lesions
2004	24 exception points for T2 lesions • No exception points for T1 lesions
2005	22 exception points for T2 lesions • No exception points for T1 lesions
2015	Lab MELD score at time of listing for T2 lesions • 28 exception points after 6 months • Maximum of 34 MELD exception points
2017	AFP < 1000 ng/mL required for active listing
2018	Establishment of national exception review board HCC exception points will be based upon median MELD at transplant (−3 points) in local donor service area.

Additional changes to HCC MELD exception policy were adopted in 2015 to delay the assignment of HCC exception points for 6 months (with restaging imaging and serum AFP required every 3 months). After 6 months listing with their natural MELD score, patients with T2 HCC are granted 28 exception points. Scores are increased every 3 months thereafter if the patient has not been transplanted, to a maximum score of 34. The primary objective of this policy change was to attempt to equalize transplant rates between patients with HCC and non-HCC diagnoses [8]. In addition, the delay in granting of the HCC exception for 6 months allowed for observation of tumor biology and dropout of patients who progressed beyond T2 criteria. This observation period has the potential of excluding patients with higher potential recurrence rates after transplantation and mitigates the seemingly counterintuitive principle that patients with HCC transplanted in UNOS regions of shorter waiting time actually have inferior survival outcomes to patients transplanted in regions with longer waiting times [9]. Presumably, longer waiting time imposes a type of natural selection on patients with more aggressive tumors and may provide an opportunity for liver-directed therapy as a bridging or neoadjuvant therapy. Furthermore, extending waiting time for transplant among HCC patients provides more equity in transplant rates among patients with HCC and non-HCC diagnoses [10].

The most recent changes to HCC exception policy require that patients with T2 tumors have a serum AFP level less than 1000 ng/mL at the time of listing. Patients with AFP levels greater than 1000 ng/mL may be treated and can be listed if the AFP level drops to less than 500 ng/mL. This policy change is an attempt to utilize a biomarker as measure of tumor biology. While not perfect, significantly elevated AFP (>1000 ng/mL) is associated with increased posttransplant recurrence and diminished survival [11]. Other biomarkers (PIVKA II, AFP-L3, glypican 3, and others) may provide additional fidelity in predicting tumor recurrence, but none have been adequately validated in transplant populations.

Disparities in Access to Transplantation for HCC

In the United States, concern has risen in the transplant community about the variation in access within geographic regions of the country. From an allocation standpoint, the country is divided into 11 geographic regions and 58 donor service areas (local areas of variable size served by a single donor service area). The boundaries of these regions and donor service areas were drawn based on historical precedent and proximity rather than population-based metrics. Thus, substantial variation in donor supply and transplant demand may exist between and within UNOS regions. This creates significant disparity in allocation MELD at time of transplant [12] and profound difference in the utilization of MELD exception scores including those applied for HCC patients [13]. Redrawing of the boundaries ("redistricting") utilized for liver transplant allocation has been debated [14], and in 2018 UNOS will execute important policy initiatives to address these inequities including reform of regional exception score variation through the establishment of a national exception review process and adjusting allocation to give priority to patients within proximity to donor hospitals regardless of regional boundaries. These initiatives are expected to improve disparity in allocation MELD score at time of transplant and limit variation in access of HCC patients to transplant but may not address differences in center behavior (differences in donor and recipient selection) that could perpetuate differences in allocation MELD at time of transplant [15].

Even greater differences exist in access to advanced therapies for HCC, including transplant, by race and ethnicity. Black and Hispanic patients in the United States are far less likely to receive definitive surgical therapy for HCC, including resection and transplant. Black patients are particularly disadvantaged in access to liver transplantation for HCC, with individual patients more than 50% less likely to be transplanted than similar White patients [16]. These disparities in access to transplant translate to inferior survival outcomes among Black and Hispanic patients with HCC [17]. Addressing race/ethnicity disparities in access to transplant for HCC is challenging but will likely require public health initiatives to improve access of minority populations to subspecialty care earlier in the course of their disease.

Eligibility for Transplant Beyond Milan Criteria

Numerous efforts have been made to expand eligibility criteria for liver transplantation beyond Milan criteria, although none have been universally accepted in a manner to drive organ allocation. Llovet and colleagues first popularized the analogy of the European Metroticket (Fig. 3.1), associating the further "distance" from Milan criteria with the higher "price" of posttransplant

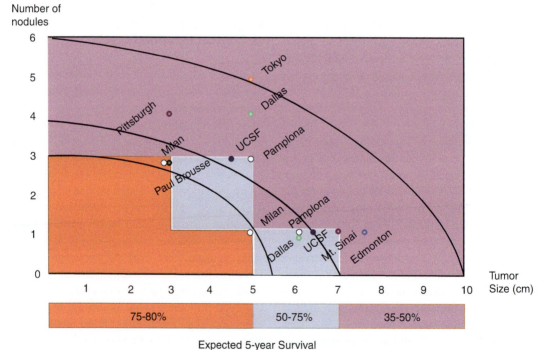

Fig. 3.1 The "Metroticket" model of HCC tumor size and number relative to posttransplant survival, used from Yao with permission [18]. Individual HCC eligibility criteria are designated by their name and associated circle. For example, the Milan criteria (solitary tumor ≤5 cm, 2–3 nodules none larger than 3 cm) would be expected to yield 75–80% 5-year posttransplant survival. Used with permission from Yao FY. Liver transplantation for hepatocellular carcinoma: beyond the Milan criteria. Am J Transplant. Wiley/Blackwell (10.1111); 2008 Oct;8(10):1982–9 [15]

recurrence [18]. Alternative criteria may be evaluated on the balance between expanding eligibility for transplant to additional patients with HCC and the increased risk of recurrent disease. Consensus in the transplant community has generally established 60% 5-year overall posttransplant survival as the lowest acceptable survival to balance the utility of transplant for HCC with other diagnoses [19].

Among alternative criteria for transplant eligibility among HCC patients, only the University of California-San Francisco (UCSF) criteria have been prospectively validated with acceptable outcomes [11, 20]. UCSF criteria extend Milan criteria by modestly extending tumor volume criteria (one tumor ≤6.5 cm, three nodules at most with the largest ≤4.5 cm, and total tumor diameter ≤8 cm). These criteria were generated retrospectively based on explant pathology, but prospective validation using preoperative imaging documented a low overall recurrence rate of 10% at 5 years, with only 15% of patients found to exceed UCSF criteria on explant pathology [20]. Despite these excellent outcomes, there has not been support from the community to change UNOS/OPTN policy to extend selection criteria for HCC candidates.

Downstaging Therapy

While extension of HCC eligibility criteria at the time of transplant has not been endorsed broadly in the United States, liver-directed therapy to downstage patients beyond Milan criteria such that they meet UNOS T2 criteria at the time of transplant has been increasingly utilized. Despite this increasing experience and expert opinion supporting the use of downstaging to expand access to transplantation, there is no consensus about the most effective modality for liver-directed therapy [21, 22]. A recent systematic review of published series of downstaging suggested that up to 60% of candidates will be successfully downstaged to within Milan criteria, but no clear advantage was demonstrated according to liver-directed therapy modality (transarterial chemoembolization versus transarterial radioembolization) [23]. Critically important to the establishment of uniform downstaging strategies is the utilization of standard criteria for measuring response to therapy by imaging. The modified RECIST (mRECIST) criteria were created by expert consensus convened by the American Association for the Study of Liver Diseases (AASLD) and remain the gold standard for evaluating response to therapy on contrast-enhanced CT or MRI [24]. The extent of residual viable tumor, rather than measurement of treatment cavity or previous tumor size, is utilized to determine the amount of residual disease. Response to therapy should be observed for at least 3 months prior to consideration of active listing for transplant. Patients who maintain residual tumor volume within Milan criteria or less after downstaging therapy are appropriate for listing and should be monitored for intrahepatic and extrahepatic progression every 3 months until transplant.

Controversy exists over whether or not there is an "outer limit" to tumors appropriate for downstaging. UNOS recently considered a policy revision to define eligibility criteria for downstaging, including patients with a solitary lesion less than 8 cm, those with 2–3 lesions each less than 5 cm and total tumor diameter not exceeding 8 cm, and those with 4–5 lesions each less than 3 cm with total diameter not exceeding 8 cm [7]. However, no consensus could be reached in the community, and examples exist of patients with extensive tumor being successfully downstaged to transplant with liver-directed therapy, often in multiple sessions, and an appropriate period of observation [25]. Most centers and experts agree that tumor thrombus is a relative contraindication to downstaging therapy, although limited cases with prolonged observation suggest that even those patients may be downstaged in some instances [26].

Living Donor Liver Transplantation for HCC

Living donor liver transplantation (LDLT) offers the opportunity to improve timely access to transplantation to patients in the United States and is the primary form of liver transplantation in Asian countries with limited access to deceased donor organs. Among patients with end-stage liver disease, LDLT appears to offer equivalent or even superior recipient survival outcomes [27], likely reflecting the benefit of access to transplant earlier in the patient's disease course when recovery from transplant may be easier. However, among HCC patients, LDLT appears to be associated with an increased risk of HCC recurrence post-transplant [28]. Explanations for inferior outcomes among HCC patients treated with LDLT include differences in pretransplant therapies (such as decreased use of liver-directed therapy), differences in patient selection (potential tendency to consider patients beyond Milan criteria for LDLT), and expedited transplant via LDLT such that a period of observation of tumor behavior does not occur [29]. The most appropriate selection criteria for selection HCC patient appropriate for LDLT have not been established, but utilization of some observation period (3–6 months) after diagnosis of HCC prior to LDLT may eliminate the possibility of transplanting patients with particularly unfavorable tumor biology and increased recurrence risk [21].

As LDLT is not regulated by the same policy criteria as deceased donor allocation, transplant centers have considered utilization of LDLT for HCC patients with tumors outside Milan criteria. This practice avoids the ethical quandary faced in deceased donor transplantation for patients with advanced HCC, where use of a scarce deceased donor organ potentially deprives other patients (including non-HCC patients) with better survival outcomes from transplant. However, recipient selection in LDLT should consider the risks of hepatectomy to the donor, such that a certain minimum expected recipient outcome should be expected to justify donor risk [30]. Most centers appear to extrapolate expected minimum acceptable recipient survival outcomes (50–60% 5-year overall survival) from deceased donor transplantation to LDLT, but no clear standard has been established by consensus in the field. As in deceased donor liver transplantation, extension of LDLT to HCC patients beyond Milan criteria is associated with increased recurrence rates but comparable overall survival [31]. Ongoing prospective study is required, but it does appear that LDLT may provide a clinical opportunity to cautiously extend HCC eligibility criteria for transplant without the ramifications for other listed patients and the need for extensive policy revision.

Summary

Liver transplantation is the definitive therapy for select patients with end-stage liver disease and HCC. The Milan criteria remain the most durable and appropriate selection criteria for HCC candidates for transplantation and are therefore incorporated in organ allocation policy for HCC. Extending transplant to patients with HCC beyond Milan criteria may be considered through the use of pretransplant downstaging therapy and appropriate periods of observation prior to transplant. The optimal therapy for downstaging has not been determined and may include a combination of liver-directed therapy in some patients. LDLT is an effective alternative source of donor organs for HCC patients, and ongoing work is needed to refine recipient selection criteria for LDLT among HCC candidates.

References

1. Kim WR, Lake JR, Smith JM, Skeans MA, Schladt DP, Edwards EB, et al. OPTN/SRTR 2015 Annual data report: liver. Am J Transplant. 2017;17(Suppl 1):174–251.
2. Starzl TE, Marchioro TL, Vonkaulla KN, Hermann G, Brittain RS, Waddell WR. Homotransplantation of the liver in humans. Surg Gynecol Obstet. 1963;117:659–76. NIH Public Access.
3. Iwatsuki S, Gordon RD, Shaw BW, Starzl TE. Role of liver transplantation in cancer therapy. Ann Surg. 1985;202(4):401–7.
4. Mazzaferro V, Regalia E, Doci R, Andreola S, Pulvirenti A, Bozzetti F, et al. Liver transplantation for the treatment of small hepatocellular carcinomas in patients with cirrhosis. N Engl J Med. 1996;334(11):693–700.
5. Kamath PS, Wiesner RH, Malinchoc M, Kremers W, Therneau TM, Kosberg CL, et al. A model to predict survival in patients with end-stage liver disease. Hepatology. 2001;33(2):464–70.
6. Malinchoc M, Kamath PS, Gordon FD, Peine CJ, Rank J, Borg ter PC. A model to predict poor survival

7. Rich NE, Parikh ND, Singal AG. Hepatocellular carcinoma and liver transplantation: changing patterns and practices. Curr Treat Options Gastroenterol. 2017;15(2):296–304.
8. Heimbach JK, Hirose R, Stock PG, Schladt DP, Xiong H, Liu J, et al. Delayed hepatocellular carcinoma model for end-stage liver disease exception score improves disparity in access to liver transplant in the United States. Hepatology. 2015;61(5):1643–50.
9. Halazun KJ, Patzer RE, Rana AA, Verna EC, Griesemer AD, Parsons RF, et al. Standing the test of time: outcomes of a decade of prioritizing patients with hepatocellular carcinoma, results of the UNOS natural geographic experiment. Hepatology. 2014;60(6):1957–62.
10. Schlansky B, Chen Y, Scott DL, Austin D, Naugler WE. Waiting time predicts survival after liver transplantation for hepatocellular carcinoma: a cohort study using the United Network for Organ Sharing registry. Liver Transpl. 2014;20(9):1045–56.
11. Yao F. Liver transplantation for hepatocellular carcinoma: expansion of the tumor size limits does not adversely impact survival. Hepatology. 2001;33(6):1394–403.
12. Yeh H, Smoot E, Schoenfeld DA, Markmann JF. Geographic inequity in access to livers for transplantation. Transplantation. 2011;91(4):479–86.
13. Massie AB, Caffo B, Gentry SE, Hall EC, Axelrod DA, Lentine KL, et al. MELD exceptions and rates of waiting list outcomes. Am J Transplant. 2011;11(11):2362–71. https://doi.org/10.1111/j.1600-6143.2011.03735.x.
14. Gentry SE, Massie AB, Cheek SW, Lentine KL, Chow EH, Wickliffe CE, et al. Addressing geographic disparities in liver transplantation through redistricting. Am J Transplant. 2013;13(8):2052–8.
15. Croome KP, Lee DD, Burns JM, Keaveny AP, Taner CB. Intra-regional MELD score variation in liver transplantation: disparity in our own backyard. Liver Transpl. 2018;24(4):1–32.
16. Sonnenday CJ, Dimick JB, Schulick RD, Choti MA. Racial and geographic disparities in the utilization of surgical therapy for hepatocellular carcinoma. J Gastrointest Surg. 2007;11(12):1636–46; discussion 1646.
17. Mathur AK, Osborne NH, Lynch RJ, Ghaferi AA, Dimick JB, Sonnenday CJ. Racial/ethnic disparities in access to care and survival for patients with early-stage hepatocellular carcinoma. Arch Surg. 2010;145(12):1158–63.
18. Yao FY. Liver transplantation for hepatocellular carcinoma: beyond the Milan criteria. Am J Transplant. 2008;8(10):1982–9.
19. Volk ML, Vijan S, Marrero JA. A novel model measuring the harm of transplanting hepatocellular carcinoma exceeding Milan criteria. Am J Transplant. 2008;8(4):839–46. https://doi.org/10.1111/j.1600-6143.2007.02138.x.
20. Yao FY, Xiao L, Bass NM, Kerlan R, Ascher NL, Roberts JP. Liver transplantation for hepatocellular carcinoma: validation of the UCSF-expanded criteria based on preoperative imaging. Am J Transplant. 2007;7(11):2587–96. https://doi.org/10.1111/j.1600-6143.2007.01965.x.
21. Clavien P-A, Lesurtel M, Bossuyt PM, Gores GJ, Langer B, Perrier A. Recommendations for liver transplantation for hepatocellular carcinoma: an international consensus conference report. Lancet Oncol. 2012;13(1):e11–22.
22. Heimbach JK, Kulik LM, Finn RS, Sirlin CB, Abecassis MM, Roberts LR, et al. AASLD guidelines for the treatment of hepatocellular carcinoma. Hepatology. 2018;67:358–80.
23. Parikh ND, Waljee AK, Singal AG. Downstaging hepatocellular carcinoma: a systematic review and pooled analysis. Liver Transpl. 2015;21(9):1142–52. 6 ed.
24. Lencioni R, Llovet JM. Modified RECIST (mRECIST) assessment for hepatocellular carcinoma. Semin Liver Dis. 2010;30(1):52–60.
25. Chapman WC, Majella Doyle MB, Stuart JE, Vachharajani N, Crippin JS, Anderson CD, et al. Outcomes of neoadjuvant transarterial chemoembolization to downstage hepatocellular carcinoma before liver transplantation. Ann Surg. 2008;248(4):617–25. Transactions of the ... Meeting of the American Surgical Association.
26. Dendy MS, Camacho JC, Ludwig JM, Krasinskas AM, Knechtle SJ, Kim HS. Infiltrative hepatocellular carcinoma with portal vein tumor thrombosis treated with a single high-dose Y90 radioembolization and subsequent liver transplantation without a recurrence. Transplant Direct. 2017;3(9):e206.
27. Olthoff KM, Abecassis MM, Emond JC, Kam I, Merion RM, Gillespie BW, et al. Outcomes of adult living donor liver transplantation: comparison of the adult-to-adult living donor liver transplantation cohort study and the national experience. Liver Transpl. 2011;17(7):789–97.
28. Fisher RA, Kulik LM, Freise CE, Lok ASF, Shearon TH, Brown RS, et al. Hepatocellular carcinoma recurrence and death following living and deceased donor liver transplantation. Am J Transplant. 2007;7(6):1601–8. https://doi.org/10.1111/j.1600-6143.2007.01802.x.
29. Kulik LM, Fisher RA, Rodrigo DR, Brown RS, Freise CE, Shaked A, et al. Outcomes of living and deceased donor liver transplant recipients with hepatocellular carcinoma: results of the A2ALL cohort. Am J Transplant. 2012;12(11):2997–3007. https://doi.org/10.1111/j.1600-6143.2012.04272.x.
30. Volk ML, Marrero JA, Lok AS, Ubel PA. Who decides? Living donor liver transplantation for advanced hepatocellular carcinoma. Transplantation. 2006;82(9):1136–9.
31. Llovet JM, Pavel M, Rimola J, Diaz MA, Colmenero J, Saavedra-Perez D, et al. Pilot study of living donor liver transplantation for patients with hepatocellular carcinoma exceeding Milan criteria (Barcelona clinic liver cancer extended criteria). Liver Transpl. 2018;24(3):369–79.

Surgical Approach in Hepatocellular Carcinoma: Resection Versus Transplantation

Vikrom K. Dhar and Shimul A. Shah

Introduction

Hepatocellular carcinoma (HCC) is the fifth most common cancer and second leading cause of cancer-related mortality worldwide [1, 2]. With an increase in the prevalence of risk factors including hepatitis C virus (HCV) and nonalcoholic steatohepatitis (NASH)-induced cirrhosis, the incidence of HCC in the United States continues to rise each year [3]. Without treatment, patients suffering from this malignancy have a median survival of less than 1 year [4–9]. While surgical resection (SR) and liver transplantation (LT) represent the only curative treatment options for HCC, the decision regarding which operation is optimal remains highly controversial [10, 11]. Patient-specific factors including tumor characteristics, underlying hepatic function, socioeconomic status, and functional performance as well as infrastructural factors including regional resources and organ availability all play a significant role in determining appropriate management for eligible surgical candidates. In this chapter, we provide an overview of the surgical approaches available in the management of HCC with an emphasis on appropriate patient selection and outcomes for SR and LT.

Preoperative Assessment

Diagnosis

HCC is most commonly discovered incidentally on radiographic imaging performed for other indications. Diagnosis can often be made without any requirement for tissue biopsy and is based on key features identified on triple-phase computed tomography (CT) scanning or gadolinium-enhanced magnetic resonance imaging (MRI) [12]. Detection of a hypervascular hepatic lesion in the arterial phase with washout during the portal venous or delayed phases is characteristic [12]. While some patients are found to have an elevated alpha-fetoprotein (AFP) level, AFP is not a definitive marker. In cases where radiographic imaging is inconclusive, tissue biopsy may be considered in order to obtain histologic confirmation. When obtaining tissue biopsy, consideration must be given to potential seeding of tumor along the needle tract, as development of metastases may preclude surgical intervention.

V. K. Dhar
Department of Surgery, University of Cincinnati College of Medicine, Cincinnati Research in Outcomes and Safety in Surgery (CROSS), Cincinnati, OH, USA
e-mail: dharvk@ucmail.uc.edu

S. A. Shah (✉)
Division of Transplantation, Department of Surgery, University of Cincinnati College of Medicine, Cincinnati Research in Outcomes and Safety in Surgery (CROSS), Cincinnati, OH, USA
e-mail: shimul.shah@uc.edu

Given the association between HCC and cirrhosis, screening regimens have been proposed for use in cirrhotic patients. Such protocols have employed monitoring of AFP levels in conjunction with radiographic surveillance by ultrasound, CT, or MRI every 6–12 months in high-risk patient populations [12, 13]. The goal of successful surveillance is to detect HCC at an early stage of disease, allowing patients to undergo potentially curative surgical treatments prior to development of metastases. Due to a lack of quality data, however, no formal consensus guidelines exist for standardized screening protocols in these patients [12, 13].

Surgical Candidacy

Once the diagnosis of HCC is made, thorough evaluation of disease characteristics including number of tumors, tumor size, and liver function based on Child-Pugh class or Model for End-Stage Liver Disease (MELD) score is critical. While SR and LT remain the sole options for curative treatment, only 25–40% of HCC patients in the United States ultimately undergo surgery [14–16]. Associated medical comorbidities and risks related to chronic liver disease or cirrhosis may impact patients' eligibility for operative intervention. Furthermore, current criteria for surgical candidacy are relatively strict.

The Barcelona Clinic Liver Cancer (BCLC) system is one of the most widely used staging systems for HCC disease, classifying patients into either early, intermediate, advanced, or terminal stages [17]. Surgical management of HCC is often limited to early-stage cancers that satisfy the Milan criteria, first established by Mazzaferro et al. in 1996 [18]. By selecting patients with a solitary tumor ≤5 cm in diameter or ≤3 tumors each ≤3 cm in size, reduced tumor recurrence and mortality rates have been achieved [18, 19]. Conversely, HCC patients with disease beyond Milan criteria or intermediate stage BCLC classification were traditionally referred for nonoperative management. With improvements in complex liver surgery over the past two decades, these patients are increasingly being considered for surgical resection [20]. Additionally, significant improvements have been made to locoregional therapies, such as ablation and embolization, as well as to novel targeted systemic therapies aimed at reducing tumor burden in patients with locally advanced disease [21]. High-risk patients previously thought to be ineligible for curative surgical treatment have recently been shown to undergo significant tumor downstaging [22, 23]. Indications for surgical intervention continue to evolve, and recent studies have explored expansion of candidacy for both SR and LT [24]. As a result of these advances, treatment options for HCC are numerous, and attempts to create standardized management algorithms have been difficult.

Surgical Resection

Resection is considered a primary treatment modality for non-cirrhotic patients with early-stage HCC that satisfies the Milan criteria. Patients with well-compensated cirrhosis (Child-Pugh class A) without evidence of portal hypertension, as seen in Fig. 4.1, are also considered for resection [25, 26]. Additionally, patients with HCC disease that has advanced beyond Milan criteria, but remains resectable with adequate hepatic reserve, are also appropriate candidates for resection [20, 24]. In patients presenting with advanced cirrhosis (Child-Pugh class B and class C), SR is typically contraindicated. Furthermore, in patients with extensive multifocal disease involving the main portal vein or inferior vena cava, surgical treatment is contraindicated.

Appropriate selection of patients for SR is dependent on tumor factors, liver anatomy, underlying hepatic function, and size of the remnant liver. In patients with inadequate functional reserve, hepatic regeneration is impaired, and normalization of liver function is slow or even absent. The presence of portal hypertension significantly increases risk for massive hemorrhage during resection. Furthermore, portal hypertension may be exacerbated following SR due to an increase in blood flow through the resultant noncompliant vascular bed. While well-compensated

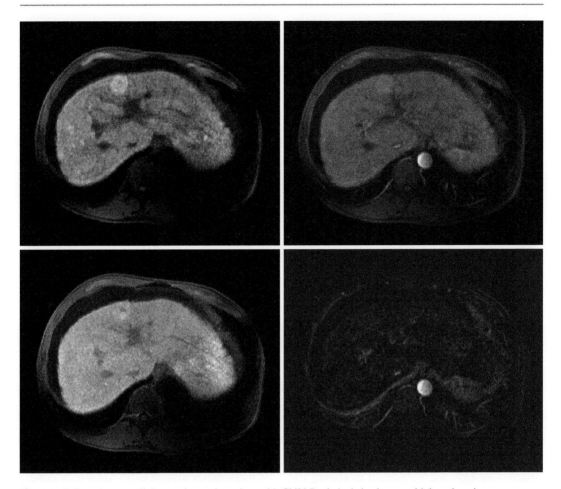

Fig. 4.1 Solitary hepatocellular carcinoma in patient with Child-Pugh A cirrhosis on multiphase imaging

cirrhotic patients are eligible for resection, consideration must be given that these patients may have undiagnosed portal hypertension. Beyond radiographic evidence, exam findings of splenomegaly, ascites, or esophageal varices should increase suspicion for portal hypertension. Laboratory findings may reveal platelet counts of less than 100,000/μL. In equivocal cases, hepatic venous catheterization may be utilized to assess hepatic venous pressures, with a pressure gradient of greater than 10 mmHg being associated with poor outcomes following resection [27]. When assessing hepatic reserve, CT imaging can be used for volumetric analysis in order to estimate the size of the liver remnant. Standardized future liver remnant (FLR) volume is an established measurement used to assess the percentage of total estimated liver volume remaining following resection. Current guidelines recommend sFLR volumes of at least 20% in patients without any underlying liver disease. In HCC patients with cirrhosis, sFLR volumes of greater than 40% are recommended [28]. In cases where remnant size is inadequate, percutaneous transhepatic portal vein embolization (PVE) has been shown to be efficacious in inducing compensatory hepatocyte hypertrophy and improving eligibility for resection [29–31]. In PVE, a branch of the portal venous system that is anatomically relevant to the location of the tumor is occluded resulting in compensatory hypertrophy of the contralateral liver remnant and an increase in volume ranging from 8 to 27% [29]. In a meta-analysis of over 1000 patients, Abulkhir et al. reported a post-PVE resection rate of 85% with a morbidity rate of 2.2% and no mortality [29].

With regard to surgical technique, much debate exists regarding the impact of anatomic versus nonanatomic resection on outcomes for patients with HCC. Despite similar rates of morbidity and mortality, anatomic resection has been shown to have more favorable rates of 5-year OS and DFS compared to nonanatomic resection. In a meta-analysis of 18 studies involving over 9000 patients, patients undergoing anatomic resection had significantly improved 5-year OS (RR 1.14, $p < 0.01$) and 5-year DFS (RR 1.38, $p < 0.01$) compared to nonanatomic resection. Of note, patients undergoing nonanatomic resection Hepatocellular carcinoma (HCC):surgical resection (SR): were found to have more advanced hepatic dysfunction and higher prevalence of cirrhosis, likely affected survival and recurrence rates [32]. The ability to perform anatomic vs. nonanatomic resection largely depends on the location of lesion, liver reserve, and degree of hepatic dysfunction assessed preoperatively.

Outcomes

Improvements in recent decades with regard to patient selection, surgical technique, and perioperative care have led to reduced morbidity and mortality for all patients undergoing complex liver resection. Regionalization of liver resections to high volume centers has also been shown to positively impact both perioperative and long-term outcomes, with reported mortality rates of less than 4% [33–36]. With respect to HCC, similar perioperative mortality rates have been reported at 3–5%, attributed to refinements in patient selection and improvements in technique [37]. Regarding long-term outcomes, 5-year overall survival (OS) rates for patients undergoing SR have been shown to range from 27 to 70% [11, 38–53]. Recurrence rates, however, remain significantly elevated for patients undergoing SR, attributing to the fact that the remnant liver may continue to harbor malignant potential. In multiple studies, 5-year disease-free survival (DFS) for patients undergoing SR has been shown to range between 18 and 57%. Due to high recurrence rates, use of locoregional therapies to reduce tumor burden, re-resection in selected patients, and utilization of salvage LT following index resection have all been studied as possible treatment modalities for HCC recurrence following SR [54–56]. Factors associated with worsening survival include major vascular invasion and multifocal HCC disease [57, 58].

Liver Transplantation

Traditionally, LT has been considered standard of care for HCC patients with decompensated cirrhosis as both the tumor and underlying liver disease are addressed with this operation. Furthermore, patients with multifocal, unresectable disease or inadequate hepatic reserve are more appropriate for LT compared to SR. In 1996, Mazzaferro et al. described the Milan criteria to establish eligibility of HCC patients for liver transplantation [18]. By selecting patients with a single lesion ≤5 cm or ≤3 tumors no greater than 3 cm, no evidence of vascular invasion, and no regional nodal or extrahepatic metastases, 5-year survival rates of up to 75% have been demonstrated [18, 19, 59]. Such survival rates are similar to those for patients undergoing LT for cirrhosis without HCC. Since then, criteria expanding eligibility for LT have been proposed. The UCSF criteria, established by Yao et al. in 2001, considered patients with a single lesion ≤6.5 cm or ≤3 tumors each no greater than 4.5 cm and a total tumor size ≤8 cm appropriate for LT, achieving 5-year survival rates of 75% [60]. With regard to organ allocation and exception points, HCC patients with 1 tumor >2 and <5 cm or 2–3 tumors with the largest being <3 cm in size receive a MELD score of 22. Furthermore, patients receive an additional 3 MELD score points every 3 months they continue to meet the above HCC staging criteria, accounting for a 10% increase in mortality risk with each step-wise increase in MELD. Due to the benefit that HCC patients receive on the waiting list, allocation policies are investigating whether HCC patients are over-prioritized when placed on the waiting list for LT. By implementing these MELD exception points, dropout rates associated with disease progression while on the waiting list are thought to be reduced.

Outcomes

When comparing overall survival of appropriately selected HCC patients undergoing LT to those undergoing LT for nonmalignant etiologies, similar survival rates have been achieved. Five-year OS rates following LT range from 41 to 78%, while 5-year DFS rates range from 54 to 98% [11, 38–53, 61]. Prognostic factors that have been shown to adversely affect overall and recurrence-free survival include tumor size >5 cm, lymph node involvement, vascular invasion, bilobar hepatic involvement, and histologic grade [61, 62]. Additionally, the impact on pretransplant AFP levels has been well studied [63]. While no large randomized controlled trials have been performed comparing outcomes of LT with other therapeutic modalities for early-stage HCC, many retrospective studies and multicenter experiences have demonstrated equivalent or improved survival with LT [11, 38–53]. One must recognize that results after LT are highly selected due to watchful waiting on the list and monitoring of tumor status.

Surgical Resection vs. Liver Transplantation

Due to the significant heterogeneity of clinical and pathophysiological characteristics found in HCC patients, determining the optimal surgical treatment is complex and depends on appropriate patient selection and risk stratification. In addition to disease-related factors, surgeon specialty and training have been shown to significantly influence choice of therapy [64]. Further compounding this controversy is the fact that no randomized controlled trials comparing SR with LT have been performed. Level 1 evidence supporting either treatment modality does not exist, with the majority of studies consisting of single or multicenter institutional experiences.. In a review of SR versus LT for HCC patients by the Cochrane Collaboration, the authors concluded that no overall recommendation or refutation of one intervention over the other could be made [65].

When framing the issue of SR versus LT, it is important to understand that particular subsets of HCC patients are considered to be more appropriate for one surgical intervention compared to the other. In patients with severe cirrhosis (Child-Pugh class B or class C) and early-stage HCC, LT is considered primary treatment as transplantation allows for treatment of HCC as well as any underlying liver pathology. In patients with no cirrhosis or well-compensated cirrhosis and resectable HCC disease that is beyond Milan criteria, SR is more appropriate. The greatest controversy exists regarding the subgroup of HCC patients with well-compensated Child-Pugh class A cirrhosis and early-stage disease within Milan criteria. While this population represents a small percentage of HCC patients overall, significant variability in choice of therapy exists. Surgeon preference, organ availability, and hospital resources are the primary factors that determine utilization of SR versus LT for these patients.

Multiple meta-analyses have been undertaken that directly evaluate outcomes between SR and LT (Table 4.1) [28, 66–69]. Many of these have demonstrated favorable outcomes for patients undergoing LT compared to SR, with improved 5-year OS and DFS rates. In their review of ten series comparing over 1700 patients, Dhir et al. demonstrated that LT was associated with a statistically significant improvement in 5-year OS compared to SR (OR 0.58, 95% CI 0.36–0.94, $p = 0.03$) in patients with early-stage HCC [68]. When comparing patients with well-compensated cirrhosis, this survival advantage persisted (OR 0.54, 95% CI 0.38–0.77, $p < 0.01$). Proneth et al. performed a review of 70 studies that demonstrated increased 5-year OS (60.9% vs. 49.4%, $p < 0.01$) as well as increased 5-year DFS (58.0% vs. 33.9%, $p < 0.01$) for LT compared to SR [66]. Rahman et al. reported 5-year DFS rates ranging from 54 to 84% for LT compared to 18–56% for SR [67]. Finally, in a review of ten studies, Rahbari et al. reported that even though SR was found to have comparable 5-year OS rates to LT in some series, a majority of studies determined

Table 4.1 Overview of selected studies reporting overall survival and disease-free survival after surgical resection and liver transplantation

Author	Tumor burden	Child-Pugh class	ITT	SR (n)	LT (n)	5-year OS SR	5-year OS LT	5-year DFS SR	5-year DFS LT
Squires et al. [38]	Milan	A, B, C	No	45	131	44	66	23	85
Koniaris et al. [39]	Milan	N/A	Yes	26	73	63	41	52	46
Lee et al. [40]	Milan + beyond	A, B	No	82	48	58	78	57	89
Facciuto et al. [41]	Milan + beyond	A, B, C	Yes	51	106	57	53	NA	NA
Baccarani et al. [44]	Milan	A, B, C	Yes	38	48	27	72	37	98
Bellavance et al. [43]	Milan	A	No	245	134	46	66	40	82
Del Gaudio et al. [42]	Milan	A, B, C	Yes	80	293	66	58	41	54
Cillo et al. [46]	Milan + beyond	A, B, C	Yes	131	40	31	63	24	91
Shah et al. [11]	Milan	A, B	Yes	121	140	56	64	56	60
Poon [45]	Milan	A, B, C	Yes	204	43	60	44	44	84
Margarit et al. [47]	Milan	A	No	37	36	70	65	39	56
Bigourdan et al. [48]	Milan	A	Yes	20	17	36	71	40	80
Adam et al. [49]	Milan + beyond	A, B, C	Yes	98	195	50	61	18	58
Shabahang et al. [50]	Milan + beyond	A, B, C	No	44	65	37	66	36	66
De Carlis et al. [51]	Milan + beyond	A, B, C	No	154	121	40	60	38	74
Figueras et al. [52]	Milan + beyond	A, B, C	No	35	85	51	60	31	60
Llovet et al. [53]	Milan	A, B, C	Yes	77	87	51	69	NA	NA

DFS disease-free survival, *ITT* intention-to-treat, *LT* liver transplantation, *OS* overall survival, *SR* surgical resection

that LT was associated with significantly higher 5-year DFS [69].

The key consideration with regard to studies reporting outcomes for LT is that many only include HCC patients who actually receive a transplant. Patients who are initially listed for transplant but develop tumor progression and become ineligible for LT ultimately do not undergo operative intervention and are thus excluded from analyses. In essence, utilizing LT selects out patients with "bad" biology, and reported survival rates following transplantation may be falsely elevated. When intention-to-treat (ITT) analysis is performed, accounting for disease progression and mortality associated with time spent on transplant waiting lists, the 5-year OS between SR and LT is found to be comparable. In their series, Llovet et al. reported a dropout rate of 23% for patients on the waiting list for LT resulting in a decrease of 2-year OS from 84 to 54% [53]. Dhir et al., when analyzing only studies that included ITT analysis, found no statistically significant difference between patients undergoing SR and LT (OR 0.60, 95% CI 0.29–1.24, $p = 0.17$) [68]. Similarly, when selecting case-control studies that included ITT data for patients undergoing LT, Proneth et al. found that the difference in 5-year OS between SR and LT patients was no longer statistically significant (OR 0.84, 95% CI 0.48–1.48, $p = 0.55$) [66].

When restricting their meta-analysis to ITT studies, Rahman et al. found there was no significant difference in 5-year OS between SR and LT (OR 1.19, 95% CI 0.78–1.80, $p = 0.42$) [67].

Further complicating the matter is that many of these studies examining outcomes between SR and LT compare heterogeneous patient populations with different stages of HCC disease and varying levels of underlying liver function. Many studies examining outcomes following SR have included patients with HCC disease beyond Milan criteria or with vascular invasion, likely contributing to higher recurrence rates and worse outcomes. Conversely, some studies have included patients without any underlying liver disease, potentially contributing to more favorable outcomes for resection. In their evaluation of patients with well-compensated cirrhosis and early-stage HCC within Milan criteria, Koniaris et al. found that SR was associated with a 5-year OS rate of 63% compared to 41% for patients undergoing LT ($p = 0.04$), concluding that resection was associated with a survival advantage [39]. Despite utilizing ITT analysis, the study included patients without underlying cirrhosis in the SR group, likely affecting the comparison and skewing the results in favor of SR.

Despite the impact of intention-to-treat analyses on OS outcomes, recurrence rates remain significantly increased for patients undergoing SR. As a result, these patients are shown to suffer lower DFS rates compared to those undergoing LT. In a recent study, utilizing propensity score matching to balance baseline clinical and pathological characteristics, patients undergoing SR achieved comparable OS rates to those undergoing LT; however, DFS remained higher for LT patients [70]. When examining studies performing ITT analysis, Rahman et al. demonstrated that 5-year DFS was statistically significantly higher in LT patients compared to SR patients (54% vs. 49%, $p = 0.05$ with OR 0.76, 95% CI 0.57–1.00, $p = 0.05$) [67]. Furthermore, studies have demonstrated significantly higher 10-year OS (OR 0.44, 95% CI 0.34–0.58, $p < 0.001$) and 10-year DFS (OR 0.27, 95% CI 0.10–0.76, $p = 0.01$) for patients undergoing LT compared to SR [67].

Ultimately, proponents of LT argue that transplantation offers a clear benefit over resection due to higher rates of OS and DFS reported in many studies. Despite the purported survival advantage of LT for appropriately selected HCC patients, however, a significant proportion of patients do not receive a graft. A lack of standardized screening regimens results in few patients with cirrhosis being diagnosed at an early enough stage to be eligible as a candidate for LT. Even if diagnosed with early-stage HCC, many live in Eastern Asian countries where viable LT programs are rare and costs are prohibitive. Lack of organ availability due to a shortage of donors also complicates the issue. For these reasons, SR has been proposed as an appropriate treatment modality in early-stage HCC with the thought that resection is immediately available for patients without need for waiting lists or delays in intervention due to organ availability. Proponents of SR also argue that the higher rate of recurrence seen following resection may be salvaged by either re-resection in patients with adequate hepatic reserve or subsequent LT.

Resection followed by salvage transplantation has emerged as a potential treatment algorithm for patients with HCC. By utilizing resection as a bridging therapy, need for organs can be minimized, and disease progression while on the waiting list can theoretically be avoided. There remains significant controversy, however, with regard to appropriate management of recurrence following resection for patients with HCC. Some studies report similar outcomes for patients who undergo resection followed by salvage transplantation compared to patients who undergo liver transplantation as index operation, while others report inferior outcomes. Zhu et al. performed a meta-analysis of 14 studies and found that salvage LT was associated with comparable 5-year OS, though 5-year DFS was better in patients undergoing primary LT [56]. Hu et al. demonstrated no difference in 5-year survival rates between patients undergoing primary LT and those undergoing salvage transplantation [71]. Consideration must be given, however, that patients who undergo resection may lose their listing status, thus precluding subsequent transplantation.

In summary, appropriately selected patients with early-stage HCC and no evidence of vascular invasion can be considered for either SR or LT (Fig. 4.2). There is a lack of studies comparing SR and LT that utilize appropriate ITT analyses as well as propensity matching to ensure equivalent patient populations. Proponents of LT point to higher recurrence rates associated with SR, while surgeons favoring SR argue that shortage of donors, risk of disease progression during long waiting list times, and long-term complications associated with posttransplant immunosuppression are reasons to consider SR over LT (Table 4.2). As a result, both surgical modalities currently remain viable treatment options for early-stage HCC patients with well-compensated cirrhosis until further, more well-designed studies are undertaken.

Conflicts of Interest There are no conflicts of interest to disclose.

Table 4.2 Considerations for surgical resection versus liver transplantation in HCC

Surgical resection	Liver transplantation
5-year OS ~30–70%	5-year OS ~40–80%
5-year DFS ~20–60%	5-year DFS ~45–98%
Higher risk of intrahepatic recurrence	Lower risk of intrahepatic recurrence
Requires adequate hepatic and functional reserve	Limited donor availability
No waiting list required	Time on waiting list allows for disease progression

DFS disease-free survival, *OS* overall survival

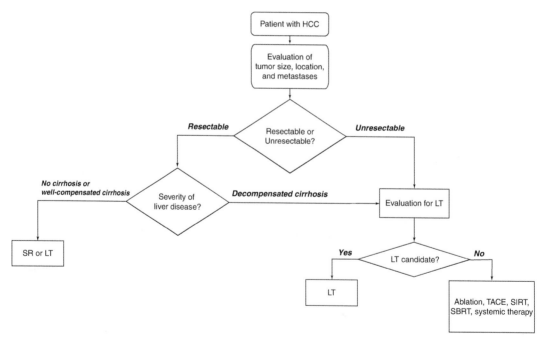

Fig. 4.2 Treatment algorithm for patients with hepatocellular carcinoma. *HCC* hepatocellular carcinoma, *LT* liver transplantation, *SBRT* stereotactic body radiotherapy, *SIRT* selective internal radiation therapy, *SR* surgical resection, *TACE* transarterial chemoembolization

References

1. Ferlay J, Soerjomataram I, Dikshit R, Eser S, Mathers C, Rebelo M, et al. Cancer incidence and mortality worldwide: sources, methods and major patterns in GLOBOCAN 2012. Int J Cancer. 2015;136(5):E359–86.
2. Jemal A, Bray F, Center MM, Ferlay J, Ward E, Forman D. Global cancer statistics. CA Cancer J Clin. 2011;61(2):69–90.
3. Ryerson AB, Eheman CR, Altekruse SF, Ward JW, Jemal A, Sherman RL, et al. Annual report to the nation on the status of cancer, 1975-2012, featuring the increasing incidence of liver cancer. Cancer. 2016;122(9):1312–37.
4. El-Serag HB, Siegel AB, Davila JA, Shaib YH, Cayton-Woody M, McBride R, et al. Treatment and outcomes of treating of hepatocellular carcinoma among Medicare recipients in the United States: a population-based study. J Hepatol. 2006;44(1):158–66.
5. Okuda K, Ohtsuki T, Obata H, Tomimatsu M, Okazaki N, Hasegawa H, et al. Natural history of hepatocellular carcinoma and prognosis in relation to treatment. Study of 850 patients. Cancer. 1985;56(4):918–28.
6. Pawarode A, Tangkijvanich P, Voravud N. Outcomes of primary hepatocellular carcinoma treatment: an 8-year experience with 368 patients in Thailand. J Gastroenterol Hepatol. 2000;15(8):860–4.
7. Rabe C, Pilz T, Klostermann C, Berna M, Schild HH, Sauerbruch T, et al. Clinical characteristics and outcome of a cohort of 101 patients with hepatocellular carcinoma. World J Gastroenterol. 2001;7(2):208–15.
8. Schoniger-Hekele M, Muller C, Kutilek M, Oesterreicher C, Ferenci P, Gangl A. Hepatocellular carcinoma in Central Europe: prognostic features and survival. Gut. 2001;48(1):103–9.
9. Yeung YP, Lo CM, Liu CL, Wong BC, Fan ST, Wong J. Natural history of untreated nonsurgical hepatocellular carcinoma. Am J Gastroenterol. 2005;100(9):1995–2004.
10. Hoofnagle JH. Hepatocellular carcinoma: summary and recommendations. Gastroenterology. 2004;127(5 Suppl 1):S319–23.
11. Shah SA, Cleary SP, Tan JC, Wei AC, Gallinger S, Grant DR, et al. An analysis of resection vs transplantation for early hepatocellular carcinoma: defining the optimal therapy at a single institution. Ann Surg Oncol. 2007;14(9):2608–14.
12. Bruix J, Sherman M, American Association for the Study of Liver Diseases. Management of hepatocellular carcinoma: an update. Hepatology. 2011;53(3):1020–2.
13. Kansagara D, Papak J, Pasha AS, O'Neil M, Freeman M, Relevo R, et al. Screening for hepatocellular carcinoma in chronic liver disease: a systematic review. Ann Intern Med. 2014;161(4):261–9.
14. Bilimoria MM, Lauwers GY, Doherty DA, Nagorney DM, Belghiti J, Do KA, et al. Underlying liver disease, not tumor factors, predicts long-term survival after resection of hepatocellular carcinoma. Arch Surg. 2001;136(5):528–35.
15. Lau WY. Future perspectives for hepatocellular carcinoma. HPB (Oxford). 2003;5(4):206–13.
16. Llovet JM, Fuster J, Bruix J, Barcelona-Clinic Liver Cancer Group. The Barcelona approach: diagnosis, staging, and treatment of hepatocellular carcinoma. Liver Transpl. 2004;10(2 Suppl 1):S115–20.
17. Llovet JM, Burroughs A, Bruix J. Hepatocellular carcinoma. Lancet. 2003;362(9399):1907–17.
18. Mazzaferro V, Regalia E, Doci R, Andreola S, Pulvirenti A, Bozzetti F, et al. Liver transplantation for the treatment of small hepatocellular carcinomas in patients with cirrhosis. N Engl J Med. 1996;334(11):693–9.
19. Clavien PA, Lesurtel M, Bossuyt PM, Gores GJ, Langer B, Perrier A, et al. Recommendations for liver transplantation for hepatocellular carcinoma: an international consensus conference report. Lancet Oncol. 2012;13(1):e11–22.
20. Hsu CY, Liu PH, Hsia CY, Lee YH, Nagaria TS, Lee RC, et al. Surgical resection is better than transarterial chemoembolization for patients with hepatocellular carcinoma beyond the Milan criteria: a prognostic nomogram study. Ann Surg Oncol. 2016;23(3):994–1002.
21. Kloeckner R, Ruckes C, Kronfeld K, Worns MA, Weinmann A, Galle PR, et al. Selective internal radiotherapy (SIRT) versus transarterial chemoembolization (TACE) for the treatment of intrahepatic cholangiocellular carcinoma (CCC): study protocol for a randomized controlled trial. Trials. 2014;15:311.
22. Lei J, Wang W, Yan L. Downstaging advanced hepatocellular carcinoma to the Milan criteria may provide a comparable outcome to conventional Milan criteria. J Gastrointest Surg. 2013;17(8):1440–6.
23. Murali AR, Romero-Marrero C, Miller C, Aucejo F, Levitin A, Gill A, et al. Predictors of successful downstaging of hepatocellular carcinoma outside Milan criteria. Transplantation. 2016;100(11):2391–7.
24. Zaydfudim VM, Vachharajani N, Klintmalm GB, Jarnagin WR, Hemming AW, Doyle MB, et al. Liver resection and transplantation for patients with hepatocellular carcinoma beyond Milan criteria. Ann Surg. 2016;264(4):650–8.
25. Jarnagin WR. Management of small hepatocellular carcinoma: a review of transplantation, resection, and ablation. Ann Surg Oncol. 2010;17(5):1226–33.
26. Truty MJ, Vauthey JN. Surgical resection of high-risk hepatocellular carcinoma: patient selection, preoperative considerations, and operative technique. Ann Surg Oncol. 2010;17(5):1219–25.
27. Bruix J, Castells A, Bosch J, Feu F, Fuster J, Garcia-Pagan JC, et al. Surgical resection of hepatocellular carcinoma in cirrhotic patients: prognostic value of preoperative portal pressure. Gastroenterology. 1996;111(4):1018–22.
28. Dhir M, Melin AA, Douaiher J, Lin C, Zhen WK, Hussain SM, et al. A review and update of treatment options and controversies in the manage-

ment of hepatocellular carcinoma. Ann Surg. 2016;263(6):1112–25.
29. Abulkhir A, Limongelli P, Healey AJ, Damrah O, Tait P, Jackson J, et al. Preoperative portal vein embolization for major liver resection: a meta-analysis. Ann Surg. 2008;247(1):49–57.
30. Azoulay D, Castaing D, Krissat J, Smail A, Hargreaves GM, Lemoine A, et al. Percutaneous portal vein embolization increases the feasibility and safety of major liver resection for hepatocellular carcinoma in injured liver. Ann Surg. 2000;232(5):665–72.
31. Wakabayashi H, Ishimura K, Okano K, Izuishi K, Karasawa Y, Goda F, et al. Is preoperative portal vein embolization effective in improving prognosis after major hepatic resection in patients with advanced-stage hepatocellular carcinoma? Cancer. 2001;92(9):2384–90.
32. Cucchetti A, Cescon M, Ercolani G, Bigonzi E, Torzilli G, Pinna AD. A comprehensive meta-regression analysis on outcome of anatomic resection versus nonanatomic resection for hepatocellular carcinoma. Ann Surg Oncol. 2012;19(12):3697–705.
33. Andreou A, Vauthey JN, Cherqui D, Zimmitti G, Ribero D, Truty MJ, et al. Improved long-term survival after major resection for hepatocellular carcinoma: a multicenter analysis based on a new definition of major hepatectomy. J Gastrointest Surg. 2013;17(1):66–77; discussion.
34. Fan ST, Mau Lo C, Poon RT, Yeung C, Leung Liu C, Yuen WK, et al. Continuous improvement of survival outcomes of resection of hepatocellular carcinoma: a 20-year experience. Ann Surg. 2011;253(4):745–58.
35. Li GZ, Speicher PJ, Lidsky ME, Darrabie MD, Scarborough JE, White RR, et al. Hepatic resection for hepatocellular carcinoma: do contemporary morbidity and mortality rates demand a transition to ablation as first-line treatment? J Am Coll Surg. 2014;218(4):827–34.
36. Yang T, Zhang J, Lu JH, Yang GS, Wu MC, Yu WF. Risk factors influencing postoperative outcomes of major hepatic resection of hepatocellular carcinoma for patients with underlying liver diseases. World J Surg. 2011;35(9):2073–82.
37. Fong ZV, Tanabe KK. The clinical management of hepatocellular carcinoma in the United States, Europe, and Asia: a comprehensive and evidence-based comparison and review. Cancer. 2014;120(18):2824–38.
38. Squires MH 3rd, Hanish SI, Fisher SB, Garrett C, Kooby DA, Sarmiento JM, et al. Transplant versus resection for the management of hepatocellular carcinoma meeting Milan criteria in the MELD exception era at a single institution in a UNOS region with short wait times. J Surg Oncol. 2014;109(6):533–41.
39. Koniaris LG, Levi DM, Pedroso FE, Franceschi D, Tzakis AG, Santamaria-Barria JA, et al. Is surgical resection superior to transplantation in the treatment of hepatocellular carcinoma? Ann Surg. 2011;254(3):527–37; discussion 37–8.
40. Lee KK, Kim DG, Moon IS, Lee MD, Park JH. Liver transplantation versus liver resection for the treatment of hepatocellular carcinoma. J Surg Oncol. 2010;101(1):47–53.
41. Facciuto ME, Rochon C, Pandey M, Rodriguez-Davalos M, Samaniego S, Wolf DC, et al. Surgical dilemma: liver resection or liver transplantation for hepatocellular carcinoma and cirrhosis. Intention-to-treat analysis in patients within and outwith Milan criteria. HPB (Oxford). 2009;11(5):398–404.
42. Del Gaudio M, Ercolani G, Ravaioli M, Cescon M, Lauro A, Vivarelli M, et al. Liver transplantation for recurrent hepatocellular carcinoma on cirrhosis after liver resection: University of Bologna experience. Am J Transplant. 2008;8(6):1177–85.
43. Bellavance EC, Lumpkins KM, Mentha G, Marques HP, Capussotti L, Pulitano C, et al. Surgical management of early-stage hepatocellular carcinoma: resection or transplantation? J Gastrointest Surg. 2008;12(10):1699–708.
44. Baccarani U, Isola M, Adani GL, Benzoni E, Avellini C, Lorenzin D, et al. Superiority of transplantation versus resection for the treatment of small hepatocellular carcinoma. Transpl Int. 2008;21(3):247–54.
45. Poon RT. Optimal initial treatment for early hepatocellular carcinoma in patients with preserved liver function: transplantation or resection? Ann Surg Oncol. 2007;14(2):541–7.
46. Cillo U, Vitale A, Brolese A, Zanus G, Neri D, Valmasoni M, et al. Partial hepatectomy as first-line treatment for patients with hepatocellular carcinoma. J Surg Oncol. 2007;95(3):213–20.
47. Margarit C, Escartin A, Castells L, Vargas V, Allende E, Bilbao I. Resection for hepatocellular carcinoma is a good option in child-turcotte-pugh Class A patients with cirrhosis who are eligible for liver transplantation. Liver Transpl. 2005;11(10):1242–51.
48. Bigourdan JM, Jaeck D, Meyer N, Meyer C, Oussoultzoglou E, Bachellier P, et al. Small hepatocellular carcinoma in child A cirrhotic patients: hepatic resection versus transplantation. Liver Transpl. 2003;9(5):513–20.
49. Adam R, Azoulay D, Castaing D, Eshkenazy R, Pascal G, Hashizume K, et al. Liver resection as a bridge to transplantation for hepatocellular carcinoma on cirrhosis: a reasonable strategy? Ann Surg. 2003;238(4):508–18; discussion 18–9.
50. Shabahang M, Franceschi D, Yamashiki N, Reddy R, Pappas PA, Aviles K, et al. Comparison of hepatic resection and hepatic transplantation in the treatment of hepatocellular carcinoma among cirrhotic patients. Ann Surg Oncol. 2002;9(9):881–6.
51. De Carlis L, Giacomoni A, Pirotta V, Lauterio A, Slim AO, Bondinara GF, et al. Treatment of HCC: the role of liver resection in the era of transplantation. Transplant Proc. 2001;33(1–2):1453–6.
52. Figueras J, Jaurrieta E, Valls C, Ramos E, Serrano T, Rafecas A, et al. Resection or transplantation for hepatocellular carcinoma in cirrhotic patients: outcomes based on indicated treatment strategy. J Am Coll Surg. 2000;190(5):580–7.

53. Llovet JM, Fuster J, Bruix J. Intention-to-treat analysis of surgical treatment for early hepatocellular carcinoma: resection versus transplantation. Hepatology. 1999;30(6):1434–40.
54. Llovet JM, Schwartz M, Mazzaferro V. Resection and liver transplantation for hepatocellular carcinoma. Semin Liver Dis. 2005;25(2):181–200.
55. Sala M, Fuster J, Llovet JM, Navasa M, Sole M, Varela M, et al. High pathological risk of recurrence after surgical resection for hepatocellular carcinoma: an indication for salvage liver transplantation. Liver Transpl. 2004;10(10):1294–300.
56. Zhu Y, Dong J, Wang WL, Li MX, Lu Y. Short- and long-term outcomes after salvage liver transplantation versus primary liver transplantation for hepatocellular carcinoma: a meta-analysis. Transplant Proc. 2013;45(9):3329–42.
57. Jarnagin W, Chapman WC, Curley S, D'Angelica M, Rosen C, Dixon E, et al. Surgical treatment of hepatocellular carcinoma: expert consensus statement. HPB (Oxford). 2010;12(5):302–10.
58. Nathan H, Schulick RD, Choti MA, Pawlik TM. Predictors of survival after resection of early hepatocellular carcinoma. Ann Surg. 2009;249(5):799–805.
59. Forner A, Llovet JM, Bruix J. Hepatocellular carcinoma. Lancet. 2012;379(9822):1245–55.
60. Yao FY, Ferrell L, Bass NM, Watson JJ, Bacchetti P, Venook A, et al. Liver transplantation for hepatocellular carcinoma: expansion of the tumor size limits does not adversely impact survival. Hepatology. 2001;33(6):1394–403.
61. Kluger MD, Salceda JA, Laurent A, Tayar C, Duvoux C, Decaens T, et al. Liver resection for hepatocellular carcinoma in 313 Western patients: tumor biology and underlying liver rather than tumor size drive prognosis. J Hepatol. 2015;62(5):1131–40.
62. Lewin M, Gelu-Simeon M, Ostos M, Boufassa F, Sobesky R, Teicher E, et al. Imaging features and prognosis of hepatocellular carcinoma in patients with cirrhosis who are coinfected with human immunodeficiency virus and hepatitis C virus. Radiology. 2015;277(2):443–53.
63. Duvoux C, Roudot-Thoraval F, Decaens T, Pessione F, Badran H, Piardi T, et al. Liver transplantation for hepatocellular carcinoma: a model including alpha-fetoprotein improves the performance of Milan criteria. Gastroenterology. 2012;143(4):986–94 e3; quiz e14–5.
64. Nathan H, Bridges JF, Schulick RD, Cameron AM, Hirose K, Edil BH, et al. Understanding surgical decision making in early hepatocellular carcinoma. J Clin Oncol. 2011;29(6):619–25.
65. Taefi A, Abrishami A, Nasseri-Moghaddam S, Eghtesad B, Sherman M. Surgical resection versus liver transplant for patients with hepatocellular carcinoma. Cochrane Database Syst Rev. 2013;(6):CD006935.
66. Proneth A, Zeman F, Schlitt HJ, Schnitzbauer AA. Is resection or transplantation the ideal treatment in patients with hepatocellular carcinoma in cirrhosis if both are possible? A systematic review and meta-analysis. Ann Surg Oncol. 2014;21(9):3096–107.
67. Rahman A, Assifi MM, Pedroso FE, Maley WR, Sola JE, Lavu H, et al. Is resection equivalent to transplantation for early cirrhotic patients with hepatocellular carcinoma? A meta-analysis. J Gastrointest Surg. 2012;16(10):1897–909.
68. Dhir M, Lyden ER, Smith LM, Are C. Comparison of outcomes of transplantation and resection in patients with early hepatocellular carcinoma: a meta-analysis. HPB (Oxford). 2012;14(9):635–45.
69. Rahbari NN, Mehrabi A, Mollberg NM, Muller SA, Koch M, Buchler MW, et al. Hepatocellular carcinoma: current management and perspectives for the future. Ann Surg. 2011;253(3):453–69.
70. Shen JY, Li C, Wen TF, Yan LN, Li B, Wang WT, et al. Liver transplantation versus surgical resection for HCC meeting the Milan criteria: a propensity score analysis. Medicine (Baltimore). 2016;95(52):e5756.
71. Hu Z, Wang W, Li Z, Ye S, Zheng SS. Recipient outcomes of salvage liver transplantation versus primary liver transplantation: a systematic review and meta-analysis. Liver Transpl. 2012;18(11):1316–23.

Locoregional Therapies in the Management of Hepatocellular Carcinoma

Alexa O. Levey, R. Mitch Ermentrout, Zachary L. Bercu, and Darren D. Kies

Introduction

Hepatocellular carcinoma (HCC) is the most common primary liver malignancy in the world, with over 14 million cases in 2012 and an expected growth to 22 million over the next 20 years [1–3]. It develops secondary to intrinsic liver diseases such as viral hepatitis, alcoholic cirrhosis, steatohepatitis, biliary cirrhosis, or other rarer causes. It represents the third most common etiology of cancer-related deaths in the world and the seventh most common etiology in the United States [3, 4]. As most patients have concomitant chronic liver disease leading to the development of HCC, management of the disease becomes more complicated. Staging and treatment options are impacted not only by the extent of the tumor but also by the patient's liver function and performance status. Because the majority of patients present with unresectable disease, locoregional therapies, including image-guided percutaneous ablation and image-guided trans-

A. O. Levey · R. M. Ermentrout · Z. L. Bercu
Department of Radiology, Division of Interventional Radiology and Image-Guided Medicine, Emory University School of Medicine, Atlanta, GA, USA
e-mail: alexa.levey@emory.edu;
robert.mitchell.ermentrout@emory.edu;
zachary.louis.bercu@emory.edu

D. D. Kies (✉)
Piedmont South Imaging,
Newnan, GA, USA
e-mail: dkies@emory.edu

catheter tumor therapies, play an important role in the management of patients with HCC.

The decision to proceed with locoregional therapy in the treatment of HCC is framed around the most widely used and well-validated system—the Barcelona Clinic Liver Cancer (BCLC) group diagnostic and treatment strategy [5]. First published in 1999 and subsequently updated, the system provides a framework to stratify patients based on the extent of tumor, their liver function, and performance status. Curative therapies are recommended for those with very early- and early-stage disease (BCLC 0 and A), while only palliative therapies are available for those with intermediate and advanced-stage disease (BCLC B and C). Terminal stage HCC (BCLC D) has a dismal prognosis, and only supportive care is recommended. Locoregional therapies are included as treatment options in both the curative and palliative arms of the BCLC guidelines. Ablation is recommended for the treatment of very early-stage HCC in patients that are not liver transplant candidates and also for early-stage HCC when associated diseases preclude liver transplantation. Chemoembolization is recommended for intermediate-stage hepatocellular carcinoma.

While the BCLC guidelines provide a framework for the management of patients with HCC, there are some limitations. In practice, locoregional therapies play a much larger and important role in the management of all stages of HCC. Percutaneous ablation and image-guided transcatheter tumor therapies are widely used as a bridge to liver transplantation. Bridging therapy diminishes the dropout rate of patients on the transplant list by preventing disease progression and improves outcomes by lowering HCC recurrence rates and improving survival following liver transplantation [6–9]. Furthermore, local therapies can be used to move patients from the palliative arm of the BCLC guidelines into the curative arm by downstaging to either resection or liver transplantation [10, 11]. Finally, locoregional therapies are also being used for the palliative management of advanced-stage HCC and in highly selected terminal-stage patients, whose performance status is maintained despite poor liver function [12]. These practical additions to the BCLC guidelines are shown below (Fig. 5.1).

Image-Guided Percutaneous Ablation for HCC

For patients with BCLC 0 and BCLC A HCC, ablation is an effective and potentially curative treatment for patients that are not eligible for resection or liver transplant. Ablation also plays a role in combination with other liver-directed therapies for patients with more advanced-stage HCC. We will discuss the mechanism, advantages, disadvantages, complications, and relative outcomes associated with cryoablation, radiofrequency ablation, microwave ablation, and irreversible electroporation in HCC.

Cryoablation

Since the early nineteenth century, cryoablation was initially used in the treatment of breast and gynecologic cancers [13]. With improved

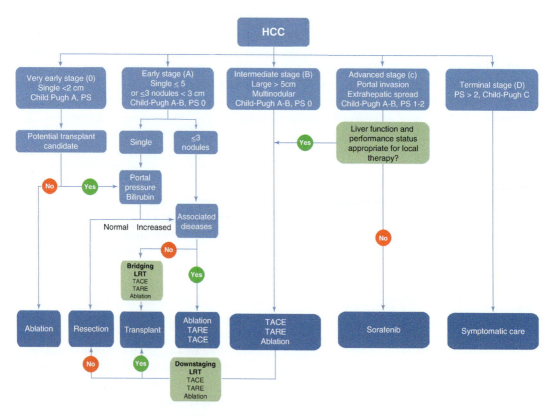

Fig. 5.1 An enhanced version of the BCLC guidelines that reflect the integration of locoregional therapies into the management of HCC, with particular emphasis on advanced-stage HCC, bridging therapy, and downstaging therapy

imaging and the development of needle-like applicators, cryoablation began to be used for the treatment of solid organ cancers via open surgery, laparoscopy, and percutaneous techniques.

Modern technique utilizes real-time ultrasound and/or CT guidance for placement of the needle-shaped probes, typically 15–17 gauges, into the targeted tumor [14]. A gas with low freezing point such as argon, nitric oxide, or liquid nitrogen is circulated through the needle. Rapid expansion of the gas into a closed chamber at the tip of the probe causes a highly endothermic reaction and subsequent formation of a predictably shaped ball of ice surrounding the probe, which can be visualized with real-time imaging. Cell death occurs at $-20°$ C, with apoptosis potentiated by the combination of at least two rapid freezing and active thawing cycles. A single probe can form an approximately 3 cm ice ball, so multiple evenly spaced probes are generally used to treat larger lesions with at least a 1 cm margin of normal tissue.

Cryoablation has been shown to be efficacious in treating patients with unresectable HCC or recurrent HCC [15]. In comparison to radiofrequency ablation, there is less procedural pain [16] and decreased heat sink effect and can be used to treat lesions larger than 3 cm with lower rates of local recurrence [17]. Additionally, the ability to see the ice ball form in real time allows clinicians to see the treatment zone in real time and ensure adequate ablation.

Cryoablation can be more expensive, and unlike RFA, not all systems allow for tract ablation, which may increase the risk of postoperative bleeding and increase the risk of tract seeding [16]. Of particular concern is the risk of cryoshock, a phenomenon in which patients treated with cryoablation experience a precipitous drop in platelet count and develop disseminated intravascular coagulation. While the incidence of cryoshock is only approximately 1%, mortality in these patients can be as high as 28% [14]. Risk of cryoshock increases with larger volume of ablation, and since the main advantage of cryoablation is the ability to achieve larger ablation zones, the risk of cryoshock is likely higher in these patients. More commonly, but still with low occurrence rates, patients may develop a pneumothorax, biliary injury, or infection as a result of the procedure.

Radiofrequency Ablation

Radiofrequency current was first used, and is still used today, to cut and coagulate living tissue in the early nineteenth century, thanks to the work of Harvey Cushing and W.T. Bovie [13]. Then, cardiologists began using this technology to treat arrhythmias in a minimally invasive manner. Initially limited by small ablation zones, newer probes and improved energy delivery systems have allowed for radiofrequency to be used to treat tumors such as HCC.

Real-time imaging guidance is used to advance the typically needle-like probe into the lesion of interest. Some systems include an array of evenly spaced tines that emerge from the tip of the probe to envelop the tumor. Probes can be monopolar or bipolar, and they require placement of a grounding pad on the patients' thighs to form a closed-loop circuit. Then, alternating electric current with a frequency ranging from 375 to 500 kHz is passed into the probe tip with the goal of heating tissue in contact with the probe and adjacent to the probe by passive frictional heating. A temperature of at least $50°$ C is needed to cause immediate cell death.

Like many ablative techniques, RFA can be performed under conscious sedation and as an outpatient procedure. Studies have reported lower complication rates with RFA than with surgical resection, ranging from 2.4 to 13.1% and 9 to 22%, respectively [18]. Some studies, including a randomized controlled trial by Chen et al., have shown no significant difference in survival of patients with small HCC treated with RFA versus surgical resection, which may make this lower-risk procedure a better option for some patients [19].

One limitation of RFA is the so-called heat sink effect. Vessels larger than 3.0 mm that are near the ablation zone can decrease passive frictional heating of the adjacent tissues, causing incomplete tumor ablation and positive treatment margins [20, 21]. To combat the "heat sink effect," new probes with local cooling mechanisms at the probe tip have come on the market to decrease charring. Additionally, vessels that may interfere with treatment can be embolized preoperatively.

Other disadvantages of this technique are related to tumor location and tract seeding. RFA in the capsular or subcapsular region of the liver can be painful and may require general anesthesia [16]. Finally, tract seeding is the spread of malignancy outside the liver into adjacent structures or the peritoneum due to percutaneous puncture of the liver tumor. This is a dreaded complication and can lead to patient removal from the liver transplantation waitlist. The reported incidence of this complication is as high as 4% and is increased in patients treated with RFA who have subcapsular lesions, increased number of probes used during the procedure, and increased number of total treatment sessions [22]. Due to this risk, tracts are now more routinely coagulated at the completion of the procedure, which has significantly decreased this risk.

The most common complication with RFA is hemorrhage, with less than 1% of patients having severe enough bleeding to need a transfusion [23]. Even less commonly, patients may experience skin burns from incorrect use of grounding pads during the procedure and develop a pneumothorax, pleural effusion, biliary injury, bowel injury, infection, or tumor seeding.

Microwave Ablation

Percutaneous microwave ablation takes advantage of the fact that the majority of tissues in the human body are composed at least partly of water and that water is a dipole. When an alternating electric current of 900–2500 MHz is applied within the tumor, water molecules within the tissue will flip back and forth to reorient with the applied electric field. This constant flipping increases the kinetic energy of the water molecules that is dissipated as friction and heat within the surrounding tissue, causing coagulation necrosis by active heating.

Single or multiple 13–17 gauge microwave antennas, which are generally needle-like but comes in a variety of designs, are inserted into the tumor under image guidance. The antenna is coupled to a device that measures local tissue temperature so intra-tumoral temperature can be monitored in real time, as well as a cooling system to decrease shaft heating. Then, a generator is turned on that produces electromagnetic waves at a typical frequency of 915 MHz. Once tissue temperature reaches 60° C or higher, coagulation necrosis occurs and the treatment is complete. This technology affects primarily water molecules, so one major advantage of this technique is that it can be used in high-risk places, such as near blood vessels, bowel, or components of the biliary system [24, 25]. Since the degree of heating created increases proportionally to the square of the number of antennas placed, overlap of electromagnetic fields creates a larger zone of ablation in a smaller amount of time [20]. Heating in this method is an active process, so MWA is not limited by electrical conductivity of a tissue and is less affected by heat sink from nearby vessels. This process allows for treatment of larger tissue, unlike RFA where treatment of larger tumors is limited by increased tissue impedance and local charring. Furthermore, because there is no need for grounding pads, there is a lower risk for local skin burns. Complications are similar to that of RFA and include hemorrhage, pleural effusion, pneumothorax, bowel injury, infection, burning of the skin, and local tumor seeding.

Irreversible Electroporation

IRE is a newer technique that employs the use of high voltage (1000–3000 V) applied over micro-milliseconds to create defects in the lipid bilayer of cells that leads to cell death [14]. Since only cells within this electric field are susceptible to these effects, surrounding structures are preserved during treatment [25]. Unlike the other ablative methods, IRE requires neuromuscular blockade to prevent movement during voltage delivery, so patients must be under general anesthesia for the procedure [26].

Tumor dimensions are calculated and used to determine the number and spacing of probes needed to create an adequate ablation zone [26]. Single/bipolar/multipolar 19-gauge probes are placed around the tumor under image guidance, ensuring probe placement is within 10° of parallel. The voltage setting for each probe is based on the distance between probes, with a maximum distance of around 2.5 cm. Then, the computer-controlled pulse generator delivers 3000 V to the probes in approximately 9 sets of 10 pulses lasting from 20 to 100 ms per pulse [27]. To prevent arrhythmias, pulse delivery is synchronized with an EKG to ensure delivery during the myocardial refractory period, which is attained when the pulse rate is less than 115 bpm. As the pulses are delivered, the amount of current delivered to the tissue is being monitored and should increase overtime as ablated tissue resistance decreases. If current flow exceeds 48A, the generator stops pulse delivery and recharges [27].

The treatment effect of IRE is on the lipid bilayer of cell membranes, thereby sparing the extracellular matrix from damage and allowing for earlier treatment evaluation with imaging. In other techniques where the parenchyma undergoes fibrosis/scarring, imaging posttreatment is usually delayed several weeks to allow for differentiation between contrast enhancements from residual tumor to posttreatment change. Therefore, residual tumor can be detected and treated in a more expeditious manner. One study also showed that patients without severe cirrhosis or prior chemoembolization treatment actually regenerated liver after the procedure [27]. In addition to preservation of the extracellular matrix of tissues within the treatment zone, the absence of direct heating in this technique prevents damage of surrounding structures such as the biliary system and bowel.

Performing IRE is technically difficult, and if probes are not placed precisely within 10° of parallel, reversible electroporation occurs, which can lead to tumor recurrence [26]. In the liver, overlying ribs and close proximity to other organ systems make this exceptionally difficult. Since this procedure also requires the use of multiple probes, there is an increased risk of subcapsular hematoma and local tumor seeding as compared to other ablative techniques [27]. Additionally, IRE requires the use of general anesthesia while other ablative techniques can usually be performed under conscious sedation. Complications from IRE are related to the delivery of high voltage and use of multiple probes and include pneumothorax, pain, and cardiac arrhythmias.

Outcomes

The major downside of surgical resection as compared to ablative therapy is the increased complication rates of up to 21.4% and longer hospital stay, which may lead to increased overall cost to the patient [18, 28]. As well, some patients are not surgical candidates due to tumor size, degree of cirrhosis, and additional comorbidities, so it is important to review the efficacy of ablation alone in the treatment of HCC.

RFA: Most studies have shown the best results of RFA when used to treat HCC lesions <3.0 cm, with up to 74% of treated lesions showing no residual disease in explanted livers at the time of liver transplantation [16, 29]. With regard to survival, patients with HCC measuring ≤3 cm have a 5-year survival of 60% of more [14, 30]. When tumors demonstrate arterial-portal shunting, patients treated with RFA may have small satellite lesions that remain/occur adjacent to the treated tumor that are occult on follow-up imaging and therefore may be left untreated.

MWA: Zhi-Yu et al. initially demonstrated that microwave ablation can be used in the treatment of HCC lesions in high-risk areas where RFA may be difficult [21]. Additionally, Graf et al. found microwave thermal ablation to be more efficacious than RFA in treating tumors <5 cm, with an overall 5-year survival of around 46–50% when treating tumors of this size [31]. Given the technical advantages with respect to the lack of undertreatment due to heat sink and charring, microwave ablation has supplanted RFA as the preferred modality in many centers.

CRYO: With the success of RFA, cryoablation is used less often in the treatment of HCC compared to other tumors due to the risk of cryo-shock without the benefit of increased survival rates. Survival rates at 5 years have been reported as high as 55% in tumor less than 5 cm [14].

IRE: As a growing form of treatment, little research has been done in evaluating efficacy of IRE in the treatment of HCC, but preliminary research has been promising. One study showed a complete response to therapy in 15/18 HCC lesions treated with IRE with the greatest success in lesions ≤2.3 cm, and another showed local recurrence-free survival at 6 months and 12 months of 90% and 50% in HCC tumors ranging from 1.3 to 4.5 cm [26, 27].

Ablation as a Bridge to Liver Transplantation

Ablation can be used as a bridge to liver transplantation or as a method for downgrading a patient so that they become eligible for transplantation or resection. While transplantation is the first option for patients with Child's B or C cirrhosis and tumors that confine to Milan criteria, increased wait times on the transplant list decreased overall 5-year survival by 10–20% if patients are on the waitlist for 6–12 months [14]. Furthermore, the dropout rate from the transplant list during this waiting period of 6–12 months can be as high as 10–30% secondary to disease progression and falling out of Milan criteria. As such, local regional therapies, including RFA, play an important role in preventing patient dropout from the transplant waitlist. In patients treated with RFA on the transplant list, there is improved overall survival, disease-free survival, and cancer mortality [23]. Patients treated with RFA are more likely to get a transplant due to decreased dropout rates [32] and have similar outcomes with regard to tumor recurrence, survival, and disease-free survival posttransplant as those patients transplanted who remained within Milan criteria while on the waitlist [33].

Ablation vs Resection

Radiofrequency ablation is the most studied local regional therapy, and its efficacy has been compared to that of surgical resection in randomized controlled trials. As such, we will focus on RFA in this section. In patients with Child's A cirrhosis or better treated with RFA versus surgical resection for a single HCC ≤5 cm, one randomized controlled trial showed equivalent disease-free and overall survival over a 4-year period when accounting for tumor size, with significantly less complications and shorter hospital stays in the group treated with RFA [19]. When looking at patients with Child's A/B cirrhosis who had no more than two tumors that measured less than 4 cm, another trial found that there was no significant difference in 3-year overall recurrence rate, overall survival, and recurrence-free survival between patients treated with RFA or surgery [28]. Similar rates of survival were also found in patients with no more than three tumors measuring ≤3 cm [34].

Conversely, another trial by Huang et al. randomized patients who met Milan criteria to RFA or surgical resection and found that overall survival rates and recurrence-free survival rates were statistically higher in surgical resection group, even when accounting for differences in tumor size and degree of cirrhosis [35].

Given different findings in randomized controlled trials, the decision of whether ablation can be used to treat a small HCC alone versus pursuing surgical resection is still very controversial. Surgical resection is more invasive and associated with higher complication rates but may lead to longer disease-free survival. On the other hand, many trials have shown RFA to have a better safety profile and to be equally as efficacious with regard to survival in lesions measuring less than 3 cm but with the risk of leaving behind imaging occult satellite lesions after treatment. As such, the decision of whether to treat a patient with ablation or surgical resection for a small FOCAL HCC should be decided by a multidisciplinary team of clinicians on a case-by-case basis.

Combination Therapies: RFA and TACE

One of the more studied combination therapies for the treatment of HCC is that of RFA and TACE. TACE delivers targeted chemotherapy and induces ischemic necrosis to the tissue. The latter reduces the "heat sink effect" which normally limits the effectiveness of RFA, making the two treatments synergistic [36]. This synergy can create larger ablation zones and lead to better control of micrometastases, which are often seen on liver explantation at the time of transplantation in patients treated with RFA alone [36].

With regard to survival, one study looking at the treatment patients with either a single HCC ≤ 7 cm or three tumors ≤ 3 cm found that survival and disease-free survival at 4 years was significantly higher in patients treated with combination therapy versus RFA alone [37]. Furthermore, some studies have found similar overall survival and disease-free survival in patients with tumors meeting Milan criteria treated with RFA + TACE versus hepatectomy [38]. Given the improved safety profile of locoregional therapy as compared to surgery, combination therapy may be a better option for patients who are poor surgical candidates.

Image-Guided Transcatheter Tumor Therapies for Hepatocellular Carcinoma

Image-guided transcatheter tumor therapies have been in use for quite some time. The first transarterial embolization (TAE) of a liver tumor was reported in 1979 with infusion of gelatin sponge [39]. In the most basic sense, the technique for all image-guided transcatheter tumor therapies is similar and requires radiologic guidance for the infusion of an embolic agent directly into the hepatic artery. This can be done from a whole liver or lobar approach via infusion into the common, proper, or lobar hepatic arteries or, in more selective fashion, from a segmental or subsegmental approach. The embolic agent may be utilized alone, which is called transarterial embolization (TAE) or bland embolization, or embolization may be proceeded by infusion of single or multiple chemotherapeutic agents alone or as an oily chemotherapeutic emulsion, which is called conventional transarterial chemoembolization (cTACE). Alternatively, chemotherapy can also be loaded directly onto the embolic agent, which is called drug-eluting embolic transarterial chemoembolization (DEE-TACE). Finally, radiopharmaceuticals can be deposited onto the surface or incorporated directly into the embolic agent prior to infusion, and this is called transarterial radioembolization (TARE).

cTACE

Conventional transarterial chemoembolization (cTACE) is considered the standard of care for multinodular HCC. This stems in large part from two highly cited studies by Lo and LLovett [40, 41], both published in 2002, which demonstrated a clear survival advantage for cTACE versus symptomatic/supportive care. The technique has been refined over time as evolving catheter and imaging technology have allowed more distal or selective administration of the chemotherapeutic agent into the target vasculature.

The procedure is accomplished by first performing a thorough evaluation of the visceral arterial anatomy with diagnostic angiography. Typically this is done with a 4 or 5 French angiographic catheter from either a transfemoral or transradial approach. At a minimum, the celiac axis and superior mesenteric artery need to be thoroughly evaluated, as anatomic variants of the hepatic arterial supply are frequent. Furthermore, depending on the size and location, HCC can often parasitize blood flow from adjacent structures, such as the diaphragm or adjacent abdominal viscera. These vessels must be identified prior to embolization to ensure adequate tumor treatment. Following the diagnostic angiogram, feeding vessels to the liver tumor are identified and selected with a 0.010–0.021″ guidewire and a 2–3 French microcatheter placed coaxially through the base catheter. As eluded above, selectivity is key—this maximizes drug delivery to the tumor and spares as much functional liver tissue as possible. Once the catheter is in position, one or more chemotherapeutic agents with or without ethiodized oil are infused into the vessel along with or followed by an embolic agent until near or complete stasis is achieved. Most operators utilize ethiodized oil as an integral component of the chemotherapeutic suspension, as it is drug carrying and tumor seeking and serves as an embolic agent itself [42]. Controversy still exists whether single-drug or multiple-drug chemoembolization is more efficacious. The most common single drug in use is doxorubicin, and the most common multiple-drug regimens include doxorubicin, cisplatin, and mitomycin C. There is also no standard with regard to the particulate embolic agent of choice. Gelatin sponge, polyvinyl alcohol particles, and tris-acryl gelatin microspheres have all been used.

For small isolated tumors, cTACE can be accomplished in a single setting. However for larger tumors with complex vascularity or with multifocal disease involving both lobes of the liver, several cTACE procedures may be needed to complete a treatment cycle.

Following cTACE, patients typically develop post-embolization syndrome, which is a constellation of symptoms including fever, abdominal pain, nausea, malaise, and loss of appetite. While the exact cause of post-embolization syndrome is unknown, it is thought to be the results of tumor ischemia and chemotherapeutic cytotoxicity resulting in intra- and extrahepatic inflammation [43]. Symptoms range in severity but typically are managed with a short inpatient hospital stay and supportive measures. Less frequent complications of therapy include liver abscess, liver decompensation, and access site complications. While there is no standard schedule with regard to posttreatment follow-up imaging assessment, usually a contrast-enhanced CT or MRI is obtained at 1–3 months. Further follow-up imaging or therapy is dictated by the imaging response.

Drug-Eluting Embolic Transarterial Chemoembolization

Drug-eluting embolics (DEEs) are a group of embolic agents that can be directly loaded with chemotherapy and then delivered through a catheter into a vascular tumor such as HCC. Once delivered into the tumor, the chemotherapy is slowly released over a time frame of minutes to hours. Drug-eluting embolics (DEEs) represent the next evolution of technique for TACE. The rationale for the development of DEEs was to minimize potential toxicities and improve survival rates of the TACE procedure by improving drug delivery and lowering systemic levels of chemotherapy. DEEs were first developed around 2005, and clinical reports demonstrating safety and efficacy were published in 2006. There are several DEEs currently on the market, and they come in varying sizes from 30 to 700 μm. A review of all the commercially available DEEs is beyond the scope of this chapter; however, it is worth noting that there is no prospective randomized data to show that one particular brand or size DEE is superior to the other. Similar to cTACE, DEE-TACE is performed by first thoroughly evaluating the hepatic vasculature and identifying tumor-feeding vessels. Once selective catheterization is achieved, the DEEs are mixed with iodinated contrast and delivered directly into the blood vessel. The endpoint of the embolization occurs with vascular stasis or complete delivery of the intended dose of chemotherapy. Doxorubicin is the most common chemotherapy utilized for DEE-TACE in patients with HCC. An image from a DEE-TACE is shown in Fig.

Two large well-designed prospective randomized studies comparing DEE-TACE and cTACE were performed in Europe to test the hypothesis that DEE-TACE is superior to cTACE. The PRECISION V trial randomized 212 patients with HCC that were unsuitable for resection or percutaneous ablation (BCLC A/B) and with well-preserved liver function (Child-Pugh A/B) and performance status (ECOG 0/1) to receive doxorubicin via DEE-TACE or cTACE [44]. The primary endpoints of the study were tumor response rate and serious adverse events. While the DEE group did show a trend toward improved tumor response, it did not reach statistical significance ($P = 0.11$). A subgroup analysis of patients with more advanced disease (Child-Pugh B, ECOG 1, bilobar disease, and/or recurrent disease) did show a significant increase in objective response ($P = 0.038$) with DEE-TACE compared to cTACE. With regard to safety, there was a significant reduction in serious liver toxicity ($P < 0.001$) and a lower rate of doxorubicin-related side effects ($P = 0.0001$) with DEE-TACE as compared to cTACE.

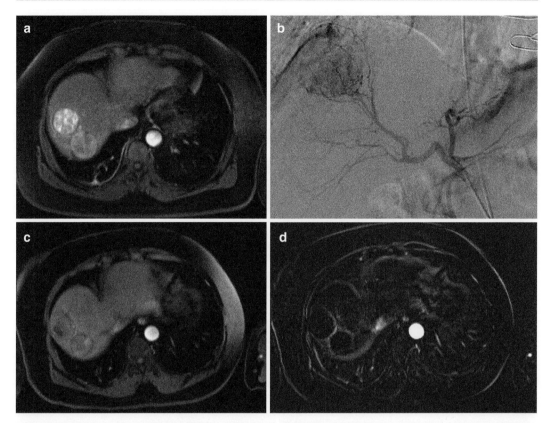

Fig. 5.2 A 62-year-old male with hepatitis C cirrhosis, well-preserved liver function, and performance status. (**a**) Arterial phase T1 weighted MRI demonstrates two enhancing tumors in the right hepatic lobe. Washout was present on venous phase imaging (not shown), consistent with multinodular HCC. (**b**) Proper hepatic artery angiogram from a transradial approach demonstrates the vascular nature of HCC; the two tumors are seen partially overlapping each other in the right hepatic lobe. Each tumor was embolized using DEE-TACE with doxorubicin over two sessions. (**c**) 12-month follow-up MRI arterial phase with subtraction (**d**) shows no internal enhancement, consistent with a complete response

The PRECISION ITALIA study randomized 177 patient to DEE-TACE or cTACE and was similar in design to PRECISION V [45]. The primary endpoint in the ITALIA study was 2-year overall survival, and no statistical difference was found between the two groups ($P = 0.949$). However, post-procedural abdominal pain was more frequent and severe after cTACE ($P < 0.001$). The reduction of post-embolization pain, liver toxicity, and doxorubicin-related side effects allows for many centers, including the authors, to perform DEE-TACE as an outpatient procedure with low complication and readmission rates [46].

The next evolution of DEE, radiopaque DEE, were recently developed and became commercially available in 2016. LC Bead LUMI™ (BTG) incorporates a radiopaque iodine moiety into the bead allowing direct and persistent visualization of the embolic under fluoroscopy and computed tomography. In theory, this should provide increased control and optimization of the embolization, as well as provide added assurance that tumor coverage was complete. More research and experience is needed to see the full impact of radiopaque DEEs on the management of patient with HCC. One interesting application of this technology is for combination therapy in difficult to ablate lesions (Fig. 5.3). One can mark a tumor by first performing DEE-TACE with LC Bead LUMI™. With improved visualization of the tumor, percutaneous CT-guided ablation can then be performed with improved targeting and efficiency.

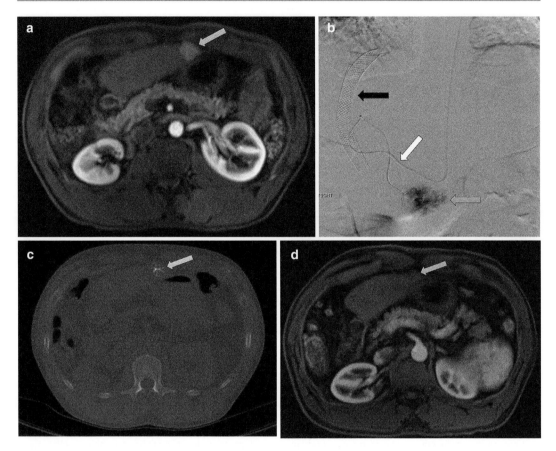

Fig. 5.3 52 year-old male with hepatitis C cirrhosis with previous history of transjugular intrahepatic portosystemic shunt (TIPS) is found to have an unresectable solitary hepatocellular carcinoma (HCC). He is Child-Pugh A6 with a performance status score of 1. (**a**) Magnetic resonance image (MRI) with arterial phase contrast demonstrates a solitary 2.6 cm segment 3 HCC (gray arrow). (**b**) Static angiographic image demonstrates a transradial catheter in the common hepatic artery (white arrow). Contrast injection is performed from a subsegmental hepatic artery demonstrating tumor blush in segment 3 (gray arrow). Incidentally noted is the prior TIPS (black arrow). Embolization was performed using radiopaque drug-eluting beads coated with doxorubicin. (**c**) 3-month follow-up non-contrast computed tomography (CT) image with bone window demonstrates complete staining of the intratumoral arteries (gray arrow). This lesion was subsequently treated with percutaneous microwave ablation. (**d**) 6-month follow-up MRI with arterial phase contrast demonstrates absence of enhancement and decreased size of patient's segment 3 HCC, compatible with complete response on imaging

Transarterial Radioembolization for HCC

Transarterial radioembolization (TARE) is the intra-arterial administration of microspheres labeled with the radiopharmaceutical yttrium-90. The term radioembolization is a bit of a misnomer, as the procedure often does not induce an embolic effect on the tumor vasculature. The arterial blood flow allows a means to deliver a concentrated dose of radiation directly into a tumor. To reflect this fact, other descriptive terms for the procedure have been used in the literature, including selective internal radiation therapy (SIRT); however, TARE remains the current preferred terminology. There are two microspheres commercially available. SIR-Spheres® (Sirtex) are biocompatible polymer resin microspheres loaded with yttrium-90. They range in size between 20 and 60 μm with a median diameter of 32.5 μm. They are FDA approved for the treatment of unresectable colorectal cancer liver metastases with adjuvant intrahepatic arterial chemotherapy (FUDR) and used off-label for the treatment of HCC. TheraSphere® (BTG) are yttrium-90 glass microspheres with a mean diameter of 20–30 µm. The device has a humanitarian device exemption from the FDA for the treatment of unresectable HCC with or without portal vein tumor thrombus (PVT). While there are subtle differences in size, specific gravity, and the administration of each device, the most important difference between glass and resin microspheres is the activity per sphere. At calibration, the activity of a single glass microsphere is approximately 50 times greater than resin (2500 Bq vs 50 Bq). Thus, far less microspheres are necessary to deliver a given dose of radiation with TheraSphere® when compared to SIR-Spheres®, and this can be beneficial when the prevention of vascular stasis is crucial or when a high dose of radioactivity is desired in a small volume of tissue.

TARE procedures are always preceded by a visceral angiographic mapping study and calculation of the liver-lung shunt. The liver-lung shunt is calculated by delivering technetium 99 MAA into the target liver volume and determining the percentage of activity within the lungs using a gamma camera. This percentage is then used in treatment planning and dosimetry calculations. The lungs can tolerate up to 30 Gray of radiation (Gy) in a single setting and 50 Gy lifetime. Above these limits, there is an increased risk of pulmonary complications, particularly pulmonary fibrosis. For patients with high liver-lung shunt values that preclude safe delivery of the radiation, several techniques have been utilized to try and reduce the degree of pulmonary shunting. Hepatic venous balloon occlusion, pre-TARE bland embolization, and external beam radiation have all been used with varying results [47, 48]. However there are also some retrospective studies suggesting that high liver-lung shunt values are predictors of poor outcomes [49] and that shunt reduction techniques with subsequent TARE may not be beneficial to the patient.

Additionally, high-quality visceral angiography is crucial to safely perform TARE, as nontarget embolization via visceral branches arising from the hepatic arteries can lead to complications, the most potentially problematic being bowel ulceration. During the mapping procedure, cone-beam CT angiography can be utilized to aid in the identification of these anatomic variants. If visceral branches are identified that are at risk of nontarget embolization, these branches can be prophylactically occluded with embolization coils during the mapping procedure. Balloon occlusion microcatheters and anti-reflux microcatheters have also been used to prevent nontarget embolization [50].

TARE can be performed at differing levels of selectivity in the liver to accomplish different goals. Patients with locally advanced disease with or without PVT or with multifocal bilobar disease will typically receive lobar treatment. If both lobes of the liver are to be treated, sessions are typically spaced anywhere from 4 to 12 weeks apart to allow time for the reassessment of the patient's liver function and performance status.

Lobar TARE can be performed as an alternative to portal vein embolization (PVE) prior to surgical resection because it typically results in a similar but to a somewhat slower degree (4 vs. 12 weeks) of contralateral liver hypertrophy [51]. Radiation doses are typically escalated from 120 to 150 Gy for this technique. One clear advantage of radiation lobectomy over PVE is that the primary tumor receives a therapeutic dose of y90, which theoretically should provide local tumor control, while the liver remnant grows in preparation for the planned hepatic resection. A second potential advantage is the slightly prolonged time to hypertrophy, which allows a biological test of time for the patient's tumor. Patients that progress to unresectable disease while hypertrophy occurs were likely not great candidates for hepatic resection in the first place. Finally, delivering a lobar dose of y90 microspheres to the right or left hepatic artery is much simpler than most techniques of portal vein embolization.

TARE can also be performed in a selective fashion for focal hepatic masses. This technique is referred to as selective TARE or radiation segmentectomy and involves the delivery of a lobar dose of y90 microspheres into 2 or less contiguous hepatic segments. This effectively escalates the dose to achieve ablative levels of radiation. The local control rates for radiation segmentectomy of focal hepatic masses more closely resemble that of percutaneous ablation as opposed to TACE [52]. There is growing literature showing higher local control rates and complete pathologic response on explant or resection specimens with selective TARE, which may possibly solidify TARE as a standard treatment option for patients with HCC [53, 54]. Images from a radiation segmentectomy procedure are shown in Fig. 5.4.

Bland Transarterial Embolization (TAE)

As discussed earlier, TAE was the original means for treating vascular liver tumors. While cTACE is still considered the standard for transcatheter embolic treatments, there are groups questioning the efficacy of adding chemotherapy to the embolization procedure. Proponents of bland embolization point out that in Llovet's pivotal study, there were in fact three treatment arms: cTACE, TAE, and best supportive care (BSC). Because the study was stopped early due to superiority of cTACE over BSC, accrual was not sufficient to show statistical differences between the TAE and BSC arms. cTACE was then quickly adopted as the standard of care, and while very limited

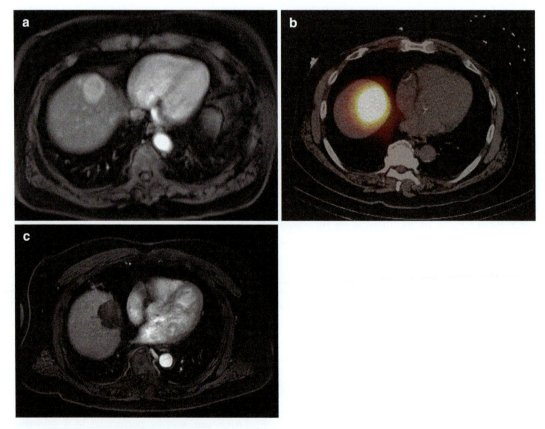

Fig. 5.4 57-year-old female with hepatitis C cirrhosis being evaluated for liver transplant. (**a**) Arterial phase T1-weighted MRI demonstrates an enhancing mass in the right hepatic lobe and a small adjacent satellite nodule. Washout was present on venous phase imaging (not shown), consistent with a diagnosis of HCC. (**b**) Bremsstrahlung SPECT/CT image after injection of glass microspheres show excellent deposition of radioactivity into the lesion. (**c**) 12-month follow-up MRI arterial phase shows no internal enhancement, consistent with a complete response

research was put toward further exploration of TAE, there are still several groups who continue to investigate the efficacy of bland embolization. The rationale for this is simple—eliminating chemotherapy, lipiodol, or drug-eluting embolics simplifies the procedure and provides significant cost savings. Perhaps the most well-known proponent of bland embolization is the group from the Memorial Sloan Kettering Cancer Center in New York. In 2016, Brown et al. published a randomized trial of 101 patients comparing doxorubicin DEE-TACE and bland embolization that showed no statistical difference in response rates, median PFS, and overall survival [55]. More work is needed to validate these results, but the implications could have a profound impact on how we treat HCC in the future.

Controversies

Despite the fact that local therapies have maintained an integral role in the treatment of HCC, multiple controversies of treatment paradigms still exist. As discussed above, there is still considerable debate over which method of chemoembolization is the most effective and whether the chemotherapy is even necessary. Perhaps the biggest current controversy in the treatment algorithm of HCC is the role of TARE with regard to HCC. As discussed earlier, it is not currently a recognized treatment option in the standard BCLC guidelines, but it is widely used in the treatment of HCC at multiple stages at most tertiary referral centers (Fig. 5.1). This particularly applies to locally advanced HCC because TARE is often used as an alternative to sorafenib in BCLC C patients with preserved liver function and performance status. Several studies demonstrate improvements in survival with TARE that meet or exceed that of sorafenib [56–58].

The SARAH trial was an investigator-initiated multicenter prospective trial comparing efficacy and safety of sorafenib and TARE with resin microspheres [59]. While the TARE arm showed no significant improvement in overall survival, it did show reduced severity and frequency of side effects and was better tolerated and associated with a better quality of life. The failure of the study to reach statistical significance with regard to survival was somewhat surprising; however, the design of the study was such that many of the patients in the TARE were heavily pretreated, particularly with TACE. There are ongoing trials evaluating the efficacy of TARE compared to sorafenib in first-line setting for BCLC C patients. The SIRveNIB trial is a phase III multicenter randomized trial comparing resin TARE and sorafenib in patients with locally advanced HCC. The STOP-HCC trial is an international phase III trial evaluating the efficacy and safety of glass TARE for unresectable HCC in patients that will be treated with sorafenib. The YES-P trial is an open-label, prospective, multicenter, randomized, phase III clinical trial evaluating glass TARE versus sorafenib for the treatment of advanced HCC with portal vein thrombosis (PVT).

Another area of controversy with regard to catheter-directed therapy is the choice between TACE and TARE, which is often influenced by institutional biases, by local expertise, and to a lesser degree by hard science. Prior to 2016, there were no randomized trials comparing the two techniques. Retrospective studies of TACE or TARE largely showed clinical equivalence [60]; however, due to the heterogeneity of the literature, making a true evidence-based decision on treatment options is difficult. Thus, it was with great anticipation that Salem et al. published the results of the PREMIERE trial in 2016 [53]. This single-center, prospective randomized trial was designed to compare the outcomes of cTACE and TARE with glass microspheres. There were difficulties with accrual that led to the early termination of the study, which points to the difficulty of conducting prospective studies in this patient population. Despite this, 45 patients were randomized to the two treatment arms. The primary outcome of time to progression (TTP) clearly favored TARE, where the median TTP was not met (>26 months vs. 6.8 months with cTACE, $P = 0.0012$). Secondary outcomes of imaging response, successful bridge to transplantation, and overall survival (OS) were not statistically significant. It is possible that the failure to reach statistical significance with regard to OS could be due to the small sample size. Regardless, this is interesting data, and more work is needed to clearly inform clinicians on the most appropriate local therapy for their patients.

Approach to the Transplant Patient

No discussion of local therapy and HCC would be complete without time spent on the approach to potential liver transplant candidates. Using local therapy as a bridge to liver transplant is widely accepted and proven to decrease dropout rates. Data also suggests improved outcomes and survival in patients who receive locoregional therapy prior to undergoing liver tranplantation [61]. The question of what technique to use however remains widely debated. There are some centers, including the authors, who tend to avoid percutaneous ablation in potential transplant candidates due to the small but real risk of intraperitoneal bleeding and tumor seeding. Despite this risk, with good technique and patient selection, there are centers that have shown ablation can be used successfully as a bridge to liver transplantation. For catheter-directed therapies, as discussed above, the choice between TACE, TARE, and even TAE is a hot topic. The results of the PREMIERE trial will likely lead to an increased utilization of TARE for bridging therapy.

Downstaging therapy typically involves taking BCLC B and C patients that are outside of transplant criteria and using locoregional techniques to bring them within the Milan criteria for liver transplantation. Again, with many techniques at your disposal, the authors recommend an aggressive approach for this patient population, as the survival benefit you afford a patient with successful downstaging and transplantation is immense.

In summary, locoregional therapies play a large role in the curative and palliative treatment options of patient with HCC. One can only predict that this role will continue to grow as technology improves, techniques are refined, and research matures.

References

1. Stuver S, Trichopoulos D. Cancer of the liver and biliary tract. In: Adami HO, Hunter D, Trichopoulos D, editors. Textbook of cancer epidemiology. 2nd ed. New York: Oxford University Press; 2008.
2. Stewart BW, Wild CP, editors. World cancer report 2014. Lyon, France: International Agency for Research on Cancer; 2014.
3. Ghouri YA, Milan I, Rowe JH. Review of hepatocellular carcinoma: epidemiology, etiology, and carcinogenesis. J Carcinog. 2017;16:1.
4. World Health Organization, International Agency for Research on Cancer. Estimated cancer incidence, mortality and prevalence worldwide in 2012. http://www.globocan.iarc.fr/PAges/fact_sheets_population.aspx.
5. Llovet JM, Brú C, Bruix J. Prognosis of hepatocellular carcinoma: the BCLC staging classification. Semin Liver Dis. 1999;19(3):329–38.
6. Llovet JM, et al. Intention-to-treat analysis of surgical treatment for early hepatocellular carcinoma: resection versus transplantation. Hepatology. 1990;30:1434–40.
7. Yao FY, et al. Liver transplantation for hepatocellular carcinoma: analysis of survival according to the intention-to-treat principle and dropout from the waiting list. Liver Transpl. 2002;8:873–83.
8. Lesurtel M, et al. Transarterial chemoembolization as a bridge to liver transplantation for hepatocellular carcinoma: an evidence-based analysis. Am J Transpl. 2006;6:2644–50.
9. Heckman JT, et al. Bridging locoregional therapy for hepatocellular carcinoma prior to liver transplantation. Ann Surg Onc. 2008;15(11):3169–77.
10. Yao FT, et al. A prospective study on downstaging of hepatocellular carcinoma prior to liver transplantation. Liver Transpl. 2005;11(12):1505–14.
11. Yao FT, et al. Downstaging of hepatocellular cancer before liver transplant: long-term outcome compared to tumors within Milan criteria. Hepatology. 2015;61:1968–77.
12. Vilgrain V, Pereira H, Assenat E, Guiu B, Ilonca AD, Pageaux GP, Sibert A, Bouattour M, Lebtahi R, Allaham W, Barraud H, Laurent V, Mathias E, Bronowicki JP, Tasu JP, Perdrisot R, Silvain C, Gerolami R, Mundler O, Seitz JF, Vidal V, Aubé C, Oberti F, Couturier O, Brenot-Rossi I, Raoul JL, Sarran A, Costentin C, Itti E, Luciani A, Adam R, Lewin M, Samuel D, Ronot M, Dinut A, Castera L, Chatellier G, SARAH Trial Group. Efficacy and safety of selective internal radiotherapy with yttrium-90 resin microspheres compared with sorafenib in locally advanced and inoperable hepatocellular carcinoma (SARAH): an open-label randomised controlled phase 3 trial. Lancet Oncol. 2017;18(12):1624–36.
13. Scudamore CH, et al. Liver tumor ablation techniques. J Investig Surg. 1997;10(4):157–64.

14. Padma S, et al. Liver tumor ablation: percutaneous and open approaches. J Surg Oncol. 2009;100(8):619–34.
15. Chen HW, et al. Ultrasound-guided percutaneous cryotherapy of hepatocellular carcinoma. Int J Surg. 2011;9(2):188–91.
16. McCarley JR, Soulen MC. Percutaneous ablation of hepatic tumors. Semin Intervent Radiol. 2010;27(3):255–60.
17. Bilchik AJ, et al. Cryosurgical ablation and radiofrequency ablation for unresectable hepatic malignant neoplasms: a proposed algorithm. Arch Surg. 2000;135(6):657–62; discussion 662–4.
18. Molla N, et al. The role of interventional radiology in the management of hepatocellular carcinoma. Curr Oncol. 2014;21(3):e480–92.
19. Chen MS, et al. A prospective randomized trial comparing percutaneous local ablative therapy and partial hepatectomy for small hepatocellular carcinoma. Ann Surg. 2006;243(3):321–8.
20. Lubner MG, et al. Microwave tumor ablation: mechanism of action, clinical results, and devices. J Vasc Interv Radiol. 2010;21(8 Suppl):S192–203.
21. Santambrogio R, et al. Comparison of laparoscopic microwave to radiofrequency ablation of small hepatocellular carcinoma (</=3 cm). Ann Surg Oncol. 2017;24(1):257–63.
22. Jaskolka JD, et al. Needle tract seeding after radiofrequency ablation of hepatic tumors. J Vasc Interv Radiol. 2005;16(4):485–91.
23. Gervais DA, et al. Society of interventional radiology position statement on percutaneous radiofrequency ablation for the treatment of liver tumors. J Vasc Interv Radiol. 2009;20(7 Suppl):S342–7.
24. Zhi-Yu H, et al. A clinical study of thermal monitoring techniques of ultrasound-guided microwave ablation for hepatocellular carcinoma in high-risk locations. Sci Rep. 2017;7:41246.
25. Rempp H, et al. The current role of minimally invasive therapies in the management of liver tumors. Abdom Imaging. 2011;36(6):635–47.
26. Cannon R, et al. Safety and early efficacy of irreversible electroporation for hepatic tumors in proximity to vital structures. J Surg Oncol. 2013;107(5):544–9.
27. Thompson KR, et al. Investigation of the safety of irreversible electroporation in humans. J Vasc Interv Radiol. 2011;22(5):611–21.
28. Feng K, et al. A randomized controlled trial of radiofrequency ablation and surgical resection in the treatment of small hepatocellular carcinoma. J Hepatol. 2012;57(4):794–802.
29. Lu DS, et al. Radiofrequency ablation of hepatocellular carcinoma: treatment success as defined by histologic examination of the explanted liver. Radiology. 2005;234(3):954–60.
30. Salmi A, et al. Efficacy of radiofrequency ablation of hepatocellular carcinoma associated with chronic liver disease without cirrhosis. Int J Med Sci. 2008;5(6):327–32.
31. Graf D, et al. Multimodal treatment of hepatocellular carcinoma. Eur J Intern Med. 2014;25(5):430–7.
32. Sheth RA, et al. Role of locoregional therapy and predictors for dropout in patients with hepatocellular carcinoma listed for liver transplantation. J Vasc Interv Radiol. 2015;26(12):1761–8. quiz 1768.
33. Ravaioli M, et al. Liver transplantation for hepatocellular carcinoma: results of down-staging in patients initially outside the Milan selection criteria. Am J Transplant. 2008;8(12):2547–57.
34. Hasegawa K, et al. Surgical resection vs. percutaneous ablation for hepatocellular carcinoma: a preliminary report of the Japanese nationwide survey. J Hepatol. 2008;49(4):589–94.
35. Huang J, et al. A randomized trial comparing radiofrequency ablation and surgical resection for HCC conforming to the Milan criteria. Ann Surg. 2010;252(6):903–12.
36. Vasnani R, et al. Radiofrequency and microwave ablation in combination with transarterial chemoembolization induce equivalent histopathologic coagulation necrosis in hepatocellular carcinoma patients bridged to liver transplantation. Hepatobiliary Surg Nutr. 2016;5(3):225–33.
37. Peng Z-W, Zhang Y-J, Chen M-S, Xu L, Liang H-H, Lin X-J, Guo R-P, Zhang Y-Q, Lau WY. Radiofrequency ablation with or without transcatheter arterial chemoembolization in the treatment of hepatocellular carcinoma: a prospective randomized trial. J Clin Oncol. 2013;31(4):426–32.
38. Bholee AK, et al. Radiofrequency ablation combined with transarterial chemoembolization versus hepatectomy for patients with hepatocellular carcinoma within Milan criteria: a retrospective case-control study. Clin Transl Oncol. 2017;19(7):844–52.
39. Wheeler G, Melia W, Dubbins P, Jones B, Nunnerley H, Johnson P, et al. Non-operative arterial embolization in primary liver tumours. Br Med J. 1979;ii:242–4.
40. Llovet JM, Real MI, Montaña X, Planas R, Coll S, Aponte J, Ayuso C, Sala M, Muchart J, Solà R, Rodés J, Bruix J, Barcelona Liver Cancer Group. Arterial embolisation or chemoembolisation versus symptomatic treatment in patients with unresectable hepatocellular carcinoma: a randomised controlled trial. Lancet. 2002;359(9319):1734–9.
41. Lo CM, Ngan H, Tso WK, Liu CL, Lam CM, Poon RT, Fan ST, Wong J. Randomized controlled trial of transarterial lipiodol chemoembolization for unresectable hepatocellular carcinoma. Hepatology. 2002;35(5):1164–71.
42. Takayasu K, Shima Y, Muramatsu Y, Moriyama N, Yamada T, Makuuchi M, Hasegawa H, Hirohashi S. Hepatocellular carcinoma: treatment with intraarterial iodized oil with and without chemotherapeutic agents. Radiology. 1987;163(2):345–51.
43. Dhand S, Gupta R. Hepatic transcatheter arterial chemoembolization complicated by postembolization syndrome. Semin Intervent Radiol. 2011;28(2):207–11.
44. Lammer J, et al. Prospective randomized study of doxorubicin-eluting-bead embolization in the treat-

ment of HCC: results of the PRECISION V study. Cardiovasc Intervent Radiol. 2010;33(1):41–52.
45. Golfieri R, Giampalma E, Renzulli M, Cioni R, Bargellini I, Bartolozzi C, Breatta AD, Gandini G, Nani R, Gasparini D, Cucchetti A, Bolondi L, Trevisani F, Precision Italia Study Group. Randomised controlled trial of doxorubicin-eluting beads vs conventional chemoembolisation for hepatocellular carcinoma. Br J Cancer. 2014;111(2):255–64.
46. Nasser F, Cavalcante RN, Galastri FL, de Rezende MB, Felga GG, Travassos FB, De Fina B, Affonso BB. Safety and feasibility of same-day discharge of patients with hepatocellular carcinoma treated with transarterial chemoembolization with drug-eluting beads in a liver transplantation program. J Vasc Interv Radiol. 2014;25(7):1012–7.
47. Ward TJ, et al. Management of high hepatopulmonary shunting in patients undergoing hepatic radioembolization. J Vasc Interv Radiol. 2015;26(12):1751–60.
48. Young L, et al. Hepatopulmonary shunt reduction using external beam radiation therapy prior to yttrium-90 radioembolization of HCC. J Vasc Interv Radiol. 2017;28(2):S76.
49. Sandow T, et al. Elevated lung shunt fraction as a prognostic indicator for disease progression and metastasis in hepatocellular carcinoma. J Vasc Interv Radiol. 2016;27(6):804–11.
50. Morshedi MM, Bauman M, Rose SC, Kikolski SG. Yttrium-90 resin microsphere radioembolization using an antireflux catheter: an alternative to traditional coil embolization for nontarget protection. Cardiovasc Interv Radiol. 2015;38(2):381–8.
51. Vouche M, Lewandowski RJ, Atassi R, Memon K, Gates VL, Ryu RK, Gaba RC, Mulcahy MF, Baker T, Sato K, Hickey R, Ganger D, Riaz A, Fryer J, Caicedo JC, Abecassis M, Kulik L, Salem R. Radiation lobectomy: time-dependent analysis of future liver remnant volume in unresectable liver cancer as a bridge to resection. J Hepatol. 2013;59(5):1029–36.
52. Vouche M, Habib A, Ward TJ, et al. Unresectable solitary hepatocellular carcinoma not amenable to radiofrequency ablation: multicenter radiology-pathology correlation and survival of radiation segmentectomy. Hepatology. 2014;60(1):192–201.
53. Salem R, Gordon AC, Mouli S, Hickey R, Kallini J, Gabr A, Mulcahy MF, Baker T, Abecassis M, Miller F, Yaghmai V, Sato K, Desai K, Thornburg B, Benson AB, Rademaker A, Ganger D, Kulik L, Lewandowski RJ. Y90 Radioembolization significantly prolongs time to progression compared with chemoembolization in patients with hepatocellular carcinoma. Gastroenterology. 2016;151(6):1155–1163.e2.
54. Arepally A et al. Society of interventional radiology annual meeting, Washington, DC; 2017.
55. Brown KT, Do RK, Gonen M, Covey AM, Getrajdman GI, Sofocleous CT, Jarnagin WR, D'Angelica MI, Allen PJ, Erinjeri JP, Brody LA, O'Neill GP, Johnson KN, Garcia AR, Beattie C, Zhao B, Solomon SB, Schwartz LH, DeMatteo R, Abou-Alfa GK. Randomized trial of hepatic artery embolization for hepatocellular carcinoma using doxorubicin-eluting microspheres compared with embolization with microspheres alone. J Clin Oncol. 2016;34(17):2046–53.
56. Mazzaferro V, Sposito C, Bhoori S, et al. Yttrium-90 radioembolization for intermediate-advanced hepatocellular carcinoma: a phase 2 study. Hepatology. 2013;57(5):1826–37.
57. Salem R, Lewandowski RJ, Mulcahy MF, et al. Radioembolization for hepatocellular carcinoma using yttrium-90 microspheres: a comprehensive report of long-term outcomes. Gastroenterology. 2010;138(1):52–64.
58. Sangro B, Carpanese L, Cianni R, et al. Survival after yttrium-90 resin microsphere radioembolization of hepatocellular carcinoma across Barcelona clinic liver cancer stages: a European evaluation. Hepatology. 2011;54(3):868–78.
59. Vilgrain V, Pereira H, Assenat E, Guiu B, Ilonca AD, Pageaux GP, Sibert A, Bouattour M, Lebtahi R, Allaham W, Barraud H, Laurent V, Mathias E, Bronowicki JP, Tasu JP, Perdrisot R, Silvain C, Gerolami R, Mundler O, Seitz JF, Vidal V, Aubé C, Oberti F, Couturier O, Brenot-Rossi I, Raoul JL, Sarran A, Costentin C, Itti E, Luciani A, Adam R, Lewin M, Samuel D, Ronot M, Dinut A, Castera L, Chatellier G, SARAH Trial Group. Efficacy and safety of selective internal radiotherapy with yttrium-90 resin microspheres compared with sorafenib in locally advanced and inoperable hepatocellular carcinoma (SARAH): an open-label randomised controlled phase 3 trial. Lancet Oncol. 2017;18(12):1624–36.
60. Fidelman N, Kerlan RK Jr. Transarterial chemoembolization and (90)Y radioembolization for hepatocellular carcinoma: review of current applications beyond intermediate-stage disease. AJR Am J Roentgenol. 2015;205(4):742–52.
61. Kokabi N, Duszak R, Xing M, et al. Cancer-directed therapy and potential impact on survivals in nonresected hepatocellular carcinoma: SEER-Medicare population study. Future Oncol. 2017;13(24):2021–33.

Role of Radiation Therapy in Hepatocellular Carcinoma

Emma B. Holliday, Eugene J. Koay, and Christopher H. Crane

Introduction

The incidence of hepatocellular carcinoma (HCC) is increasing in the United States [1]. Transplant and surgical resection are considered to be the only curative options for patients with HCC [2]; however, a minority of patients are anatomically and medically eligible for a curative surgical resection at diagnosis [3] or meet criteria for liver transplant. The National Comprehensive Cancer Network guidelines list ablation, arterially directed therapies, and external beam radiation therapy (EBRT) as locoregional therapy options for those patients for whom resection is not feasible or a bridge to transplant is desired [4]. EBRT is recommended with the category of 2B (based on lower-level evidence, with consensus that the intervention is appropriate). European guidelines and consensus statements likewise assign EBRT the lowest recommendation with the lowest level of evidence [5]. Additionally, the Korean Practice Guidelines for the Management of HCC recommend RT in one of the following five settings: (1) patients with Child-Pugh A or B liver function with the volume of liver receiving ≥30 Gray (Gy) is ≤60% (V30 < 60%); (2) patients who are ineligible for liver transplant, surgical resection, radiofrequency ablation (RFA), percutaneous ethanol injection (PEI), or transcatheter arterial chemoembolization (TACE); (3) patients with an incomplete response to TACE; (4) patients with portal venous invasion; or (5) patients with symptoms from primary or metastatic HCC requiring palliation [6].

Historically, only a minority of patients have been referred for radiation therapy (RT), despite meeting one of the criteria above. Data from the Surveillance, Epidemiology, and End Results (SEER) suggest that only 9% of Medicare patients diagnosed with HCC between 1998 and 2007 were even seen by a radiation oncologist despite the fact that only 20% of patients in that cohort had early-stage disease [7]. Similar patterns were shown in a survey of Italian radiotherapy centers, 73% of which had an active multidisciplinary liver tumor board. Results from the survey study showed approximately 10% of Italian radiotherapy centers utilized liver-directed radiotherapy for primary liver tumors, and the majority of respondents considered liver-directed radiotherapy as a third-line choice when other therapies were not medically or technically suitable [8]. There are several factors that likely influence the low utilization of RT for patients with HCC. One likely contributing factor is the lack of high-quality prospective, randomized evidence showing a benefit to radiation therapy over the standard of care, sorafenib, for unresectable HCC. Additionally, concerns regarding radiation-induced liver disease (RILD) and other toxicities associated with EBRT may also dampen general enthusiasm for the modality [9]. However, more recent data demonstrate that radiation can be delivered safely to higher doses leading to durable long-term local control (LC) using more conformal techniques. In patients with solitary lesions and well-compensated cirrhosis, implementation of this treatment modality has translated into improved overall survival (OS) rates.

3D Conformal and Intensity-Modulated Radiation Therapy

Background and Rationale

3D conformal radiation therapy (3DCRT) technique involves multiple radiation fields that converge to provide coverage of the tumor target while reducing the exposure of the adjacent healthy liver, bowel, and other normal organs to high-dose radiation. The advent of computed tomography (CT) imaging and computerized treatment planning systems allowed for more accurate delineation and dose prescription to the tumor. Additionally, the dose to nearby normal organs, especially the liver itself, could be more precisely quantified leading to an accurate pretreatment determination of the safety of treatment and minimal long-term complications of treatment.

Retrospective Data

Retrospective studies from Asia have shown a 1-year OS of 45–70% with standard or hypofractionated conformal radiation and further emphasized the importance of baseline liver function on the risk of RILD as well as OS [10–12]. A Korean study retrospectively evaluated 398 patients with HCC, 78% of whom had stage III–IV disease. The majority of patients received ≥45Gy, median survival was 12 months, and 2-year OS was 27.9% [10]. A smaller Japanese study of 44 patients with unresectable HCC who either failed or were unsuitable for TACE reported a response rate of 61.4% and 1- and 2-year OS rates of 60.5% and 40.3%, respectively, with doses ranging from 39.6 to 60Gy (median 50.4Gy) [12]. A Chinese study of 128 patients with technically or medically inoperable HCC treated with 3DCRT ± TACE utilized a hypofractionated approach consisting of a mean of 53.6Gy given with a mean fraction size of 4.88Gy. One- and two-year OS rates were similar to the Japanese study at 65% and 43%, respectively. However, 19 patients developed fatal liver toxicity, the majority of whom had Child-Pugh B liver disease pretreatment [11]. Therefore these retrospective studies suggest that high-dose radiation may be an effective option for patients with inoperable HCC as long as it is delivered safely, particularly in the setting of patients with poor liver function.

Prospective Studies

High-dose 3DCRT was first described by Dawson and colleagues at the University of Michigan in the early 2000s with phase II trials evaluating radiation and concurrent hepatic artery floxuridine for patients with unresectable HCC [13–15]. Patients receiving a median of 60.75Gy in 1.5Gy twice daily fractions had a median survival of 15.8 months, 1-year LC, and OS of 81% and 57%, respectively, which were significantly higher than historical controls. One patient in this cohort suffered a treatment-related death, and 9% of patients developed grade 3 or 4 toxicities [14]. A subsequent European prospective, phase II trial also demonstrated the safety and efficacy of high-dose conformal radiation for patients with small HCC tumors medically unsuitable for standard curative therapies and reported a 1-year LC of 76% for patients with Child-Pugh A and B disease using a regimen of 66Gy in 33 fractions. Patients with Child-Pugh B disease had higher rates of toxicity with 22% of patient developing a grade 4 toxicity [16]. Few studies exist comparing the efficacy of EBRT with other established treatment modalities, but a recent meta-analysis showed adding EBRT to TACE did provide a better tumor response and survival compared with TACE alone [17]. Additionally, a comparative retrospective study suggested a survival benefit when adding EBRT for patients with HCC and either portal vein or inferior vena cava tumor thrombi [18].

Stereotactic Body Radiotherapy

Background and Rationale

Stereotactic body radiotherapy (SBRT), also called stereotactic ablative body radiotherapy (SABR), is defined as the delivery of high doses of radiation in a small number (typically 1–5) of fractions utilizing advanced imaging techniques to conform the radiation beam in three planes with a high degree of precision. Delivery of SBRT requires onboard imaging integrated onto the treatment machine for advanced image-guided radiation therapy (IGRT). First described for brain and lung tumors [19], SBRT utilization is increasing for patients with HCC, and both US and Korean guidelines recommend SBRT as an alternative to ablation and embolization when these techniques have failed or cannot be performed [4, 6]. SBRT can also be utilized for tumor downsizing or as bridging therapy for patients awaiting liver transplantation [20, 21]. It has also been studied in combination with transarterial hepatic chemoembolization (TACE) for more advanced tumors [17]. As more data indicate the efficacy and curative potential of SBRT for patients with HCC and its role is expanded to larger tumors, there is a greater need to optimize its safe delivery.

Retrospective Data

The first reported use of SBRT for liver tumors came from the Karolinska Hospital in 1995 where a mean total dose of 41Gy was given in a mean fraction size of 14.2Gy. Plans were intentionally heterogeneous, with the center of the tumor given approximately 50% higher dose than the periphery. LC was excellent at 80% during the follow-up period [22].

Since then, there have been many single-institution as well as multi-institutional experiences of SBRT for HCC. Two-year LC ranges from 59% to 100%, and 2-year OS ranges from 45% to 67%, and the wide variation stems from differences in tumor size, radiation dose, and the patient's pretreatment liver function [23–33]. The best results have come from series of patients with small tumors, <5 cm or even <2 cm, where local control nears 100% [29, 33]. Fewer studies have evaluated SBRT in patients with larger tumors or poor liver function. In one series in which all patients had Child-Pugh B6 or B7 liver function and 76% of patients had tumor vascular thrombi, the dose used was only 30Gy in six fractions, and the median survival was only 7.9 months [30]. Several studies have shown a dose-response relationship [28], with a BED $\geq$ 100 associated with increases in both LC and OS [31]. Several studies have also looked at SBRT in combination with other therapies, or in a heavily pretreated patient population. A study from the University of Alabama also looked at SBRT for patients who had undergone TACE for tumors $\geq$3 cm and found that the addition of SBRT to TACE provides a survival advantage [34].

Prospective Studies

One of the early phase I/II studies was performed in the Netherlands. Eight patients with HCC (two had Child-Pugh B liver function) were included in the 25-patient cohort. Three fractions of 12.5Gy each were given to all the HCC patients except for one patient with Child-Pugh B liver function and a tumor >4 cm who received five fractions of 5Gy each. One of the patients with Child-Pugh B liver function developed liver failure after treatment and ultimately died. The 1-year local control for HCC was only 80%, and this was thought to be because of the lower dose given to larger HCC tumors in patients with poor liver function. The 1- and 2-year OS for HCC patients were 75% and 40%, respectively [35]. Since then, several phase I–II, prospective studies have been published, and reported 1-year LC ranged from 44 to 100% and 1-year OS ranged from 42 to 77% [36–44]. Details of these selected prospective trials for SBRT in HCC can be found in Table 6.1. Patients enrolled on these studies

Table 6.1 Prospective studies describing the using of stereotactic body radiation therapy for hepatocellular carcinoma

1st author, year of publication	# patients	Tumor size	Tumor extent	% Child-Pugh B	Prior therapies	#Fractions × fractional dose in Gy	1-yr LC	1-yr OS	RILD	Grade 3+ toxicity
Mendez Romero, 2006 [35]	25 (8 with HCC)	Allowed 3 lesions ≤7 cm each (median was 3.2 cm)	38% TVT for HCC pts	25% for HCC pts	–	3 × 12.5 if CPA or CPB with HCC <4 cm 5 × 5 if CPB with HCC ≥4 cm	94% for all pts	75% for HCC pts	1 of 8 HCC pts	1 grade 5 in HCC pt who had CPB
Tse, 2008 [36]	41 (31 with HCC)	Median tumor volume 173 mL range 9–1913 mL	52% TVT 10% EHD for HCC pts	0%	61% any prior therapy for HCC pts	6 × 4 to 6 × 6	65% for all pts	48% for HCC pts	None	12%
Cárdenes, 2010 [37]	17	Allowed ≤6 cm	18% TVT	40%	23.5% any prior therapy	4 × 9 to 4 × 12 (for CPA) 3 × 8.6 to 3 × 14 (for CPB)	100%	75% (100% for CPA and 60% for CPB)	3 pts, all with CPB disease, 2 had prior TACE	12%
Price, 2012 [38]	26 (all with HCC)	Allowed 3 lesions sum ≤6 cm	12% TVT 8% EHD	46%	27% any prior therapy	3 × 9 to 3 × 16 5 × 8 for CPB	96%	77%	None	None reported
Kang, 2012 [39]	47 (all HCC)	Median 2.9 cm range 1.3–8 cm	5% TVT	13%	All received TACE prior to RT	3 × 14 to 3 × 20	2 yr was 95%	2 yr was 68.7%	None	10% including 2 pts with perforated gastric ulcer
Bujold, 2013 [40]	102 (all HCC) from 2 prospective trials	Median 7.2 cm range 1.4–23.1	55% TVT 12% EHD	0%	52% any prior therapy	6 × 4 to 6 × 9	87%	55%	None	30% and 7 of 102 with potential treatment-related death

(continued)

Table 6.1 (continued)

1st author, year of publication	# patients	Tumor size	Tumor extent	% Child-Pugh B	Prior therapies	#Fractions × fractional dose in Gy	1-yr LC	1-yr OS	RILD	Grade 3+ toxicity
Brade, 2016 [41]	16 (all with HCC) with neoadj, concurrent and adj sorafenib	Median 3.5 cm for low Veff cohort and 8.7 cm for high Veff cohort	63% TVT 19% EHD	0%	38% any prior therapy	6 × 5 to 6 × 8.5	44%	44%	None	2 pts died of probably tumor-related bleeding
Takeda, 2016 [42]	101 (all HCC) + optional TACE prior	Median 2.3 cm range 1–4 cm	3% TVT	9%	64% any prior therapy	5 × 7 (11%) 5 × 6 (89%)	3 yr was 96.3%	3 yr was 66.7%	None	6 of 101
Kim, 2016 [43]	18 (all with HCC)	Median 2 cm (cumulative) range 1–4.4 cm	0% TVT	0%	83% any prior therapy	4 × 9 to 4 × 15 Escalating doses	2 yr was 71.3%	2 yr was 69.3%	None	5 of 18 (all hematologic, no GI toxicities)
Weiner, 2016 [44]	26 (12 with HCC, 12 with IHC 2 with bi-phenotypic)	Mean tumor diameter was 5 cm	27% TVT	12%	8% prior surgery, 4% prior RFA, 31% prior TACE, 35% prior chemo	5 × 8 to 5 × 11 (median 5 × 11)	91%	42%	2 of 26	6 of 26

HCC hepatocellular carcinoma, *LC* local control, *OS* overall survival, *RILD* radiation-induced liver disease, *CP* Child-Pugh, *TACE* transcatheter arterial chemoembolization, *neoadj* neoadjuvant, *adj* adjuvant, *GI* gastrointestinal, *RFA* radiofrequency ablation, *IHC* intrahepatic cholangiocarcinoma, *TVT* tumor vascular thrombosis, *EHD* extrahepatic disease, *Gy* Gray, *yr* year, *pt* patient had all been treated previously with other modalities, but otherwise considerable heterogeneity exists regarding tumor size, tumor extent, dose and fractionation, as well as underlying liver function. SBRT has been evaluated in combination with TACE [39, 42] as well as with sorafenib [41]. Brade and colleagues recently published the findings from their phase I trial evaluating neoadjuvant, concurrent, and adjuvant sorafenib with SBRT for HCC and reported that significant toxicities occurred and seemed to depend on both the irradiated volume and the dose of sorafenib. Patients with locally advanced HCC and Child-Pugh A liver disease were stratified by low versus high volume of irradiated liver (<30% vs 30–60%), and the dose of sorafenib was escalated from 200 mg daily to 400 mg twice daily. Response rates and time to progression were promising, but dose-limiting toxicities included a lower GI bleed, bowel obstruction, and fatal tumor hemorrhage. Therefore, the authors concluded sorafenib should not be given concurrently with SBRT, at least to larger volumes that include GI mucosal irradiation [41]. Retrospective data suggest sorafenib can be safely given after SBRT [45], and this is being further studied in the Radiation Therapy Oncology Group (RTOG) 1112 randomized controlled trial comparing sorafenib alone versus SBRT followed by sorafenib for locally advanced HCC.

Proton Beam Radiotherapy

Background and Rationale

Conformal fractionated radiation and SBRT have both been shown to confer a high percentage of local control for patients with HCC. However, the goal of delivering an ablative dose of radiation to the tumor must be weighed against the need to respect the radiation tolerance of the adjacent normal liver. Details regarding RILD and the specific dose-volume constraints derived to ensure patients have adequate functional liver after radiation are outlined in the next section. However, radiation technologies and modalities that allow dose sparing to normal liver as especially for patients with low anatomic or functional liver reserve after prior liver-directed therapies or as a result of underlying liver disease are areas of active investigation.

The unique physical properties of proton beam radiation (PBR) make it uniquely suited for the treatment of liver tumors, particularly when sparing dose to adjacent normal liver is desired. The mass and charge of a proton particle allow it to lose speed as it moves through the body toward its target. By altering the energy given to the proton by the cyclotron, the depth at which the proton delivers its maximum dose can be precisely calculated. After this point of maximum dose delivery (known as the Bragg peak), the proton stops within tissue, eliminating exit dose to more distal tissues [46]. Thus, PBR can offer a better therapeutic ratio particularly for HCC patients who might otherwise have unacceptable hepatic toxicities with photon-based radiation.

Retrospective Data

The majority of the early data on the use of PBR for HCC has come from Japan, where HCC is endemic. Results from hypofractionated regimens (16–25 fractions) to ablative doses for large tumors are similar to those after surgical resection, with 5-year LC and OS rates of 90% and 50%, respectively. The group at the University of Tsukuba has published extensively on the utilization of PBR in order to safely treat larger tumors to larger doses per fraction, beginning with a large retrospective review of 165 patients with HCC treated with PBR from 1985 to 1998. Five-year LC and OS were excellent at 86.9% and 23.5%, respectively, with only five patients experiencing significant chronic toxicities, all of whom were treated prior to motion management being introduced in 1995. It should also be noted that patients were treated with large doses per fraction 3–4 days per week given the logistical time constraints on the proton beam [47]. The same group published on a more recent cohort of 318 patients with HCC treated between 2001 and 2007. This patient cohort was slightly more favorable with fewer Child-Pugh B and C patients and more patients who received other liver-directed therapies prior to PBR, and the 5-year OS was better 44.6%. Treatment regimens were more standardized in this cohort with patients with peripheral tumors away from the gastrointestinal mucosa and porta hepatis receiving 66Gy(RBE) (Gy-relative biologic effectiveness, assuming a RBE of 1.1 for protons compared with photons) in 10 fractions, tumors within 2 cm of the porta hepatis receiving 72.6Gy(RBE) in 22 fractions, and tumor within 2 cm of the gastrointestinal mucosa receiving 77Gy(RBE) in 35 fractions. These regimens were very well tolerated with no reported cases of RILD and few serious toxicities [48]. Other case series from Asian centers show similar outcomes [49, 50], which have been shown to vary based on patient and tumor characteristics including liver function, disease burden, and tumor vascular thrombosis. Encouraging response rates and acceptable toxicity profiles were seen as well when PBR was used for advanced HCC with portal vein tumor thrombus [51]. A more recent report showed feasible and promising results from a risk-adapted simultaneous integrated boost technique using PBR for patients with HCC and tumor vascular thrombosis. Median OS was 34.4 months in this cohort of 41 patients treated with 50-66Gy(RBE) in 10 fractions depending on gross tumor volume and distance from GI mucosa [52].

Prospective Studies

Mizumoto and colleagues reported on 266 patients treated on three prospective protocols developed at the Proton Medical Research Center in Tsukuba, including 66GyE in 10 fractions for tumors >2 cm away from the portal region, 72.6GyE in 22 fractions for tumors within 2 cm of the hilum, and further reduction to 77GyE in 35 fractions for tumors adjacent to the GI tract. The majority of the tumors were less than 5 cm. The average 3-year local control and OS were 87% and 61%, respectively, with no significant differences in local control among the three different fractionation schemes used. Toxicity rates were low, suggesting appropriate selection of dose and fractionation based on tumor location can improve the therapeutic ratio [53]. Long-term outcomes for patients treated at Tsukuba were recently reported and showed favorable long-term control with no grade 3 or higher toxicities. This update also showed 5-year LC and OS of 90% and 34%, respectively, for patients with portal vein tumor thrombi, suggesting PBR may be a viable treatment strategy for this subset of patients with historically poor outcomes [54].

In the United States, a phase II trial from Loma Linda evaluated PBT in 76 patients with inoperable HCC and cirrhosis. Eighteen patients in this cohort eventually underwent liver transplant, and 33% of those explants showed a pathologic complete response after 63Gy(RBE) delivered over a 3-week period [55]. Additionally, a multi-institutional phase II study of high-dose hypofractionated proton beam therapy for liver tumors included 44 HCC patients with median tumor size of 5.0 cm and tumor vascular thrombosis present in 29.5%. Planned dose was 67.5GyE in 15 fractions for peripheral tumors and 58.05GyE in 15 fractions for central tumors. Dose de-escalation was allowed in order to meet liver constraints. Median dose delivered was 58 GyE (range 40.5–67.5). LC and OS for this group at 2 years were 94.8% and 63.2%, respectively. Importantly, very few grade 3 toxicities and no grade 4–5 toxicities were observed [56]. The only randomized clinical trial involving PBR for HCC is currently underway at Loma Linda. Patients with HCC who met either Milan or San Francisco transplant criteria were randomized to PBR or TACE. In the PBR arm, the dose was 70.2Gy(RBE) in 15 fractions over 3 weeks. Interim analysis was reported recently, and the 2-year OS was 59% for the cohort with no difference between the groups. Approximately 1/3 of the patients in each arm went on to transplant, and pathologic complete response after PBR was 25% compared with 10% after TACE, though the difference was not statistically significant. There was a trend toward improved LC in the PBR arm (88% vs 45% at 2 years; $p = 0.06$). There were fewer hospitalization days also after PBR when compared with TACE, which the author suggests may indicate reduced toxicity [57].

There are no definitive data on the optimal dose for control of HCC, but collectively retrospective and prospective studies discussed above suggest that dose escalation above BED of 80Gy(RBE) is associated with excellent outcomes and can be safely accomplished using proton beam therapy. While patients with relatively small, isolated tumors with well-compensated cirrhosis represent ideal candidates for ablative dose escalation, proton therapy may also be used for select candidates with larger tumors or Child-Pugh class B/C liver disease in whom maximum non-diseased liver sparing is essential for adequate function post-treatment. A summary of selected studies using PBR for HCC can be found in Table 6.2.

Toxicities

Radiation-Induced Liver Disease

Pathophysiology
Much of the early trepidation toward using EBRT for HCC stemmed from fear of causing liver failure from RILD, also called radiation hepatitis in earlier studies. RILD was first described as anicteric hepatomegaly and thought to be caused by retrograde congestion [58].

Clinical Presentation
Symptoms of RILD are non-specific and typically include fatigue, right upper quadrant pain, and discomfort related to ascites and hepatomegaly. Portal hypertension can come from obstruction of the central vein, and subsequent splenic sequestration can lead to profound thrombocytopenia. Classic RILD occurs 2–8 weeks after completion of radiation [59] and is associated with findings of elevated alkaline phosphatase above twice the normal/pretreatment level. Typically transaminases, ammonia, and bilirubin remain normal [60]. Nonclassic RILD occurs between 1 week and 3 months after completion of radiation and involves elevated transaminases up to five times the upper limit of normal or a decline in liver function as defined by a worsening of the Child-Pugh score by 2+ points in the absence of classic RILD. One potential confounding condition is the reactivation of hepatitis B by radiation and resulting injury to hepatocytes which can also cause elevation of transaminases and ascites [60]. Jaundice and elevated bilirubin is not a common symptom of RILD and may indicate ascending cholangitis or a malfunctioning biliary stent, if one is present [9].

Diagnosis and Work-Up
In addition to laboratory examinations, an ultrasound and paracentesis can be useful in the work-up of suspected RILD to exclude other causes of ascites. Computed tomography (CT) and magnetic resonance imaging (MRI) can provide insight as to the location of abnormal-appearing liver which can be compared with the area of irradiated liver from the radiation treatment plan [61, 62]. Ultimately, diagnostic laparoscopy and biopsy may be necessary to diagnose RILD as it is a diagnosis of exclusion [9]. Pathologic features of veno-occlusive disease around the central vein are commonly seen upon pathologic examination [63].

Treatment and Prognosis
Unfortunately, there is no way to halt the progression or reverse RILD, so therapies are given only to treat the symptoms. Diuretics or therapeutic paracenteses can be given to manage symptoms of ascites, platelets can be given to correct thrombocytopenia, and steroids can help reduce hepatic congestion [61]. Some studies have shown an improvement with anticoagulation and thrombolytic therapy [64, 65]. Despite best supportive measures, most patients with RILD eventually die. One study showed that grade 3 or higher elevation in transaminases, a pretreatment Child-Pugh score of 8 or higher, or grade 3 or higher thrombocytopenia predicted a higher risk of fatal hepatic failure within 12 months [66].

Dose-Volume Constraints for Prevention of Liver Toxicity

Mean Liver Dose Constraints
In the 1960s, Ingold et al. reported ascites and hepatomegaly in 1 of 8 patients who received 30–35Gy and 12 of 27 patients who received >35Gy to the liver [67]. In the 1980s, studies of whole liver irradiation for pancreas cancer

Table 6.2 Studies describing the using of proton beam radiation therapy for hepatocellular carcinoma

1st Author, year of publication	A.1.1. # patients	A.1.2. Study design	A.1.3. Tumor size in cm	A.1.4. Tumor extent	A.1.5. Child-pugh B	A.1.6. Prior therapy	A.1.7. Dose in GyRBE/# fractions	A.1.8. 1-yr LC	A.1.9. 1-yr OS	A.1.10. RILD	A.1.11. Grade 3+ toxicity
Chiba, 2005 [47]	162	RS	Median 3.8 Range 1.5–14.5	6% TVT	38% (6% CPC)	–	Median 72/4.5 Range 50–88/2.9–6 3–4 d per wk	5 yr 86.9%	5 yr 23.5%	None	5 of 162 (stenosis of CBD, infected biloma, gastric or colon ulcers, all treated before motion management introduced in 1995)
Nakayama, 2009 [48]	318	RS	–	19% TVT	24% (2% CPC)	57%	77/35 if <2 cm from GIM 72.6/22 if <2 cm from PH 66/10 if >2 cm from PH and GIM	1 yr	1 yr 89.5% 3 yr 64.7% 5 yr 44.6%	None	7 of 318 (colon hemorrhage, 6pts with G3 hematologic toxicities)
Fukumitsu, 2009 [89]	51	PS	Allowed <10 (88.2% ≤5), >2 cm from PH or GIM	–	20%	64.7%	66/10	3 yr 94.5% 5 yr 87.8%	3 yr 49.2% 5 yr 38.7%	None	One pt with G3 pneumonitis, 3 with rib fractures treated conservatively
Kawashima, 2011 [49]	30	RS	Median 4.5 Range 2.5–8.2	70% TVT	22%	60%	Median 76/20	3 yr 97% 5 yr 93%	3 yr 56% 5 yr 25%	None	One pt with hemorrhagic duodenitis, one with colonic bleed requiring surgery
Komatsu, 2011 [50]	343 (242 received PBR, 101 received carbon)	RS	71% were <5 cm, 23% were 5–10 cm and 6% were >10 cm	26% TVT	23% PBR pts (1% CPC)	47%	52.8–84/4–38	5 yr 90.2 for PBR	5 yr 38% for PBR	4 pts	8 of 242 PBR pts developed chronic G3+ toxicities: hematologic, gastric ulcer, pneumonitis, 5 pts with refractory skin ulcers (1 requiring skin transplant)

(continued)

Table 6.2 (continued)

1st Author, year of publication	A.1.1. # patients	A.1.2. Study design	A.1.3. Tumor size in cm	A.1.4. Tumor extent	A.1.5. Child-pugh B	A.1.6. Prior therapy	A.1.7. Dose in GyRBE/# fractions	A.1.8. 1-yr LC	A.1.9. 1-yr OS	A.1.10. RILD	A.1.11. Grade 3+ toxicity
Mizumoto, 2011 [53]	266	PS	Median 3.4 range 0.6–1.3	–	23% (1% CPC)	63%	77/35 if <2 cm from GIM 72.6/22 if <2 cm from PH 66/10 if >2 cm from PH and GIM	1 yr 98% 3 yr 87% 5 yr 81%	1 yr 87% 3 yr 61% 5 yr 48%	None	1 with G3 radiation dermatitis, 6 with perforation, bleeding, or inflammation of the GIM
Bush, 2011 [55]	76	PS	Mean 5.5	No EHD	47%	–	63/15	–	Median PFS was 36 mo	None	None
Lee, 2014 [51]	27	RS	–	59% main PVTT	33.3%	77.8%	50–66/20–22	–	1 yr 55.6% 2 yr 33.3%	None	None
Hong, 2016 [56]	92 (44 with HCC, 37 with IHC)	PS	Median 5.0 range 1.9–12	29.5% TVT in HCC pts	20.5%	–	67.5/15 58.05/15	2 yr LC 94.8% for HCC pts	1 yr 69.7% 2 yr 46.5%	None	1 of 44 HCC pts developed G3 thrombocytopenia

HCC hepatocellular carcinoma, *LC* local control, *OS* overall survival, *RILD* radiation-induced liver disease, *PBR* proton beam radiation, *RS* retrospective, *PS* prospective, *CPC* Child-Pugh C, *d* days, *wk* week, *mo* month, *yr* year, *pt* patient, *G3* grade 3, *PH* porta hepatis, *GIM* gastrointestinal mucosa, *TVT* tumor vascular thrombus, *PVTT* portal vein tumor thrombus, *PFS* progression-free survival, *IHC* intrahepatic cholangiocarcinoma, *btwn* between, *TACE* transcatheter arterial chemoembolization demonstrated that mean liver doses in excess of 30Gy could lead to liver failure [68]. Emami and colleagues reported the mean liver dose expected to produce a 5% risk of liver failure within 5 years of treatment to be 30Gy in 2Gy fractions [69]. The 30Gy threshold was also significant in a population of patients with liver metastases treated with hyperfractionated EBRT on a prospective trial. No patient receiving 27–30Gy in 1.5Gy twice daily fractions developed severe RILD, while nearly 10% of patients receiving 33Gy in 1.5Gy twice daily fractions developed severe RILD [70].

A volume effect for the liver was demonstrated when studies showed much higher doses could be safely applied when only part of the liver was being treated [15]. This suggested that the older toxicity prediction models may overestimate the risk of liver toxicity for patients who are not undergoing whole liver irradiation [71]. For this reason, the Lyman-Kutcher-Burman model for normal tissue complication probability (NTCP) model was favored instead. Using the NTCP model, Dawson and colleagues found no cases of RILD when the mean liver dose was kept below 31Gy.

Additionally, they suggested patients with primary liver disease, such as HCC, may have a lower threshold for developing RILD when compared to patients with hepatic metastases treated with radiation [13]. Subsequent work showed that Child-Pugh score (A vs B) also significantly affected the fractional dose dependence of the normalized total dose, an expression proposed to convert NTCP data between different dose/fractionation Schemes [72]. Higher sensitivity of cirrhotic liver to irradiation could be linked to active proliferation of fibrotic tissue with loss of hepatic functional reserve. As a result, cirrhotic liver volume obtained from the volumetric imaging used for radiation treatment planning may not adequately represent functional hepatic parenchyma, and CT-based dose-volume constraints applied to non-cirrhotic liver may be inappropriate. Therefore, prediction of RILD by the NTCP model for patients with advanced cirrhosis can be underestimated [73].

The Quantitative Analysis of Normal Tissue Effects in the Clinic (QUANTEC) organ-specific paper for the liver recommends the following mean liver dose constraints for patients with HCC and other primary liver tumors: <28Gy in 2Gy fractions, <18Gy for six-fraction SBRT regimens, and <13Gy for three-fraction SBRT regimens. When patients have a Child-Pugh B liver disease, it is recommended to reduce the mean liver dose to <6Gy in regimens using 4–6Gy fraction sizes [74]. It should be mentioned that when calculating the mean liver dose, the gross tumor volume is subtracted from the total liver volume before determining whether a radiation plan meets the above constraints.

Relative Volume Constraints

In addition to mean liver dose, the percentage of the liver volume receiving greater than 30Gy (V30) has also been shown to be significantly associated with RILD. Early studies suggest that when the whole liver receives 18Gy in standard fractionation, the V30 should be limited to 30% [68]. More recent studies evaluating partial liver radiation suggest that the V30 should be limited to 28–60% to decrease the risk of RILD [75–77].

Absolute Volume Constraints

When conducting a trial of SBRT for liver metastases, the University of Colorado utilized a critical volume model to reduce the risk of liver toxicity. Borrowing data from surgical series, an absolute volume of 700 cc of healthy, functioning liver was deemed necessary for the best chance at maintaining normal liver function. For the University of Colorado's prospective trial, the maximum dose allowed to the critical volume of 700 cc was 15Gy in three fractions [78], and no RILD has been reported when using this constraint [79].

Technical Considerations for Treatment Planning and Delivery

To begin radiation treatment planning, a CT simulation is first performed in order to create a reproducible setup for daily treatment as well as to obtain CT images for treatment planning.

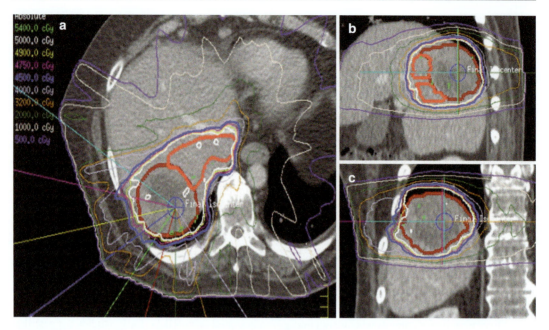

Fig. 6.1 Panels **a**, **b**, and **c** show representative axial, sagittal, and coronal images for a patient with hepatocellular carcinoma (red bold outline) and a portal venous tumor thrombus (pink bold outline) treated with stereotactic body radiotherapy to a total dose of 50 Gray in 5 fractions using intensity-modulated radiation therapy. The patient was enrolled on an ongoing clinical trial, Radiation Therapy Oncology Group 1112, and all protocol constraints were met. The patient was NPO 3 h prior to each day's treatment. Radiation was delivered using a breath-hold technique. Daily CT-on-rails was used for daily alignment with setup to tumor and liver shape

Accurate radiation delivery depends on the ability to manage motion of the tumor during treatment and to reliably identify and target the tumor on a daily basis. The liver moves with respiration, mostly in the craniocaudal direction [80]. If treatment while the patient is free-breathing is desired, a 4DCT must be obtained after which the tumor must be contoured in all phases of the respiratory cycle and the target volume enlarged to encompass all possible positions of the tumor. This often leads to a prohibitively large target volume, particularly when large doses per fraction are employed. An alternative is to plan and treat the patient with them holding their breath, which decreases variation in tumor position to approximately 2–4 mm [81, 82]. Another option is to treat with respiratory gating in which the radiation beam is only turned on during specific phases of the respiratory cycle [83]. Abdominal compression can minimize liver motion with respiration but can also cause variable deformation of the liver and move the adjacent bowel closer to the tumor target [84]. Difference in gastric filling may impact liver shape and position, particularly the left liver [85]. Therefore, patients are advised to have nothing to eat or drink for 3 h prior to the simulation appointment as well as for each daily treatment.

Daily image guidance is paramount to precise radiation delivery, and there are several ways this can be done. Radiopaque fiducials can be implanted in or near the tumor and identified either with daily X-ray and/or CT imaging on the treatment machine [86, 87]. The advantage of this method is that most linear accelerators have the necessary onboard imaging technology, but the disadvantage is that it requires an invasive procedure to place the fiducials, and the fiducials could migrate prior to or during treatment. An alternative to fiducial placement is to align to soft tissue, with onboard CT-on-rails or cone-beam CT imaging which also allows monitoring of daily tumor regression, changes in liver shape, and day-to-day bowel motion (Fig. 6.1) [85]. MRI-based treatment planning and daily image guidance will allow for improved visualization of

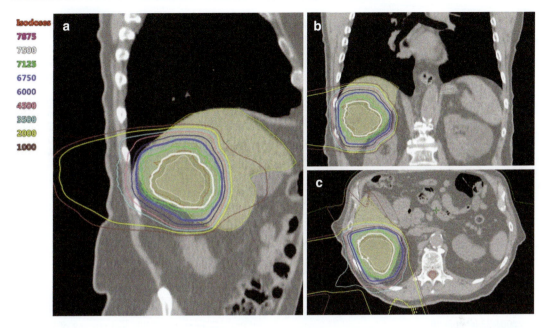

Fig. 6.2 Panels **a**, **b**, and **c** show representative sagittal, coronal, and axial images for a patient with hepatocellular carcinoma treated with proton beam radiotherapy to a total dose of 75 Gray (relative biological effectiveness) in 15 fractions. Note the conformal coverage of the target (red-shaded volume) with the prescription dose line (white bold outline) as well as the rapid falloff of radiation dose distal to the target. Nontarget liver and abdominal viscera received doses that were well below constraints. The patient was NPO 3 h prior to each day's treatment. Radiation was delivered using a breath-hold technique. Three carbon fiducials were placed prior to treatment and were used daily for alignment using kilovoltage X-ray imaging on the treatment machine

the tumors within the liver and will improve daily setup accuracy in the future [88]. All of these imaging modalities have the best resolution with a breath-hold technique (Fig. 6.2).

Future Directions and Ongoing Studies

RTOG 1112 (NCT01730937) is a randomized, phase III trial comparing sorafenib alone with SBRT followed by sorafenib for patients with HCC. The primary endpoint of this trial is to see if SBRT improves OS compared to the standard of care, sorafenib alone. Patients must be unsuitable for transplant, surgical resection, RFA, and TACE. Patients are eligible as long as they don't have any one HCC >15 cm or the total max sum of HCC >20 cm or more than five discrete intraparenchymal HCC foci. Tumor thrombus is allowed, but extrahepatic metastases or malignant nodes >3 cm in maximum diameter are not allowed. RTOG 1112 is currently accruing and hopefully will provide insight as to the benefit SBRT can provide patients with inoperable HCC over sorafenib alone. Additionally, single-institutional trials are currently evaluating the safety and efficacy of the combination of SRBT with ipilimumab (NCT02239900) or crystalline nanoparticles (NCT02721056) for advanced liver tumors.

Summary

Radiation has emerged as an effective treatment option for patients with HCC. Long-term tumor control rates appear to be comparable to ablation and surgical resection, and toxicity rates from modern series are acceptable, particularly given the common comorbidity profile of this patient population. This may be due to advances in radiation delivery techniques which allow for higher doses to be given more precisely with a lower risk of adverse toxicity to the uninvolved liver and other nearby critical structures. More conformal techniques using IMRT or proton therapy can help to achieve this goal. SBRT and hypofractionated regimens also appear promising and allow shorter courses without compromising safety.

References

1. Altekruse SF, McGlynn KA, Reichman ME. Hepatocellular carcinoma incidence, mortality, and survival trends in the United States from 1975 to 2005. J Clin Oncol Off J Am Soc Clin Oncol. 2009;27(9):1485–91.
2. Poon RT, Fan ST, Lo CM, Ng IO, Liu CL, Lam CM, et al. Improving survival results after resection of hepatocellular carcinoma: a prospective study of 377 patients over 10 years. Ann Surg. 2001;234(1):63–70.
3. Bruix J, Llovet JM. Prognostic prediction and treatment strategy in hepatocellular carcinoma. Hepatology (Baltimore MD). 2002;35(3):519–24.
4. National comprehensive cancer network guidelines-hepatobiliary cancers [Internet]. [cited 2017 Jan 2]. https://www.nccn.org/professionals/physician_gls/pdf/hepatobiliary.pdf.
5. Rim CH, Seong J. Application of radiotherapy for hepatocellular carcinoma in current clinical practice guidelines. Radiat Oncol J. 2016;34(3):160–7.
6. Korean Liver Cancer Study Group (KLCSG), National Cancer Center, Korea (NCC). 2014 KLCSG-NCC Korea practice guideline for the management of hepatocellular carcinoma. Gut Liver. 2015;9(3):267–317.
7. Hyder O, Dodson RM, Nathan H, Herman JM, Cosgrove D, Kamel I, et al. Referral patterns and treatment choices for patients with hepatocellular carcinoma: a United States population-based study. J Am Coll Surg. 2013;217(5):896–906.
8. Dionisi F, Guarneri A, Dell'Acqua V, Leonardi M, Niespolo R, Macchia G, et al. Radiotherapy in the multidisciplinary treatment of liver cancer: a survey on behalf of the Italian Association of Radiation Oncology. Radiol Med (Torino). 2016;121(9):735–43.
9. Benson R, Madan R, Kilambi R, Chander S. Radiation induced liver disease: a clinical update. J Egypt Natl Cancer Inst. 2016;28(1):7–11.
10. Seong J, Park HC, Han KH, Chon CY. Clinical results and prognostic factors in radiotherapy for unresectable hepatocellular carcinoma: a retrospective study of 158 patients. Int J Radiat Oncol Biol Phys. 2003;55(2):329–36.
11. Liang S-X, Zhu X-D, Lu H-J, Pan C-Y, Li F-X, Huang Q-F, et al. Hypofractionated three-dimensional conformal radiation therapy for primary liver carcinoma. Cancer. 2005;103(10):2181–8.
12. Liu M-T, Li S-H, Chu T-C, Hsieh C-Y, Wang A-Y, Chang T-H, et al. Three-dimensional conformal radiation therapy for unresectable hepatocellular carcinoma patients who had failed with or were unsuited for transcatheter arterial chemoembolization. Jpn J Clin Oncol. 2004;34(9):532–9.
13. Dawson LA, Normolle D, Balter JM, McGinn CJ, Lawrence TS, Ten Haken RK. Analysis of radiation-induced liver disease using the Lyman NTCP model. Int J Radiat Oncol Biol Phys. 2002;53(4):810–21.
14. Ben-Josef E, Normolle D, Ensminger WD, Walker S, Tatro D, Ten Haken RK, et al. Phase II trial of high-dose conformal radiation therapy with concurrent hepatic artery floxuridine for unresectable intrahepatic malignancies. J Clin Oncol Off J Am Soc Clin Oncol. 2005;23(34):8739–47.
15. Dawson LA, McGinn CJ, Normolle D, Ten Haken RK, Walker S, Ensminger W, et al. Escalated focal liver radiation and concurrent hepatic artery fluorodeoxyuridine for unresectable intrahepatic malignancies. J Clin Oncol Off J Am Soc Clin Oncol. 2000;18(11):2210–8.
16. Mornex F, Girard N, Beziat C, Kubas A, Khodri M, Trepo C, et al. Feasibility and efficacy of high-dose three-dimensional-conformal radiotherapy in cirrhotic patients with small-size hepatocellular carcinoma non-eligible for curative therapies--mature results of the French phase II RTF-1 trial. Int J Radiat Oncol Biol Phys. 2006;66(4):1152–8.
17. Meng M-B, Cui Y-L, Lu Y, She B, Chen Y, Guan Y-S, et al. Transcatheter arterial chemoembolization in combination with radiotherapy for unresectable hepatocellular carcinoma: a systematic review and meta-analysis. Radiother Oncol J Eur Soc Ther Radiol Oncol. 2009;92(2):184–94.
18. Zeng Z-C, Fan J, Tang Z-Y, Zhou J, Qin L-X, Wang J-H, et al. A comparison of treatment combinations with and without radiotherapy for hepatocellular carcinoma with portal vein and/or inferior vena cava tumor thrombus. Int J Radiat Oncol Biol Phys. 2005;61(2):432–43.
19. Song DY, Kavanagh BD, Benedict SH, Schefter T. Stereotactic body radiation therapy. Rationale, techniques, applications, and optimization. Oncology (Williston Park). 2004;18(11):1419–30, 1432, 1435–6.
20. Katz AW, Chawla S, Qu Z, Kashyap R, Milano MT, Hezel AF. Stereotactic hypofractionated radiation therapy as a bridge to transplantation for hepatocellular carcinoma: clinical outcome and pathologic correlation. Int J Radiat Oncol Biol Phys. 2012;83(3):895–900.
21. O'Connor JK, Trotter J, Davis GL, Dempster J, Klintmalm GB, Goldstein RM. Long-term outcomes of stereotactic body radiation therapy in the treatment of hepatocellular cancer as a bridge to transplantation. Liver Transpl. 2012;18(8):949–54.
22. Blomgren H, Lax I, Näslund I, Svanström R. Stereotactic high dose fraction radiation therapy of extracranial tumors using an accelerator. Clinical

experience of the first thirty-one patients. Acta Oncol. 1995;34(6):861–70.
23. Choi BO, Choi IB, Jang HS, Kang YN, Jang JS, Bae SH, et al. Stereotactic body radiation therapy with or without transarterial chemoembolization for patients with primary hepatocellular carcinoma: preliminary analysis. BMC Cancer. 2008;8:351.
24. Goyal K, Einstein D, Yao M, Kunos C, Barton F, Singh D, et al. Cyberknife stereotactic body radiation therapy for nonresectable tumors of the liver: preliminary results. HPB Surg. 2010;2010:8.
25. Seo YS, Kim M-S, Yoo SY, Cho CK, Choi CW, Kim JH, et al. Preliminary result of stereotactic body radiotherapy as a local salvage treatment for inoperable hepatocellular carcinoma. J Surg Oncol. 2010;102(3):209–14.
26. Kwon JH, Bae SH, Kim JY, Choi BO, Jang HS, Jang JW, et al. Long-term effect of stereotactic body radiation therapy for primary hepatocellular carcinoma ineligible for local ablation therapy or surgical resection. Stereotactic radiotherapy for liver cancer. BMC Cancer. 2010;10:475.
27. Andolino DL, Johnson CS, Maluccio M, Kwo P, Tector AJ, Zook J, et al. Stereotactic body radiotherapy for primary hepatocellular carcinoma. Int J Radiat Oncol Biol Phys. 2011;81(4):e447–53.
28. Jang WI, Kim M-S, Bae SH, Cho CK, Yoo HJ, Seo YS, et al. High-dose stereotactic body radiotherapy correlates increased local control and overall survival in patients with inoperable hepatocellular carcinoma. Radiat Oncol. 2013;8:250.
29. Yoon SM, Lim Y-S, Park MJ, Kim SY, Cho B, Shim JH, et al. Stereotactic body radiation therapy as an alternative treatment for small hepatocellular carcinoma. PLoS One. 2013;8(11):e79854.
30. Culleton S, Jiang H, Haddad CR, Kim J, Brierley J, Brade A, et al. Outcomes following definitive stereotactic body radiotherapy for patients with child-Pugh B or C hepatocellular carcinoma. Radiother Oncol. 2014;111(3):412–7.
31. Scorsetti M, Comito T, Cozzi L, Clerici E, Tozzi A, Franzese C, et al. The challenge of inoperable hepatocellular carcinoma (HCC): results of a single-institutional experience on stereotactic body radiation therapy (SBRT). J Cancer Res Clin Oncol. 2015;141(7):1301–9.
32. Su T-S, Liang P, Lu H-Z, Liang J, Gao Y-C, Zhou Y, et al. Stereotactic body radiation therapy for small primary or recurrent hepatocellular carcinoma in 132 Chinese patients. J Surg Oncol. 2016;113(2):181–7.
33. Su T-S, Lu H-Z, Cheng T, Zhou Y, Huang Y, Gao Y-C, et al. Long-term survival analysis in combined transarterial embolization and stereotactic body radiation therapy versus stereotactic body radiation monotherapy for unresectable hepatocellular carcinoma >5 cm. BMC Cancer. 2016;16(1):834.
34. Jacob R, Turley F, Redden DT, Saddekni S, Aal AKA, Keene K, et al. Adjuvant stereotactic body radiotherapy following transarterial chemoembolization in patients with non-resectable hepatocellular carcinoma tumours of ≥ 3 cm. HPB. 2015;17(2):140–9.
35. Méndez Romero A, Wunderink W, Hussain SM, De Pooter JA, Heijmen BJM, Nowak PCJM, et al. Stereotactic body radiation therapy for primary and metastatic liver tumors: a single institution phase i-ii study. Acta Oncol. 2006;45(7):831–7.
36. Tse RV, Hawkins M, Lockwood G, Kim JJ, Cummings B, Knox J, et al. Phase I study of individualized stereotactic body radiotherapy for hepatocellular carcinoma and intrahepatic cholangiocarcinoma. J Clin Oncol Off J Am Soc Clin Oncol. 2008;26(4):657–64.
37. Cárdenes HR, Price TR, Perkins SM, Maluccio M, Kwo P, Breen TE, et al. Phase I feasibility trial of stereotactic body radiation therapy for primary hepatocellular carcinoma. Clin Transl Oncol. 2010;12(3):218–25.
38. Price TR, Perkins SM, Sandrasegaran K, Henderson MA, Maluccio MA, Zook JE, et al. Evaluation of response after stereotactic body radiotherapy for hepatocellular carcinoma. Cancer. 2012;118(12):3191–8.
39. Kang J-K, Kim M-S, Cho CK, Yang KM, Yoo HJ, Kim JH, et al. Stereotactic body radiation therapy for inoperable hepatocellular carcinoma as a local salvage treatment after incomplete transarterial chemoembolization. Cancer. 2012;118(21):5424–31.
40. Bujold A, Massey CA, Kim JJ, Brierley J, Cho C, Wong RKS, et al. Sequential phase I and II trials of stereotactic body radiotherapy for locally advanced hepatocellular carcinoma. J Clin Oncol Off J Am Soc Clin Oncol. 2013;31(13):1631–9.
41. Brade AM, Ng S, Brierley J, Kim J, Dinniwell R, Ringash J, et al. Phase 1 trial of sorafenib and stereotactic body radiation therapy for hepatocellular carcinoma. Int J Radiat Oncol Biol Phys. 2016;94(3):580–7.
42. Takeda A, Sanuki N, Tsurugai Y, Iwabuchi S, Matsunaga K, Ebinuma H, et al. Phase 2 study of stereotactic body radiotherapy and optional transarterial chemoembolization for solitary hepatocellular carcinoma not amenable to resection and radiofrequency ablation. Cancer. 2016;122(13):2041–9.
43. Kim JW, Seong J, Lee IJ, Woo JY, Han K-H. Phase I dose escalation study of helical intensity-modulated radiotherapy-based stereotactic body radiotherapy for hepatocellular carcinoma. Oncotarget. 2016;7(26):40756–66.
44. Weiner AA, Olsen J, Ma D, Dyk P, DeWees T, Myerson RJ, et al. Stereotactic body radiotherapy for primary hepatic malignancies - report of a phase I/II institutional study. Radiother Oncol. 2016;121(1):79–85.
45. Horgan AM, Dawson LA, Swaminath A, Knox JJ. Sorafenib and radiation therapy for the treatment of advanced hepatocellular carcinoma. J Gastrointest Cancer. 2012;43(2):344–8.
46. Lawrence JH, Tobias CA, Born JL, Linfoot JA, Kling RP, Gottschalk A. Alpha and proton heavy particles and the bragg peak in therapy. Trans Am Clin Climatol Assoc. 1964;75:111–6.

47. Chiba T, Tokuuye K, Matsuzaki Y, Sugahara S, Chuganji Y, Kagei K, et al. Proton beam therapy for hepatocellular carcinoma: a retrospective review of 162 patients. Clin Cancer Res. 2005;11(10):3799–805.
48. Nakayama H, Sugahara S, Tokita M, Fukuda K, Mizumoto M, Abei M, et al. Proton beam therapy for hepatocellular carcinoma: the University of Tsukuba experience. Cancer. 2009;115(23):5499–506.
49. Kawashima M, Kohno R, Nakachi K, Nishio T, Mitsunaga S, Ikeda M, et al. Dose-volume histogram analysis of the safety of proton beam therapy for unresectable hepatocellular carcinoma. Int J Radiat Oncol Biol Phys. 2011;79(5):1479–86.
50. Komatsu S, Fukumoto T, Demizu Y, Miyawaki D, Terashima K, Sasaki R, et al. Clinical results and risk factors of proton and carbon ion therapy for hepatocellular carcinoma. Cancer. 2011;117(21):4890–904.
51. Lee SU, Park J-W, Kim TH, Kim Y-J, Woo SM, Koh Y-H, et al. Effectiveness and safety of proton beam therapy for advanced hepatocellular carcinoma with portal vein tumor thrombosis. Strahlenther Onkol. 2014;190(9):806–14.
52. Kim DY, Park J-W, Kim TH, Kim BH, Moon SH, Kim SS, et al. Risk-adapted simultaneous integrated boost-proton beam therapy (SIB-PBT) for advanced hepatocellular carcinoma with tumour vascular thrombosis. Radiother Oncol. 2017;122(1):122–9.
53. Mizumoto M, Okumura T, Hashimoto T, Fukuda K, Oshiro Y, Fukumitsu N, et al. Proton beam therapy for hepatocellular carcinoma: a comparison of three treatment protocols. Int J Radiat Oncol Biol Phys. 2011;81(4):1039–45.
54. Fukuda K, Okumura T, Abei M, Fukumitsu N, Ishige K, Mizumoto M, et al. Long-term outcomes of proton beam therapy in patients with previously untreated hepatocellular carcinoma. Cancer Sci. 2017;108(3):497–503.
55. Bush DA, Kayali Z, Grove R, Slater JD. The safety and efficacy of high-dose proton beam radiotherapy for hepatocellular carcinoma: a phase 2 prospective trial. Cancer. 2011;117(13):3053–9.
56. Hong TS, Wo JY, Yeap BY, Ben-Josef E, McDonnell EI, Blaszkowsky LS, et al. Multi-institutional phase II study of high-dose hypofractionated proton beam therapy in patients with localized, unresectable hepatocellular carcinoma and intrahepatic cholangiocarcinoma. J Clin Oncol Off J Am Soc Clin Oncol. 2016;34(5):460–8.
57. Bush DA, Smith JC, Slater JD, Volk ML, Reeves ME, Cheng J, et al. Randomized clinical trial comparing proton beam radiation therapy with transarterial chemoembolization for hepatocellular carcinoma: results of an interim analysis. Int J Radiat Oncol Biol Phys. 2016;95(1):477–82.
58. Reed GB, Cox AJ. The human liver after radiation injury. A form of veno-occlusive disease. Am J Pathol. 1966;48(4):597–611.
59. Mornex F, Gérard F, Ramuz O, Van Houtte P. Late effects of radiations on the liver. Cancer Radiother. 1997;1(6):753–9.
60. Lawrence TS, Robertson JM, Anscher MS, Jirtle RL, Ensminger WD, Fajardo LF. Hepatic toxicity resulting from cancer treatment. Int J Radiat Oncol Biol Phys. 1995;31(5):1237–48.
61. Guha C, Kavanagh BD. Hepatic radiation toxicity: avoidance and amelioration. Semin Radiat Oncol. 2011;21(4):256–63.
62. Unger EC, Lee JK, Weyman PJ. CT and MR imaging of radiation hepatitis. J Comput Assist Tomogr. 1987;11(2):264–8.
63. da Silveira EBV, Jeffers L, Schiff ER. Diagnostic laparoscopy in radiation-induced liver disease. Gastrointest Endosc. 2002;55(3):432–4.
64. Lightdale CJ, Wasser J, Coleman M, Brower M, Tefft M, Pasmantier M. Anticoagulation and high dose liver radiation: a preliminary report. Cancer. 1979;43(1):174–81.
65. Bearman SI, Lee JL, Barón AE, McDonald GB. Treatment of hepatic venocclusive disease with recombinant human tissue plasminogen activator and heparin in 42 marrow transplant patients. Blood. 1997;89(5):1501–6.
66. Sanuki N, Takeda A, Oku Y, Eriguchi T, Nishimura S, Aoki Y, et al. Influence of liver toxicities on prognosis after stereotactic body radiation therapy for hepatocellular carcinoma. Hepatol Res. 2015;45(5):540–7.
67. Ingold JA, Reed GB, Kaplan HS, Bagshaw MA. Radiation hepatitis. Am J Roentgenol Radium Therapy, Nucl Med. 1965;93:200–8.
68. Austin-Seymour MM, Chen GT, Castro JR, Saunders WM, Pitluck S, Woodruff KH, et al. Dose volume histogram analysis of liver radiation tolerance. Int J Radiat Oncol Biol Phys. 1986;12(1):31–5.
69. Emami B, Lyman J, Brown A, Coia L, Goitein M, Munzenrider JE, et al. Tolerance of normal tissue to therapeutic irradiation. Int J Radiat Oncol Biol Phys. 1991;21(1):109–22.
70. Russell AH, Clyde C, Wasserman TH, Turner SS, Rotman M. Accelerated hyperfractionated hepatic irradiation in the management of patients with liver metastases: results of the RTOG dose escalating protocol. Int J Radiat Oncol Biol Phys. 1993;27(1):117–23.
71. Lawrence TS, Ten Haken RK, Kessler ML, Robertson JM, Lyman JT, Lavigne ML, et al. The use of 3-D dose volume analysis to predict radiation hepatitis. Int J Radiat Oncol Biol Phys. 1992;23(4):781–8.
72. Tai A, Erickson B, Li XA. Extrapolation of normal tissue complication probability for different fractionations in liver irradiation. Int J Radiat Oncol Biol Phys. 2009;74(1):283–9.
73. Xu Z-Y, Liang S-X, Zhu J, Zhu X-D, Zhao J-D, Lu H-J, et al. Prediction of radiation-induced liver disease by Lyman normal-tissue complication probability model in three-dimensional conformal radiation therapy for primary liver carcinoma. Int J Radiat Oncol Biol Phys. 2006;65(1):189–95.
74. Pan CC, Kavanagh BD, Dawson LA, Li XA, Das SK, Miften M, et al. Radiation-associated liver injury. Int J Radiat Oncol Biol Phys. 2010;76(3 Suppl):S94–100.

75. Kim TH, Kim DY, Park J-W, Kim SH, Choi J-I, Kim HB, et al. Dose-volumetric parameters predicting radiation-induced hepatic toxicity in unresectable hepatocellular carcinoma patients treated with three-dimensional conformal radiotherapy. Int J Radiat Oncol Biol Phys. 2007;67(1):225–31.
76. Liang S-X, Zhu X-D, Xu Z-Y, Zhu J, Zhao J-D, Lu H-J, et al. Radiation-induced liver disease in three-dimensional conformal radiation therapy for primary liver carcinoma: the risk factors and hepatic radiation tolerance. Int J Radiat Oncol Biol Phys. 2006;65(2):426–34.
77. Yamada K, Izaki K, Sugimoto K, Mayahara H, Morita Y, Yoden E, et al. Prospective trial of combined transcatheter arterial chemoembolization and three-dimensional conformal radiotherapy for portal vein tumor thrombus in patients with unresectable hepatocellular carcinoma. Int J Radiat Oncol Biol Phys. 2003;57(1):113–9.
78. Schefter TE, Kavanagh BD, Timmerman RD, Cardenes HR, Baron A, Gaspar LE. A phase I trial of stereotactic body radiation therapy (SBRT) for liver metastases. Int J Radiat Oncol Biol Phys. 2005;62(5):1371–8.
79. Kavanagh BD, Schefter TE, Cardenes HR, Stieber VW, Raben D, Timmerman RD, et al. Interim analysis of a prospective phase I/II trial of SBRT for liver metastases. Acta Oncol. 2006;45(7):848–55.
80. Schuppan D, Afdhal NH. Liver cirrhosis. Lancet. 2008;371(9615):838–51.
81. Eccles C, Brock KK, Bissonnette J-P, Hawkins M, Dawson LA. Reproducibility of liver position using active breathing coordinator for liver cancer radiotherapy. Int J Radiat Oncol Biol Phys. 2006;64(3):751–9.
82. Dawson LA, Brock KK, Kazanjian S, Fitch D, McGinn CJ, Lawrence TS, et al. The reproducibility of organ position using active breathing control (ABC) during liver radiotherapy. Int J Radiat Oncol Biol Phys. 2001;51(5):1410–21.
83. Briere TM, Beddar S, Balter P, Murthy R, Gupta S, Nelson C, et al. Respiratory gating with EPID-based verification: the MDACC experience. Phys Med Biol. 2009;54(11):3379–91.
84. Heinzerling JH, Anderson JF, Papiez L, Boike T, Chien S, Zhang G, et al. Four-dimensional computed tomography scan analysis of tumor and organ motion at varying levels of abdominal compression during stereotactic treatment of lung and liver. Int J Radiat Oncol Biol Phys. 2008;70(5):1571–8.
85. Crane CH, Koay EJ. Solutions that enable ablative radiotherapy for large liver tumors: fractionated dose painting, simultaneous integrated protection, motion management, and computed tomography image guidance. Cancer. 2016;122(13):1974–86.
86. Wurm RE, Gum F, Erbel S, Schlenger L, Scheffler D, Agaoglu D, et al. Image guided respiratory gated hypofractionated stereotactic body radiation therapy (H-SBRT) for liver and lung tumors: initial experience. Acta Oncol. 2006;45(7):881–9.
87. Brock KK, Dawson LA. Adaptive management of liver cancer radiotherapy. Semin Radiat Oncol. 2010;20(2):107–15.
88. van de Lindt TN, Schubert G, van der Heide UA, Sonke J-J. An MRI-based mid-ventilation approach for radiotherapy of the liver. Radiother Oncol. 2016;121(2):276–80.
89. Fukumitsu N, Sugahara S, Nakayama H, Fukuda K, Mizumoto M, Abei M, Shoda J, Thono E, Tsuboi K, Tokuuye K. A prospective study of hypofractionated proton beam therapy for patients with hepatocellular carcinoma. Int J Radiat Oncol Biol Phys. 2009;74(3):831–6. https://doi.org/10.1016/j.ijrobp.2008.10.073.

Medical Therapy Options for Advanced Disease in Hepatocellular Carcinoma

Imane El Dika and Ghassan K. Abou-Alfa

Introduction

Advanced hepatocellular carcinoma (HCC) is defined by the presence of multicentric unresectable disease, major vessel involvement, or extrahepatic spread. Eighty percent of HCC cases arise in preneoplastic cirrhotic liver, either due to hepatitis B or C, alcoholic cirrhosis, nonalcoholic steatohepatitis (NASH), metabolic diseases (hemochromatosis, alpha-1 antitrypsin deficiency), or toxin exposure (aflatoxins). Treatment and outcome highly depend on the residual liver function in the context of cirrhosis, defined by Child-Pugh score [1]. Treatment of HCC has significantly shifted forward during the last decade, with the advance in sophisticated diagnostics and development of new therapeutics. Molecular signature and correlatives of response are also being explored.

I. El Dika
Memorial Sloan Kettering Cancer Center,
New York, NY, USA
e-mail: eldikai@mskcc.org

G. K. Abou-Alfa (✉)
Memorial Sloan Kettering Cancer Center,
New York, NY, USA

Weil Cornel Medical College, New York, NY, USA
e-mail: abou-alg@mskcc.org

Tyrosine Kinase Inhibitors

In HCC, a net excess of angiogenic factors produced by tumor cells, vascular endothelial cells, immune cells, and pericytes leads to the activation and recruitment of endothelial cells and pericytes [2]. Sorafenib is an oral multikinase inhibitor that inhibits VEGFR1, VEGFR2, VEGFR3, PDGFR-α, PDGFR-β, c-KIT, Raf-1, and BRAF. Early evidence of clinical antitumor activity was observed from a phase II study of 137 patients with advanced HCC; time to progression (TTP) was 4.2 months and OS 9.2 months [3]. In a randomized phase III trial [4], patients who received sorafenib showed a 10.7-month median overall survival compared to 7.9 months for patients who received placebo (HR = 0.69; $p < 0.001$). While benefit from sorafenib is observed across patients regardless of disease stage and etiology, an improved benefit of sorafenib in patients with hepatitis C virus (HCV)-induced HCC was observed. The superior activity of sorafenib in HCV-induced HCC might be due to high RAF kinase activity driven by HCV core protein-1, in this subgroup [5]. Sorafenib was thus approved for the treatment of inoperable HCC. This led to several antiangiogenic agents and tyrosine kinase inhibitors to be evaluated in advanced HCC.

Sunitinib malate inhibits multiple kinases including VEGFR-1, VEGFR-2, and VEGFR-3, PDGFR-α and PDGFR-β, KIT, FMS-like tyrosine kinase 3, colony-stimulating factor receptor type 1, and RET. In a phase II study of sunitinib, ORR was 2.9%, median PFS was 3.9 months (95% CI, 2.6–6.9 months), and OS was 9.8 months (95% CI, 7.4 months to not available) [6]. The randomized phase III trial comparing sunitinib to sorafenib in the first line was terminated early for futility and safety reasons [7]. Sunitinib was significantly inferior to sorafenib with median OS of 7.9 versus 10.2 months (two-sided $p = 0.0014$). Brivanib is a selective dual inhibitor of VEGF and FGF receptors, both implicated in HCC tumorigenesis and angiogenesis; a phase III study randomized 395 patients with advanced HCC who progressed on/after or were intolerant to sorafenib to receive brivanib 800 mg orally once per day or placebo. Median OS was 9.4 months for brivanib and 8.2 months for placebo ([HR], 0.89; 95.8% CI, 0.69–1.15; $p = 0.3307$) [8].

Lenvatinib is an oral inhibitor of VEGFR1–3, FGFR1–4, PDGFR-α, RET, and KIT. A phase II single-arm study including 46 patients was conducted at sites across Japan and Korea. The median TTP was 7.4 months [95% confidence interval (CI), 5.5–9.4], 37% had partial response, and 41% had stable disease (ORR, 37%; DCR, 78%). Median OS was 18.7 months (95% CI, 12.7–25.1). The most common any-grade adverse events were hypertension, palmar-plantar erythrodysesthesia syndrome, decreased appetite, and proteinuria [9]. An open-label, phase III trial (NCT01761266), comparing lenvatinib versus sorafenib in first-line treatment of patients with unresectable HCC, was completed and has met its primary endpoint of non-inferiority with OS of 13.6 vs 12.3 months and HR 0.92 (0.79–1.06). It showed statistically significant improvement for PFS, 7.4 vs 3.7 months; HR, 0.66 (0.57–0.77); TTP, 8.9 vs 3.7 months; HR, 0.63 (0.53–0.73); and ORR, 24% vs 9%, $p < 0.00001$ [10].

Ramucirumab, a recombinant IgG1 monoclonal antibody and VEGF receptor-2 antagonist, was assessed in the second line in a randomized phase III trial. Median OS was 9.2 months (95% CI 8.0–10.6) versus 7.6 months (6.0–9.3) for the placebo group (HR 0.87 [95% CI 0.72–1.05]; $p = 0.14$) [11]. Patients with Child-Pugh B disease had significant adverse liver events, so investigators stopped enrolment of patients with Child-Pugh B disease, and they were excluded from analysis. Prespecified tests for OS identified baseline AFP concentration as the only clinically relevant factor with an interaction with treatment ($p = 0.027$). In patients with AFP $\geq$400 ng/mL, median OS was 7.8 months (95% CI 5.8–9.3) for the ramucirumab versus 4.2 months (3.7–4.8) for placebo. Elevated AFP has been associated with elevated VEGFR expression, increased angiogenesis, and poor prognosis in hepatocellular carcinoma [12]. A follow-up study evaluated ramucirumab in patients with of $\geq$ 400ng/ml showed an improvement in overall survival to 8.5 months versus 7.3 months for placebo (HR 0.710; 95% CI 0.531, 0.949; $p =.0199$). and reference Zhu, A. et al. J Clin Oncol 36, 2018 (suppl; abstr 4003).

Regorafenib, a TKI that targets TIE-2, FGFR, c-kit, and RET in addition to VEGF, PDGFR, and RAF-MEK-ERK, showed significant improvement in overall survival (10.6 vs 7.8 months; $p < 0.001$) and progression-free survival (3.1 vs 1.5 months; $p < 0.001$) after progression on sorafenib in a randomized, international, multicenter, phase III trial RESORCE [13]. OS benefit was observed across subgroup populations, including Asian vs non-Asian, AFP level, and hepatitis B- or C-related HCC. On April 27, 2017, the US Food and Drug Administration expanded the indications of regorafenib to include the treatment of patients with HCC who have been previously treated with sorafenib.

c-Met and HGF are the most common deregulated pathways in HCC. Patients with c-Met overexpression have a poorer prognosis compared to the general population. Targeting Met has been an increasingly interesting approach in HCC. Tivantinib, a selective Met inhibitor, demonstrated antitumor activity in a phase II second-line trial [14]. The benefit was more notable in patients with c-Met-positive tumors, and subsequently a phase III trial evaluating tivantinib in select Met-positive population in the second-line setting was conducted and recently reported. Primary endpoint of OS was not met [15]. Median OS (95% CI) was 8.4 months (6.8–10.0) in the tivantinib arm and 9.1 m (7.3–10.4) in the placebo arm, HR = 0.97 (0.75–1.25), and p = 0.81. Median PFS (95% CI) was, respectively, 2.1 m (1.9–3.0) vs 2 m (1.9–3.6), HR = 0.96 (0.75–1.22), p = 0.72 [15]. Cabozantinib has both anti-Met and antiangiogenic activity and has shown activity against HCC in the preclinical and early clinical studies. In the phase II randomized discontinuation study of cabozantinib, median OS time for all 41 treated patients from the initial cabozantinib dose was 11.5 months (95% CI = 7.3–15.6 months) [16]. A randomized phase III trial evaluating cabozantinib regardless of Met status showed an overall survival of 10.2 mo for cabozantinib vs 8 months for placebo (HR 0.76, 95% CI 0.63-0.92; p = 0.0049). Median PFS was 5.2 months for cabozantinib vs 1.9 months for cabozantinib (HR 0.44, 95% CI 0.36-0.52; p < 0.001), and reference Abou-Alfa, GK, et al. Journal of Clinical Oncology 36, no. 4_suppl (February 1 2018) 207-207.

Immunotherapy

Checkpoint Inhibition

Emerging data are available for checkpoint inhibitors acting on the CTLA-4 and PD-1 checkpoint pathways in HCC. The CTLA-4 pathway inhibits the activation of T cells, specifically Tregs. A phase II study of tremelimumab, a CTLA-4-blocking antibody, demonstrated a partial response (PR) of 17.6%, a disease control rate (DCR) of 76.4%, and a TTP of 6.48 months in HCV-induced HCC patients [17]. Tremelimumab is now being evaluated as single agent and in combination with durvalumab (previously MEDI4736) in a phase II trial. Nivolumab is a human monoclonal antibody that targets the PD-1 cell surface membrane receptor. Nivolumab was well tolerated in the phase I/II trial, demonstrating antitumor activity across different etiologies. The median OS was 70% at 9 months and 62% at 12 months [18]. In the dose expansion part of the study, nivolumab at 3 mg/kg demonstrated an OS rates for all patients at 6 and 9 months of 82.5% and 70.8%, respectively. The most recently reported ORR was 20% (95% CI 15–26) in 214 patients treated in the dose expansion phase; DCR was 64% (95% CI 58–71). Responses were observed across etiologies and regardless of tumor PD-L1 expression. ORRs of 23% (95% CI 13–36) and 21% (95% CI 11–34) were observed in the uninfected sorafenib-naive and sorafenib-treated patients, respectively [19]. A randomized phase III trial comparing nivolumab to sorafenib in the first-line setting (NCT02576509) is currently underway. Pembrolizumab is also being studied in the second line after progression on sorafenib. Immunotherapy is associated with rare but notable risk of serious adverse events, including severe colitis, pneumonitis, nephrotoxicity, hepatotoxicity, and other immune-related adverse events, which might require hospitalization and high-dose immunosuppressive therapy, with eventual discontinuation of the drug.

Vaccine Therapy

Vaccine therapy was recently described and is currently looked at in HCC. JX-594 is a targeted oncolytic poxvirus designed to selectively replicate in and destroy cancer cells with cell-cycle abnormalities and EGFR-RAS pathway activation. Intratumoral injection was shown to be safe and induce tumor response in a small cohort [20]. A randomized phase II dose-ranging study was initiated to evaluate the safety and antitumor efficacy of Pexa-Vec administered at high dose versus low dose in 30 patients with advanced HCC [21]. All patients experienced flu-like symptoms consisting of fever, chills, rigors, nausea, or vomiting within 24 h of JX-594. Four patients responded to treatment based on modified RECIST (one complete response, three partial responses). Furthermore, overall survival was significantly longer in the high-dose arm compared with the low-dose arm (median 14.1 months versus 6.7 months, p-value 0.020). In contrast, a phase IIb clinical trial in HCC patients who failed sorafenib therapy (n = 129) was recently completed and did not achieve the primary endpoint of prolonging overall survival in Pexa-Vec-treated patients when compared to patients treated with best supportive care in this patient population [22]. This study was critiqued for the poor performance of the eligible patients. Based on preliminary preclinical and clinical data that suggests a complementary antitumor effects of a sequential combination of Pexa-Vec followed by sorafenib possibly by targeting the tumor vasculature via different mechanisms [23], a randomized phase III study (PHOCUS) comparing vaccine therapy combined to sorafenib vs sorafenib alone in the first-line setting is currently underway (NCT02562755).

CAR T Cell Therapy

Immunotherapy based on T cells modified with a chimeric antigen receptor (CAR) has been demonstrated as a promising strategy for cancer treatment. CAR T cells can specifically recognize tumor-associated antigen and eliminate tumor cells in a nonmajor histocompatibility complex-restricted manner. Several pilot clinical trials using CAR T cells have recently been reported with promising clinical outcomes. AFP is a secreted glycoprotein commonly expressed in HCC and was studied as a potential target for CAR T cell therapy [24]. This study demonstrated that AFP-CAR T cells targeting intracellular/secreted solid tumor antigens can elicit an antitumor response while being specific to the target antigen complex in cell lines. In vivo activity was tested in liver cancer xenograft models, and a reduction in tumor size was demonstrated. Potential off-target/off-tumor toxicity resulting from the cross-reactivity of these receptors with nonidentical sequence-related HLA-I-binding peptides presented by vital cells is one limitation to this strategy [25]. GPC3 is an attractive liver cancer-specific target because it is highly expressed in HCC with limited expression in normal tissues. Phase I studies of GPC-3 naked antibody [26] failed to demonstrate efficacy in HCC. Results from a phase I study of GPC-3-derived peptide vaccine [27] suggest that GPC3-targeted T cells could be potential agents for HCC treatment. The GPC3-targeted CAR T cells were shown to efficiently kill GPC3-positive HCC cells but not GPC3-negative cells in vitro [28]. These cytotoxic activities seemed to be positively correlated with GPC3 expression levels in the target cells. The survival of the mice bearing established orthotopic Huh-7 xenografts was significantly prolonged by the treatment with the third-generation GPC3-targeted CAR T cells. The cytotoxic activity of CAR T cell was also evaluated in three PDX models in vivo [29]. Glypican 3 (GPC3)-CAR T cells efficiently suppressed tumor growth in PDX3 and impressively eradicated tumor cells from PDX1 and PDX2, in which GPC3 proteins were highly expressed. AFP is not as sensitive or specific as GPC3 in HCC, and future directions are mostly geared to target GPC3 in the upcoming studies. Success of this approach partly depends on safer antigen selection, CAR sensitivity, and possibly combined antigen targeting.

Chemotherapy

Prior to the sorafenib era, cytotoxic systemic and hepatic arterial chemotherapies were the accepted therapeutic choices for advanced HCC. Anthracyclines, 5-FU, and platinum were widely studied agents, among which doxorubicin has been thought of as the most promising, yielding response rates of up to 20% and median survival of 4 months [30]. Interferons with immunomodulatory and antiproliferative effects on tumor cells have shown modest activity in HCC [31] which justified its combination to chemotherapy. Cisplatin, interferon, doxorubicin, and fluorouracil (PIAF) used in combination have shown promise in a phase II study with median overall survival (OS) of 5.9 months [32]. This led to the study of doxorubicin versus PIAF phase III trial in patients with unresectable HCC [33]; most patients were hepatitis B positive and have Child-Pugh score A cirrhosis. The overall response rates (ORR) were 10.5% (95% CI = 3.9–16.9%) in the doxorubicin group and 20.9% (95% CI = 12.5–29.2%) in the PIAF group ($p = 0.058$). The median survival was 6.83 months in the doxorubicin group and 8.67 months in the PIAF group. There was no difference in the HR of OS between treatment groups (HR = 0.97; 95% CI = 0.71–1.32). PIAF was associated with significantly higher myelotoxicity, and nearly 40% of the study population developed hepatitis that was attributed to HBV reactivation. FOLFOX was also studied extensively. A randomized open-label controlled trial was conducted in Asia to compare FOLFOX (5-FU and oxaliplatin) to doxorubicin [34], in patients who were ineligible for curative resection or local treatment. Median OS was 6.4 months with FOLFOX (95% CI, 5.30–7.03) and 4.97 months with doxorubicin (95% CI, 4.23–6.03; $p = 0.07$). Although the primary endpoint of OS was not met, a trend toward improved OS may suggest a benefit in this population. With the development of targeted therapy, namely, the multikinase inhibitor sorafenib, a rationale that sorafenib may help induce apoptosis and thus increase the cytotoxicity of chemotherapeutic agents led to the evaluation of the two in combination. Doxorubicin and sorafenib combination evaluated in a phase II trial [35] suggested a superiority to doxorubicin alone. When compared to sorafenib alone in a phase III randomized study, the combination resulted in higher toxicity and no improvement in OS or PFS [36].

Combination Local and Systemic Therapy

Several efforts are carried out to optimize efficacy of local and systemic approaches. Sometimes management depends on the approach of multidisciplinary specialists involved in the treatment of HCC. TACE causes increased hypoxia leading to an upregulation in hypoxia-inducible factor-1 (HIF-1), which in turn upregulates VEGF and PDGFR and increases tumor angiogenesis. This angiogenic surge leads to the contemplation that adding sorafenib therapy to TACE might improve outcomes [37]. In a phase II, open-label trial investigating the safety and efficacy of the combination of sorafenib and conventional TACE in patients from the Asia-Pacific region with intermediate HCC, 63.3% of patients achieved either partial response or stable disease [38]. A randomized trial did not show improvement in time to progression with TACE plus sorafenib vs TACE alone in intermediate-stage multifocal HCC with no extrahepatic disease [39]. TACE 2, another multicenter, randomized, phase III trial performed in the United Kingdom, also compared sorafenib added to DEB TACE versus placebo in 294 patients and showed no benefit in progression-free survival or overall survival [40]. We are waiting for the outcome of the same approach evaluated in the randomized study, ECOG 1208 (NCT01004978). Challenges to this approach include timing of antiangiogenic therapy and assessment of response and efficacy.

It is also thought that ablative therapies induce a peripheral immune response which may enhance the effect of immune modulating agents [41]. Tremelimumab has been studied in combination with radio-frequency ablation [42] with favorable safety profile and outcome. Six-week tumor biopsies showed a clear increase in $CD8^+$ T cells in patients showing a clinical benefit only. Multiple studies of combined immune checkpoint inhibition and ablative therapies are ongoing: nivolumab and TACE (NCT03143270), tremelimumab and durvalumab in combination with ablative therapies (TACE, radio-frequency ablation, and cryoablation) (NCT02821754), and a study of Y90 radio-embolization with nivolumab in the Asian population (NCT03033446).

References

1. Pugh RN, Murray-Lyon IM, Dawson JL, Pietroni MC, Williams R. Transection of the oesophagus for bleeding oesophageal varices. Br J Surg. 1973;60(8):646–9.
2. Zhu AX, Duda DG, Sahani DV, Jain RK. HCC and angiogenesis: possible targets and future directions. Nat Rev Clin Oncol. 2011;8(5):292–301.
3. Abou-Alfa GK, Schwartz L, Ricci S, Amadori D, Santoro A, Figer A, et al. Phase II study of sorafenib in patients with advanced hepatocellular carcinoma. J Clin Oncol. 2006;24(26):4293–300.
4. Llovet JM, Ricci S, Mazzaferro V, Hilgard P, Gane E, Blanc JF, et al. Sorafenib in advanced hepatocellular carcinoma. N Engl J Med. 2008;359(4):378–90.
5. Giambartolomei S, Covone F, Levrero M, Balsano C. Sustained activation of the Raf/MEK/Erk pathway in response to EGF in stable cell lines expressing the Hepatitis C Virus (HCV) core protein. Oncogene. 2001;20(20):2606–10.

6. Zhu AX, Sahani DV, Duda DG, di Tomaso E, Ancukiewicz M, Catalano OA, et al. Efficacy, safety, and potential biomarkers of sunitinib monotherapy in advanced hepatocellular carcinoma: a phase II study. J Clin Oncol. 2009;27(18):3027–35.
7. Cheng AL, Kang YK, Lin DY, Park JW, Kudo M, Qin S, et al. Sunitinib versus sorafenib in advanced hepatocellular cancer: results of a randomized phase III trial. J Clin Oncol. 2013;31(32):4067–75.
8. Llovet JM, Decaens T, Raoul JL, Boucher E, Kudo M, Chang C, et al. Brivanib in patients with advanced hepatocellular carcinoma who were intolerant to sorafenib or for whom sorafenib failed: results from the randomized phase III BRISK-PS study. J Clin Oncol. 2013;31(28):3509–16.
9. Ikeda K, Kudo M, Kawazoe S, Osaki Y, Ikeda M, Okusaka T, et al. Phase 2 study of lenvatinib in patients with advanced hepatocellular carcinoma. J Gastroenterol. 2017;52(4):512–9.
10. Ann-Lii Cheng RSF, Qin S, et al. Phase III trial of lenvatinib (LEN) vs sorafenib (SOR) in first-line treatment of patients (pts) with unresectable hepatocellular carcinoma (uHCC). J Clin Oncol. 2017;35(15 Suppl):abstr 4001.
11. Zhu AX, Park JO, Ryoo BY, Yen CJ, Poon R, Pastorelli D, et al. Ramucirumab versus placebo as second-line treatment in patients with advanced hepatocellular carcinoma following first-line therapy with sorafenib (REACH): a randomised, double-blind, multicentre, phase 3 trial. Lancet Oncol. 2015;16(7):859–70.
12. Yamashita T, Forgues M, Wang W, Kim JW, Ye Q, Jia H, et al. EpCAM and alpha-fetoprotein expression defines novel prognostic subtypes of hepatocellular carcinoma. Cancer Res. 2008;68(5):1451–61.
13. Bruix J, Qin S, Merle P, Granito A, Huang YH, Bodoky G, et al. Regorafenib for patients with hepatocellular carcinoma who progressed on sorafenib treatment (RESORCE): a randomised, double-blind, placebo-controlled, phase 3 trial. Lancet (London, England). 2017;389(10064):56–66.
14. Santoro A, Rimassa L, Borbath I, Daniele B, Salvagni S, Van Laethem JL, et al. Tivantinib for second-line treatment of advanced hepatocellular carcinoma: a randomised, placebo-controlled phase 2 study. Lancet Oncol. 2013;14(1):55–63.
15. Rimassa L, Assenat E, Peck-Radosavljevic M, Zagonel V, Pracht M, Caremoli ER, et al. Second-line tivantinib (ARQ 197) vs placebo in patients (Pts) with MET-high hepatocellular carcinoma (HCC): results of the METIV-HCC phase III trial. J Clin Oncol. 2017;35(15 Suppl):4000.
16. Kelley RK, Verslype C, Cohn AL, Yang TS, Su WC, Burris H, et al. Cabozantinib in hepatocellular carcinoma: results of a phase 2 placebo-controlled randomized discontinuation study. Ann Oncol. 2017;28(3):528–34.
17. Sangro B, Gomez-Martin C, de la Mata M, Inarrairaegui M, Garralda E, Barrera P, et al. A clinical trial of CTLA-4 blockade with tremelimumab in patients with hepatocellular carcinoma and chronic hepatitis C. J Hepatol. 2013;59(1):81–8.
18. El-Khoueiry AB, Sangro B, Yau T, Crocenzi TS, Kudo M, Hsu C, et al. Nivolumab in patients with advanced hepatocellular carcinoma (CheckMate 040): an open-label, non-comparative, phase 1/2 dose escalation and expansion trial. Lancet (London, England). 2017;389(10088):2492–502.
19. Melero I, Sangro B, Yau TC, Hsu C, Kudo M. Nivolumab dose escalation and expansion in patients with advanced hepatocellular carcinoma (HCC): the CheckMate 040 study. J Clin Oncol. 2017;35(Suppl 4S):abstract 226.
20. Park BH, Hwang T, Liu TC, Sze DY, Kim JS, Kwon HC, et al. Use of a targeted oncolytic poxvirus, JX-594, in patients with refractory primary or metastatic liver cancer: a phase I trial. Lancet Oncol. 2008;9(6):533–42.
21. Heo J, Reid T, Ruo L, Breitbach CJ, Rose S, Bloomston M, et al. Randomized dose-finding clinical trial of oncolytic immunotherapeutic vaccinia JX-594 in liver cancer. Nat Med. 2013;19(3):329–36.
22. Burke JM, Breitbach C, Patt RH, Lencioni R, Homerin M, Limacher J-M, et al. Phase IIb randomized trial of JX-594, a targeted multimechanistic oncolytic vaccinia virus, plus best supportive care (BSC) versus BSC alone in patients with advanced hepatocellular carcinoma who have failed sorafenib treatment (TRAVERSE). J Clin Oncol. 2012;30(15 Suppl):abstr TPS4152.
23. Heo J, Breitbach CJ, Moon A, Kim CW, Patt R, Kim MK, et al. Sequential therapy with JX-594, a targeted oncolytic poxvirus, followed by sorafenib in hepatocellular carcinoma: preclinical and clinical demonstration of combination efficacy. Mol Ther. 2011;19(6):1170–9.
24. Liu H, Xu Y, Xiang J, Long L, Green S, Yang Z, et al. Targeting alpha-fetoprotein (AFP)-MHC complex with CAR T-cell therapy for liver cancer. Clin Cancer Res. 2017;23(2):478–88.
25. Wang Z, Wu Z, Liu Y, Han W. New development in CAR-T cell therapy. J Hematol Oncol. 2017;10(1):53.
26. Zhu AX, Gold PJ, El-Khoueiry AB, Abrams TA, Morikawa H, Ohishi N, et al. First-in-man Phase I study of GC33, a novel recombinant humanized antibody against Glypican-3, in patients with advanced hepatocellular carcinoma. Clin Cancer Res. 2013;19(4):920–8.
27. Sawada Y, Yoshikawa T, Nobuoka D, Shirakawa H, Kuronuma T, Motomura Y, et al. Phase I trial of a Glypican-3–derived peptide vaccine for advanced hepatocellular carcinoma: immunologic evidence and potential for improving overall survival. Clin Cancer Res. 2012;18(13):3686–96.
28. Gao H, Li K, Tu H, Pan X, Jiang H, Shi B, et al. Development of T cells redirected to glypican-3 for the treatment of hepatocellular carcinoma. Clin Cancer Res. 2014;20(24):6418–28.

29. Jiang Z, Jiang X, Chen S, Lai Y, Wei X, Li B, et al. Anti-GPC3-CAR T cells suppress the growth of tumor cells in patient-derived xenografts of hepatocellular carcinoma. Front Immunol. 2016;7:690.
30. Hochster HS, Green MD, Speyer J, Fazzini E, Blum R, Muggia FM. 4′Epidoxorubicin (epirubicin): activity in hepatocellular carcinoma. J Clin Oncol. 1985;3(11):1535–40.
31. Lai CL, Lau JY, Wu PC, Ngan H, Chung HT, Mitchell SJ, et al. Recombinant interferon-alpha in inoperable hepatocellular carcinoma: a randomized controlled trial. Hepatology (Baltimore, MD). 1993;17(3):389–94.
32. Leung TW, Patt YZ, Lau WY, Ho SK, Yu SC, Chan AT, et al. Complete pathological remission is possible with systemic combination chemotherapy for inoperable hepatocellular carcinoma. Clin Cancer Res. 1999;5(7):1676–81.
33. Yeo W, Mok TS, Zee B, Leung TW, Lai PB, Lau WY, et al. A randomized phase III study of doxorubicin versus cisplatin/interferon alpha-2b/doxorubicin/fluorouracil (PIAF) combination chemotherapy for unresectable hepatocellular carcinoma. J Natl Cancer Inst. 2005;97(20):1532–8.
34. Qin S, Bai Y, Lim HY, Thongprasert S, Chao Y, Fan J, et al. Randomized, multicenter, open-label study of oxaliplatin plus fluorouracil/leucovorin versus doxorubicin as palliative chemotherapy in patients with advanced hepatocellular carcinoma from Asia. J Clin Oncol. 2013;31(28):3501–8.
35. Abou-Alfa GK, Johnson P, Knox JJ, Capanu M, Davidenko I, Lacava J, et al. Doxorubicin plus sorafenib vs doxorubicin alone in patients with advanced hepatocellular carcinoma: a randomized trial. JAMA. 2010;304(19):2154–60.
36. Abou-Alfa GK. Phase III randomized study of sorafenib plus doxorubicin versus sorafenib in patients with advanced hepatocellular carcinoma (HCC): CALGB 80802 (Alliance). J Clin Oncol. 2016;34(Suppl 4S):abstr 192.
37. Abou-Alfa GK. TACE and sorafenib: a good marriage? J Clin Oncol. 2011;29(30):3949–52.
38. Chung YH, Han G, Yoon JH, Yang J, Wang J, Shao GL, et al. Interim analysis of START: study in Asia of the combination of TACE (transcatheter arterial chemoembolization) with sorafenib in patients with hepatocellular carcinoma trial. Int J Cancer. 2013;132(10):2448–58.
39. Lencioni R, Llovet JM, Han G, Tak WY, Yang J, Guglielmi A, et al. Sorafenib or placebo plus TACE with doxorubicin-eluting beads for intermediate stage HCC: the SPACE trial. J Hepatol. 2016;64(5):1090–8.
40. Meyer T, Fox R, Ma YT, Ross PJ, James MW, Sturgess R, et al. Sorafenib in combination with transarterial chemoembolisation in patients with unresectable hepatocellular carcinoma (TACE 2): a randomised placebo-controlled, double-blind, phase 3 trial. Lancet Gastroenterol Hepatol. 2017;2(8):565–75.
41. Waitz R, Solomon SB, Petre EN, Trumble AE, Fasso M, Norton L, et al. Potent induction of tumor immunity by combining tumor cryoablation with anti-CTLA-4 therapy. Cancer Res. 2012;72(2):430–9.
42. Duffy AG, Ulahannan SV, Makorova-Rusher O, Rahma O, Wedemeyer H, Pratt D, et al. Tremelimumab in combination with ablation in patients with advanced hepatocellular carcinoma. J Hepatol. 2017;66(3):545–51.

Guidelines for Resection of Intrahepatic Cholangiocarcinoma

Richard Tang, Nicholas Latchana, Amir A. Rahnemai-Azar, and Timothy M. Pawlik

Introduction

Cholangiocarcinoma (CCA) is a neoplasm of the biliary tract epithelium and is commonly categorized according to anatomic location into intrahepatic (ICC), perihilar, and extrahepatic subtypes (Fig. 8.1). The distinction is important as each variant differs in clinical presentation, as well as diagnostic and prognostic attributes. ICC is the least common subtype and arises from malignant proliferation of epithelial cells located proximal to the second-degree bile ducts. ICC is also the second most common primary liver neoplasm after hepatocellular carcinoma (HCC) and accounts for 15% of primary hepatic tumors [1]. The incidence and mortality of ICC continues to rise in the United States [2].

Most cases are not detected prior to the onset of symptoms, which usually manifest in the seventh decade of life [3]. Unfortunately, the majority of patients present at advanced stages when the tumor has already metastasized or progressed locally to involve adjacent vital structures [4, 5]. Hepatitis B, hepatitis C, cirrhosis, choledochal cysts, hepatolithiasis, hepatic flukes (*Clonorchis sinensis*, *Opisthorchis viverrini*), primary sclerosing cholangitis, obesity, and alcohol and nitrosamine ingestion are some of the known risk factors for the development of ICC [6, 7].

Surgical resection with negative microscopic margins (R0 resection) remains the mainstay of curative therapy. The 5-year overall survival (OS) of patients following surgical resection is dependent on several factors and usually varies from 11 to 40% [8–12]. Unfortunately, only 30–40% of patients with ICC (stages 1 and 2) are amenable to surgical resection at the time of diagnosis [4, 6, 13]. Unresectable lesions have a poor prognosis with a median survival of 7–12 months and a 3-year OS of 3% [14, 15].

Herein, we will review the current management of ICC while highlighting the role of surgery.

Clinical Presentation

ICC is diagnosed incidentally in 19–43% of cases; patients usually only develop nonspecific symptoms at advanced stages of the disease [16, 17]. Biliary obstruction is the most frequent presentation; however, patients can also manifest with unexplained weight loss, malaise, abdominal discomfort, palpable abdominal

R. Tang · N. Latchana · T. M. Pawlik (✉)
Department of Surgery, The Ohio State University Wexner Medical Center, Columbus, OH, USA
e-mail: Tim.Pawlik@osumc.edu

A. A. Rahnemai-Azar
Department of Surgery, University of Washington Medical Center, Seattle, WA, USA

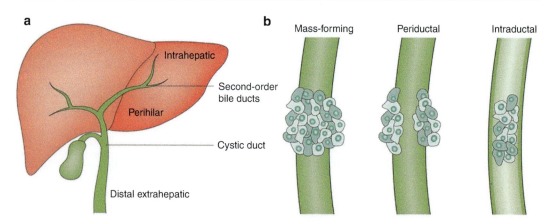

Fig. 8.1 Classification of cholangiocarcinoma. (**a**) CCAs are classified according to the anatomical location into intrahepatic (ICC), perihilar, and extrahepatic subtypes. (**b**) Three different pathologic patterns of ICC growth

mass, and hepatomegaly. The diagnosis of ICC is usually made based upon a combination of clinical, laboratory, and radiologic data (Fig. 8.2) [4, 18].

Imaging

Dynamic cross-sectional imaging is essential for characterizing intrahepatic masses and preoperative planning. Computed tomography (CT) and magnetic resonance imaging (MRI) can help in distinguishing ICC from HCC. On CT scan, ICC appears as a hypodense mass in the unenhanced phase with progressive and heterogeneous enhancement on arterial, venous, and delayed phases [4, 19]. In contrast, homogeneous arterial phase enhancement followed by portal venous and delayed phase washout is more characteristic of HCC (Fig. 8.3) [20]. Less specific radiological features of ICC include homogeneous low-attenuation masses with irregular peripheral enhancement, lobulated morphology, hepatic capsular retraction, local vascular invasion, and proximal biliary dilation [21]. On MRI, ICC is typically hypointense on T1-weighted and hyperintense on T2-weighted images [22]. Similar to CT scan, peripheral enhancement followed by progressive concentric filling of the tumor with contrast in the arterial and delayed phases of contrast-enhanced MRI is suggestive of ICC.

Ultrasonography (US) may also identify, localize, and determine the extent of intrahepatic masses while ruling out other etiologies. On US, ICC typically appears as a hypoechoic mass that may be associated with intrahepatic ductal dilatation. However, these features are not specific to ICC [23]. The role of fluorodeoxyglucose (FDG)-positron emission tomography (FDG-PET) in the evaluation of ICC remains controversial. FDG-PET with CT has a sensitivity and specificity up to 95% and 83% in detecting ICC, respectively [24]. However, the sensitivity of FDG-PET is not superior to CT or MRI for detecting primary tumors as increased FDG avidity can also be seen in other intrahepatic malignancies or inflammatory/infectious processes. Notably, the diagnostic yield of PET scan is higher for mass-forming ICC than infiltrating tumors. Also, FDG-PET has a sensitivity and specificity of 80% and 92% for detecting lymph node metastases (LNM) [24].

Biomarkers

Currently tumor markers have a very limited role in the diagnosis of ICC. Although CA 19-9 is the most commonly used tumor biomarker, it only has a modest accuracy in distinguishing ICC from HCC with a sensitivity of 62% and specificity of 63% [25]. Notably, patients with unresectable ICC tend to have higher CA 19-9 levels compared with patients who have resect-

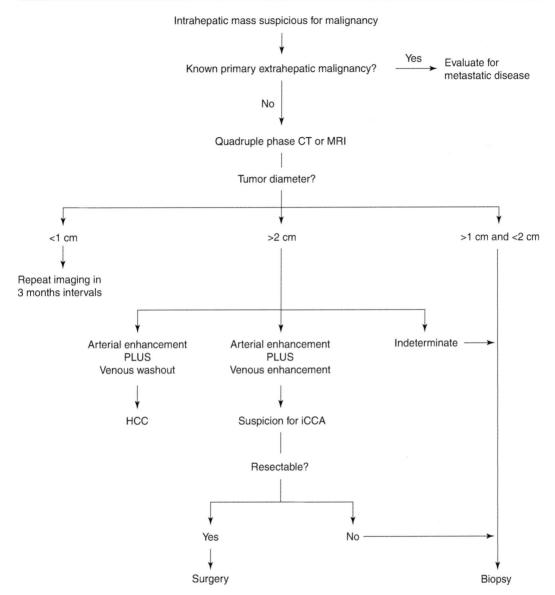

Fig. 8.2 Algorithm for diagnostic evaluation of intrahepatic cholangiocarcinoma. (Adapted from Blechacz et al. "Cholangiocarcinoma: Current Knowledge and New Developments." "Copyright © 2017 by The Korean Society of Gastroenterology, the Korean Society of Gastrointestinal Endoscopy, the Korean Society of Neurogastroenterology and Motility, Korean College of Helicobacter and Upper Gastrointestinal Research, Korean Association the Study of Intestinal Diseases, the Korean Association for the Study of the Liver, Korean Pancreatobiliary Association, and Korean Society of Gastrointestinal Cancer. This is an Open Access article distributed under the terms of the Creative Commons Attribution Non-Commercial License (http://creativecommons.org/licenses/by-nc/4.0) which permits unrestricted non-commercial use, distribution, and reproduction in any medium, provided the original work is properly cited")

able disease [25]. CA 19-9 elevation is also associated with other gastrointestinal and gynecologic malignancies as well as benign biliary diseases, further limiting its application as an ICC-specific biomarker. Therefore, the majority of studies examining CA 19-9 as a biomarker for the detection of CCA have noted suboptimal accuracy, with wide variation of reported sensitivity (38–93%) and specificity (67–98%) [26–28].

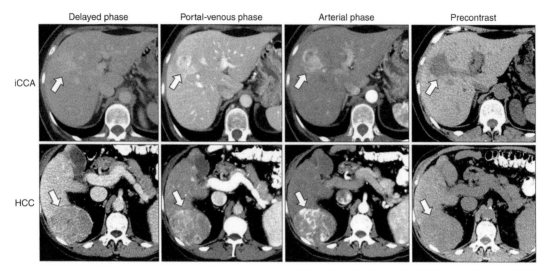

Fig. 8.3 Hepatocellular versus intrahepatic cholangiocarcinoma on dynamic CT imaging. Adapted with permission from Blechaz, et al. Images courtesy of Dr. Janio Szklaruk, MD Anderson Cancer Center, Houston, TX, USA

Carcinoembryonic antigen (CEA), an effective marker for colorectal cancer, has a low diagnostic yield in ICC. Recent advances have elucidated molecular and genetic characteristics of ICC and offer the potential for molecular-based diagnosis. However, the clinical applicability of most existing markers such as mucins, 14-3-3 protein, and serum cytokeratin 19 fragments (CYFRA 21-1) is limited due to a lack of adequate sensitivity and specificity [29–32].

Pathology

If clinical presentation, laboratory analyses, and imaging modalities are inconclusive or yield contradictory results, tissue biopsy can be performed to confirm the diagnosis. The pathologic confirmation is not routinely recommended for lesions that appear resectable based on preoperative investigations [4, 6]. Tissue diagnosis is, however, necessary before starting systemic chemo- or radiotherapies.

ICC needs to be distinguished from benign lesions, such as peribiliary glands, reactive ductular proliferation, biliary microhamartomas, and bile duct adenomas [33]. The most common histologic features of ICC are adenocarcinoma with tubular and/or papillary structures with variable fibrous stroma [34]. ICC cannot be readily differentiated from metastatic adenocarcinoma of extrahepatic primary tumors based on histopathology alone and requires further immunohistochemical evaluation. ICCs are predominantly mass-forming lesions, whereas perihilar cholangiocarcinomas typically have periductal-infiltrating morphologic patterns.

Staging

The seventh edition of the American Joint Committee on Cancer/Union for International Cancer Control (AJCC/UICC) staging system, which was published in 2010, introduced a distinct ICC TNM classification in recognition of biologic behavior and prognostic differences between ICC and HCC (Table 8.1) [35]. Using the seventh edition as a baseline, multi-institutional studies have subsequently refined the staging system and have proposed several changes. For instance, in stage 2b (patients with multiple tumors), it is clinically difficult to distinguish multifocal disease from tumors with intrahepatic metastases or satellite lesions [4, 6]. In addition, a study by Hyder et al. demonstrated that tumor size is an important factor with nonlinear threshold effect on postsurgical ICC outcome [8].

Table 8.1 Staging of intrahepatic cholangiocarcinoma

Primary tumor (T)			
TX	Primary tumor cannot be assessed		
T0	No evidence of primary tumor		
Tis	Carcinoma in situ (intraductal tumor)		
TI	Solitary tumor without vascular invasion		
T2a	Solitary tumor with vascular invasion		
T2b	Multiple tumors, with or without vascular invasion		
T3	Tumor perforating the visceral peritoneum or involving the local extra hepatic structures by direct invasion		
T4	Tumor with periductal invasion		
Regional lymph nodes (N)			
NX	Regional lymph nodes cannot be assessed		
N0	No regional lymph node metastasis		
N1	Regional lymph node metastasis present		
Distant metastasis (M)			
M0	No distant metastasis		
M1	Distant metastasis present		
Stage grouping			
Stage 0	Tis	N0	M0
Stage I	TI	N0	M0
Stage II	T2	N0	M0
Stage III	T3	N0	M0
Stage IVA	T4	N0	M0
	Any T	N1	M0
Stage IVB	Any T	Any N	M1

Adapted with permission from Eckel et al.

The eighth edition, published in late 2016, took some of these refinements into account, and several changes were made to ICC staging in the eighth edition. Specifically, in the eighth edition staging, the T1 category was revised to account for the prognostic impact of tumor size (T1a $\leq$ 5 cm vs. T1b > 5 cm). Regional lymph node metastases in the hilar, peri-duodenal, and peripancreatic nodes are considered N1 disease, whereas distant lymphatic involvement of celiac, periaortic, or caval nodes is considered M1 disease.

Biliary Decompression

The role of preoperative biliary drainage remains controversial, and the current data is mainly limited to the experience derived from the management of perihilar cholangiocarcinoma. Biliary drainage is indicated in septic patients with suspected cholangitis and may also help to improve their hepatic function (e.g., coagulopathy, renal failure) and relieve symptoms (e.g., pruritus) [36]. Proponents of preoperative biliary drainage claim improved hepatic function, optimization of nutritional parameters, and reduction of cholangitis and postoperative liver failure as advantages of this strategy. However, in a recent multicenter retrospective study, preoperative biliary drainage was not associated with improved postoperative outcomes [37]. In contrast, opponents believe that biliary drainage increases the risk of tumor seeding (with transabdominal drain placement), cholangitis, pancreatitis, and perioperative infection and may also lengthen postoperative hospital stay [38, 39].

Due to a reported 1.4–5% risk of tumor seeding of the drain track with percutaneous biliary drainage, endoscopic retrograde cholangiopancreatography (ERCP) is widely advocated as the preferred choice [40, 41]. However, endoscopic stent occlusion rate has been reported to be as high as 60%. Furthermore, unsuccessful attempts with endoscopic decompression place patients at risk for contamination of undrained areas (due to retrograde injection of contrast) and cause delays in treatment [42]. Several groups are investigating the utility of alternate preoperative drainage methods such as nasobiliary drainage. Overall, data is sparse for biliary drainage in the setting of ICC and remains at the discretion of the clinician based on the clinical condition of the patient.

Indications for Resection

Resection should be considered in patients with disease who have potentially resectable tumors and adequate performance status (Fig. 8.4). Resectable tumors are defined as lesions that can be completely removed with negative histologic margins (R0) and leave sufficient liver remnant. Preoperative cross-sectional imaging using contrast-enhanced multi-detector CT (MDCT scan) and/or magnetic resonance imaging/magnetic resonance cholangiopancreatography (MRI/ MRCP) plays a key role in the assessment of tumor resectability [4, 6].

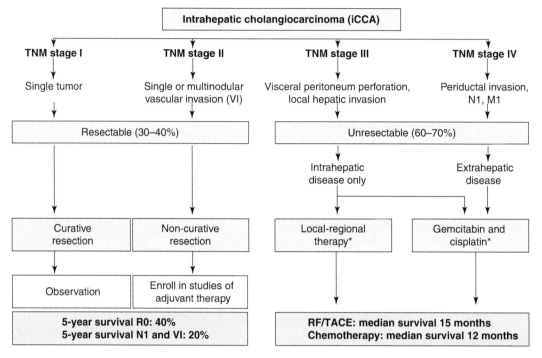

Fig. 8.4 Algorithm for management of intrahepatic cholangiocarcinoma. Adapted with permission from Bridgewater et al.

Evidence of extrahepatic disease, including involvement of other organs or distant LNs (i.e., celiac and the para-aortic nodes), is a contraindication to resection. Bilateral, multifocal, and multicentric diseases are also considered as relative contraindications for surgical resection [4, 35, 43]. Multifocal/multicentric tumors are detected in up to 44% of patients and reported to be associated with worse survival [13, 44]. This may be in part attributed to the presence of occult metastatic dissemination. There are no data to address the prognostic relevance of true peri-tumoral satellite lesions versus multifocal disease.

An adequate future liver remnant (FLR) includes a minimum of two contiguous segments with adequate inflow, outflow, and biliary drainage. A patient with a normal underlying liver requires at least a 20% FLR to prevent postoperative liver failure. The percentage increases to 30% for patients who had steatosis or steatohepatitis and to 40% in patients with underlying cirrhosis [45, 46]. Patients with ICC who do not meet FLR requirements may benefit from additional preoperative procedures to induce hypertrophy of the FLR such as portal vein embolization or even associating liver partition and portal vein ligation for staged hepatectomy (ALPPS) [43, 47, 48].

The rate of achieving R0 resection can be as high as 85% with an aggressive surgical approach that often involves a major or extended hepatectomy combined with concurrent bile duct or vascular resection [4, 49]. However, due to delayed diagnosis, only 30–40% of patients with ICC are amenable to surgical resection at the time of diagnosis [4, 6]. In part, because of the technical complexity of an R0 resection in some cases, only a subset of patients who could benefit from surgery are even offered resection. For example, in one study, only 91 of 248 patients (37%) with localized potentially resectable disease underwent surgery [50].

Orthotopic liver transplantation (OLT) has a very limited role in management of patients with ICC. The reported survival of patients with ICC following OLT is markedly less than cirrhotic patients undergoing transplantation [51,

52]. Recently, an international multicentric cohort study reported outcomes for OLT in cirrhotic patients noted to have very early, incidental ICC (single tumor ≤2 cm). In this study, the reported 5-year actuarial survival and incidence of recurrence among 15 patients with very early ICC (total of 48 patients with ICC) were 65% and 18%, respectively [53]. OLT is not considered a standard therapy for ICC at this time and should only be offered to highly selected patients and in expert centers using designed clinical protocols.

Staging Laparoscopy

The role of routine staging laparoscopy in the surgical management of ICC is still controversial, with a diagnostic yield ranging from 27% to 38% [54, 55]. Staging laparoscopy is generally recommended in patients at high risk for occult metastatic disease, including those with multicentric disease, high preoperative serum CA 19-9 levels, potential vascular invasion, and suspicion of peritoneal disease spread [4, 6, 56]. Selective use of laparoscopic ultrasonography can further increase the yield of diagnostic laparoscopy in selected patients as intrahepatic metastases or extensive vascular invasion might be detected sonographically.

Neoadjuvant Therapy

There is very limited evidence regarding the use of neoadjuvant therapy prior to surgical resection for cholangiocarcinoma. A small case series demonstrated increased surgical resectability for extrahepatic cholangiocarcinoma following neoadjuvant chemoradiation [57]. Likewise, the application of neoadjuvant therapy in ICC patients is limited to a few series that reported conversion of the large, locally advanced unresectable tumors to potentially resectable lesions [50, 58]. Therefore, neoadjuvant therapy has insufficient evidence to support a therapeutic benefit in the setting of ICC and cannot be recommended for routine use.

Adjuvant Therapy

Due to rarity of the tumor, the data on adjuvant therapy for ICC are mainly derived from studies that examine a broad category of patients with advanced biliary tract cancers. Bektas et al. in a single center experience of 221 patients with ICC demonstrated that adjuvant chemotherapy did not improve patient survival ($P = 0.55$) [14]. Similarly, in a systematic review of 57 ICC-specific studies (4756 patients), the application of adjuvant chemotherapy and/or radiotherapy was not associated with any improvement in recurrence-free survival (RFS) or overall survival (OS) [59].

Takada et al. evaluated the role of postoperative chemotherapy with 5-FU, doxorubicin, and mitomycin in 508 patients with resected pancreatobiliary malignancy and failed to show any statistically significant survival benefit. The same results were achieved when the data were stratified to include only 118 patients with bile duct cancer (5-year survival rate of 26.7% in treatment group vs. 24.1% in control group; $p = NS$) [60]. In an international European trial (ESPAC)-3, the use of adjuvant therapy was not associated with a survival advantage in all patients with periampullary malignancies or in the subset of patients with bile duct cancer [61]. However, a meta-analysis of data of 6712 patients with biliary tract cancer who underwent curative-intent surgery revealed that chemo- and chemoradiotherapy are associated with better survival than radiation therapy alone ($p = 0.02$) [62].

The major limitation of these studies included the broad categories of patients with biliary tract cancers. Recently, several ICC-focused studies have demonstrated a survival benefit of adjuvant therapy in patients who had positive LNs and/or margins. Patients with R1 resection (resection with positive microscopic margins) conclude that almost 14% of ICC patients who underwent curative-intent surgery and had a worse 5-year survival (13% vs. 49% in R0 resection group; $p = 0.01$) [63]. McNamara et al. evaluated 296 patients with biliary tumors (17% ICC) and noted that adjuvant chemotherapy alone or chemoradiation for patients with R1 resection was associated with improved DFS (13.8 vs. 10.4 months in a group without therapy, $p = 0.07$) and OS (37.7 vs. 21 months in a group without therapy, $p = 0.01$) [64]. Notably, there was no DFS or OS benefit in individuals with R0 resection following adjuvant therapy. Patients with node-positive disease have also been suggested to potentially benefit from adjuvant therapy. Approximately 27–47% of patients with ICC are found to have a node-positive disease following surgical intervention with a 5-year OS of 0–30% [13, 63]. The number of involved LNs is an important prognostic factor, and patients with more than three positive LNs have a worse prognosis [65]. In a study of 90 patients with resected ICC and concurrent regional LNM, Jiang et al. showed that adjuvant external beam radiation was associated with improved survival (19.5 vs. 9.5 months; $p = 0.01$) [66]. Similarly, National Cancer Database (NCDB) analysis of 2751 patients with ICC demonstrated a significant OS benefit for chemotherapy in patients with N1 disease (19.8 vs. 10.7 months in patients who did not receive adjuvant therapy; $p < 0.001$) [67]. These results were further validated by another NCDB study that noted an association of adjuvant therapy with improved survival among patients with positive nodes or margins [68].

Currently, until the outcomes of ongoing studies (e.g., BILACP, PRODIGE-12, ACTICCA, ASCOT, BCAT) that are investigating the efficacy of adjuvant therapy in biliary neoplasms become available, enrollment in clinical trials remains the best approach. Adjuvant therapy is usually recommended for the management of patients with positive surgical margins (R1 or R2 resection), LNM, or patients predicted to have a high risk of recurrence based on preoperative work-up (e.g., vascular invasion, large tumors, multicentricity) [4, 5]. Therefore, regional lymphadenectomy is strongly suggested in addition to hepatectomy due to the strong prognostic value of LN involvement and its potential role in assigning high-risk patients for adjuvant therapy.

Outcome and Recurrence

Reported 5-year OS after surgical resection of ICC ranges between 11 and 40% and is dependent on several factors [4, 8, 9]. Unfortunately, even after R0 resection, disease recurrence is high, with some series reporting 60% and 80% recurrence at median follow-up of 21 months and 5 years, respectively [69, 70]. Tumor recurrence is the leading cause of death in ICC patients who underwent surgical resection. The liver is the most common location of tumor recurrence (64%). However, extrahepatic recurrence to the lymphatic basins, peritoneum, and lung is not uncommon [70–73]. Multiple tumors, LN metastasis, large tumor size (>5 cm), high-grade histology, and vascular invasion were defined as independent factors of tumor recurrence.

Limited data exist on the treatment of recurrent disease after primary resection of ICC. Several series reported successful resection of recurrent lesions in 8.5–30% of patients [74–76]. Similar to resection of primary ICC, the application of surgical therapy is considered according to the feasibility of R0 resection and the status of FLR. In recent years, emerging modalities such as radiofrequency ablation (RFA), transarterial chemoembolization (TACE), and transarterial radioembolization (TARE) using yttrium-90 (Y-90) tagged glass or resin microspheres have been reported to be effective and safe in the treatment of recurrent ICC. Kim et al. reported a median OS of 27.4 months in 20 patients with recurrent ICC who underwent RFA [77]. In another study, Sulpice et al. demonstrated a survival benefit of TARE with Y-90 in management of intrahepatic recurrent lesions [78].

Overall, chemotherapy and RFA remain the mainstay of therapy for individuals with recurrent ICC. Surgery is considered only in minority of patients with resectable recurrent disease. While comparative outcomes of different approaches are still unknown, strategies combining resection and ablation are gaining popularity.

Management of Locally Advanced or Metastatic Disease

Several locoregional treatment strategies including hepatic artery-based therapies, radiation therapy, and ablation can be considered in the management of locally advanced inoperable

ICC. A recent meta-analysis of 657 patients with inoperable ICC showed that transarterial chemoinfusion (TACI) offered reasonable outcomes in terms of tumor response and OS (22.8 months in TACI vs. 13.9, 12.4, and 12.3 months in Y90, TACE, and drug-eluting TACE, respectively), but therapy was limited due to toxicity [79].

Thermal ablation is another potential modality to treat small (<3 cm) locally advanced unresectable ICC [80, 81]. Future randomized clinical trials are required to establish first-line locoregional treatment options in patients with unresectable ICC and investigate the value of these therapies in comparison and in combination with systemic therapies.

Likewise, there is still no definitive consensus regarding the standard chemotherapy regimen to treat patients with ICC. Overall, the combination of gemcitabine plus cisplatin (or oxaliplatin as a potentially better-tolerated agent) has been recommended as first-line chemotherapy by several investigators [4, 5, 82]. Valle et al. in a phase 3 trial (ABC-02) of 410 patients with locally advanced biliary tract cancers (58% CCA) demonstrated that gemcitabine plus cisplatin was associated with a survival advantage over the gemcitabine alone group (11.7 months vs. 8.1 months, respectively; $p < 0.001$) without additional toxicity [82]. The PFS also was better (combination therapy group median 8.0 months vs. gemcitabine-only arm median 5.0 months) ($p < 0.001$). Similarly, Okusaka et al. in a randomized trial of 84 Japanese patients with advanced BTC (33% ICC) reported the advantage of gemcitabine plus cisplatin combination therapy over gemcitabine alone regimen [83]. Other ongoing trials are currently investigating the clinical efficacy of different chemotherapy regimens like gemcitabine plus S-1 compared with current standard therapy.

Considering the limited benefit of conventional chemotherapy in the management of unresectable or metastatic ICC, identifying ICC-specific biomarkers will assist in guiding emerging molecular-targeted therapies and personalized medicine. For example, ponatinib (nonselective pan-FGFR inhibitor), everolimus (mTOR inhibitor), and selumetinib (MEK1/MEK2 inhibitor) have shown promising results in early trials [84–86]. More studies are being conducted to investigate the efficacy of other targeted therapies (ClinicalTrials.gov identifier: NCT02053376, NCT02272998, NCT02318329, NCT02381886, NCT01915498).

> **Conclusion**
>
> ICC is a rare malignancy with an increasing incidence and a high case fatality. Although R0 resection offers the only potential for cure in ICC patients, prognosis remains relatively poor with a high disease recurrence. Furthermore, many patients are not surgical candidates because of the delayed diagnosis. While evidence to support the use of neoadjuvant therapy prior to surgical resection does not exist, adjuvant therapy is recommended in individuals with non-R0 resection and N1 disease. For inoperable tumors, current standard first-line chemotherapy (gemcitabine plus cisplatin) is associated with a survival of less than a year. New advances in genomic profiling have contributed to a better understanding of the landscape of molecular alterations in ICC and offer hope for the development of novel targeted therapies.

References

1. Eckel F, Brunner T, Jelic S, Group EGW. Biliary cancer: ESMO clinical practice guidelines for diagnosis, treatment and follow-up. Ann Oncol. 2010;21(Suppl 5):v65–9.
2. Saha SK, Zhu AX, Fuchs CS, Brooks GA. Forty-year trends in cholangiocarcinoma incidence in the U.S.: intrahepatic disease on the rise. Oncologist. 2016;21(5):594–9.
3. Aljiffry M, Abdulelah A, Walsh M, Peltekian K, Alwayn I, Molinari M. Evidence-based approach to cholangiocarcinoma: a systematic review of the current literature. J Am Coll Surg. 2009;208(1):134–47.
4. Weber SM, Ribero D, O'Reilly EM, Kokudo N, Miyazaki M, Pawlik TM. Intrahepatic cholangiocarcinoma: expert consensus statement. HPB (Oxford). 2015;17(8):669–80.
5. Banales JM, Cardinale V, Carpino G, Marzioni M, Andersen JB, Invernizzi P, et al. Expert consensus document: cholangiocarcinoma: current knowledge and future perspectives consensus statement from the European network for the study of cholangiocarcinoma (ENS-CCA). Nat Rev Gastroenterol Hepatol. 2016;13(5):261–80.

6. Bridgewater J, Galle PR, Khan SA, Llovet JM, Park JW, Patel T, et al. Guidelines for the diagnosis and management of intrahepatic cholangiocarcinoma. J Hepatol. 2014;60(6):1268–89.
7. Lang H, Sotiropoulos GC, Fruhauf NR, Domland M, Paul A, Kind EM, et al. Extended hepatectomy for intrahepatic cholangiocellular carcinoma (ICC): when is it worthwhile? Single center experience with 27 resections in 50 patients over a 5-year period. Ann Surg. 2005;241(1):134–43.
8. Hyder O, Marques H, Pulitano C, Marsh JW, Alexandrescu S, Bauer TW, et al. A nomogram to predict long-term survival after resection for intrahepatic cholangiocarcinoma: an eastern and western experience. JAMA Surg. 2014;149(5):432–8.
9. Nathan H, Pawlik TM, Wolfgang CL, Choti MA, Cameron JL, Schulick RD. Trends in survival after surgery for cholangiocarcinoma: a 30-year population-based SEER database analysis. J Gastrointest Surg. 2007;11(11):1488–96; discussion 96–7.
10. Shimada K, Sano T, Nara S, Esaki M, Sakamoto Y, Kosuge T, et al. Therapeutic value of lymph node dissection during hepatectomy in patients with intrahepatic cholangiocellular carcinoma with negative lymph node involvement. Surgery. 2009;145(4):411–6.
11. Nakagohri T, Kinoshita T, Konishi M, Takahashi S, Gotohda N. Surgical outcome and prognostic factors in intrahepatic cholangiocarcinoma. World J Surg. 2008;32(12):2675–80.
12. Uenishi T, Kubo S, Yamazaki O, Yamada T, Sasaki Y, Nagano H, et al. Indications for surgical treatment of intrahepatic cholangiocarcinoma with lymph node metastases. J Hepato-Biliary-Pancreat Surg. 2008;15(4):417–22.
13. Ruzzenente A, Conci S, Valdegamberi A, Pedrazzani C, Guglielmi A. Role of surgery in the treatment of intrahepatic cholangiocarcinoma. Eur Rev Med Pharmacol Sci. 2015;19(15):2892–900.
14. Bektas H, Yeyrek C, Kleine M, Vondran FW, Timrott K, Schweitzer N, et al. Surgical treatment for intrahepatic cholangiocarcinoma in Europe: a single center experience. J Hepatobiliary Pancreat Sci. 2015;22(2):131–7.
15. Tao R, Krishnan S, Bhosale PR, Javle MM, Aloia TA, Shroff RT, et al. Ablative radiotherapy doses lead to a substantial prolongation of survival in patients with inoperable intrahepatic cholangiocarcinoma: a retrospective dose response analysis. J Clin Oncol. 2016;34(3):219–26.
16. Weber SM, Jarnagin WR, Klimstra D, DeMatteo RP, Fong Y, Blumgart LH. Intrahepatic cholangiocarcinoma: resectability, recurrence pattern, and outcomes. J Am Coll Surg. 2001;193(4):384–91.
17. Morimoto Y, Tanaka Y, Ito T, Nakahara M, Nakaba H, Nishida T, et al. Long-term survival and prognostic factors in the surgical treatment for intrahepatic cholangiocarcinoma. J Hepato-Biliary-Pancreat Surg. 2003;10(6):432–40.
18. Blechacz B. Cholangiocarcinoma: current knowledge and new developments. Gut Liver. 2017;11(1):13–26.
19. Valls C, Guma A, Puig I, Sanchez A, Andia E, Serrano T, et al. Intrahepatic peripheral cholangiocarcinoma: CT evaluation. Abdom Imaging. 2000;25(5):490–6.
20. Rimola J, Forner A, Reig M, Vilana R, de Lope CR, Ayuso C, et al. Cholangiocarcinoma in cirrhosis: absence of contrast washout in delayed phases by magnetic resonance imaging avoids misdiagnosis of hepatocellular carcinoma. Hepatology. 2009;50(3):791–8.
21. Han JK, Choi BI, Kim AY, An SK, Lee JW, Kim TK, et al. Cholangiocarcinoma: pictorial essay of CT and cholangiographic findings. Radiographics. 2002;22(1):173–87.
22. Miller G, Schwartz LH, D'Angelica M. The use of imaging in the diagnosis and staging of hepatobiliary malignancies. Surg Oncol Clin N Am. 2007;16(2):343–68.
23. Galassi M, Iavarone M, Rossi S, Bota S, Vavassori S, Rosa L, et al. Patterns of appearance and risk of misdiagnosis of intrahepatic cholangiocarcinoma in cirrhosis at contrast enhanced ultrasound. Liver Int. 2013;33(5):771–9.
24. Annunziata S, Caldarella C, Pizzuto DA, Galiandro F, Sadeghi R, Giovanella L, et al. Diagnostic accuracy of fluorine-18-fluorodeoxyglucose positron emission tomography in the evaluation of the primary tumor in patients with cholangiocarcinoma: a meta-analysis. Biomed Res Int. 2014;2014:247693.
25. Patel AH, Harnois DM, Klee GG, LaRusso NF, Gores GJ. The utility of CA 19-9 in the diagnoses of cholangiocarcinoma in patients without primary sclerosing cholangitis. Am J Gastroenterol. 2000;95(1):204–7.
26. Charatcharoenwitthaya P, Enders FB, Halling KC, Lindor KD. Utility of serum tumor markers, imaging, and biliary cytology for detecting cholangiocarcinoma in primary sclerosing cholangitis. Hepatology. 2008;48(4):1106–17.
27. Singh S, Tang SJ, Sreenarasimhaiah J, Lara LF, Siddiqui A. The clinical utility and limitations of serum carbohydrate antigen (CA19-9) as a diagnostic tool for pancreatic cancer and cholangiocarcinoma. Dig Dis Sci. 2011;56(8):2491–6.
28. Leelawat K, Narong S, Wannaprasert J, Ratanashu-ek T. Prospective study of MMP7 serum levels in the diagnosis of cholangiocarcinoma. World J Gastroenterol. 2010;16(37):4697–703.
29. Wongkham S, Silsirivanit A. State of serum markers for detection of cholangiocarcinoma. Asian Pac J Cancer Prev. 2012;13 Suppl:17–27.
30. Uenishi T, Yamazaki O, Tanaka H, Takemura S, Yamamoto T, Tanaka S, et al. Serum cytokeratin 19 fragment (CYFRA21-1) as a prognostic factor in intrahepatic cholangiocarcinoma. Ann Surg Oncol. 2008;15(2):583–9.
31. Lumachi F, Lo Re G, Tozzoli R, D'Aurizio F, Facomer F, Chiara GB, et al. Measurement of serum carcinoembryonic antigen, carbohydrate antigen 19-9, cytokeratin-19 fragment and matrix metalloproteinase-7 for detecting cholangiocarcinoma: a preliminary case-control study. Anticancer Res. 2014;34(11):6663–7.

32. Kashihara T, Ohki A, Kobayashi T, Sato T, Nishizawa H, Ogawa K, et al. Intrahepatic cholangiocarcinoma with increased serum CYFRA 21-1 level. J Gastroenterol. 1998;33(3):447–53.
33. Goodman ZD. Neoplasms of the liver. Mod Pathol. 2007;20(Suppl 1):S49–60.
34. Nakanuma Y, Sato Y, Harada K, Sasaki M, Xu J, Ikeda H. Pathological classification of intrahepatic cholangiocarcinoma based on a new concept. World J Hepatol. 2010;2(12):419–27.
35. Edge SB, Compton CC. The American Joint Committee on Cancer: the 7th edition of the AJCC cancer staging manual and the future of TNM. Ann Surg Oncol. 2010;17(6):1471–4.
36. Sarmiento JM, Nagorney DM. Hepatic resection in the treatment of perihilar cholangiocarcinoma. Surg Oncol Clin N Am. 2002;11(4):893–908, viii–ix.
37. Gouma DJ. Multicentre European study of preoperative biliary drainage for hilar cholangiocarcinoma (Br J Surg 2013; 100: 274-283). Br J Surg. 2013;100(2):283–4.
38. Figueras J, Llado L, Valls C, Serrano T, Ramos E, Fabregat J, et al. Changing strategies in diagnosis and management of hilar cholangiocarcinoma. Liver Transpl. 2000;6(6):786–94.
39. Gomez D, Patel PB, Lacasia-Purroy C, Byrne C, Sturgess RP, Palmer D, et al. Impact of specialized multi-disciplinary approach and an integrated pathway on outcomes in hilar cholangiocarcinoma. Eur J Surg Oncol. 2014;40(1):77–84.
40. Chapman WC, Sharp KW, Weaver F, Sawyers JL. Tumor seeding from percutaneous biliary catheters. Ann Surg. 1989;209(6):708–13; discussion 13–5.
41. Belghiti J, Ogata S. Preoperative optimization of the liver for resection in patients with hilar cholangiocarcinoma. HPB (Oxford). 2005;7(4):252–3.
42. Walter T, Ho CS, Horgan AM, Warkentin A, Gallinger S, Greig PD, et al. Endoscopic or percutaneous biliary drainage for Klatskin tumors? J Vasc Interv Radiol. 2013;24(1):113–21.
43. Ribero D, Pinna AD, Guglielmi A, Ponti A, Nuzzo G, Giulini SM, et al. Surgical approach for long-term survival of patients with intrahepatic cholangiocarcinoma: a multi-institutional analysis of 434 patients. Arch Surg. 2012;147(12):1107–13.
44. Spolverato G, Kim Y, Alexandrescu S, Popescu I, Marques HP, Aldrighetti L, et al. Is hepatic resection for large or multifocal intrahepatic cholangiocarcinoma justified? Results from a multi-institutional collaboration. Ann Surg Oncol. 2015;22(7):2218–25.
45. Abdalla EK. Portal vein embolization (prior to major hepatectomy) effects on regeneration, resectability, and outcome. J Surg Oncol. 2010;102(8):960–7.
46. Abdalla EK, Adam R, Bilchik AJ, Jaeck D, Vauthey JN, Mahvi D. Improving resectability of hepatic colorectal metastases: expert consensus statement. Ann Surg Oncol. 2006;13(10):1271–80.
47. de Santibanes E, Clavien PA. Playing play-Doh to prevent postoperative liver failure: the "ALPPS" approach. Ann Surg. 2012;255(3):415–7.
48. Schadde E, Ardiles V, Robles-Campos R, Malago M, Machado M, Hernandez-Alejandro R, et al. Early survival and safety of ALPPS: first report of the international ALPPS registry. Ann Surg. 2014;260(5):829–36; discussion 36–8
49. Ebata T, Yokoyama Y, Igami T, Sugawara G, Takahashi Y, Nimura Y, et al. Hepatopancreatoduodenectomy for cholangiocarcinoma: a single-center review of 85 consecutive patients. Ann Surg. 2012;256(2):297–305.
50. Tan JC, Coburn NG, Baxter NN, Kiss A, Law CH. Surgical management of intrahepatic cholangiocarcinoma--a population-based study. Ann Surg Oncol. 2008;15(2):600–8.
51. Ghali P, Marotta PJ, Yoshida EM, Bain VG, Marleau D, Peltekian K, et al. Liver transplantation for incidental cholangiocarcinoma: analysis of the Canadian experience. Liver Transpl. 2005;11(11):1412–6.
52. Shimoda M, Farmer DG, Colquhoun SD, Rosove M, Ghobrial RM, Yersiz H, et al. Liver transplantation for cholangiocellular carcinoma: analysis of a single-center experience and review of the literature. Liver Transpl. 2001;7(12):1023–33.
53. Sapisochin G, Facciuto M, Rubbia-Brandt L, Marti J, Mehta N, Yao FY, et al. Liver transplantation for "very early" intrahepatic cholangiocarcinoma: international retrospective study supporting a prospective assessment. Hepatology. 2016;64(4):1178–88.
54. D'Angelica M, Fong Y, Weber S, Gonen M, DeMatteo RP, Conlon K, et al. The role of staging laparoscopy in hepatobiliary malignancy: prospective analysis of 401 cases. Ann Surg Oncol. 2003;10(2):183–9.
55. Goere D, Wagholikar GD, Pessaux P, Carrere N, Sibert A, Vilgrain V, et al. Utility of staging laparoscopy in subsets of biliary cancers : laparoscopy is a powerful diagnostic tool in patients with intrahepatic and gallbladder carcinoma. Surg Endosc. 2006;20(5):721–5.
56. Weber SM, DeMatteo RP, Fong Y, Blumgart LH, Jarnagin WR. Staging laparoscopy in patients with extrahepatic biliary carcinoma. Analysis of 100 patients. Ann Surg. 2002;235(3):392–9.
57. McMasters KM, Tuttle TM, Leach SD, Rich T, Cleary KR, Evans DB, et al. Neoadjuvant chemoradiation for extrahepatic cholangiocarcinoma. Am J Surg. 1997;174(6):605–8; discussion 8–9.
58. Hashimoto K, Tono T, Nishida K, Nonaka R, Tsunashima R, Fujie Y, et al. A case of curatively resected advanced intrahepatic cholangiocellular carcinoma through effective response to neoadjuvant chemotherapy. Gan To Kagaku Ryoho. 2014;41(12):2083–5.
59. Mavros MN, Economopoulos KP, Alexiou VG, Pawlik TM. Treatment and prognosis for patients with intrahepatic cholangiocarcinoma: systematic review and meta-analysis. JAMA Surg. 2014;149(6):565–74.
60. Takada T, Nimura Y, Katoh H, Nagakawa T, Nakayama T, Matsushiro T, et al. Prospective randomized trial of 5-fluorouracil, doxorubicin, and mitomycin C for non-resectable pancreatic and biliary carcinoma: multicenter randomized trial. Hepato-Gastroenterology. 1998;45(24):2020–6.

61. Neoptolemos JP, Moore MJ, Cox TF, Valle JW, Palmer DH, McDonald AC, et al. Effect of adjuvant chemotherapy with fluorouracil plus folinic acid or gemcitabine vs observation on survival in patients with resected periampullary adenocarcinoma: the ESPAC-3 periampullary cancer randomized trial. JAMA. 2012;308(2):147–56.
62. Horgan AM, Amir E, Walter T, Knox JJ. Adjuvant therapy in the treatment of biliary tract cancer: a systematic review and meta-analysis. J Clin Oncol. 2012;30(16):1934–40.
63. Murakami Y, Uemura K, Sudo T, Hashimoto Y, Nakashima A, Kondo N, et al. Prognostic factors after surgical resection for intrahepatic, hilar, and distal cholangiocarcinoma. Ann Surg Oncol. 2011;18(3):651–8.
64. McNamara MG, Walter T, Horgan AM, Amir E, Cleary S, McKeever EL, et al. Outcome of adjuvant therapy in biliary tract cancers. Am J Clin Oncol. 2015;38(4):382–7.
65. Nakagawa T, Kamiyama T, Kurauchi N, Matsushita M, Nakanishi K, Kamachi H, et al. Number of lymph node metastases is a significant prognostic factor in intrahepatic cholangiocarcinoma. World J Surg. 2005;29(6):728–33.
66. Jiang W, Zeng ZC, Tang ZY, Fan J, Zhou J, Zeng MS, et al. Benefit of radiotherapy for 90 patients with resected intrahepatic cholangiocarcinoma and concurrent lymph node metastases. J Cancer Res Clin Oncol. 2010;136(9):1323–31.
67. Miura JT, Johnston FM, Tsai S, George B, Thomas J, Eastwood D, et al. Chemotherapy for surgically resected intrahepatic cholangiocarcinoma. Ann Surg Oncol. 2015;22(11):3716–23.
68. Sur MD, In H, Sharpe SM, Baker MS, Weichselbaum RR, Talamonti MS, et al. Defining the benefit of adjuvant therapy following resection for intrahepatic cholangiocarcinoma. Ann Surg Oncol. 2015;22(7):2209–17.
69. Hyder O, Hatzaras I, Sotiropoulos GC, Paul A, Alexandrescu S, Marques H, et al. Recurrence after operative management of intrahepatic cholangiocarcinoma. Surgery. 2013;153(6):811–8.
70. Tabrizian P, Jibara G, Hechtman JF, Franssen B, Labow DM, Schwartz ME, et al. Outcomes following resection of intrahepatic cholangiocarcinoma. HPB (Oxford). 2015;17(4):344–51.
71. Ercolani G, Vetrone G, Grazi GL, Aramaki O, Cescon M, Ravaioli M, et al. Intrahepatic cholangiocarcinoma: primary liver resection and aggressive multimodal treatment of recurrence significantly prolong survival. Ann Surg. 2010;252(1):107–14.
72. Endo I, Gonen M, Yopp AC, Dalal KM, Zhou Q, Klimstra D, et al. Intrahepatic cholangiocarcinoma: rising frequency, improved survival, and determinants of outcome after resection. Ann Surg. 2008;248(1):84–96.
73. Yamamoto M, Takasaki K, Otsubo T, Katsuragawa H, Katagiri S. Recurrence after surgical resection of intrahepatic cholangiocarcinoma. J Hepato-Biliary-Pancreat Surg. 2001;8(2):154–7.
74. Cherqui D, Tantawi B, Alon R, Piedbois P, Rahmouni A, Dhumeaux D, et al. Intrahepatic cholangiocarcinoma. Results of aggressive surgical management. Arch Surg. 1995;130(10):1073–8.
75. Sotiropoulos GC, Lang H, Broelsch CE. Surgical management of recurrent intrahepatic cholangiocellular carcinoma after liver resection. Surgery. 2005;137(6):669–70.
76. Konstadoulakis MM, Roayaie S, Gomatos IP, Labow D, Fiel MI, Miller CM, et al. Fifteen-year, single-center experience with the surgical management of intrahepatic cholangiocarcinoma: operative results and long-term outcome. Surgery. 2008;143(3):366–74.
77. Kim JH, Won HJ, Shin YM, Kim PN, Lee SG, Hwang S. Radiofrequency ablation for recurrent intrahepatic cholangiocarcinoma after curative resection. Eur J Radiol. 2011;80(3):e221–5.
78. Sulpice L, Rayar M, Boucher E, Pracht M, Meunier B, Boudjema K. Treatment of recurrent intrahepatic cholangiocarcinoma. Br J Surg. 2012;99(12):1711–7.
79. Boehm LM, Jayakrishnan TT, Miura JT, Zacharias AJ, Johnston FM, Turaga KK, et al. Comparative effectiveness of hepatic artery based therapies for unresectable intrahepatic cholangiocarcinoma. J Surg Oncol. 2015;111(2):213–20.
80. Fu Y, Yang W, Wu W, Yan K, Xing BC, Chen MH. Radiofrequency ablation in the management of unresectable intrahepatic cholangiocarcinoma. J Vasc Interv Radiol. 2012;23(5):642–9.
81. Haidu M, Dobrozemsky G, Schullian P, Widmann G, Klaus A, Weiss H, et al. Stereotactic radiofrequency ablation of unresectable intrahepatic cholangiocarcinomas: a retrospective study. Cardiovasc Intervent Radiol. 2012;35(5):1074–82.
82. Valle J, Wasan H, Palmer DH, Cunningham D, Anthoney A, Maraveyas A, et al. Cisplatin plus gemcitabine versus gemcitabine for biliary tract cancer. N Engl J Med. 2010;362(14):1273–81.
83. Okusaka T, Nakachi K, Fukutomi A, Mizuno N, Ohkawa S, Funakoshi A, et al. Gemcitabine alone or in combination with cisplatin in patients with biliary tract cancer: a comparative multicentre study in Japan. Br J Cancer. 2010;103(4):469–74.
84. Bekaii-Saab T, Phelps MA, Li X, Saji M, Goff L, Kauh JS, et al. Multi-institutional phase II study of selumetinib in patients with metastatic biliary cancers. J Clin Oncol. 2011;29(17):2357–63.
85. Borad MJ, Champion MD, Egan JB, Liang WS, Fonseca R, Bryce AH, et al. Integrated genomic characterization reveals novel, therapeutically relevant drug targets in FGFR and EGFR pathways in sporadic intrahepatic cholangiocarcinoma. PLoS Genet. 2014;10(2):e1004135.
86. Costello BA, Borad MJ, Qi Y, Kim GP, Northfelt DW, Erlichman C, et al. Phase I trial of everolimus, gemcitabine and cisplatin in patients with solid tumors. Investig New Drugs. 2014;32(4):710–6.

Regional Liver-Directed Therapies for Intrahepatic Cholangiocarcinoma

Nikitha Murali, Lynn Jeanette Savic, Nariman Nezami, Julius Chapiro, and Jean-François Geschwind

Introduction

Intrahepatic cholangiocarcinoma (ICC) is the second most common primary liver cancer after hepatocellular carcinoma, representing about 10% of all cholangiocarcinomas [1]. Incidence levels have been rising over the past 15 years across Europe, North America, and Asia [2, 3]. Though a majority of patients develop ICC de novo, risk factors such as infectious agents (viral hepatitis, liver flukes), biliary tract disease (primary sclerosing cholangitis, biliary cystic disease), toxic exposures, metabolic abnormalities, cirrhosis, and lifestyle factors (smoking, alcohol abuse) increase the likelihood of developing ICC [4]. Despite improvements in the treatment, the prognosis of patients with ICC remains poor, since patients commonly present at advanced disease stages when symptoms first arise [5]. Median survival is less than 27 months, and 5-year overall survival (OS) rates range from 15 to 45% [6].

Diagnosis of ICC requires combined clinical suspicion and confirmatory laboratory, endoscopic, and radiologic data. ICC is often detected incidentally on imaging obtained for other indications. Symptoms, if they exist, usually consist of upper right quadrant discomfort, cholestasis, and weight loss. Lab work-up includes assessment of tumor markers such as carcinoembryonic antigen (CEA), alpha-fetoprotein (AFP), and carbohydrate antigen 19-9 (CA19-9). CA19-9 values are the most useful for diagnosing ICC; CA19-9 levels >100 U/mL have a sensitivity and specificity of 53% and 75–90%, respectively [5, 7]. Combined increases in CA19-9 and AFP levels would suggest a mixed hepatocellular-cholangiocarcinoma, a distinction that is important to make since the two pathologies respond differently to treatment and have markedly different outcomes [8]. Cross-sectional imaging including contrast-enhanced helical computed tomography (CT), magnetic resonance imaging (MRI)/MR cholangiopancreatography (MRCP), and position emission tomography

N. Murali
Department of Diagnostic Radiology, Yale University School of Medicine, New Haven, CT, USA
e-mail: nikitha.murali@yale.edu

L. J. Savic
Department of Diagnostic Radiology, Yale University School of Medicine, New Haven, CT, USA

Department of Radiology and Biomedical Imaging, Yale School of Medicine, New Haven, CT, USA
e-mail: lynn.savic@yale.edu

N. Nezami · J. Chapiro
Department of Diagnostic Radiology, Yale University School of Medicine, New Haven, CT, USA

Department of Radiology and Biomedical Imaging, Yale New Haven Hospital, Yale School of Medicine, New Haven, CT, USA
e-mail: nariman.nezami@yale.edu; julius.chapiro@yale.edu

J.-F. Geschwind (✉)
PreScience Labs LLC, Westport, CT, USA
e-mail: jfgeschwind@yale.edu

(PET) is used to support an ICC diagnosis [5]. Contrast CT is useful for detecting the degree of biliary obstruction, liver atrophy, and the location of tumor-adjacent vessels and organs. Triple-phase helical CT will detect ICC lesions greater than 1 cm but cannot determine resectability in a majority of patients [9, 10]. MRCP is used to assess the degree of biliary obstruction through 3-D images of the biliary tree and surrounding tissue [11]. ICC lesions have a median size between 4 and 8 cm [12]. Tumors are typically hypovascular in nature and display significant fibrosis on contrast-enhanced imaging, appearing hypoenhanced on the arterial phase [5, 13]. Substantial fibrosis reduces tumor uptake of chemotherapy [14, 15].

Cholangiocarcinoma lesions develop from epithelial cells of small intrahepatic ductules or large intrahepatic ducts proximal to the hepatic ducts and are first classified as intrahepatic or extrahepatic according to their anatomical location along the separation point of second-order bile ducts [16]. ICC is further subclassified according to macroscopic growth patterns such as intraductal infiltrative, mass forming, periductal, or a combination of mass forming and periductal [17].

The advanced nature of ICC at the typical timepoint of diagnosis precludes a majority of patients from being eligible for surgical intervention, the only curative option. Patients with unresectable tumors go on to receive some combination of chemotherapy, radiation, and locoregional treatments. Locoregional therapy refers to targeted ablation of tumors or intra-arterial embolic therapies. Three of the most commonly utilized modalities of intra-arterial therapy include conventional transarterial chemoembolization (cTACE), TACE with drug-eluting beads (DEB-TACE), and yttrium-90 radioembolization (Y90-RE) (Fig. 9.1). These treatments work by exploiting the fact that tumoral tissue is primarily vascularized by the hepatic artery, while healthy parenchyma is mainly supplied by the portal vein. A catheter is advanced through the hepatic artery in order to deliver a combination of embolic particles, radiation, and chemotherapy drugs directly into tumors. This targeted approach reduces systemic chemotherapeutic side effects while maintaining a locally tumoricidal dose of drug. Evidence underscoring the importance of local tumor control in ICC continues to grow. In this chapter, locoregional treatments and current clinical evidence supporting their use in patients with unresectable ICC will be described.

Surgical Resection

Surgical resection is the only potentially curative intervention for patients with ICC, though up to 37% of patients with resectable tumors may not be offered the option of surgical resection [18]. While the goal of resection is to remove all disease while preserving liver volume, these procedures frequently require resection of the vena cava, extrahepatic biliary tree, or bowel, depending on the size and location of the tumor [5]. Lymphadenectomy is also necessary in a majority of cases [12].

Qualification for resection primarily relies on clinical judgment of whether the necessary resection is compatible with the level of functionality of the remaining liver tissue. Other factors considered include biochemical characteristics, the presence of metastatic lesions, and lymphatic involvement [19]. Tumors that are poorly differentiated are associated with unresectable disease, while other characteristics such as tumor size, histological origin, level of vascular invasion, and perineural invasion are not individually significant predictors of resectability [20].

A multi-institutional study reported resection outcomes for ICC patients and found that although clear intraoperative surgical margins occurred in 81.1% of patients, recurrence was observed in 53.5% of cases, with most recurrences occurring in the liver remnant [21, 22]. Positive margins, lymph node metastases, advanced cirrhosis with Child-Pugh scores beyond A, and portal hypertension are associated with poor outcomes for patients after resection [19]. Liver transplantation has poor reported outcomes and is not typically recommended for ICC [19].

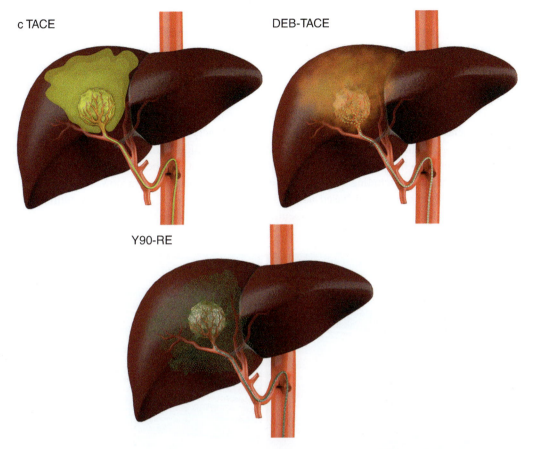

Fig. 9.1 Intra-arterial treatment visualization. This schematic demonstrates the differences between the three primary intra-arterial treatments for ICC: cTACE, DEB-TACE, and Y90-RE. cTACE involves the direct administration of a chemotherapy and Lipiodol suspension into the tumor region through the hepatic artery. DEB-TACE uses beads which release chemotherapy into the tumor vessels over time. Y90-RE utilizes the smallest microspheres which diffuse across the entire target lobe, enabling non-specific radioembolization of the tumor and surrounding area

Regional Liver-Directed Therapies

Regional therapies are the foundation of treatment for patients who are not eligible for surgical intervention, though ICC pathology presents unique technical challenges. Treatments targeting the hepatic artery may be less effective in ICC because tumors are relatively hypovascular. Fibrosis also reduces the penetrability of chemotherapy drugs [23]. As a result, locoregional therapies are both more technically challenging and less effective in ICC relative to other liver malignancies.

Of note, a meta-analysis across five major institutions in the United States demonstrated that median OS did not significantly differ among ICC patients receiving cTACE, DEB-TACE, and Y90-RE. Tumor response to treatment on follow-up imaging was the only predictor of improved survival [23]. Currently, selection of locoregional therapy is determined by clinical assessment of tumor characteristics, patient liver function and comorbidities, and treatment history. High-quality randomized studies of locoregional therapies are necessary in order to provide better evidence-driven guidelines for locoregional therapy selection.

Intra-arterial Therapies

Conventional Transarterial Chemoembolization

Background

The development of cTACE began in the 1970s as a treatment for hypervascular hepatocellular carcinoma. cTACE has since become the primary intra-arterial technique used to treat unresectable liver cancers, including ICC [24]. The therapy works through catheter-based administration of a suspension of chemotherapeutic drugs and an ethiodized contrast agent (Lipiodol) directly into tumor-supplying vasculature, typically a branch of one of the hepatic arteries. Then, an embolizing agent is administered in order to block the blood supply of the tumor, thereby inducing tumor necrosis. Embolic particles such as Gelfoam, polyvinyl alcohol (PVA), and trisacryl gelatin (TG) microspheres occlude more proximal blood vessels and further delay the washout of chemotherapy from the tumor [25]. The end result is a slow, sustained, and targeted delivery of chemotherapy with effective embolic blockade (Fig. 9.2).

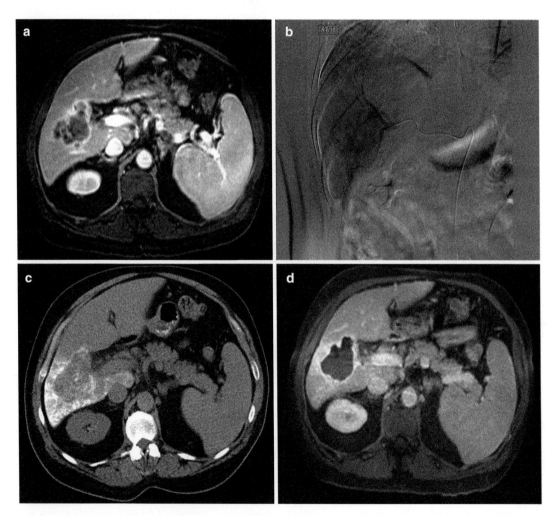

Fig. 9.2 Conventional TACE treatment in a patient diagnosed with mass-forming ICC. (**a**) Pre-treatment portal venous phase MR scan without contrast shows a tumor in the right lobe. (**b**) Digital angiography reveals diffuse blush in the right hepatic lobe. (**c**) CT scan 1 day after TACE shows Lipiodol deposition in tumor region. (**d**) Two-month follow-up MR scan shows necrosis in target lesion, indicating tumor response to treatment

In the United States and Europe, the chemotherapy combinations most frequently used for cTACE are gemcitabine and cisplatin or cisplatin, doxorubicin, and mitomycin-C [23]. Lipiodol is the primary contrast agent used and is advantageous in that it functions simultaneously as a drug transporter as well as an effective embolic agent that can penetrate tumor vasculature and reach capillaries [24]. Since Lipiodol is radiopaque on CT, it can be used to evaluate the technical success of the procedure. Lipiodol deposition on tumor has also been shown to correlate with tumor response [26].

Conventional TACE is generally well tolerated by patients. Adverse effects reported include fatigue, abdominal pain, nausea, and a transient increase in liver enzymes, often referred to as post-embolization syndrome [27–29]. Since its adoption, this technique has been applied to a wide spectrum of liver malignancies with successful results and is the mainstay therapy for patients with unresectable ICC [24, 30].

Evidence

Useful outcomes data of cTACE in ICC are limited because of a lack of standardized protocols. However, the role of cTACE in ICC as an adjuvant therapy to surgical resection and chemotherapy has been relatively well explored. One study of 125 patients compared various chemotherapy combinations with cTACE and demonstrated that patients treated with cTACE showed prolonged survival when compared to a control group who received chemotherapy alone (37.7% vs. 20.8% 5-year OS). Median OS was 5 months in patients who underwent surgical resection and 12 months in patients who received cTACE. Disease recurrence rates did not differ significantly between cTACE and resection groups [31]. Prospective trials are limited but have demonstrated that tumor downsizing is possible, resulting in resection eligibility after cTACE treatment in previously inoperable cases [30]. Another study identified a survival benefit for patients who had received systemic chemotherapy followed by cTACE compared to cTACE alone [32]. A third study of 42 patients showed good tumor response to cTACE treatment according to Response Evaluation Criteria in Solid Tumors (RECIST): 20 patients (48%) had stable disease (SD), 15 patients (36%) had progressive disease (PD), and 7 patients (17%) could not be evaluated. The median OS was 9.1 months. The choice of chemotherapy administered prior to cTACE is an important predictor of survival; gemcitabine combined with cisplatin resulted in a significant survival benefit when compared to gemcitabine alone (13.8 vs. 6.3 months) [33].

cTACE as a stand-alone treatment option for ICC has also been studied, though to a much lesser extent. As a stand-alone therapy, most studies suggest that if a tumor responds to the treatment, cTACE will produce a survival benefit. Additionally, current data shows that cTACE alone does not result in a survival benefit when compared to other intra-arterial therapies [23].

One study suggests that when compared to TACE, surgery does not result in increased survival for patients whose surgical procedure identifies positive lymph nodes or positive surgical margins. A retrospective study compared survival outcomes of 130 patients who underwent surgical resection, 32 patients who received cTACE, and 3 patients who received DEB-TACE. The median OS of surgical patients varied significantly if patients had positive lymph node status (9 months) or positive resection margin (11 months) when compared to patients with clear surgical margins (37 months). By contrast, the median OS of TACE patients (cTACE and DEB-TACE combined) was 11 months [34].

Drug-Eluting Beads Transarterial Chemoembolization

Background

TACE with drug-eluting beads (DEB-TACE) was developed in the last decade with the goal of addressing some limitations of conventional TACE, namely, challenges maintaining adequate drug dosing over time while continuing to minimize systemic toxicities. DEB microspheres aim to accomplish this by both embolizing and delivering chemotherapeutic agents in a manner similar to cTACE. The chemotherapeutic drugs are released more slowly when compared to cTACE, which could in theory make DEB-TACE a more controlled and targeted therapy [35]. The most common drug-eluting beads used in practice are DC or LC beads loaded with doxorubicin (DEBDOX). Beads are available in a range of diameters, typically 100–300 μm. Smaller beads such as the LC Bead M1 (diameter 70–150 μm) are currently being evaluated for efficacy. In theory, smaller beads can penetrate further into the tumor vessels, and initial studies have demonstrated they are more effective at delivering chemotherapy into tumors [36]. Irinotecan (DEBIRI) can also be used in place of doxorubicin [37]. Superabsorbent polymer (SAP) microspheres are another bead type that can be loaded with virtually any drug type, including irinotecan, cytotoxic antibiotics, and platinum-based agents [38] (Fig. 9.3).

Evidence

Though the safety of DEB-TACE has been validated, as with cTACE, the lack of standardized treatment protocols diminishes the utility of studies comparing outcomes of patients with varying forms of DEB-TACE treatment.

One study suggests that DEB-TACE in combination with systemic chemotherapy may be more effective than chemotherapy alone. This prospective study of seven patients with ICC found that DEB-TACE and systemic chemotherapy resulted in a higher median OS when compared to systemic chemotherapy alone (30 vs. 12.7 months), the largest reported improvement in survival rate. The patients receiving DEB-TACE received oxaliplatin-loaded beads in conjunction with systemic oxaliplatin and

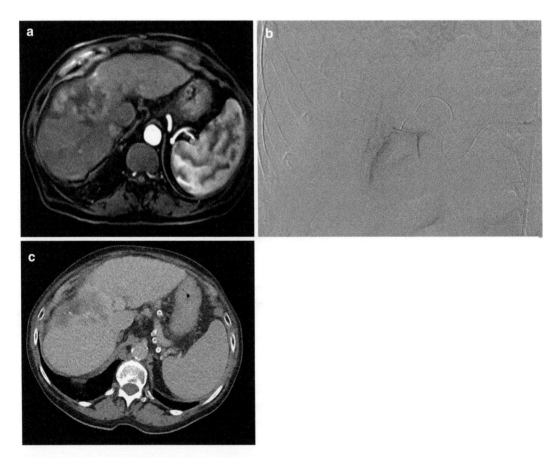

Fig. 9.3 TACE with drug-eluting beads (DEB-TACE) treatment in a patient with ICC. (**a**) Pretreatment arterial phase MR scan without contrast shows a large tumor in right hepatic lobe. (**b**) Digital angiography illustrates corresponding blush in the right lobe during treatment administration. (**c**) Post-embolization CT scan obtained 1 month after DEB-TACE treatment shows tumor reduction

gemcitabine and were compared to a historical cohort of patients receiving only systemic oxaliplatin and gemcitabine [39].

DEB-TACE has been demonstrated to result in tumor downsizing to the extent where previously unresectable ICC can be surgically removed. A multi-institutional study enrolled 24 patients with unresectable ICC who were treated with DEB-TACE. 83.3% of patients had received prior chemotherapy. The DEB-TACE treatment used DC beads loaded with doxorubicin (150 mg) and irinotecan (75 mg), and in eight patients the treatment was combined with systemic chemotherapy. Three patients were eligible for surgical resection after DEB-TACE and systemic chemotherapy [40].

A third study demonstrated good tumor response after DEB-TACE was administered following chemotherapy or surgery. This prospective study treated 11 ICC patients with DEB-TACE following systemic chemotherapy or hepatic resection. The cohort received a median of three DEB-TACE sessions per patient and used DC Beads loaded with doxorubicin (75 mg/2 mL). The tumor response of the group was 100% according to RECIST, and the median OS was 13 months. One patient had a complete response, and nine patients had a partial response to the treatment [37].

Based on current evidence, DEB-TACE has not yet been demonstrated to lead to an improved survival benefit when compared to cTACE. While one study demonstrated prolonged median OS in patients treated with DEBIRI compared to cTACE and systemic chemotherapy, a larger meta-analysis found no differences in OS comparing DEB-TACE to cTACE and other intraarterial therapies [22, 41]. Larger studies are needed to accurately evaluate the efficacy of DEB-TACE relative to cTACE and other treatment options for unresectable ICC.

Yttrium-90 Radioembolization

Background

Yttrium-90 radioembolization (Y90-RE) is a selective internal radiation therapy (SIRT) technique that uses microspheres to infuse radiolabeled particles through the hepatic artery, where the radioactive particles are trapped in the precapillary level and emit toxic ß-radiation. External beam radiation is used in a limited setting in liver malignancies because of the extreme sensitivity of liver tissue to radiation. The Y90-RE technique allows for higher levels of radiation to be used than what is permissible through external radiation, since exposure to surrounding parenchyma is limited. Target doses in Y90-RE are typically around 120 Gy [42]. Glass-based (TheraSphere®) or resin-based (SIR-Spheres®) microspheres are clinically used. Both produce similar outcomes, though glass microspheres are administered in higher doses [43, 44]. The small size of these microspheres allows them to penetrate tumors better than those used for DEB-TACE, but limits the embolic ability of the microsphere. Thus, Y90 microspheres are administered nonselectively across the entire lobes of the liver, resulting in a procedure that is less targeted than TACE but with more reproducible results [42, 45].

The nonselective administration of Y90-RE combined with the strong penetrative abilities of the particles often results in significant toxic side effects. After treatment, approximately half of patients will experience abdominal pain [46]. Up to 24% of patients may develop gastroduodenal ulcers, and this risk is significantly increased if Y90 spheres are administered close to a gastric artery, causing stasis in flow [47]. Angiographic imaging is vital in mitigating this risk; all patients are evaluated for arterial anatomical variants and arteriovenous shunting prior to Y90-RE treatment. If shunt vessels are identified, they may be sealed prior to treatment [48]. Since arteriovenous shunting to the lung is common in primary liver cancer, the risk of lung shunting is calculated prior to Y90 treatment and is used to modify the radiation dose [49] (Fig. 9.4).

Despite these toxicities, Y90-RE can be administered in patients with portal involvement, since it does not induce ischemic effects [50]. Canada was the first country to approve Y90-RE for the treatment of liver malignancies, and the United States soon followed suit, although the

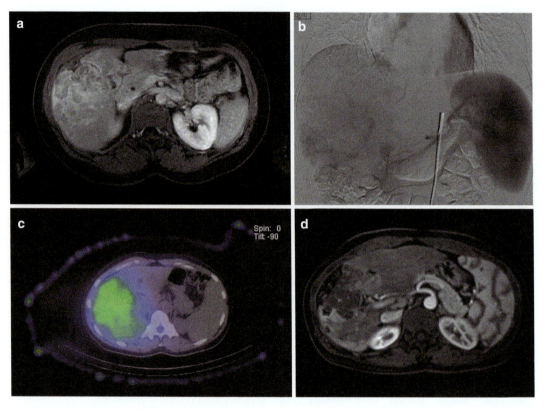

Fig. 9.4 Yttrium-90 radioembolization (Y90-RE) treatment in a patient with ICC. (**a**) Pre-treatment portal venous phase MR scan without contrast shows a tumor in right hepatic lobe. (**b**) Digital angiography illustrates diffuse blush corresponding to tumor location during treatment. (**c**) SPECT image shows diffuse area of radioembolization in green. (**d**) Post-treatment MR scan shows increased necrosis in tumor region, indicating treatment response

procedure is only FDA approved for hepatocellular carcinoma. Hence, the use of Y90-RE in ICC currently requires IRB approval in the United States [51].

Evidence

As with other intra-arterial therapies, survival outcomes reported for Y90-RE are confounded by small patient cohorts with various prior treatment histories and heterogeneous dosing regimens. The safety of Y90-RE was evaluated in a study that used SIR-Spheres to treat 33 patients with cholangiocarcinoma. Patients had various previous treatments including chemotherapy and TACE. The study showed that patients had a median OS of 20 months, time to progression (TTP) of 9.8 months, and good ECOG performance status after treatment. Patients tolerated the procedure well and reported no significant toxicities [52].

A phase I trial was conducted to identify the maximum tolerable Y90-RE dose for ICC. In this study, 17 ICC patients were treated with Y90-RE using TheraSphere in combination with a radiosensitizing agent, capecitabine. The study evaluated progressively escalating doses of Y90 and found that Y90 > 170 Gy could be used with only two patients reporting dose-limiting toxicity of abdominal pain. The study concluded that radiosensitizing agents may enhance the technical success of Y90-RE and confirmed that high doses of Y90-RE can be tolerated by patients [53].

One prospective study suggests that patients naïve to systemic chemotherapy may benefit from Y90-RE more than patients with prior chemotherapy treatment. The study examined 24 patients with unresectable ICC who were treated with TheraSphere. Twenty-nine percent of patients had prior chemotherapy, and extrahepatic and bilobar diseases were present in 33% and 67% of patients, respectively. The study reported a median OS of 14.9 months, and 77% of patients observed significant tumor response. Patients who had not received prior systemic chemotherapy had a survival benefit compared to the treated group, although this may be due to the confounding factor of initial disease severity at the time of the treatment [51].

As with cTACE and DEB-TACE, Y90-RE can also downsize ICC tumors to become eligible for resection. One study reported that of 46 ICC patients treated with Y90-RE using glass-based microspheres, 5 tumors were converted to a resectable form [46].

Ablation Therapies

Background
Ablation therapy refers to a minimally invasive procedure used to directly destroy tumor tissue primarily using thermal energy. In the context of ICC, the most common ablative therapy is radiofrequency ablation (RFA), though microwaves are also used. A radiofrequency generating electrode is inserted directly into the tumor under ultrasound image guidance [54]. When properly positioned, radiofrequency energy is delivered for a set amount of time, typically 10 min. Tissue temperature is monitored and maintained at an ideal temperature for tumor tissue destruction, typically around 105 °C. To achieve an optimal ablative margin of 0.5–1 cm, a single electrode is used for tumors less than 3 cm in diameter, and multiple or clustered electrodes are used for larger tumors [55]. Besides therapeutic efficacy, one of the primary advantages of image-guided thermal ablation is its cost-effectiveness [54].

Evidence
Modest literature is available on the use of ablative therapies for ICC, likely because ICC tumors are typically large in diameter and their central location near sensitive hilar structures limits heat application [56–58]. The reported technical success of RFA on eligible ICC lesions ranges from 80 to 100%. Tumor size is the primary factor in determining the success of RFA and its impact on survival; complete ablation in a single session is challenging for nodules larger than 4 cm [59, 60]. In patients with smaller tumors (<3 cm diameter), RFA or microwave ablation is nearly as effective as repeated hepatic resection, with significantly fewer complications [61]. The complication rate of ablative therapies is 3.9% on average, compared to a 46.9% complication rate in repeated resection [61]. In one review of 13 ICC patients treated with RFA, the progression-free survival (PFS) was 32.2 months. In this cohort, ten tumors measured less than 3 cm; five tumors were 3–5 cm. Two tumors were larger than 5 cm, and treatment failed in these tumors. The median OS was 38.5 months, and the 3- and 5-year survival rates were 51% and 15%, respectively [62]. A meta-analysis of 86 ICC patients treated with RFA found pooled 1-, 3-, and 5-year survival rates of 82, 47, and 24%, respectively. Complications occurred in five patients, with one death related to treatment complications [58].

Microwave ablation is only used in limited cases in ICC, and therefore data on its efficacy is extremely limited [55]. One study including 15 patients with a mean ICC tumor size of 3.2 cm treated with sonography-guided microwave ablation reported a 2-year survival rate of 60% [63]. Another study examined 18 patients who received either RFA or microwave ablation and reported a 3-year survival rate of 30.3%. A control group was not included [54].

The Role of Radiation Therapy

CT-guided high-dose brachytherapy (CT-HDRBT) has been used since 2002 to treat liver malignancies. It is particularly well suited to tumors that are large or near critical blood vessels which are unsuitable for ablative treatment [64, 65]. The treatment works by inserting a coaxial needle to puncture the lesion. Next, an angiography guidewire is introduced and exchanged with the needle. The guidewire is then removed and replaced with a brachytherapy catheter, which sits inside the tumor. Fluoroscopy CT is used to aid in the positioning of the catheters. The tumor is then irradiated with a high dose of iridium-192 for a maximum of 90 min [66]. Though the technique has been determined to be safe, outcomes data supporting the use of brachytherapy in ICC is scarce. One retrospective study of 15 patients receiving 27 brachytherapy treatments reported a median OS of 14 months after treatment. The median dose administered was 20 Gy, and the mean targeted tumor volume was 131 mL [64, 67].

Stereotactic body radiation therapy (SBRT) can also be used to treat small ICC tumors <5 cm in diameter. In this treatment, diagnostic imaging is first obtained to plan the procedure, including 4D imaging mapping of target lesion movement during patient respiratory cycles. Then, high doses of hypofractionated conformal external beam radiation are directed to the tumor, usually in less than five fractions. Usual doses of SBRT are 20–40 Gy and are delivered in 30–60 min sessions over the course of a week [68]. Study data of SBRT in ICC is also limited. One study followed 34 patients with intrahepatic and hilar cholangiocarcinoma receiving SBRT. The median SBRT dose was 30 Gy in three fractions. Median OS was 17 months, and PFS was 10 months. Four patients developed grade III toxicities [69]. Another retrospective dose-response study of 79 patients with large ICC tumors (7.9 cm median) treated with SBRT reported a median OS of 30 months and a 3-year OS rate of 44%. Patients in this study received an average dose of 58.05 Gy. Radiation dose was the most important prognostic factor that correlated with improved local control and OS [70].

Medical Therapy Options for Advanced Disease

Chemotherapy is the foundation of medical therapy for patients with advanced ICC and is used in patients regardless of resection eligibility. Systemic chemotherapy primarily includes fluorouracil, gemcitabine, or oxaliplatin. Gemcitabine is generally considered first-line therapy for any advanced biliary tract cancer. A recent phase III trial demonstrated that doublet therapy with gemcitabine and cisplatin resulted in improved ICC tumor response and prolonged PFS without additional toxicity when compared to gemcitabine alone. Overall survival was 11.7 months for the gemcitabine/cisplatin group compared to 8.1 months for gemcitabine alone [71].

Generally, systemic chemotherapy has demonstrated disappointing effectiveness, with a majority of regimens resulting in a median survival of 6–12 months [33]. One meta-analysis of 57 studies concluded that adjuvant chemotherapy combined with resection did not appear to increase OS or recurrence-free survival [12]. Currently, all forms of cholangiocarcinoma are treated with similar chemotherapeutic regimens. Emerging genomic sequencing data suggests that ICC contains a different genetic profile than extrahepatic bile duct and gallbladder tumors. This evidence suggests there may be room for future advances in more targeted medical therapy based on tumor genetic profile [72].

In cases when biliary obstruction is severe and the tumor is unresectable, stents can be placed through endoscopic retrograde cholangiopancreatography (ERCP) or percutaneous transhepatic cholangiography (PTC). Stents are typically plastic or metal, with plastic stents requiring replacement every 3 months [73]. Experimental therapies such as photodynamic therapy may also be considered for advanced ICC patients to restore biliary drainage. The therapy consists of intravenous administration of a photosensitizer followed by light illumination to relieve biliary blockade [74].

Conclusion

Intrahepatic cholangiocarcinoma is a relatively rare but serious cancer with poor prognosis. Surgical resection is the best curative option, but most patients are ineligible due to the advanced stage of the disease at the time of diagnosis. In this group of patients, locoregional therapies, including ablation as well as intra-arterial therapies such as cTACE, DEB-TACE, and Y90-RE, constitute the mainstay therapies. Radiation and systemic chemotherapy are used both as adjuvant and last resort therapies for advanced ICC. However, randomized trials are warranted to determine evidence-driven guidelines for the use of these therapies.

References

1. Buettner S, van Vugt JL, JN IJ, Groot Koerkamp B. Intrahepatic cholangiocarcinoma: current perspectives. Onco Targets Ther. 2017;10:1131–42.
2. Patel T. Worldwide trends in mortality from biliary tract malignancies. BMC Cancer. 2002;2:10.
3. Khan SA, Taylor-Robinson SD, Toledano MB, Beck A, Elliott P, Thomas HC. Changing international trends in mortality rates for liver, biliary and pancreatic tumours. J Hepatol. 2002;37(6):806–13.
4. Gupta A, Dixon E. Epidemiology and risk factors: intrahepatic cholangiocarcinoma. Hepatobiliary Surg Nutr. 2017;6(2):101–4.
5. Poultsides GA, Zhu AX, Choti MA, Pawlik TM. Intrahepatic cholangiocarcinoma. Surg Clin North Am. 2010;90(4):817–37.
6. Kim Y, Moris DP, Zhang XF, Bagante F, Spolverato G, Schmidt C, et al. Evaluation of the 8th edition American joint commission on cancer (AJCC) staging system for patients with intrahepatic cholangiocarcinoma: a surveillance, epidemiology, and end results (SEER) analysis. J Surg Oncol. 2017;116(6):643–50.
7. Patel T. Cholangiocarcinoma--controversies and challenges. Nat Rev Gastroenterol Hepatol. 2011;8(4):189–200.
8. Khan SA, Thomas HC, Davidson BR, Taylor-Robinson SD. Cholangiocarcinoma. Lancet. 2005;366(9493):1303–14.
9. Valls C, Guma A, Puig I, Sanchez A, Andia E, Serrano T, et al. Intrahepatic peripheral cholangiocarcinoma: CT evaluation. Abdom Imaging. 2000;25(5):490–6.
10. Tillich M, Mischinger HJ, Preisegger KH, Rabl H, Szolar DH. Multiphasic helical CT in diagnosis and staging of hilar cholangiocarcinoma. AJR Am J Roentgenol. 1998;171(3):651–8.
11. Anderson CD, Pinson CW, Berlin J, Chari RS. Diagnosis and treatment of cholangiocarcinoma. Oncologist. 2004;9(1):43–57.
12. Mavros MN, Economopoulos KP, Alexiou VG, Pawlik TM. Treatment and prognosis for patients with intrahepatic cholangiocarcinoma: systematic review and meta-analysis. JAMA Surg. 2014;149(6):565–74.
13. Savic LJ, Chapiro J, Geschwind JH. Intra-arterial embolotherapy for intrahepatic cholangiocarcinoma: update and future prospects. Hepatobiliary Surg Nutr. 2017;6(1):7–21.
14. Dodson RM, Weiss MJ, Cosgrove D, Herman JM, Kamel I, Anders R, et al. Intrahepatic cholangiocarcinoma: management options and emerging therapies. J Am Coll Surg. 2013;217(4):736–50 e4.
15. Lee JI, Campbell JS. Role of desmoplasia in cholangiocarcinoma and hepatocellular carcinoma. J Hepatol. 2014;61(2):432–4.
16. Wang K, Zhang H, Xia Y, Liu J, Shen F. Surgical options for intrahepatic cholangiocarcinoma. Hepatobiliary Surg Nutr. 2017;6(2):79–90.
17. Vijgen S, Terris B, Rubbia-Brandt L. Pathology of intrahepatic cholangiocarcinoma. Hepatobiliary Surg Nutr. 2017;6(1):22–34.
18. Tan JC, Coburn NG, Baxter NN, Kiss A, Law CH. Surgical management of intrahepatic cholangiocarcinoma--a population-based study. Ann Surg Oncol. 2008;15(2):600–8.
19. Razumilava N, Gores GJ. Cholangiocarcinoma. Lancet. 2014;383(9935):2168–79.
20. Weber SM, Jarnagin WR, Klimstra D, DeMatteo RP, Fong Y, Blumgart LH. Intrahepatic cholangiocarcinoma: resectability, recurrence pattern, and outcomes. J Am Coll Surg. 2001;193(4):384–91.
21. Endo I, Gonen M, Yopp AC, Dalal KM, Zhou Q, Klimstra D, et al. Intrahepatic cholangiocarcinoma: rising frequency, improved survival, and determinants of outcome after resection. Ann Surg. 2008;248(1):84–96.
22. Hyder O, Hatzaras I, Sotiropoulos GC, Paul A, Alexandrescu S, Marques H, et al. Recurrence after operative management of intrahepatic cholangiocarcinoma. Surgery. 2013;153(6):811–8.
23. Hyder O, Marsh JW, Salem R, Petre EN, Kalva S, Liapi E, et al. Intra-arterial therapy for advanced intrahepatic cholangiocarcinoma: a multi-institutional analysis. Ann Surg Oncol. 2013;20(12):3779–86.
24. Yamada R, Nakatsuka H, Nakamura K, Sato M, Itami M, Kobayashi N, et al. Hepatic artery embolization in 32 patients with unresectable hepatoma. Osaka City Med J. 1980;26(2):81–96.
25. Georgiades CS, Hong K, Geschwind JF. Radiofrequency ablation and chemoembolization for hepatocellular carcinoma. Cancer J. 2008;14(2):117–22.
26. Minami Y, Kudo M. Imaging modalities for assessment of treatment response to nonsurgical hepatocellular carcinoma therapy: contrast-enhanced US, CT, and MRI. Liver Cancer. 2015;4(2):106–14.
27. Cohen MJ, Levy I, Barak O, Bloom AI, Fernandez-Ruiz M, Di Maio M, et al. Trans-arterial chemoembolization is safe and effective for elderly advanced hepatocellular carcinoma patients: results from an international database. Liver Int. 2014;34(7):1109–17.
28. Vogl TJ, Naguib NN, Nour-Eldin NE, Bechstein WO, Zeuzem S, Trojan J, et al. Transarterial chemoembolization in the treatment of patients with unresectable cholangiocarcinoma: results and prognostic factors governing treatment success. Int J Cancer. 2012;131(3):733–40.
29. Pomoni M, Malagari K, Moschouris H, Spyridopoulos TN, Dourakis S, Kornezos J, et al. Post embolization syndrome in doxorubicin eluting chemoembolization with DC bead. Hepato-Gastroenterology. 2012;59(115):820–5.

30. Burger I, Hong K, Schulick R, Georgiades C, Thuluvath P, Choti M, et al. Transcatheter arterial chemoembolization in unresectable cholangiocarcinoma: initial experience in a single institution. J Vasc Interv Radiol. 2005;16(3):353–61.
31. Shen WF, Zhong W, Liu Q, Sui CJ, Huang YQ, Yang JM. Adjuvant transcatheter arterial chemoembolization for intrahepatic cholangiocarcinoma after curative surgery: retrospective control study. World J Surg. 2011;35(9):2083–91.
32. Kiefer MV, Albert M, McNally M, Robertson M, Sun W, Fraker D, et al. Chemoembolization of intrahepatic cholangiocarcinoma with cisplatinum, doxorubicin, mitomycin C, ethiodol, and polyvinyl alcohol: a 2-center study. Cancer. 2011;117(7):1498–505.
33. Gusani NJ, Balaa FK, Steel JL, Geller DA, Marsh JW, Zajko AB, et al. Treatment of unresectable cholangiocarcinoma with gemcitabine-based transcatheter arterial chemoembolization (TACE): a single-institution experience. J Gastrointest Surg. 2008;12(1):129–37.
34. Scheuermann U, Kaths JM, Heise M, Pitton MB, Weinmann A, Hoppe-Lotichius M, et al. Comparison of resection and transarterial chemoembolisation in the treatment of advanced intrahepatic cholangiocarcinoma--a single-center experience. Eur J Surg Oncol. 2013;39(6):593–600.
35. Hong K, Khwaja A, Liapi E, Torbenson MS, Georgiades CS, Geschwind JF. New intra-arterial drug delivery system for the treatment of liver cancer: preclinical assessment in a rabbit model of liver cancer. Clin Cancer Res. 2006;12(8):2563–7.
36. Lewis AL, Dreher MR, O'Byrne V, Grey D, Caine M, Dunn A, et al. DC BeadM1: towards an optimal transcatheter hepatic tumour therapy. J Mater Sci Mater Med. 2016;27(1):13.
37. Aliberti C, Benea G, Tilli M, Fiorentini G. Chemoembolization (TACE) of unresectable intrahepatic cholangiocarcinoma with slow-release doxorubicin-eluting beads: preliminary results. Cardiovasc Intervent Radiol. 2008;31(5):883–8.
38. Huppert P, Wenzel T, Wietholtz H. Transcatheter arterial chemoembolization (TACE) of colorectal cancer liver metastases by irinotecan-eluting microspheres in a salvage patient population. Cardiovasc Intervent Radiol. 2014;37(1):154–64.
39. Poggi G, Amatu A, Montagna B, Quaretti P, Minoia C, Sottani C, et al. OEM-TACE: a new therapeutic approach in unresectable intrahepatic cholangiocarcinoma. Cardiovasc Intervent Radiol. 2009;32(6):1187–92.
40. Schiffman SC, Metzger T, Dubel G, Andrasina T, Kralj I, Tatum C, et al. Precision hepatic arterial irinotecan therapy in the treatment of unresectable intrahepatic cholangiocellular carcinoma: optimal tolerance and prolonged overall survival. Ann Surg Oncol. 2011;18(2):431–8.
41. Kuhlmann JB, Euringer W, Spangenberg HC, Breidert M, Blum HE, Harder J, et al. Treatment of unresectable cholangiocarcinoma: conventional transarterial chemoembolization compared with drug eluting bead-transarterial chemoembolization and systemic chemotherapy. Eur J Gastroenterol Hepatol. 2012;24(4):437–43.
42. Salem R, Thurston KG. Radioembolization with 90Yttrium microspheres: a state-of-the-art brachytherapy treatment for primary and secondary liver malignancies. Part 1: technical and methodologic considerations. J Vasc Interv Radiol. 2006;17(8):1251–78.
43. Saxena A, Bester L, Chua TC, Chu FC, Morris DL. Yttrium-90 radiotherapy for unresectable intrahepatic cholangiocarcinoma: a preliminary assessment of this novel treatment option. Ann Surg Oncol. 2010;17(2):484–91.
44. Rafi S, Piduru SM, El-Rayes B, Kauh JS, Kooby DA, Sarmiento JM, et al. Yttrium-90 radioembolization for unresectable standard-chemorefractory intrahepatic cholangiocarcinoma: survival, efficacy, and safety study. Cardiovasc Intervent Radiol. 2013;36(2):440–8.
45. Hoffmann RT, Paprottka PM, Schon A, Bamberg F, Haug A, Durr EM, et al. Transarterial hepatic yttrium-90 radioembolization in patients with unresectable intrahepatic cholangiocarcinoma: factors associated with prolonged survival. Cardiovasc Intervent Radiol. 2012;35(1):105–16.
46. Mouli S, Memon K, Baker T, Benson AB 3rd, Mulcahy MF, Gupta R, et al. Yttrium-90 radioembolization for intrahepatic cholangiocarcinoma: safety, response, and survival analysis. J Vasc Interv Radiol. 2013;24(8):1227–34.
47. Konda A, Savin MA, Cappell MS, Duffy MC. Radiation microsphere-induced GI ulcers after selective internal radiation therapy for hepatic tumors: an underrecognized clinical entity. Gastrointest Endosc. 2009;70(3):561–7.
48. Rodriguez-Lago I, Carretero C, Herraiz M, Subtil JC, Betes M, Rodriguez-Fraile M, et al. Long-term follow-up study of gastroduodenal lesions after radioembolization of hepatic tumors. World J Gastroenterol. 2013;19(19):2935–40.
49. Mosconi C, Cappelli A, Ascanio S, Pettinari I, Modestino F, Renzulli M, et al. Yttrium-90 microsphere radioembolization in unresectable intrahepatic cholangiocarcinoma. Future Oncol. 2017;13(15):1301–10.
50. Riaz A, Awais R, Salem R. Side effects of yttrium-90 radioembolization. Front Oncol. 2014;4:198.
51. Ibrahim SM, Mulcahy MF, Lewandowski RJ, Sato KT, Ryu RK, Masterson EJ, et al. Treatment of unresectable cholangiocarcinoma using yttrium-90 microspheres: results from a pilot study. Cancer. 2008;113(8):2119–28.
52. Camacho JC, Kokabi N, Xing M, Prajapati HJ, El-Rayes B, Kim HS. Modified response evaluation criteria in solid tumors and European Association for the Study of the liver criteria using delayed-phase imaging at an early time point predict survival in patients with unresectable intrahepatic cholangiocarcinoma following yttrium-90 radioembolization. J Vasc Interv Radiol. 2014;25(2):256–65.

53. Hickey R, Mulcahy MF, Lewandowski RJ, Gates VL, Vouche M, Habib A, et al. Chemoradiation of hepatic malignancies: prospective, phase 1 study of full-dose capecitabine with escalating doses of yttrium-90 radioembolization. Int J Radiat Oncol Biol Phys. 2014;88(5):1025–31.
54. Xu HX, Wang Y, Lu MD, Liu LN. Percutaneous ultrasound-guided thermal ablation for intrahepatic cholangiocarcinoma. Br J Radiol. 2012;85(1016):1078–84.
55. Shindoh J. Ablative therapies for intrahepatic cholangiocarcinoma. Hepatobiliary Surg Nutr. 2017;6(1):2–6.
56. Slakey DP. Radiofrequency ablation of recurrent cholangiocarcinoma. Am Surg. 2002;68(4):395–7.
57. Simo KA, Halpin LE, McBrier NM, Hessey JA, Baker E, Ross S, et al. Multimodality treatment of intrahepatic cholangiocarcinoma: a review. J Surg Oncol. 2016;113(1):62–83.
58. Han K, Ko HK, Kim KW, Won HJ, Shin YM, Kim PN. Radiofrequency ablation in the treatment of unresectable intrahepatic cholangiocarcinoma: systematic review and meta-analysis. J Vasc Interv Radiol. 2015;26(7):943–8.
59. Giorgio A, Calisti G, DE Stefano G, Farella N, DI Sarno A, Amendola F, et al. Radiofrequency ablation for intrahepatic cholangiocarcinoma: retrospective analysis of a single Centre experience. Anticancer Res. 2011;31(12):4575–80.
60. Carrafiello G, Lagana D, Cotta E, Mangini M, Fontana F, Bandiera F, et al. Radiofrequency ablation of intrahepatic cholangiocarcinoma: preliminary experience. Cardiovasc Intervent Radiol. 2010;33(4):835–9.
61. Zhang SJ, Hu P, Wang N, Shen Q, Sun AX, Kuang M, et al. Thermal ablation versus repeated hepatic resection for recurrent intrahepatic cholangiocarcinoma. Ann Surg Oncol. 2013;20(11):3596–602.
62. Kim JH, Won HJ, Shin YM, Kim PN, Lee SG, Hwang S. Radiofrequency ablation for recurrent intrahepatic cholangiocarcinoma after curative resection. Eur J Radiol. 2011;80(3):e221–5.
63. Yu MA, Liang P, Yu XL, Cheng ZG, Han ZY, Liu FY, et al. Sonography-guided percutaneous microwave ablation of intrahepatic primary cholangiocarcinoma. Eur J Radiol. 2011;80(2):548–52.
64. Schnapauff D, Denecke T, Grieser C, Collettini F, Seehofer D, Sinn M, et al. Computed tomography-guided interstitial HDR brachytherapy (CT-HDRBT) of the liver in patients with irresectable intrahepatic cholangiocarcinoma. Cardiovasc Intervent Radiol. 2012;35(3):581–7.
65. Ricke J, Wust P, Wieners G, Beck A, Cho CH, Seidensticker M, et al. Liver malignancies: CT-guided interstitial brachytherapy in patients with unfavorable lesions for thermal ablation. J Vasc Interv Radiol. 2004;15(11):1279–86.
66. Ricke J, Wust P. Computed tomography-guided brachytherapy for liver cancer. Semin Radiat Oncol. 2011;21(4):287–93.
67. Koay EJ, Odisio BC, Javle M, Vauthey JN, Crane CH. Management of unresectable intrahepatic cholangiocarcinoma: how do we decide among the various liver-directed treatments? Hepatobiliary Surg Nutr. 2017;6(2):105–16.
68. Weiner AA, Olsen J, Ma D, Dyk P, DeWees T, Myerson RJ, et al. Stereotactic body radiotherapy for primary hepatic malignancies - report of a phase I/II institutional study. Radiother Oncol. 2016;121(1):79–85.
69. Mahadevan A, Dagoglu N, Mancias J, Raven K, Khwaja K, Tseng JF, et al. Stereotactic body radiotherapy (SBRT) for intrahepatic and hilar cholangiocarcinoma. J Cancer. 2015;6(11):1099–104.
70. Tao R, Krishnan S, Bhosale PR, Javle MM, Aloia TA, Shroff RT, et al. Ablative radiotherapy doses lead to a substantial prolongation of survival in patients with inoperable intrahepatic cholangiocarcinoma: a retrospective dose response analysis. J Clin Oncol. 2016;34(3):219–26.
71. Valle JW, Furuse J, Jitlal M, Beare S, Mizuno N, Wasan H, et al. Cisplatin and gemcitabine for advanced biliary tract cancer: a meta-analysis of two randomised trials. Ann Oncol. 2014;25(2):391–8.
72. Lee H, Ross JS. The potential role of comprehensive genomic profiling to guide targeted therapy for patients with biliary cancer. Therap Adv Gastroenterol. 2017;10(6):507–20.
73. Doherty B, Nambudiri VE, Palmer WC. Update on the diagnosis and treatment of cholangiocarcinoma. Curr Gastroenterol Rep. 2017;19(1):2.
74. Zoepf T, Jakobs R, Arnold JC, Apel D, Riemann JF. Palliation of nonresectable bile duct cancer: improved survival after photodynamic therapy. Am J Gastroenterol. 2005;100(11):2426–30.

Role of Radiation Therapy for Intrahepatic Cholangiocarcinoma

Sagar A. Patel, Florence K. Keane, and Theodore S. Hong

Introduction

Cholangiocarcinomas are rare malignancies arising from intrahepatic and extrahepatic bile ducts and characterized by early nodal and distant metastases. These tumors account for the second most common primary liver malignancy. They are divided into three categories based on location of origin within the biliary tree: intrahepatic, hilar, and extrahepatic. Each variant likely demonstrates a distinct biology and pattern of progression, as reflected by individual staging systems for each class [1]. While hilar tumors remain the most prevalent, the incidence of intrahepatic cholangiocarcinoma (IHC) continues to rise in the United States, accounting for approximately 15% of the 33,190 cases of liver and intrahepatic bile duct cancer diagnosed in the United States each year [2, 3]. Complete surgical resection is optimal and provides the highest chance for cure; however, there is a high rate of both local and distant relapse [4, 5]. Long-term survival is poor because of advanced presentation of disease and limited liver-directed and systemic therapies. Median 5-year overall survival for all patients is between 25 and 35%, while those who achieve margin-negative resections may be as high as 63% [6–8].

Adjuvant Therapy Following Resection

Given the high rates of recurrence despite even optimal resection, adjuvant local and systemic therapies have been explored. The survival benefit of any adjuvant strategy has never been proven in prospective, randomized trials; however, the inclusion of adjuvant therapy is widely accepted and often recommended in expert guidelines. With relatively few patients resectable at presentation, it is difficult to complete a large randomized adjuvant trial powered to show improvements in overall survival. However, in patients who are able to undergo surgery, lymph node involvement, residual disease, and vascular invasion are all associated with worse prognosis compared with R0 resections [9, 10]. Because IHC is typically confined to the liver and chemotherapy traditionally has had limited efficacy, there has been increasing interest in locoregional therapy. Furthermore, before publication of the ABC-02 trial [11], there was a lack of consensus regarding the optimal chemotherapy regimen that could be extrapolated for use in the adjuvant setting. The literature, as a result, consists mainly of single

S. A. Patel
Harvard Radiation Oncology Program, Harvard Medical School, Boston, MA, USA
e-mail: sagar_patel@alumni.harvard.edu

F. K. Keane · T. S. Hong (✉)
Department of Radiation Oncology, Massachusetts General Hospital, Boston, MA, USA
e-mail: florence.keane@mgh.harvard.edu; tshong1@partners.org

institutional series and registry analyses, and the data on the value of adjuvant therapy is mixed. Nonetheless, fluoropyrimidine-based chemoradiotherapy or chemotherapy alone is often offered to patients with any high-risk features.

Perhaps due to historical concern over hepatic tolerance and inability to deliver tumoricidal dose for intrahepatic and perihilar tumors, the use of radiation therapy in the adjuvant setting was more favored for distal extrahepatic lesions [12]. Therefore, most of the available data include a heterogeneous mix of patients with intra- and extrahepatic cholangiocarcinoma, including gallbladder cancer. In 2012, Horgan et al. published a meta-analysis [13] of 20 published institutional and registry studies to explore the impact of adjuvant therapy on survival for biliary tract cancers (tumors of the gallbladder and intrahepatic, perihilar, and distal bile duct). These studies incorporated over 6700 patients, and approximately 27% received adjuvant therapy. Notably only one study within the meta-analysis included patients with intrahepatic tumors. The majority of patients with margin-negative, node-positive disease received either chemotherapy or chemoradiotherapy, while the majority with margin-positive, node-negative disease received radiation therapy alone. There was a near-significant improvement in overall survival with the addition of any adjuvant therapy compared to surgery (OR 0.74, $p = 0.06$); there were no differences in outcomes with the use of adjuvant therapy in gallbladder and bile duct tumors. When compared to surgery alone, patients receiving adjuvant chemotherapy (OR 0.39, 95% CI 0.23–0.66) or chemoradiotherapy (OR 0.61, 95% CI 0.38–0.99) had better survival relative to those treated with adjuvant radiotherapy alone (OR 0.98, 95% CI 0.67–1.43). Furthermore, the greatest benefit of adding adjuvant therapy was observed in node-positive (OR 0.49, 95% CI 0.30–0.80) and margin-positive disease (OR 0.36, 95% CI 0.19–0.68).

While a minority of patients in this meta-analysis had intrahepatic disease, smaller institutional series have demonstrated an improvement in outcomes in those with IHC receiving adjuvant therapy. A retrospective review of 90 patients with resected IHC with involved regional lymph nodes treated at Fudan University in China between 1998 and 2008 found that median survival was 19.1 months in the 24 patients who received adjuvant radiotherapy compared to 9.5 months in the 66 patients who did not receive radiotherapy [14]. Another retrospective series of 373 patients treated at Chang Gung Memorial Hospital between 1977 and 2001 reported median overall survival of 11.7 months in the 63 patients receiving radiotherapy compared to 6.25 months in the patients who did not receive radiotherapy ($p = 0.0197$) [15]. These reports are of course limited by their retrospective nature and the fact that many of the patients did not receive systemic chemotherapy. Regardless, these data provide support for the consideration of adjuvant radiation therapy, usually with concurrent fluoropyrimidine-based chemotherapy, following resection of IHC with high-risk features.

Definitive/Palliative Therapy for Inoperable Tumors

Rates of resectability for IHC have slightly increased over time, due in part to more aggressive operative strategies and more liberal criteria for resectability. Still, approximately 70% of patients are unresectable at diagnosis due to the presence of multiple intrahepatic tumors, vascular invasion, and/or nodal/distant metastases [16]. For these patients unable to achieve optimal resection, median survival is low, ranging from 2.3 to 9 months [16, 17]. Chemotherapy became the mainstay of treatment for these patients after the ABC-02 randomized controlled trial demonstrated an improvement in overall survival from 8.1 to 11.7 months in patients with metastatic or unresectable cholangiocarcinoma who received gemcitabine and cisplatin over those who received gemcitabine alone [11].

The inclusion of radiotherapy has also been employed in patients with unresectable disease. A retrospective study of 84 patients with intrahepatic cholangiocarcinoma treated at a single institution in China demonstrated improvements in overall survival in 35 patients receiving radiotherapy with or without trans-arterial chemoembolization (TACE) compared to the 49 patients who received supportive care and/or TACE without radiotherapy. Patients were treated with 30–60 Gy in conventional 1.8–2.0 Gy fractions, and 86% of patients received ≥50Gy. Comparing the radiotherapy versus the no-radiotherapy groups, 1-year survival was 38.5% versus 16.4%, and median overall survival was 9.5 months versus 5.1 months, respectively ($p = 0.0003$) [18, 19].

Likewise, a SEER analysis of 3839 patients with unresected IHC found a median survival of 7 months compared to 3 months in patients who did and did not receive radiotherapy, respectively. While this report was a retrospective population-based analysis and the addition of chemotherapy was unknown, it did provided additional support on a possible survival benefit from radiotherapy in patients who could not receive surgery [20].

It is important to note that these data stem from patients treated with outdated radiotherapy techniques and doses that have now been shown to be insufficient for disease control, as most patients experienced local progression as the first site of disease after treatment [21]. Dose was limited by the risk of liver toxicity. Hepatic tissue tolerance within a notoriously poor patient substrate resulted in a very narrow therapeutic window; however, the delivery of tumoricidal doses of radiotherapy has become feasible with the development of modern techniques of radiation delivery, including charged particles and stereotaxy. The use of these advanced techniques has resulted in impressive local control that translated into prolonged survival, rivaling that of resection, without an increase in toxicity. Thus, the role of radiation in the management of primary liver tumors, especially intrahepatic cholangiocarcinoma, is rapidly rising. These techniques, as well as notable data supporting their use, will be discussed in subsequent sections.

Neoadjuvant Therapy with Transplantation for Hilar Cholangiocarcinoma

Cholangiocarcinoma arising at the hepatic duct bifurcation (i.e., hilar cholangiocarcinoma) characteristically arises in patients with primary sclerosing cholangitis (PSC). These patients, similar to those with severe cirrhosis, are usually not candidates for the extensive resection that would be needed to obtain negative margins. Despite the rare incidence of cholangiocarcinoma, overall, patients with PSC are at significantly higher risk with incidence reported from 4 to 20%, and majority are hilar (i.e., Klatskin tumor) [22, 23]. Liver transplantation was studied as an alternative for those patients with localized disease who were not candidates for extensive resection. Initial outcomes were poor due to high incidence of locoregional dissemination and recurrence [24, 25]. Due to the potentially long waiting time for organ transplantation, however, neoadjuvant therapy with radiation and concurrent chemotherapy was proposed in order to obtain local control and decrease risk of regional recurrence following transplant [25, 26]. The University of Nebraska and the Mayo Clinic have demonstrated that excellent survival can be achieved for highly selected patients with early stage hilar cholangiocarcinoma treated with aggressive neoadjuvant therapy leading to liver transplantation.

The University of Nebraska initially studied this multimodal technique; 17 patients with hilar cholangiocarcinoma, all presenting with obstructive cholangitis, were treated between 1987 and 2000 with chemotherapy (daily 5-FU 300 mg/m^2) and intraluminal bile duct brachytherapy (iridium-192 6000 cGy delivered over 55–60 h) while awaiting liver transplantation. Patients were only eligible if maximal tumor dimension was 2 cm without radiographic extrahepatic disease or intra/extrahepatic metastasis. The basis for these guidelines was the fact that the iridium wires use for radiotherapy had a penetration of 1 cm; therefore, tumors greater than 2 cm in diameter may not achieve optimal dose at the periphery. Notably, nine patients had PSC and/or ulcerative colitis, and three patients had decompensated cirrhosis. The most significant complication between chemoradiation and surgery was the recurrent episodes of cholangitis. Eleven patients were free of complications or tumor progression precluding surgery and underwent transplantation (median waiting time

87 days, range 15–792). The median survival was 25 months for the patients who underwent liver transplantation; 5 of these patients (45%) remained free of tumor recurrence 2.8–14.5 years after transplant [27].

In 1993, the Mayo Clinic also initiated a protocol for unresectable hilar cholangiocarcinoma due to the extent of disease and/or underlying liver disease. All patients were treated with neoadjuvant radiation (4000–4500 cGy by external beam, followed by 2000–3000 cGy intraluminal brachytherapy with iridium-192) and chemotherapy (concurrent bolus 5-FU with external beam and proactive venous infusion 5-FU with brachytherapy, which continued until surgery) followed by liver transplantation as well. This protocol differed with the additional use of external beam radiotherapy. Eligible patients had a maximal tumor diameter of 3 cm without evidence of intra-/extrahepatic metastasis. The initial publication [28] presented the first 19 patients, for which 11 patients had no evidence of progression at that the time of surgery and completed the protocol. With a median follow-up of 44 months, only 1 patient who completed the protocol developed tumor relapse. Since this publication, over 130 additional patients with unresectable hilar cholangiocarcinoma have been enrolled, and 90 patients have been reported to have favorable findings at the time of transplant. Five-year actuarial survival for all patients that began neoadjuvant therapy is 55%, and 5-year survival after transplant is 71% [29].

Delivery of Radiotherapy

The use of radiotherapy to treat intrahepatic malignancies was traditionally limited by concerns over hepatic tolerance and the resulting inability to deliver a sufficient treatment dose, particularly in patients who may have compromised overall hepatic function. However, the development of more advanced radiation techniques has enabled delivery of increased doses of radiotherapy with decreased toxicity, prompting renewed interest in the use of radiotherapy in treatment of IHC, both in the adjuvant and inoperable setting. The bulk of the data on the use of radiotherapy in intrahepatic cholangiocarcinoma are limited to small prospective trials or retrospective reviews of individual center experiences. Much of the data are extrapolated from larger studies of patients with hepatocellular carcinoma.

Historical Techniques

The initial use of liver-directed radiotherapy was primarily limited to palliative whole-liver irradiation for treatment of hepatic metastases. A retrospective review from Stanford found that 12 of 27 patients receiving ≥35 Gy to the whole liver developed radiation hepatitis [30]. A study of whole abdomen radiotherapy for ovarian cancer reported development of radiation hepatitis at even lower doses; in this series, 14 of 65 patients receiving 24.5–29.2 Gy to the whole liver in 12 fractions developed radiation hepatitis [31].

RTOG 76-09, a pilot study of whole-liver radiotherapy regimens for solitary or multiple hepatic metastases, produced promising results, as there were no incidences of radiation hepatitis in 109 patients receiving whole-liver regimens, which included 21 Gy in 7 fractions and 30 Gy in 15 fractions [32]. However, a subsequent study (RTOG 84-05) closed after 10% of the patients treated with 33Gy in 1.5Gy twice-daily fractions developed grade 3 hepatitis [33].

Conformal Techniques

The development of three-dimensional conformal radiotherapy (3D-CRT) allowed for more targeted delivery of higher doses of radiation to tumor while avoiding surrounding normal tissue. In addition, dose-volume histograms (DVH) with 3D-CRT have allowed for assessment of the interaction between dose and toxicity [34]. Initial series of toxicity in the era of 3D-CRT were largely retrospective. However, refined models of the interaction between radiotherapy dose, treatment volume, and toxicity were subsequently developed. A phase I/II dose escalation study of radiotherapy with concurrent hepatic arterial fluorodeoxyuridine enrolled 43 patients with either primary or metastatic liver tumors (18 with IHC, 9 with HCC, and 16 with colorectal metastases to the liver). Radiotherapy dose was calculated based on a maximum 10% complication risk of RILD as per the Lyman normal tissue complication probability (NTCP) model. This model assumes a sigmoid relationship between dose of uniform radiation to an organ and the probability of a complication [35]. Patients were treated to a median dose of 58.5 Gy in 1.5 Gy twice-daily fractions. The median overall survival of patients with hepatobiliary tumors was 11 months, and there was improved overall and progression-free survival for all patients receiving over 70 Gy compared with patients receiving less than 70 Gy [36, 37]. There was one case of grade 3 RILD, which resolved with supportive care. In the 18 patients with intrahepatic cholangiocarcinoma, the median survival was 16.4 months for patients treated with more than 70 Gy versus 11 months for those treated with less than 70 Gy.

This refined NTCP model described above was subsequently used in a phase II trial of hyperfractionated 3D-CRT with concurrent hepatic arterial chemotherapy [38]. A total of 128 patients (47 with liver metastases, 46 with cholangiocarcinoma, and 35 with HCC) were prescribed radiation doses according to a maximum 10–15% risk of RILD. Of note, the model was adjusted for patients with primary hepatobiliary versus metastatic tumors based on previous data showing differences in liver tolerance in patients with primary hepatobiliary disease. Median survival was 13.3 months in patients with cholangiocarcinoma, which was superior to historical controls. On multivariate analysis, tumor dose ≥75 Gy was associated with improved overall survival (23.9 months versus 14.9 months, $p < 0.01$). These early data demonstrated both the feasibility and importance of dose-escalated conformal radiotherapy to achieve tumor control.

Dose Escalation

Tao et al. [39] reported a series of patients with IHC treated with dose-escalated radiotherapy between 2002 and 2014. Among the patients, 89% received chemotherapy prior to RT. Radiation doses ranged from 35 to 100 Gy (median 58.05 Gy) in 3 to 30 fractions (median biologic equivalence dose (BED), assuming $\alpha/\beta = 10$, of 80.5 Gy, range 43.75–180 Gy). For the entire cohort, 3-year overall survival (OS) was 44%. There was a significant difference in both overall survival and local control based on BED. For patients treated with doses corresponding to a BED >80.5 Gy, 3-year OS was 73% versus 38% for patients who received doses corresponding to BED <80.5 Gy ($p = 0.02$). Three-year local control was 78% in the dose-escalated cohort versus 45% for those receiving lower doses ($p = 0.04$). This finding was independent of primary tumor size.

Dose-escalated radiotherapy was achieved with three-dimensional conformal intensity-modulated radiation therapy with 6 MV photons or passive scatter proton beam techniques. For patients who received 50.4 Gy or more, motion control and image guidance were implemented in two ways. For some cases, a fiducial-based kilovoltage image guidance for soft tissue alignment during deep inspiration breath-hold was used to minimize doses to the liver, bile duct, and GI mucosa. In other cases, an internal target volume was created, and patients were treated during free breathing with kilovoltage image-guided alignment to bone. In selected larger tumors receiving >50.4 Gy, gross tumor volume was treated with a simultaneous integrated boost (SIB); a central SIB of 75 Gy in 15 fractions or 100 Gy in 25 fractions was delivered to the center of the tumor via this technique.

This analysis demonstrated that using high radiation doses with a moderately hypofractionated approach to treat inoperable IHC improves local control, thereby resulting in a substantial survival benefit for patients. Modern techniques of radiotherapy including stereotactic delivery and charged particle therapy have enabled the ability to reach optimal tumoricidal doses for cholangiocarcinoma while still respecting normal tissue tolerances.

Stereotactic Body Radiotherapy

Stereotactic body radiotherapy (SBRT) is a delivery modality which employs rigid immobilization, motion control, and multiple conformal beams to deliver high doses of radiotherapy to a target volume with rapid dose falloff. It was first used to treat intracranial lesions in the early 1950s [40], but it was not utilized for extracranial sites until the 1990s [41, 42] given the challenges of immobilization and intrafractional tracking. The high dose per fraction of SBRT is thought to result in an ablative effect on the tumor, potentially through vascular damage. However, the precise mechanism of SBRT-induced cell death remains to be determined [43–46].

The feasibility and safety of SBRT in the treatment of liver tumors was initially assessed in patients with metastatic lesions primarily from colorectal adenocarcinoma [47–50], and local control at 1 year ranged from 71 to 95%. The use of SBRT has since expanded to include both primary and metastatic tumors confined to the liver.

A phase I dose escalation study of SBRT in 41 patients with unresectable HCC or IHC at Princess Margaret Hospital included 10 patients with IHC [51]. Patients were treated within three predefined liver effective volume (V_{eff}) strata, with three dose levels within each strata based on a 5%, 10%, or 20% risk of toxicity. With the exception of low accrual to the low V_{eff} strata, all risk levels within each strata were assessed. The median dose delivered was 36 Gy (range, 24–54 Gy) in 6 fractions. The median survival in patients with IHC was 15 months, and 1-year overall survival was 38%. There was no grade 4/5 toxicity or radiation-induced liver disease, although two patients with IHC did have transient biliary obstruction, presumably due to radiation edema. One patient experienced a gastrointestinal bleed, and one patient developed a small bowel obstruction due to tumor progression. Finally, seven patients had a decline in liver function, from Child-Pugh Class A to Child-Pugh Class B, presumably due to progression of baseline hepatic disease.

Several small phase I or II studies and retrospective reviews of SBRT for hepatic lesions have included small numbers of patients with IHC (Table 10.1). To date, there have been no randomized trials on the use of SBRT in IHC.

Charged Particle Therapy

Protons and carbon ions represent a potential modality for increasing the dose to a tumor while minimizing damage to the surrounding hepatic parenchyma. Protons have a distinct physical advantage over standard photon-based radiation. Photons deposit energy along the beam path beyond the tumor; this exit dose often leads to unwanted radiation exposure to uninvolved hepatic parenchyma, thereby increasing the risk of RILD [35, 63]. In contrast, protons have minimal exit dose, which provides a theoretical clinical benefit by allowing dose escalation without compromising normal tissue exposure. There are no randomized data on the use of charged particle therapy versus photon therapy for HCC or IHC. This modality, however, has been used effectively in the treatment of individual patients with IHC, often with dramatic shrinkage of the primary lesion (Fig. 10.1).

Recently, a multi-institutional phase II study was completed utilizing high-dose, hypofractionated proton beam therapy for localized, unresectable HCC and IHC [62]. Of the 83 evaluable patients, 44 had HCC and 39 had IHC; almost 90% of the IHC patients had no evidence of cirrhosis. For IHC patients, 34 (87%) had one lesion, 3 (8%) had two lesions, and 2 (5%) had three lesions. The median dose delivered was 58.0 GyE in 15 fractions. The average dose received by liver tissue not involved by tumor for all patients was 21.4 GyE (range 3.2–29.5 GyE). In the entire cohort, only four patients experienced at least one grade 3 treatment-related toxicity. One of the 44 HCC patients developed grade 3 thrombocytopenia; of the 39 IHC patients, one developed liver failure and ascites, one developed a stomach ulcer, and one was found to have hyperbilirubinemia. Three of the 83 patients (3.6%) had worsening Child-Turcotte-Pugh (CTP) score: two patients from A to B at 3 months, and one patient from A to B at 6 months. There were no grade 4 or 5 treatment-related toxicities. In terms of efficacy, only 4 patients developed local progression within 2 years of follow-up; 2-year local control rate

Table 10.1 The use of high-dose radiotherapy in the treatment of intrahepatic cholangiocarcinoma

Author, year of publication	Study design	No. of IHC pts	Tumor size (cm³)	Mode of RT delivery	Total dose (Gy)	No. of Fx	1 year LC	1 year OS	Toxicity
Liu et al., 2013 [52]	Retrospective	6	8.8 (0.2–222.4)	Three-dimensional conformal SBRT	20–50	3–5	93%[a]	81%[a]	None for IHC pts
Ibarra et al., 2012 [53]	Retrospective	11	80.2 (30.6–818.5)	SBRT, CyberKnife or Linac based	22–50	1–10	50%	45%	7 with grade 3 toxicities
Lanciano et al., 2012 [54]	Retrospective	4	60.9 (2.29–316)	SBRT, CyberKnife	36–60	3	92%[a]	73%[a]	None for IHC pts
Barney et al., 2012 [55]	Retrospective	6	16–412.4	IMRT or three-dimensional conformal SBRT	55 (45–60)	3 or 5	100%	73%	1 w/gr. 3 biliary stenosis; 1 w/gr. 5 liver failure[a]
Dewas et al., 2012 [56]	Retrospective	6	63 (36–112)	SBRT, CyberKnife	45 (29–45)	3 or 4	100%	NR	NR
Goyal et al., 2010 [57]	Retrospective	3	384 (80–818)	SBRT, CyberKnife	34 (24–45)	1–3	82% at 8 months	NR	None
Goodman et al., 2010 [58]	Phase I	5	32 (0.8–146.6)	SBRT, CyberKnife	18–30	1	77%[a]	71.4%[b]	None for IHC pts
Kopek et al., 2010 [59]	Prospective	1	32 (9–205)	SBRT, Linac based	45	3	84%[a]	Median 10.6 months[a]	21 w/gr. 3 elevation in liver enzymes, 6 w/GI bleed[a]
Tse et al., 2008 [51]	Phase I	10	172 (10–465)	SBRT, Linac based	36 (24–54)	6	65%	58%	2 w transient biliary obstruction, 2 w/decline to CP B
Wulf et al., 2006 [60]	Retrospective	1	53 (9–516)	SBRT, Linac based	26–37.5	1–3	100%	60%	No grade 3
Herfarth et al., 2001 [61]	Phase I/II	3	10	SBRT, Linac based	14–26	1	71%[c]	72%[c]	None
Blomgren et al., 1995 [42]	Retrospective	1	67	SBRT, microtron, or Linac based	63	3	14 months median	11 months median	NR
Tao et al., 2016 [39]	Retrospective	79	198 (12–966)	Three-dimensional conformal, IMRT, or proton	58.05 (35–100)	28 (15–30)	81% at 1 year 45% at 2 years	87% at 1 year 61% at 2 years	7 w/biliary stenosis requiring stent[d]
Hong et al., 2016 [62]	Phase II	39	133.7 (3.7–599.7)	Proton	58 (15–67.5)	15	94.1% at 2 years	69.7% at 1 year 46.5% at 2 years	3 w/ gr 3 Liver failure, hyperbilirubinemia, gastric ulcer

SBRT stereotactic body radiotherapy, *IHC* intrahepatic cholangiocarcinoma, *RT* radiotherapy, *Fx* fractions of radiotherapy, *LC* local control, *OS* overall survival, *NR* not reported, *CP B* Child-Pugh Class B cirrhosis, *GI* gastrointestinal, *pts* patients

[a]Includes entire cohort in study
[b]Includes two patients with HCC
[c]Includes 56 patients with metastatic lesions
[d]Unclear if due to radiation-induced biliary toxicity or tumor progression

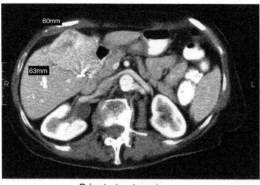
Prior to treatment

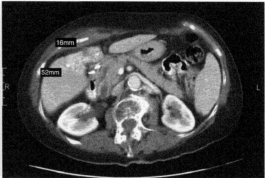
9 months after completion of proton therapy

Fig. 10.1 Axial CT slices of an intrahepatic cholangiocarcinoma lesion before and after completion of proton therapy

was 94% for patients with either HCC or IHC; however, recurrence beyond 2 years only occurred in patients with IHC, specifically in 4 additional patients. Notably, all patients who experienced local progression had received less than 60 GyE. For patients with IHC, the median progression-free survival was 8.4 months, median overall survival was 22.5 months, and 2-year overall survival was 46.5%. The impressive results of this study, especially when compared with historical data using conventionally fractionated RT for IHC, has recognized high-dose, hypofractionated proton beam therapy as an attractive modality for inoperable intrahepatic tumors, especially those that are too large for the extreme hypofractionation associated with SBRT (Table 10.1).

Radiation Therapy with Chemotherapy

The optimal integration of radiotherapy with modern-day systemic therapy for IHC remains to be determined. However, given the encouraging results seen with the addition of radiation therapy for localized, unresectable IHC, the NRG Oncology Group developed a phase III trial of gemcitabine and cisplatin with or without liver-directed radiotherapy in 2014. The estimated primary completion date is 2019.

This trial will help determine the impact of radiotherapy on outcomes in patients receiving optimal systemic therapy. Patients will receive three cycles of gemcitabine and cisplatin, followed by restaging and stratification based on tumor size (≤6 cm vs. >6 cm) and the presence or absence of satellite lesions. Patients will then be randomized to liver-directed radiotherapy (with one cycle of gemcitabine/cisplatin preceding RT and four cycles of gemcitabine/cisplatin following completion of RT) versus gemcitabine and cisplatin alone (five cycles). The inclusion of maintenance gemcitabine in either arm will be determined by the treating physicians. Selection of the prescription dose is based on the mean liver dose. Mandatory dose constraints for organs at risk in this trial are listed in Table 10.2.

Table 10.2 Dose constraints for organs at risk in NRG GI001

Organ at risk	Dose (Gy or Gy RBE)
Esophagus max (to 0.5 cc)	$D_{0.5\,cc} \leq 45$
Stomach max (to 0.5 cc)	$D_{0.5\,cc} \leq 40$
Duodenum max (to 0.5 cc)	$D_{0.5\,cc} \leq 45$
Small bowel max (to 0.5 cc)	$D_{0.5\,cc} \leq 45$
Large bowel max (to 0.5 cc)	$D_{0.5\,cc} \leq 48$
Cord +5 mm max (0.5 cc)	$D_{0.5\,cc} \leq 37.5$
Kidneys: Bilateral mean dose	$D_{0.5\,cc} \leq 12$ Gy

Note: If 1 kidney with mean dose >12 Gy, the remaining (or only) kidney must have V12Gy < 10%

Conclusion

The development of modern radiotherapy techniques has facilitated the incorporation of radiotherapy into the treatment of intrahepatic cholangiocarcinoma, specifically by allowing for dose escalation to tumor without increasing toxicity or the risk of radiation-induced liver disease. In the unresectable setting, the ability to achieve tumoricidal dose for primary cholangiocarcinoma has led to significant improvements in local control, translating into a survival benefit for patients, which is in some instances comparable to those historically reported after resection. Through the use of modern techniques, including SBRT and proton therapy, liver-directed radiotherapy has become effective and feasible. Further study is needed to determine its full potential in the treatment of IHC, as well as the optimal integration of radiotherapy with chemotherapy.

References

1. Edge S, Byrd D, Compton C, et al., editors. AJCC cancer staging manual. New York: Springer; 2010.
2. Shaib YH, Davila JA, McGlynn K, El-Serag HB. Rising incidence of intrahepatic cholangiocarcinoma in the United States: a true increase? J Hepatol. 2004;40:472–7.
3. Shaib Y, El-Serag HB. The epidemiology of cholangiocarcinoma. Semin Liver Dis. 2004;24:115–25.
4. Hasegawa S, Ikai I, Fujii H, et al. Surgical resection of hilar cholangiocarcinoma: analysis of survival and postoperative complications. World J Surg. 2007;31:1256.
5. Jarnagin WR, Ruo L, Little SA, et al. Patterns of initial disease recurrence after resection of gallbladder carcinoma and hilar cholangiocarcinoma: implications for adjuvant therapeutic strategies. Cancer. 2003;98:1689.
6. Maithel SK, Gamblin TC, Kamel I, et al. Multidisciplinary approaches to intrahepatic cholangiocarcinoma. Cancer. 2013;119:3929–42.
7. Spolverato G, Vitale A, Cuchetti A, et al. Can hepatic resection provide a long-term cure for patients with intrahepatic cholangiocarcinoma? Cancer. 2015;121:3998–4006.
8. Mavros MN, Economopoulos KP, Alexiou VG, et al. Treatment and prognosis for patients with intrahepatic cholangiocarcinoma: systematic review and meta-analysis. JAMA Surg. 2014;149:565–74.
9. Guglielmi A, et al. Intrahepatic cholangiocarcinoma: prognostic factors after surgical resection. World J Surg. 2009;33:1247–54.
10. Shimada K, et al. Clinical impact of the surgical margin status in hepatectomy for solitary mass-forming type intrahepatic cholangiocarcinoma without lymph node metastases. J Surg Oncol. 2007;96:160–5.
11. Valle J, et al. Cisplatin plus gemcitabine versus gemcitabine for biliary tract cancer. N Engl J Med. 2010;362:1273–81.
12. Nelson JW, Ghafoori AP, Willett CG, et al. Concurrent chemoradiotherapy in resected extrahepatic cholangiocarcinoma. Int J Radiat Oncol Biol Phys. 2011;81:189.
13. Horgan AM, Amir E, Walter T, et al. Adjuvant therapy in the treatment of biliary tract cancer: a systematic review and meta-analysis. J Clin Oncol. 2012;30:1934.
14. Jiang W, et al. Benefit of radiotherapy for 90 patients with resected intrahepatic cholangiocarcinoma and concurrent lymph node metastases. J Cancer Res Clin Oncol. 2010;136:1323–31.
15. Jan YY, Yeh CN, Yeh TS, Chen TC. Prognostic analysis of surgical treatment of peripheral cholangiocarcinoma: two decades of experience at Chang Gung Memorial Hospital. World J Gastroenterol. 2005;11:1779–84.
16. Endo I, et al. Intrahepatic cholangiocarcinoma: rising frequency, improved survival, and determinants of outcome after resection. Ann Surg. 2008;248:84–96.
17. Ohtsuka M, et al. Results of surgical treatment for intrahepatic cholangiocarcinoma and clinicopathological factors influencing survival. Br J Surg. 2002;89:1525–31.
18. Chen YX, et al. Determining the role of external beam radiotherapy in unresectable intrahepatic cholangiocarcinoma: a retrospective analysis of 84 patients. BMC Cancer. 2010;10:492.
19. Zeng ZC, et al. Consideration of the role of radiotherapy for unresectable intrahepatic cholangiocarcinoma: a retrospective analysis of 75 patients. Cancer J. 2006;12:113–22.
20. Shinohara ET, Mitra N, Guo M, Metz JM. Radiation therapy is associated with improved survival in the adjuvant and definitive treatment of intrahepatic cholangiocarcinoma. Int J Radiat Oncol Biol Phys. 2008;72:1495–501.
21. Crane CH, Macdonald KO, Vauthey JN, et al. Limitations of conventional doses of chemoradiation for unresectable biliary cancer. Int J Radiat Oncol Biol Phys. 2002;53:969–74.
22. Ahrendt SA, Cameron JL, Pitt HA. Current management of patients with perihilar cholangiocarcinoma. Adv Surg. 1996;30:427–52.

23. Rosen CB, Nagomey DM, Wiesner RH, et al. Cholangiocarcinoma complicating primary sclerosing cholangitis. Ann Surg. 1991;213:21–5.
24. Iwatsuki S, Todo S, Marsh JW, et al. Treatment of hilar cholangiocarcinoma (Klatskin tumors) with hepatic resection transplantation. J Am Coll Surg. 1998;187:358–64.
25. Goldstein RM, Stone M, Tillery GW, et al. Is liver transplantation indicated for cholangiocarcinoma? Am J Surg. 1993;166:768–71.
26. McMasters KM, Tuttle TM, Leach SD, et al. Neoadjuvant chemoradiation for extrahepatic cholangiocarcinoma. Am J Surg. 1997;174:605–8.
27. Sudan D, DeRoover A, Chinnakotla S, et al. Radiochemotherapy and transplantation allow long-term survival for nonresectable hilar cholangiocarcinoma. Am J Transplant. 2002;2:774–9.
28. DeVreede I, Steers JL, Burch PA, et al. Prolonged disease-free survival after orthotopic liver transplantation plus adjuvant chemoirradiation for cholangiocarcinoma. Liver Transpl. 2000;6:309–16.
29. Rosen CB, Heimbach JK, Gores GJ. Surgery for cholangiocarcinoma: the role of liver transplantation. HPB. 2008;10:186–9.
30. Ingold JA, Reed GB, Kaplan HS, Bagshaw MA. Radiation hepatitis. Am J Roentgenol Radium Ther Nucl Med. 1965;93:200–8.
31. Wharton JT, Delclos L, Gallager S, Smith JP. Radiation hepatitis induced by abdominal irradiation with the cobalt 60 moving strip technique. Am J Roentgenol Radium Therapy, Nucl Med. 1973;117:73–80.
32. Borgelt BB, Gelber R, Brady LW, Griffin T, Hendrickson FR. The palliation of hepatic metastases: results of the Radiation Therapy Oncology Group pilot study. Int J Radiat Oncol Biol Phys. 1981;7:587–91.
33. Russell AH, Clyde C, Wasserman TH, Turner SS, Rotman M. Accelerated hyperfractionated hepatic irradiation in the management of patients with liver metastases: results of the RTOG dose escalating protocol. Int J Radiat Oncol Biol Phys. 1993;27:117–23.
34. Ben-Josef E, Lawrence TS. Radiotherapy for unresectable hepatic malignancies. Semin Radiat Oncol. 2005;15:273–8.
35. Dawson LA, et al. Analysis of radiation-induced liver disease using the Lyman NTCP model. Int J Radiat Oncol Biol Phys. 2002;53:810–21.
36. McGinn CJ, et al. Treatment of intrahepatic cancers with radiation doses based on a normal tissue complication probability model. J Clin Oncol. 1998;16:2246–52.
37. Dawson LA, et al. Escalated focal liver radiation and concurrent hepatic artery fluorodeoxyuridine for unresectable intrahepatic malignancies. J Clin Oncol. 2000;18:2210–8.
38. Ben-Josef E, et al. Phase II trial of high-dose conformal radiation therapy with concurrent hepatic artery floxuridine for unresectable intrahepatic malignancies. J Clin Oncol. 2005;23:8739–47.
39. Tao R, Krishnan S, Bhosale PR, et al. Ablative radiotherapy doses lead to a substantial prolongation of survival in patients with inoperable intrahepatic cholangiocarcinoma: a retrospective dose response analysis. J Clin Oncol. 2016;34:129–226.
40. Leksell L. The stereotaxic method and radiosurgery of the brain. Acta Chir Scand. 1951;102:316–9.
41. Lax I, Blomgren H, Näslund I, Svanström R. Stereotactic radiotherapy of malignancies in the abdomen. Methodological aspects. Acta Oncol. 1994;33:677–83.
42. Blomgren H, Lax I, Näslund I, Svanström R. Stereotactic high dose fraction radiation therapy of extracranial tumors using an accelerator. Clinical experience of the first thirty-one patients. Acta Oncol. 1995;34:861–70.
43. Park C, Papiez L, Zhang S, Story M, Timmerman RD. Universal survival curve and single fraction equivalent dose: useful tools in understanding potency of ablative radiotherapy. Int J Radiat Oncol Biol Phys. 2008;70:847–52.
44. Song CW et al. Radiobiology of stereotactic body radiation therapy/stereotactic radiosurgery and the linear-quadratic model. Int J Radiat Oncol Biol Phys. 2013;87:18–9.
45. Brown JM, Carlson DJ, Brenner DJ. The tumor radiobiology of SRS and SBRT: are more than the 5 Rs involved? Int J Radiat Oncol Biol Phys. 2014;88:254–62.
46. Song CW, Kim MS, Cho LC, Dusenbery K, Sperduto PW. Radiobiological basis of SBRT and SRS. Int J Clin Oncol. 2014;19(4):570–8.
47. Méndez Romero A, et al. Stereotactic body radiation therapy for primary and metastatic liver tumors: a single institution phase i-ii study. Acta Oncol. 2006;45:831–7.
48. van der Pool AEM, et al. Stereotactic body radiation therapy for colorectal liver metastases. Br J Surg. 2010;97:377–82.
49. Rusthoven KE, et al. Multi-institutional phase I/II trial of stereotactic body radiation therapy for liver metastases. J Clin Oncol. 2009;27:1572–8.
50. Lee MT, et al. Phase I study of individualized stereotactic body radiotherapy of liver metastases. J Clin Oncol. 2009;27:1585–91.
51. Tse RV, et al. Phase I study of individualized stereotactic body radiotherapy for hepatocellular carcinoma and intrahepatic cholangiocarcinoma. J Clin Oncol. 2008;26:657–64.
52. Liu E, et al. Stereotactic body radiation therapy for primary and metastatic liver tumors. Transl Oncol. 2013;6:442–6.
53. Ibarra RA, et al. Multicenter results of stereotactic body radiotherapy (SBRT) for non-resectable primary liver tumors. Acta Oncol. 2012;51:575–83.
54. Lanciano R, et al. Stereotactic body radiation therapy for patients with heavily pretreated liver metastases and liver tumors. Front Oncol. 2012;2:23.
55. Barney MB, Olivier KR, Miller RC, Haddock MG. Clinical outcomes and toxicity using stereotactic body radiotherapy (SBRT) for advanced cholangiocarcinoma. Radiat Oncol. 2012;7:67.

56. Dewas S, et al. Prognostic factors affecting local control of hepatic tumors treated by stereotactic body radiation therapy. Radiat Oncol. 2012;7:166.
57. Goyal K, et al. Cyberknife stereotactic body radiation therapy for nonresectable tumors of the liver: preliminary results. HPB Surg. 2010;2010, pii: 309780.
58. Goodman KA, et al. Dose-escalation study of single-fraction stereotactic body radiotherapy for liver malignancies. Int J Radiat Oncol Biol Phys. 2010;78:486–93.
59. Kopek N, Holt MI, Hansen AT, Høyer M. Stereotactic body radiotherapy for unresectable cholangiocarcinoma. Radiother Oncol. 2010;94:47–52.
60. Wulf J, et al. Stereotactic radiotherapy of primary liver cancer and hepatic metastases. Acta Oncol. 2006;45:838–47.
61. Herfarth KK, et al. Stereotactic single-dose radiation therapy of liver tumors: results of a phase I/II trial. J Clin Oncol. 2001;19:164–70.
62. Hong TS, Wo JY, Beow YY, et al. A multi-institutional phase II study of high dose hypofractionated proton beam therapy in patients with localized, unresectable hepatocellular carcinoma and intrahepatic cholangiocarcinoma. J Clin Oncol. 2016;34:460–8.
63. Emami B, et al. Tolerance of normal tissue to therapeutic irradiation. Int J Radiat Oncol Biol Phys. 1991;21:109–22.

Current and Emerging Medical Therapies for Advanced Disease in Intrahepatic Cholangiocarcinoma

11

Aileen Deng and Steven Cohen

Introduction

Cholangiocarcinoma, or biliary tract cancer, is a heterogeneous group of cancers arising from different points of the biliary tree [1]. It is classified anatomically by the World Health Organization as intrahepatic or extrahepatic, of which, the latter is subdivided into perihilar and distal by the European Network for the Study of Cholangiocarcinoma [2].

Surgical resection remains the only potentially curative treatment for biliary tract cancers. Survival after surgery depends on having adequate remnant liver function, in the setting of tumor-negative margins and absence of vascular or lymph node invasion [3]. Despite resection, disease recurrence remains common, and outcome remains suboptimal. Overall, the 5-year survival after surgical resection ranges between 22 and 44% for intrahepatic, 11 and 41% for perihilar, and 27 and 37% for distal cholangiocarcinoma [2]. Unfortunately, more than 50% of patients present with advanced disease, which is associated with an overall survival of less than 12 months and a 5-year survival of less than 10% [3–6]. On average, survival ranges between 3 and 5 months with best supportive care and 6 and 12 months with palliative chemotherapy [7–9]. As only modest benefits are seen with palliative chemotherapy, further advances in medical therapies are urgently needed.

The heterogeneity and rarity of biliary tract cancer have made it challenging to study new treatment options in robust clinical trials. However, recent advances in genomic profiling have helped unravel a plethora of genomic alterations that may alter our treatment landscape. These efforts are shedding light on the disease pathogenesis as well as guiding the development of targeted agents. This chapter aims to summarize our evolving understanding of both current and emerging systemic therapies in cholangiocarcinoma.

A. Deng
Sidney Kimmel Cancer Center, Thomas Jefferson University Hospitalh, Philadelphia, PA, USA

S. Cohen (✉)
Rosenfeld Cancer Center at Abington Jefferson Health, Abington, PA, USA

Department of Medical Oncology, Sidney Kimmel Cancer Center, Thomas Jefferson University Hospital, Philadelphia, PA, USA
e-mail: Steven.cohen@jefferson.edu

Systemic Chemotherapy for Advanced Disease

In the setting of advanced (locally advanced, recurrent, or metastatic) biliary tract cancer, systemic chemotherapy is the mainstay of treatment [2]. The combination of gemcitabine and cisplatin has become the standard regimen in frontline therapy, based upon the results of two randomized trials (ABC-02, phase III and BT22, phase II) [8, 10, 11].

In the 2010 landmark of United Kingdom advanced biliary cancer (ABC)-02 trial, 410 patients with locally advanced or metastatic cholangiocarcinoma, gallbladder cancer, or ampullary cancer were randomly assigned to receive either cisplatin and gemcitabine or gemcitabine alone [8]. As compared with gemcitabine alone, cisplatin plus gemcitabine was associated with a significant improvement in both overall survival (OS) and progression-free survival (PFS) without substantial added toxicity. The median OS was 11.7 months in the combination group and 8.1 months in the gemcitabine alone group (HR 0.64, $p < 0.001$). The median PFS was 8.0 months in the combination group and 5.0 months in the gemcitabine alone group (HR 0.63, $p < 0.001$). While more neutropenia was reported with the combination of cisplatin-gemcitabine, neutropenia-associated infections were similar in both groups.

In parallel, the Japan biliary tract (BT)22 study randomized 84 patients with advanced biliary tract cancers to receive the same regimen used in the ABC-02 study [11]. Compared to gemcitabine alone, cisplatin plus gemcitabine demonstrated higher 1-year survival (the primary end point, 39% versus 31%), median OS (11.2 versus 7.7 months, HR 0.69, p 0.139), median PFS (5.8 versus 3.7 months, HR 0.66, p 0.077), and overall response rate (19.5% versus 11.9%, p 0.380).

To evaluate the efficacy of cisplatin-gemcitabine with increased statistical power, a subsequent meta-analysis of the ABC-02 and BT22 trials was published in 2014. It demonstrated improved PFS (HR 0.64; 95% CI 0.53–0.76; $p < 0.001$) and OS (HR 0.65; 95% CI 0.54–0.78; $p < 0.001$) with combination cisplatin-gemcitabine versus gemcitabine alone [12]. Similar improvements in PFS and OS were noted in intrahepatic and extrahepatic cholangiocarcinoma and gallbladder cancer. Patients with good performance status (PS 0-1) appeared most likely to benefit, while patients with poor performance status (PS 2) or ampullary tumors appeared least likely to benefit from combination chemotherapy.

To date, the ABC-02 study remains our only phase III evidence for using first-line combination chemotherapy in patients with advanced biliary tract cancers. When cisplatin is contraindicated (e.g., renal failure), the safety and efficacy of a number of alternative gemcitabine- or fluoropyrimidine (5-fluorouracil or capecitabine)-based regimens have been reported in the phase II setting [10, 13]. Due to the scarcity of phase III trials, studies have analyzed available prospective data to identify active regimens in the first-line setting [13, 14]. They supported the use of gemcitabine-based chemotherapy in the treatment of advanced biliary tract cancers.

In a meta-analysis of seven randomized trials, including the ABC-02 and BT22 studies, gemcitabine-based combination chemotherapy showed improved survival with added toxicity [14]. The overall analysis revealed that patients treated with gemcitabine-based combination chemotherapy had significantly higher disease response rates [OR 1.69; 95% CI 1.17–2.43; p 0.01], a longer PFS [mean difference 1.95; 95% CI 0.9–3.00; p 0.00], and a longer OS [mean difference 1.85; 95% CI 0.26–3.44; p 0.02] compared with the gemcitabine alone and non-gemcitabine-based chemotherapy groups. However, higher incidences of grade 3-4 hematological toxicities were noted in the gemcitabine-based combination chemotherapy group compared with those in other groups.

An analysis of 83 first- and second-line trials noted a strong trend toward improved survival with gemcitabine-based chemotherapy [13]. Compared to non-gemcitabine-based regimens, gemcitabine-based regimens showed a trend toward improved OS (9.7 versus 8.9 months, p 0.014) and a significant improvement in PFS (5.0 versus 3.8 months, p 0.003). In addition, gemcitabine-based regimens containing 5-fluorouracil demonstrated a trend toward improved OS (12.5 versus 9.5 months, p 0.047) compared to platinum agents.

For patients who progress on cisplatin and gemcitabine, there are no standard regimens in the second-line setting [2]. In the largest published retrospective study to date, with 196 patients who received second-line chemotherapy, no significant difference in PFS and OS was found between different regimens [15]. In a 2014 systematic review with 761 patients, insufficient evidence was available to recommend a second-line chemotherapy regimen [16]. Treatment with second-line chemotherapy was associated with a mean OS of 7.2 months (95% CI 6.2–8.2), PFS of 3.2 months (95% CI 2.7–3.7), response rate of 7.7% (95% CI 6.5–8.9), and disease control rate of 49.5% (95% CI 41.4–57.7).

Available results on second-line chemotherapy need to be interpreted cautiously as any perceived improvement in survival may in fact be due to selection bias. Patients who receive second-line chemotherapy have better performance status, which may account for improved outcomes [4]. As it remains unclear whether second-line chemotherapy truly benefits patients over the best supportive case (BSC) in advanced biliary tract cancers, the first randomized phase III trial is currently underway. The ongoing ABC-06 trial, which compares FOLFOX chemotherapy versus BSC after frontline cisplatin-gemcitabine, will hopefully answer this question in the near future (NCT01926236).

Currently, in clinical practice, fluoropyrimidine-based regimens are often used when patients progress on gemcitabine-based regimens. Results have differed on whether fluoropyrimidine-based doublet chemotherapy is superior to fluoropyrimidine alone [15, 17]. A good PS, disease control with first-line chemotherapy, and a low CA 19-9 level are associated with longer OS with second-line chemotherapy [15]. These prognostic factors may help clinicians to select those patients who may best benefit from second-line chemotherapy.

Adjuvant Chemotherapy

Due to the high rates of disease recurrence and poor outcomes following surgical resection, there has been ongoing interest in adjuvant therapy in biliary tract cancers. Unfortunately, randomized data on the efficacy of adjuvant treatment are scarce. Thus, current guidelines largely reflect systematic reviews and consensus statements [3]. Currently, adjuvant chemotherapy is not a standard of care for most patients with cholangiocarcinoma; however, it has been recommended for local recurrence in hilar cholangiocarcinoma due to the risks of radiation-related toxicity to the area of jejunal reconstruction [18].

The role of adjuvant therapy in cholangiocarcinoma remains uncertain. A 2014 systematic review of 14 retrospective studies and 2289 patients did not show a survival benefit with adjuvant chemotherapy or radiotherapy in intrahepatic cholangiocarcinoma [19]. Adjuvant chemotherapy (fluorouracil, gemcitabine, or oxaliplatin based) did not affect OS in five of these studies. In addition, four studies looking at the impact of adjuvant chemotherapy and/or radiotherapy did not detect a significant difference in OS or recurrence-free survival (RFS).

Randomized data on the efficacy of adjuvant chemotherapy have been limited. In 2002, a multicenter phase III trial randomized 139 patients with resected pancreaticobiliary cancers to adjuvant chemotherapy with mitomycin C and fluorouracil versus surgery alone [20]. A nonsignificant survival benefit was seen in patients with adjuvant chemotherapy following R0 resection for cholangiocarcinoma with a disease-free survival (DFS) at 5 years of 32.4% versus 15.8% with surgery alone. Gallbladder cancer appeared to derive the most benefit from adjuvant chemotherapy, with a significant increase of 8.7% in the 5-year DFS with adjuvant chemotherapy compared to surgery alone in subgroup analysis. More recently, the ESPAC-3 phase III trial evaluated adjuvant chemotherapy in 428 patients with resected peri-ampullary cancer [21]. Unfortunately, subgroup analysis failed to show survival benefit with adjuvant chemotherapy in the 393 patients with ampullary or bile duct cancers.

However, adjuvant therapy may benefit selected patients with biliary tract cancers. A 2012 systematic review and meta-analysis of adjuvant therapy in biliary tract cancer included 6712 patients and 20 studies [22]. Compared to surgery alone, adjuvant chemotherapy was associated with a trend toward improved OS (pooled OR 0.74, *p* 0.06). Patients who received adjuvant chemotherapy or chemoradiation derived greater benefit than those who received radiation alone (OR 0.39, 0.61, and 0.98, respectively, *p* 0.02). A subset analysis suggested that patients with lymph node involvement (OR 0.49, *p* 0.004) or R1 resection margins (OR 0.36, *p* 0.002) benefited the most from adjuvant chemoradiation or chemotherapy [22]. It is important to remember that these findings were derived from retrospective studies, which lacked consistency in the surgical approach as well as its reporting. In addition, it may not be applicable for all biliary tract cancers, as a very small number of intrahepatic cholangiocarcinoma cases were included. However, until better data become available, these results establish the basis to consider adjuvant chemotherapy and chemoradiation in patients with lymph node or margin positive disease [3].

There is no standard adjuvant regimen currently used in biliary tract cancers. A commonly cited study is the SWOG S0809 phase II trial, which evaluated adjuvant chemotherapy (gemcitabine plus capecitabine) followed by chemoradiation in 79 patients with extrahepatic cholangiocarcinoma and gallbladder cancer [23]. The study showed a 2-year survival of 65% and a median OS of 35 months. In R0 and R1 patients, the 2-year survival was 67% and 60%, respectively. Although this study is limited by the lack of a control arm, gemcitabine plus capecitabine is considered an effective and reasonable adjuvant approach.

Several studies are currently underway to investigate the role of adjuvant chemotherapy. Two studies where final data are pending include the French PRODIGE-12 study evaluating gemcitabine and oxaliplatin (NCT01313377) and the British BILCAP study evaluating capecitabine (NCT02170090). The ACTICCA-1 study, which began in 2014, is a multinational, randomized, controlled phase III trial that will evaluate the efficacy of adjuvant gemcitabine plus cisplatin versus surgery alone (NCT02170090) [24]. Two separate cohorts (cholangiocarcinoma and muscle invasive gallbladder carcinoma) will be included to capture any differences in treatment effects. As there remains no standard of care, patients being considered for adjuvant therapy should be evaluated for ongoing clinical trials (NCT02548195, NCT02798510).

Molecular-Targeted Therapy for Advanced Disease

Our knowledge of the genomic profiles of biliary tract cancers has rapidly evolved with the advent of new genomic profiling technology. Whole-exome and next-generation sequencing have identified multiple molecular aberrations that contribute to tumor pathogenesis [25–28]. Common genetic and epigenetic alterations in biliary tract cancers result in deregulation of DNA repair (TP53) and DNA methylation (IDH1/2), activation of complex signaling pathways (WNT-CTNNB1 and tyrosine kinase signaling pathways), and altered chromatin remodeling (SWI-SNF complex) [2].

Genomic alterations in biliary tract cancers vary by tumor location. While IDH1/IDH2 and BAP1 mutations and FGFR2 fusions are more common in intrahepatic cholangiocarcinoma, ERBB2 and p53 mutations are more frequently seen in extrahepatic cholangiocarcinoma and gallbladder cancer [4, 29–31]. While PRKACA and PRKABC fusions are exclusively found in extrahepatic tumors, EGFR, ERBB3, and PTEN mutations occur more frequently in gallbladder cancers. It has been reported that up to 83% of biliary tract cancers have clinically relevant and potentially actionable alterations [32].

The heterogeneity between different biliary tract cancers provides a strong rationale for the development of personalized molecularly targeted therapy. Ideally, treatment should be selected based upon a patient's tumor molecular profile to optimize the therapeutic benefit and to minimize unnecessary toxicity. However, moving beyond the current model of "one-size-fits all," systemic chemotherapy is challenging. Next-generation sequencing studies require core needle biopsies, whereas current biliary tract cancer biopsies are often limited to fine-needle aspirations and cytology [31]. Variation and redundancy in tumor pathways calls into the following questions: What is the right target, and is this a relevant molecular alteration in tumor proliferation [33]? Ongoing clinical trials are evaluating the effect of specific molecularly targeted therapies in biliary tract cancers. Here, we explore known molecular alterations and the targeted therapies currently under investigation.

Epidermal Growth Factor Receptor (EGFR)/HER2 and Its Signaling Pathways

The EGFR family of tyrosine kinase receptors is made of ERBB1–ERBB4 [34]. Binding of EGFR activates downstream signaling pathways important in cell differentiation, proliferation, migration, angiogenesis, and survival.

Alterations in ERBB1 (EGFR) and ERBB2 (HER2) and its downstream signaling cascades have been implicated in cholangiocarcinoma carcinogenesis [35]. EGFR and HER2 overexpression has been reported in up to 27% and 25% of biliary tract tumors, respectively [27, 31, 36]. The majority of EGFR and HER2 overexpression is due to copy number gains and rarely due to activating mutations [25]. HER2 mutations are much more common in extrahepatic and gallbladder cancers compared to intrahepatic cancers [27, 29, 31, 37]. Data suggest that EGFR overexpression is a risk factor for disease recurrence and may have prognostic significance in intrahepatic cholangiocarcinoma [36].

Completed randomized studies have not shown a benefit to targeting EGFR thus far. To date, randomized studies adding cetuximab [38, 39], erlotinib [40], or panitumumab [41] to gemcitabine and oxaliplatin have not shown an improvement in PFS or OS over chemotherapy alone. Of these studies, only one phase III study has been reported, which randomized 133 patients with metastatic biliary tract cancer to gemcitabine and oxaliplatin with or without erlotinib, an anti-EGFR tyrosine kinase inhibitor [40]. While the addition of erlotinib significantly improved objective response, it did not improve survival (median OS of 9.5 months in both arms). A subgroup analyses found that the addition of erlotinib significantly prolonged median PFS by 2.9 months [5.9 versus 3.0 months, HR 0.73 (95% CI 0.53–1.00, p 0.049)] in cholangiocarcinoma.

As KRAS mutations are known to predict resistance to EGFR inhibitors in colorectal cancer, studies have evaluated the role of KRAS as a biomarker in biliary tract cancers [27, 42, 43]. While limited retrospective data suggest that KRAS mutation is a biomarker of poor prognosis in biliary tract cancers [42], it has yet to be seen in prospective data. A KRAS mutation-stratified phase II study of gemcitabine and oxaliplatin with or without cetuximab found that KRAS mutation status did not correlate with ORR or PFS [44]. Similarly, in a randomized phase II trial of KRAS wild-type advanced biliary tract cancer, panitumumab in combination with gemcitabine and oxaliplatin demonstrated a nonsignificant improvement in PFS (5.3 versus 4.4 months, p 0.27) without any differences in OS (9.9 versus 10.2 months, p 0.42) over chemotherapy alone [41]. Subgroup analyses suggested that the addition of panitumumab may improve survival in KRAS wild-type intrahepatic cholangiocarcinoma (15.1 versus 11.8 months, p 0.13).

Although prospective data on targeting HER2 in biliary tract cancer is limited, preclinical data and case series suggest a possible role for anti-HER2 therapy in gallbladder cancer. In animal models, HER2 overexpression in the gallbladder epithelium led to gallbladder cancer and cholangiocarcinoma in 100% and 30% of transgenic mice, respectively [45]. A case series showed that patients with gallbladder cancer and HER2 amplification or overexpression achieved stable disease ($n = 3$), partial ($n = 4$), or complete responses ($n = 1$) with HER2-directed therapy (trastuzumab, lapatinib, or pertuzumab) [46]. To date, two completed phase II studies of lapatinib, a dual-HER and EGFR inhibitor, in biliary tract cancer found no response [47, 48]. However, one study did not report HER2 status, and the other found no HER2 mutations or overexpression in its enrolled patients. MyPathway is an ongoing phase IIA multi-basket study evaluating targeted therapies in tumors harboring relevant genetic alterations [49]. Its preliminary data indicate that pertuzumab and trastuzumab have activity in 11 patients with HER2-positive biliary cancer with 4 patients achieving partial response and 3 patients achieving stable disease.

Given the lack of association between KRAS status and response to EGFR inhibitors, the search for other predictive biomarkers is currently underway. A retrospective study evaluating ROS1, ALK, and c-MET (RAM) expression levels in advanced biliary tract cancer showed that chemotherapy plus cetuximab in tumors with low expression levels (IHC <3+ for all markers) was associated with an improved disease control rate (68% versus 41%, p 0.044), PFS (7.3 versus 4.9 months, p 0.026), and a nonsignificant improvement in OS (14.1 versus 9.6 months, p 0.056) compared to chemotherapy alone [50]. Implementing randomized studies with biomarker-defined subgroups will be important in evaluating potential biomarkers such as RAM expression in predicting response to EGFR inhibitors in biliary tract cancer.

Vascular Endothelial Growth Factor (VEGF)

The VEGF family includes potent factors critical in angiogenesis and vascular permeability [51]. Binding of VEGF to its receptors promotes tumor growth and metastasis [36]. VEGF overexpression has been reported in up to 60% of biliary tract cancer and has been associated with poor survival, disease recurrence, and metastasis [29, 36, 52].

Anti-VEGF agents aim to normalize tumor vasculature structure and function in a process termed vasculature normalization [51]. In addition, the combination of cytotoxic drugs and anti-VEGF agents may enhance the delivery of cytotoxic drugs to tumor cells. Various VEGF and VEGFR inhibitors have been evaluated in biliary tract cancer. To date, bevacizumab [53, 54], cediranib [55], sorafenib [56–59], sunitinib [60], and vandetanib [61] studies have not demonstrated a clear benefit to targeting VEGF or VEGFR.

Bevacizumab, a recombinant humanized monoclonal antibody against VEGF, has been studied in the phase II setting in biliary tract cancer. Bevacizumab has been combined with gemcitabine-oxaliplatin, erlotinib, and gemcitabine-capecitabine to result in a PFS and OS of 4–8 months and 10–13 months, respectively [53, 54, 62]. The combination of gemcitabine-oxaliplatin and bevacizumab yielded promising results with an overall response rate of 40% and a median PFS and OS of 7.0 and 12.7 months, respectively [53]. However, the 6-month PFS rate of 63% failed to meet its predefined endpoint of 70%. Other studies with bevacizumab showed results similar to that with standard chemotherapy. Gemcitabine-capecitabine and bevacizumab as first-line treatment for advanced biliary tract cancer noted a median PFS and OS of 8.1 months and 11.3 months, respectively [54].

Sorafenib [56–59], sunitinib [60], and vandetanib [61] have not demonstrated benefit in biliary tract cancer with response rates mostly less than 10% as monotherapy or combination therapy. Cediranib, a potent inhibitor of VEGFR, was evaluated in a phase II study that randomized patients to gemcitabine-cisplatin plus cediranib or placebo [55]. While the cediranib arm showed a higher ORR (43% versus 19%, p 0.004) and a trend toward higher OS (14.1 versus 11.9 months, HR 0.76, p 0.19) compared to the placebo arm, no significant difference was found in PFS (7.7 versus 7.4 months, HR 0.99, p 0.95).

Biomarkers that predict response to VEGF or VEGFR inhibition remain to be investigated. Increased levels of PDGFbb have been associated with a benefit from cediranib in biliary tract cancer [55]. Randomized phase III trials evaluating the efficacy of bevacizumab in combination with biomarker analyses suggest that plasma VEGF-A, expression of neuropilin-1, and tumor or plasma VEGFR1 levels may be strong biomarker candidates for predicting response to antiangiogenic agents [63].

Fibroblast Growth Factor Receptor (FGFR) 2 Fusions

The fibroblast growth factor receptor (FGFR 1-4) family of tyrosine kinase receptors activate downstream signaling pathways important in cell proliferation, differentiation, migration, and angiogenesis [29, 31, 64]. Various FGFR2 gene fusions have been identified almost exclusively in intrahepatic cholangiocarcinoma in up to 16% of tumors [27, 29, 31]. In addition, it is associated with female predilection, younger age, relatively indolent disease, and improved survival compared with biliary tumors without FGFR2 fusions [43, 65].

Preliminary antitumor activity was initially seen in patients with FGFR2-MGEA5 and FGFR2-TACC3 fusion with intrahepatic cholangiocarcinoma treated with ponatinib and pazopanib [66]. These promising results have served as the premise for targeting FGFR fusion kinase in biliary tract cancers. While a vast array of anti-FGFR agents have been developed, small molecule kinase inhibitors remain the largest class of agents. FGFR-selective small molecule kinase inhibitors such as BGJ398 [67], ARQ087 (NCT01752920), AZD4547 (NCT00979134), and JNJ42756493 (NCT01703481) are being investigated in mechanism-driven phase I trials of advanced solid tumors with FGFR genetic alterations. One exception is BGJ398, which is being evaluated in an ongoing phase II study of patients with FGFR-altered refractory advanced cholangiocarcinoma [67]. Initial data shows an impressive antitumor activity with an overall disease control rate of 82%.

FGFR nonselective small molecule kinase inhibitors such as ponatinib, pazopanib, lenvatinib, dovitinib, and regorafenib are being investigated in phase I and II studies [64]. Prolonged stable disease has been reported in a phase I study of pazopanib and gemcitabine in a patient with cholangiocarcinoma [68]. Ongoing single-arm phase II studies are evaluating the efficacy of first-line gemcitabine and pazopanib (NCT01855724), second-line regorafenib (NCT02053376, NCT02115542), and second-line ponatinib (NCT02265341) in advanced biliary cancer. Of these studies, only the ponatinib study specifies confirmation of advanced biliary cancer with FGFR2 gene fusions or FGFR pathway alterations as part of its inclusion criteria. A separate phase II study evaluating the efficacy of ponatinib in advanced solid tumors harboring FGFR genetic alterations is currently ongoing (NCT02272998).

Many small molecule kinase inhibitors lack specificity and exhibit significant off-target activity [69]. The resultant off-target toxicities may limit their use in clinical practice. Future development of FGFR-specific kinase inhibitors may help overcome these challenges. Other anti-FGFR agents such as monoclonal antibodies are in early clinical development [64]. Studies that evaluate combination therapies with single- or dual-target inhibition may hold significant promise given the genomic heterogeneity seen in cholangiocarcinoma. One such example is an ongoing phase I trial evaluating the combination of pazopanib and trametinib, a MEK inhibitor, in patients with advanced solid tumors [70].

Isocitrate Dehydrogenase (IDH) 1/IDH2 Mutations

IDH is an enzyme that converts isocitrate to alpha-ketoglutarate [4, 71, 72]. Mutations in IDH lead to the production of D-2-hydroxyglutarate (D-2-HG), an oncometabolite that inhibits alpha-ketoglutarate-dependent enzymes important in DNA methylation, epigenetic regulation, and cell signaling. IDH mutations promote biliary tract cancer development by deregulating hepatocyte nuclear factor 4α and blocking hepatocyte differentiation [73]. IDH mutations have been reported in up to 24% of intrahepatic cholangiocarcinoma and are rare in extrahepatic tumors [27, 43, 74].

Inhibitors of IDH1 (AG-120, IDH-305), IDH2 (AG-221), and pan-IDH1/2 (AG-881) are in clinical development. Preliminary results of a phase 1 study of AG-120 in IDH1 mutation-positive solid tumors are promising [75]. Of 20 patients with intrahepatic cholangiocarcinoma, 1 patient achieved partial response and 11 patients had stable disease. The clinical benefit rate, defined as lack of progression for at least 6 months, was 43% in cholangiocarcinoma and 37% in all patients. Phase I studies of AG-221 (NCT02273739), IDH-305 (NCT02381886), and AG-881 (NCT02481154) in patients with IDH-mutated advanced solid tumors are underway.

An ongoing phase III placebo-controlled study is evaluating AG-120 in previously treated cholangiocarcinoma with an IDH1 mutation (NCT02989857).

Biomarkers and alternative methods to determine response to IDH inhibitors remain areas of ongoing research. As IDH inhibitors promote tumor cell differentiation rather than direct cell death, traditional imaging-based response criteria such as RECIST may not be optimal in assessing treatment response [72]. As D-2-HG is significantly higher in patients with IDH-mutated tumors compared to those with wild-type IDH, studies are investigating the use of serum D-2-HG as a biomarker in determining disease burden and treatment response in IDH-mutated tumors [72, 76].

C-MET/Hepatocyte Growth Factor (HGF)

C-MET is a proto-oncogene that encodes a tyrosine kinase growth factor receptor called HGF receptor [77]. Binding to the HGF receptor activates multiple signaling pathways involved in proliferation, motility, migration, and invasion [77]. Alterations in c-Met are linked to tumor invasion, angiogenesis, differentiation, and proliferation [78]. C-MET overexpression has been observed in up to 60% of intrahepatic and up to 70% of extrahepatic cholangiocarcinoma [43]. It is associated with poor prognosis in intrahepatic cholangiocarcinoma and may contribute to resistance to EGFR inhibitors [77, 79].

The efficacy of c-MET inhibitors in cholangiocarcinoma remains to be seen. A number of phase I studies have evaluated tivantinib, a selective c-MET inhibitor, in advanced solid tumors (NCT00302172, NCT00612209, NCT00612703, NCT00802555, NCT00827177, NCT00874042). Encouraging clinical activity with a disease control rate of 82% was observed in 11 patients with biliary tract cancer treated with tivantinib in different phase 1 studies [80]. Stable disease, partial response, and complete response were seen in 8 (73%), 1 (9%), and 0 (0%) patients with biliary tract cancer, respectively. In a phase II study of cabozantinib, a dual VEGFR and c-MET inhibitor, in advanced cholangiocarcinoma, showed limited activity and significant toxicity in unselected patients [81]. A planned correlative study found tumor MET overexpression (2+ or 3+ by IHC) in 4 of 10 patients with sufficient tissue for testing. Although one patient with 3+ tumor MET expression stayed on treatment for 278 days, MET expression by immunohistochemistry did not correlate with PFS (p 0.38) or OS (p 0.17) in the 10 patients evaluated. Ongoing studies of MET inhibitors in cholangiocarcinoma are underway. A double-blind, randomized phase II trial is evaluating gemcitabine and cisplatin plus either VEGFR inhibitor ramucirumab, c-MET inhibitor merestinib, or placebo in advanced biliary tract cancer [82]. A phase 1 study is evaluating merestinib in advanced solid tumors including cholangiocarcinoma (NCT01285037).

C-MET-driven patient selection may be the key to response in c-MET-targeted therapies. Characterizing c-Met alterations with consistent and validated methods is needed. Detecting c-MET overexpression via immunohistochemistry is likely to vary widely as different IHC detection antibodies target different c-MET domains [83]. Defining those antibodies specific to detecting c-MET expression is a necessary step in developing accurate predictive biomarkers.

Mitogen-Activated ERK Kinase (MEK) Pathway

The RAS/RAF/MEK/ERK pathway (also known as the MAPK/ERK pathway) is one of the key signaling pathways in normal cell proliferation, survival, and differentiation [84, 85]. In this pathway, multiple signals activate RAS (KRAS, NRAS, HRAS), which sequentially turns on RAF (BRAF, CRAF, and ARAF), MEK (MEK1, MEK2), and ERK kinases. Importantly, RAS is the most frequently mutated oncogene in human cancers with KRAS mutations reported in up to 60% of cholangiocarcinoma [43]. KRAS mutations are more common in hilar tumors compared to intrahepatic tumors and are associated with poor prognosis [42]. Mutations in BRAF, the RAF isoform, are also highly oncogenic and have been found in up to 22% of cholangiocarcinoma [31, 43, 86].

MEK inhibitors are showing promising activity in phase I/II studies. The MEK1/MEK2 inhibitor selumetinib was evaluated in a phase II study in 28 patients with advanced biliary tract cancer [87]. While the overall response rate was only 12%, 17 patients (68%) had stable disease leading to a disease control rate of 80% [87]. Of those patients with stable disease, 44% had stable disease for at least 4 months and 12% had stable disease for >1 year. In the ABC-04 phase 1b study of selumetinib in combination with gemcitabine-cisplatin in advanced biliary tract cancer, eight patients were evaluable for objective response: three patients achieved partial response, and eight patients achieved stable disease; median PFS was 6.4 months [88]. Another MEK1/MEK2 inhibitor binimetinib was evaluated in combination with gemcitabine-cisplatin in a phase I study in untreated advanced biliary cancer [89]. Of the 12 enrolled patients, partial response and stable disease were seen in 6 (50%) and 4 (33%) patients, respectively, and median PFS and OS were 6.4 and 9.1 months, respectively. Significant activity with prolonged and complete response has been reported in the phase I/II study of the MEK1/MEK2 inhibitor MEK162 in combination with gemcitabine-cisplatin in untreated advanced biliary cancer [90]. Of the 35 patients included in the phase II analysis, median PFS and OS were 6 and 21 months, respectively. The overall response rate was 36% with 2 patients achieving a CR and remaining on study for over 24 months. A number of ongoing studies are evaluating trametinib (NCT02042443, NCT02034110), selumetinib (NCT02151084), and MEK162 (NCT01828034, NCT02773459) in biliary tract cancer.

PI3K/AKT/mTOR Pathway

The PI3K signaling pathway regulates cell growth and survival. It remains one of the most dysregulated pathways in cancer, where it is critical in tumor metabolism, growth, and survival [91]. Increased PI3K signaling can be caused by mutations or amplifications of key signaling components or loss of PTEN [92]. It can also be due to genetic alterations of upstream receptor tyrosine kinases. Aberrant PI3K pathway activation has been implicated in gallbladder tumorigenesis [93]. In addition, preclinical data suggest that the combination of PTEN loss and KRAS activation results in rapid biliary tumorigenesis [94].

PI3K inhibitors are in early clinical development. Several phase I studies have evaluated BKM120, an oral PI3K inhibitor in advanced solid tumors [95–98]. BKM120 was combined with mFOLFOX6 in 17 patients with refractory solid tumors [98]. Of those patients evaluable for response, one patient with intrahepatic cholangiocarcinoma sustained stable disease for 26 weeks. The study reported significant toxicity with 76% of patients experiencing grade 3/4 adverse events, most commonly cytopenias, fatigue, and hyperglycemia. Another study of BKM120 monotherapy, which included 1 patient with gallbladder cancer, had 7 patients (20%) on therapy for at least 8 months [96].

Everolimus, a mTOR inhibitor, has been studied in both the frontline and refractory settings in advanced biliary tract cancer. In a phase II study in 39 patients with refractory biliary tract cancer, although the ORR was only 5.1%, DCR was 44.7% with 1 patient achieving a partial response at 2 months and 1 patient sustaining a complete response for 8 months [99]. Median PFS and OS were 3.2 and 7.7 months, respectively. Of note, 32.4% and 25% of patients who remained alive after the first month of treatment were alive after 12 and 15 months of therapy, respectively. Everolimus monotherapy as first-line treatment in advanced biliary tract cancer showed DCR, median PFS, and OS of 56%, 6.0 months, 9.5 months, respectively [100]. A biomarker-driven trial evaluated everolimus in PIK3CA altered and/or PTEN loss advanced refractory solid tumors [101]. Although the study did not demonstrate antitumor activity with everolimus, it included one patient with cholangiocarcinoma who achieved disease control.

Immunotherapy

The immune system can detect and destroy abnormal cells via tumor-specific or tumor-associated antigens (TAA) to prevent the development of cancer [35]. However, cancer cells can sometimes avoid detection and destruction by the immune system by reducing TAA expression or suppressing the host immune response. As some immune cells retain the ability to detect and invade tumor, the characteristics of immune infiltration have been studied in various cancers. Tumor infiltration by mediators of the adaptive immune response has been correlated with better prognosis in biliary tract cancer [102]. The presence of dendritic cells, CD4+ T cells, CD8+ T cells, or plasma cells within the biliary tumor is predictive of improved OS [103–106].

Immunotherapies aim to strengthen the immune response against cancer cells. Manipulation of the immune response has historically involved vaccination, autologous cell transfer, and immunomodulatory therapy [107]. To date, the completed clinical trials of immunotherapy in biliary tract cancer have mostly involved peptide-based or dendritic cell-based vaccines to sensitize the immune system against TAA.

While peptide-based vaccines have yet to show definite efficacy, dendritic cell-based vaccines appear efficacious against biliary tract cancer. In a phase I/II study of anti-MUC1 dendritic cell-based vaccine as adjuvant therapy in resected pancreatic and biliary tumors, 4 of 12 patients are alive and without evidence of disease recurrence after 4 years [108]. Of these patients, one patient had resected intrahepatic cholangiocarcinoma. In a retrospective study of anti-WT1 and/or anti-MUC1 dendritic cell-based vaccine in 65 patients with biliary tract cancer, the median survival time after the first vaccination was significantly higher with chemotherapy than without chemotherapy (8.2 versus 5.3 months, p 0.016) [109].

Adoptive autologous cell transfer, where patient's own lymphocytes are used after an ex vivo "priming" event, has been applied to biliary tract cancer therapy with clinical efficacy [107]. In a proof-of-concept study, whole-exome sequencing was used to isolate, expand, and reintroduce tumor-infiltrating lymphocytes (TILs) to treat a 43-year-old woman with poorly differentiated intrahepatic cholangiocarcinoma [110]. After identifying an ERBB2-interacting protein mutation (ERBB2IP^{E805G}) that was recognized by a subpopulation of CD4+ TILs, the patient received an infusion of TILs with 25% ERBB2IP^{E805G}-reactive TILs after nonmyeloid ablative chemotherapy. Tumor regression was observed after 2 months, and stable disease was reported for over 12 months. Later on, after disease progression, tumor regression was again achieved with a second dose of TILs with 95% ERBB2IP^{E805G}-reactive TILs. In another study that investigated adjuvant immunotherapy with vaccine and activated T-cell transfer in intrahepatic cholangiocarcinoma, median PFS and OS were significantly higher with adjuvant immunotherapy at 18.3 and 31.9 months, respectively, compared to surgery alone at 7.7 and 17.4 months, respectively (p 0.005 and 0.022, respectively) [111].

Immunomodulatory therapy is not well studied in biliary tract cancer. Interim results of KEYNOTE-028 of pembrolizumab in advanced biliary tract cancer reported an ORR 17% with 4 (17%) patients achieving a partial response and 4 (17%) patients maintaining stable disease [112]. In addition to promising antitumor activity, a subset of patients achieved durable responses of >40 weeks. Studies with immunomodulatory agents such as pembrolizumab (KEYNOTE-158, NCT02703714), nivolumab (NCT02829918), ipilimumab plus nivolumab (NCT01853618, NCT02834013), and tremelimumab plus durvalumab (NCT02821754) in biliary tract cancer are underway.

Conclusion

Biliary tract cancer is a heterogeneous group of rare and aggressive cancers. Due to the high incidence of advanced and recurrence disease, along with the suboptimal response to conventional chemotherapy, prognosis remains poor. Advances in genomic profiling have begun to shed light on the diverse genomic landscape of this disease and its multiple targetable alterations. Much work remains in investigating predictive and prognostic biomarkers and determining the efficacy of targeted agents. Future studies that incorporate molecular profiling and correlative studies will be necessary if we want to better understand and change the trajectory of this disease.

References

1. Edge SB, American Joint Committee on Cancer, American Cancer Society, editors. AJCC cancer staging handbook: from the AJCC cancer staging manual. 7th ed. New York: Springer; 2010. 718 p.
2. Banales JM, Cardinale V, Carpino G, Marzioni M, Andersen JB, Invernizzi P, et al. Expert consensus document: cholangiocarcinoma: current knowledge and future perspectives consensus statement from the European Network for the Study of Cholangiocarcinoma (ENS-CCA). Nat Rev Gastroenterol Hepatol. 2016;13(5):261–80.
3. Abou-Alfa GK, Andersen JB, Chapman W, Choti M, Forbes SJ, Gores GJ, et al. Advances in cholangiocarcinoma research: report from the third cholangiocarcinoma foundation annual conference. J Gastrointest Oncol. 2016;7(6):819–27.
4. Chong DQ, Zhu AX, Chong DQ, Zhu AX. The landscape of targeted therapies for cholangiocarcinoma: current status and emerging targets. Oncotarget. 2016;7(29):46750–67.
5. Anderson CD, Pinson CW, Berlin J, Chari RS. Diagnosis and treatment of cholangiocarcinoma. Oncologist. 2004;9(1):43–57.
6. Anand MGAC, Purl CP, Dhar BA. The value of molecular biomarkers in biliary tract cancer in the era of targeted therapy. J Clin Exp Hepatol. 2011;1(1):2.
7. Park J, Kim M-H, Kim K, Park DH, Moon S-H, Song TJ, et al. Natural history and prognostic factors of advanced cholangiocarcinoma without surgery, chemotherapy, or radiotherapy: a large-scale observational study. Gut Liver. 2009;3(4):298–305.
8. Valle J, Wasan H, Palmer DH, Cunningham D, Anthoney A, Maraveyas A, et al. Cisplatin plus gemcitabine versus gemcitabine for biliary tract cancer. N Engl J Med. 2010;362(14):1273–81.
9. Glimelius B, Hoffman K, Sjödén P-O, Jacobsson G, Sellström H, Enander L-K, et al. Chemotherapy improves survival and quality of life in advanced pancreatic and biliary cancer. Ann Oncol. 1996;7(6):593–600.
10. Benson AB, D'Angelica MI, Abrams TA, Are C, Bloomston PM, Chang DT, et al. Hepatobiliary cancers, version 2.2014. J Natl Compr Cancer Netw. 2014;12(8):1152–82.
11. Okusaka T, Nakachi K, Fukutomi A, Mizuno N, Ohkawa S, Funakoshi A, et al. Gemcitabine alone or in combination with cisplatin in patients with biliary tract cancer: a comparative multicentre study in Japan. Br J Cancer. 2010;103(4):469–74.
12. Valle JW, Furuse J, Jitlal M, Beare S, Mizuno N, Wasan H, et al. Cisplatin and gemcitabine for advanced biliary tract cancer: a meta-analysis of two randomised trials. Ann Oncol. 2014;25(2):391–8.
13. Ulahannan SV, Rahma OE, Duffy AG, Makarova-Rusher OV, Kurtoglu M, Liewehr DJ, et al. Identification of active chemotherapy regimens in advanced biliary tract carcinoma: a review of chemotherapy trials in the past two decades. Hepatic Oncol. 2015;2(1):39.
14. Liu H, Zhang Q-D, Li Z-H, Zhang Q-Q, Lu L-G. Efficacy and safety of gemcitabine-based chemotherapies in biliary tract cancer: a meta-analysis. World J Gastroenterol. 2014;20(47):18001–12.
15. Brieau B, Dahan L, De Rycke Y, Boussaha T, Vasseur P, Tougeron D, et al. Second-line chemotherapy for advanced biliary tract cancer after failure of the gemcitabine-platinum combination: a large multicenter study by the Association des Gastro-Entérologues Oncologues. Cancer. 2015;121(18):3290–7.
16. Lamarca A, Hubner RA, Ryder WD, Valle JW. Second-line chemotherapy in advanced biliary cancer: a systematic review. Ann Oncol. 2014;25(12):2328–38.
17. Walter T, Horgan AM, McNamara M, McKeever L, Min T, Hedley D, et al. Feasibility and benefits of second-line chemotherapy in advanced biliary tract cancer: a large retrospective study. Eur J Cancer. 2013;49(2):329–35.
18. Mansour JC, Aloia TA, Crane CH, Heimbach JK, Nagino M, Vauthey J-N. Hilar cholangiocarcinoma: expert consensus statement. HPB. 2015;17(8):691–9.
19. Mavros MN, Economopoulos KP, Alexiou VG, Pawlik TM. Treatment and prognosis for patients with intrahepatic cholangiocarcinoma: systematic review and meta-analysis. JAMA Surg. 2014;149(6):565–74.
20. Takada T, Amano H, Yasuda H, Nimura Y, Matsushiro T, Kato H, et al. Is postoperative adjuvant chemotherapy useful for gallbladder carcinoma? A phase III multicenter prospective randomized controlled trial in patients with resected pancreaticobiliary carcinoma. Cancer. 2002;95(8):1685–95.
21. Neoptolemos JP, Moore MJ, Cox TF, Valle JW, Palmer DH, McDonald AC, et al. Effect of adjuvant chemotherapy with fluorouracil plus folinic acid or gemcitabine vs observation on survival in patients with resected periampullary adenocarcinoma: the ESPAC-3 periampullary cancer randomized trial. JAMA. 2012;308(2):147–56.
22. Horgan AM, Amir E, Walter T, Knox JJ. Adjuvant therapy in the treatment of biliary tract cancer: a systematic review and meta-analysis. J Clin Oncol. 2012;30(16):1934–40.
23. Ben-Josef E, Guthrie KA, El-Khoueiry AB, Corless CL, Zalupski MM, Lowy AM, et al. SWOG S0809: a phase II intergroup trial of adjuvant capecitabine

and gemcitabine followed by radiotherapy and concurrent capecitabine in extrahepatic cholangiocarcinoma and gallbladder carcinoma. J Clin Oncol Off J Am Soc Clin Oncol. 2015;33(24):2617–22.
24. Stein A, Arnold D, Bridgewater J, Goldstein D, Jensen LH, Klümpen H-J, et al. Adjuvant chemotherapy with gemcitabine and cisplatin compared to observation after curative intent resection of cholangiocarcinoma and muscle invasive gallbladder carcinoma (ACTICCA-1 trial)—a randomized, multidisciplinary, multinational phase III trial. BMC Cancer. 2015;15:564. http://www.ncbi.nlm.nih.gov/pmc/articles/PMC4520064/
25. Andersen JB. Molecular pathogenesis of intrahepatic cholangiocarcinoma. J Hepatobiliary Pancreat Sci. 2015;22(2):101–13.
26. Yoo KH, Kim NKD, Kwon WI, Lee C, Kim SY, Jang J, et al. Genomic alterations in biliary tract cancer using targeted sequencing. Transl Oncol. 2016;9(3):173.
27. Churi CR, Shroff R, Wang Y, Rashid A, Kang HC, Weatherly J, et al. Mutation profiling in cholangiocarcinoma: prognostic and therapeutic implications. PLoS One. 2014;9(12):e115383. http://www.ncbi.nlm.nih.gov/pmc/articles/PMC4275227/
28. Ross JS, Wang K, Gay L, Al-Rohil R, Rand JV, Jones DM, et al. New routes to targeted therapy of intrahepatic cholangiocarcinomas revealed by next-generation sequencing. Oncologist. 2014;19(3):235–42.
29. Lee H, Ross JS. The potential role of comprehensive genomic profiling to guide targeted therapy for patients with biliary cancer. Therap Adv Gastroenterol. 2017;10(6):507–20. https://doi.org/10.1177/1756283X17698090.
30. Jain A, Javle M. Molecular profiling of biliary tract cancer: a target rich disease. J Gastrointest Oncol. 2016;7(5):797.
31. Jain A, Kwong LN, Javle M. Genomic profiling of biliary tract cancers and implications for clinical practice. Curr Treat Options in Oncol. 2016;17(11):58.
32. Lee H, Wang K, Johnson A, Jones DM, Ali SM, Elvin JA, et al. Comprehensive genomic profiling of extrahepatic cholangiocarcinoma reveals a long tail of therapeutic targets. J Clin Pathol. 2016;69(5):403–8.
33. Fisher SB, Fisher KE, Maithel SK. Molecular targeted therapy for biliary tract malignancy: defining the target. Hepatobiliary Surg Nutr. 2012;1(1):53.
34. Sirica AE. Role of ErbB family receptor tyrosine kinases in intrahepatic cholangiocarcinoma. World J Gastroenterol. 2008;14(46):7033.
35. Merla A, Liu KG, Rajdev L. Targeted therapy in biliary tract cancers. Curr Treat Options in Oncol. 2015;16(10):48.
36. Yoshikawa D, Ojima H, Iwasaki M, Hiraoka N, Kosuge T, Kasai S, et al. Clinicopathological and prognostic significance of EGFR, VEGF, and HER2 expression in cholangiocarcinoma. Br J Cancer. 2008;98(2):418–25.
37. Nakamura H, Arai Y, Totoki Y, Shirota T, Elzawahry A, Kato M, et al. Genomic spectra of biliary tract cancer. Nat Genet. 2015;47(9):1003–10.
38. Malka D, Cervera P, Foulon S, Trarbach T, de la Fouchardière C, Boucher E, et al. Gemcitabine and oxaliplatin with or without cetuximab in advanced biliary-tract cancer (BINGO): a randomised, open-label, non-comparative phase 2 trial. Lancet Oncol. 2014;15(8):819–28.
39. Chen L-T, Chen J-S, Chao Y, Tsai C-S, Shan Y-S, Hsu C, et al. KRAS mutation status-stratified randomized phase II trial of GEMOX with and without cetuximab in advanced biliary tract cancer (ABTC): the TCOG T1210 trial. J Clin Oncol. 2013;31(Suppl; abstr):4018. http://meetinglibrary.asco.org/content/116810-132
40. Lee J, Park SH, Chang H-M, Kim JS, Choi HJ, Lee MA, et al. Gemcitabine and oxaliplatin with or without erlotinib in advanced biliary-tract cancer: a multicentre, open-label, randomised, phase 3 study. Lancet Oncol. 2012;13(2):181–8.
41. Leone F, Marino D, Cereda S, Filippi R, Belli C, Spadi R, et al. Panitumumab in combination with gemcitabine and oxaliplatin does not prolong survival in wild-type KRAS advanced biliary tract cancer: a randomized phase 2 trial (Vecti-BIL study). Cancer. 2016;122(4):574–81.
42. Yokoyama M, Ohnishi H, Ohtsuka K, Matsushima S, Ohkura Y, Furuse J, et al. KRAS mutation as a potential prognostic biomarker of biliary tract cancers. Jpn Clin Med. 2016;7:33–9.
43. Javle M, Bekaii-Saab T, Jain A, Wang Y, Kelley RK, Wang K, et al. Biliary cancer: utility of next-generation sequencing for clinical management. Cancer. 2016;122(24):3838–47.
44. Chen JS, Hsu C, Chiang NJ, Tsai CS, Tsou HH, Huang SF, et al. A KRAS mutation status-stratified randomized phase II trial of gemcitabine and oxaliplatin alone or in combination with cetuximab in advanced biliary tract cancer. Ann Oncol. 2015;26(5):943–9.
45. Kiguchi K, Carbajal S, Chan K, Beltrán L, Ruffino L, Shen J, et al. Constitutive expression of ErbB-2 in gallbladder epithelium results in development of adenocarcinoma. Cancer Res. 2001;61(19):6971–6.
46. Javle M, Churi C, Kang HC, Shroff R, Janku F, Surapaneni R, et al. HER2/neu-directed therapy for biliary tract cancer. J Hematol Oncol. 2015;8:58. https://www-ncbi-nlm-nih-gov.proxy1.lib.tju.edu/pmc/articles/PMC4469402/
47. Peck J, Wei L, Zalupski M, O'Neil B, Villalona Calero M, Bekaii-Saab T. HER2/neu may not be an interesting target in biliary cancers: results of an early phase II study with lapatinib. Oncology. 2012;82(3):175–9.
48. Ramanathan RK, Belani CP, Singh DA, Tanaka M, Lenz H-J, Yen Y, et al. A phase II study of lapatinib in patients with advanced biliary tree and hepatocellular cancer. Cancer Chemother Pharmacol. 2009;64(4):777–83.

49. Javle MM, Hainsworth JD, Swanton C, Burris HA, Kurzrock R, Sweeney C, et al. Pertuzumab + trastuzumab for HER2-positive metastatic biliary cancer: preliminary data from MyPathway. J Clin Oncol. 2017;35(Suppl 4S; abstract):402. http://meetinglibrary.asco.org/content/176131-195
50. Chiang N-J, Hsu C, Chen J-S, Tsou H-H, Shen Y-Y, Chao Y, et al. Expression levels of ROS1/ALK/c-MET and therapeutic efficacy of cetuximab plus chemotherapy in advanced biliary tract cancer. Sci Rep. 2016;6:25369. https://www-ncbi-nlm-nih-gov.proxy1.lib.tju.edu/pmc/articles/PMC4853728/
51. Goel S, Duda DG, Xu L, Munn LL, Boucher Y, Fukumura D, et al. Normalization of the vasculature for treatment of cancer and other diseases. Physiol Rev. 2011;91(3):1071–121.
52. Oyasiji T, Zhang J, Kuvshinoff B, Iyer R, Hochwald SN. Molecular targets in biliary carcinogenesis and implications for therapy. Oncologist. 2015;20(7):742.
53. Zhu AX, Meyerhardt JA, Blaszkowsky LS, Kambadakone AR, Muzikansky A, Zheng H, et al. Efficacy and safety of gemcitabine, oxaliplatin, and bevacizumab in advanced biliary-tract cancers and correlation of changes in 18-fluorodeoxyglucose PET with clinical outcome: a phase 2 study. Lancet Oncol. 2010;11(1):48–54.
54. Iyer RV, Groman A, Ma WW, Malhotra U, Iancu D, Grande C, et al. Gemcitabine (G), capecitabine (C) and bevacizumab (BV) in patients with advanced biliary cancers (ABC): final results of a multicenter phase II study. J Clin Oncol. 2015;33(Suppl; abstr):4078. http://meetinglibrary.asco.org/content/148921-156
55. Valle JW, Wasan H, Lopes A, Backen AC, Palmer DH, Morris K, et al. Cediranib or placebo in combination with cisplatin and gemcitabine chemotherapy for patients with advanced biliary tract cancer (ABC-03): a randomised phase 2 trial. Lancet Oncol. 2015;16(8):967–78.
56. Bengala C, Bertolini F, Malavasi N, Boni C, Aitini E, Dealis C, et al. Sorafenib in patients with advanced biliary tract carcinoma: a phase II trial. Br J Cancer. 2010;102(1):68–72.
57. El-Khoueiry AB, Rankin C, Siegel AB, Iqbal S, Gong I-Y, Micetich KC, et al. S0941: a phase 2 SWOG study of sorafenib and erlotinib in patients with advanced gallbladder carcinoma or cholangiocarcinoma. Br J Cancer. 2014;110(4):882.
58. Moehler M, Maderer A, Schimanski C, Kanzler S, Denzer U, Kolligs FT, et al. Gemcitabine plus sorafenib versus gemcitabine alone in advanced biliary tract cancer: a double-blind placebo-controlled multicentre phase II AIO study with biomarker and serum programme. Eur J Cancer. 2014;50(18):3125–35.
59. Lee JK, Capanu M, O'Reilly EM, Ma J, Chou JF, Shia J, et al. A phase II study of gemcitabine and cisplatin plus sorafenib in patients with advanced biliary adenocarcinomas. Br J Cancer. 2013;109(4):915–9.
60. Yi JH, Thongprasert S, Lee J, Doval DC, Park SH, Park JO, et al. A phase II study of sunitinib as a second-line treatment in advanced biliary tract carcinoma: a multicentre, multinational study. Eur J Cancer. 2012;48(2):196–201.
61. Santoro A, Gebbia V, Pressiani T, Testa A, Personeni N, Arrivas Bajardi E, et al. A randomized, multicenter, phase II study of vandetanib monotherapy versus vandetanib in combination with gemcitabine versus gemcitabine plus placebo in subjects with advanced biliary tract cancer: the VanGogh study. Ann Oncol. 2015;26(3):542–7.
62. Lubner SJ, Mahoney MR, Kolesar JL, LoConte NK, Kim GP, Pitot HC, et al. Report of a multicenter phase II trial testing a combination of biweekly bevacizumab and daily Erlotinib in patients with unresectable biliary cancer: a phase II consortium study. J Clin Oncol. 2010;28(21):3491.
63. Lambrechts D, Lenz H-J, de Haas S, Carmeliet P, Scherer SJ. Markers of response for the antiangiogenic agent bevacizumab. J Clin Oncol. 2013;31(9):1219–30.
64. Ang C. Role of the fibroblast growth factor receptor axis in cholangiocarcinoma. J Gastroenterol Hepatol. 2015;30(7):1116–22.
65. Graham RP, Barr Fritcher EG, Pestova E, Schulz J, Sitailo LA, Vasmatzis G, et al. Fibroblast growth factor receptor 2 translocations in intrahepatic cholangiocarcinoma. Hum Pathol. 2014;45(8):1630–8.
66. Borad MJ, Champion MD, Egan JB, Liang WS, Fonseca R, Bryce AH, et al. Integrated genomic characterization reveals novel, therapeutically relevant drug targets in FGFR and EGFR pathways in sporadic intrahepatic cholangiocarcinoma. PLoS Genet. 2014;10(2):e1004135.
67. Javle MM, Shroff RT, Zhu A, Sadeghi S, Choo S, Borad MJ, et al. A phase 2 study of BGJ398 in patients (pts) with advanced or metastatic FGFR-altered cholangiocarcinoma (CCA) who failed or are intolerant to platinum-based chemotherapy. J Clin Oncol. 2016;34(Suppl 4S; abstr):335. http://meetinglibrary.asco.org/content/159420-173
68. Plummer R, Madi A, Jeffels M, Richly H, Nokay B, Rubin S, et al. A phase I study of pazopanib in combination with gemcitabine in patients with advanced solid tumors. Cancer Chemother Pharmacol. 2013;71(1):93–101.
69. Gudernova I, Vesela I, Balek L, Buchtova M, Dosedelova H, Kunova M, et al. Multikinase activity of fibroblast growth factor receptor (FGFR) inhibitors SU5402, PD173074, AZD1480, AZD4547 and BGJ398 compromises the use of small chemicals targeting FGFR catalytic activity for therapy of short-stature syndromes. Hum Mol Genet. 2016;25(1):9–23.
70. Phase I study determining the safety and tolerability of combination therapy with pazopanib, a VEGFR/PDGFR/Raf inhibitor, and GSK1120212, a MEK inhibitor, in advanced solid tumors enriched with patients with advanced differentiated thyroid can-

cer, soft tissue sarcoma, and cholangiocarcinoma—AdisInsight [Internet]. [cited 24 Apr 2017]. http://adisinsight.springer.com/trials/700205728#disabled
71. Dang L, Yen K, Attar EC. IDH mutations in cancer and progress toward development of targeted therapeutics. Ann Oncol. 2016;27(4):599–608.
72. Fujii T, Khawaja MR, DiNardo CD, Atkins JT, Janku F. Targeting isocitrate dehydrogenase (IDH) in cancer. Discov Med. 2016;21(117):373–80.
73. Saha SK, Parachoniak CA, Ghanta KS, Fitamant J, Ross KN, Najem MS, et al. Mutant IDH inhibits HNF-4α to block hepatocyte differentiation and promote biliary cancer. Nature. 2014;513(7516):110–4.
74. Borger DR, Tanabe KK, Fan KC, Lopez HU, Fantin VR, Straley KS, et al. Frequent mutation of isocitrate dehydrogenase (IDH)1 and IDH2 in cholangiocarcinoma identified through broad-based tumor genotyping. Oncologist. 2012;17(1):72–9.
75. Pharmaceuticals A. Agios announces data from dose-escalation phase 1 study of AG-120 in patients with IDH1 mutant positive advanced solid tumors [Internet]. GlobeNewswire News Room. 2015 [cited 25 Apr 2017]. http://globenewswire.com/news-release/2015/11/08/784897/10155627/en/Agios-Announces-Data-from-Dose-Escalation-Phase-1-Study-of-AG-120-in-Patients-with-IDH1-Mutant-Positive-Advanced-Solid-Tumors.html
76. Yen KE, Bittinger MA, Su SM, Fantin VR. Cancer-associated IDH mutations: biomarker and therapeutic opportunities. Oncogene. 2010;29(49):6409–17.
77. Organ SL, Tsao M-S. An overview of the c-MET signaling pathway. Ther Adv Med Oncol. 2011;3(1 Suppl):S7–19.
78. Socoteanu MP, Mott F, Alpini G, Frankel AE. c-Met targeted therapy of cholangiocarcinoma. World J Gastroenterol. 2008;14(19):2990.
79. Miyamoto M, Ojima H, Iwasaki M, Shimizu H, Kokubu A, Hiraoka N, et al. Prognostic significance of overexpression of c-Met oncoprotein in cholangiocarcinoma. Br J Cancer. 2011;105(1):131–8.
80. Chai: 739P| Phase 1 experience of tivantinib in patients...—Google Scholar [Internet]. [cited 27 Apr 2017]. https://scholar.google.com/scholar_lookup?title=Phase%201%20experience%20of%20tivantinib%20in%20patients%20with%20hepatocellular%20carcinoma%20(HCC)%20or%20biliary%20tract%20cancer%20(BTC)&author=Chai,+F.&author=Abbadessa,+G.&author=Savage,+R.&author=Zahir,+H.&author=Chen,+Y.&author=Lamar,+M.&author=Kazakin,+J.&author=Ferrari,+D.&author=von+Roemeling,+R.&author=Schwartz,+B.&publication_year=2012&journal=Ann.+Oncol.&volume=23&pages=245
81. Goyal L, Zheng H, Yurgelun MB, Abrams TA, Allen JN, Cleary JM, et al. A phase 2 and biomarker study of cabozantinib in patients with advanced cholangiocarcinoma. Cancer. 2017;123(11):1979–88.
82. Sama AR, Denlinger CS, Vogel A, He AR, Bousmans N, Zhang W, et al. Gemcitabine and cisplatin plus ramucirumab or merestinib or placebo in first-line treatment for advanced or metastatic biliary tract cancer: a double-blind, randomized phase II trial. J Clin Oncol. 2017;35(Suppl 4S; abstract):TPS509. http://meetinglibrary.asco.org/content/176544-195
83. Zhang Y, Du Z, Zhang M. Biomarker development in MET-targeted therapy. Oncotarget. 2016;7(24):37370–89.
84. Roberts PJ, Der CJ. Targeting the Raf-MEK-ERK mitogen-activated protein kinase cascade for the treatment of cancer. Oncogene. 2007;26(22):3291–310.
85. McArthur G. Exploring the pathway: the RAS/RAF/MEK/ERK pathway in cancer: combination therapies and overcoming feedback [Internet]. ASCO annual meeting. 2015 [cited 27 Apr 2017]. https://am.asco.org/exploring-pathway-rasrafmekerkpathway-cancer-combination-therapies-and-overcoming-feedback
86. Tannapfel A, Sommerer F, Benicke M, Katalinic A, Uhlmann D, Witzigmann H, et al. Mutations of the BRAF gene in cholangiocarcinoma but not in hepatocellular carcinoma. Gut. 2003;52(5):706–12.
87. Bekaii-Saab T, Phelps MA, Li X, Saji M, Goff L, Kauh JSW, et al. Multi-institutional phase II study of selumetinib in patients with metastatic biliary cancers. J Clin Oncol Off J Am Soc Clin Oncol. 2011;29(17):2357–63.
88. Bridgewater J, Lopes A, Beare S, Duggan M, Lee D, Ricamara M, et al. A phase 1b study of Selumetinib in combination with cisplatin and gemcitabine in advanced or metastatic biliary tract cancer: the ABC-04 study. BMC Cancer. 2016;16:153.
89. Lowery MA, O'Reilly EM, Harding JJ, Salehi E, Hollywood E, Bradley M, et al. A phase I trial of binimetinib in combination with gemcitabine (G) and cisplatin (C) patients (pts) with untreated advanced biliary cancer (ABC). J Clin Oncol. 2015;33(Suppl; abstr):e15125. http://meetinglibrary.asco.org/content/152744-156
90. Lowery MA, O'Reilly EM, Harding JJ, Yu KH, Cercek A, Hollywood E, et al. A phase I/II trial of MEK162 in combination with gemcitabine (G) and cisplatin (C) for patients (pts) with untreated advanced biliary cancer (ABC). J Clin Oncol. 2017;35(Suppl 4S; abstract):290. http://meetinglibrary.asco.org/content/177293-195
91. Yuan TL, Cantley LC. PI3K pathway alterations in cancer: variations on a theme. Oncogene. 2008;27(41):5497–510.
92. Courtney KD, Corcoran RB, Engelman JA. The PI3K pathway as drug target in human cancer. J Clin Oncol. 2010;28(6):1075–83.
93. Lunardi A, Webster KA, Papa A, Padmani B, Clohessy JG, Bronson RT, et al. Role of aberrant PI3K pathway activation in gallbladder tumorigenesis. Oncotarget. 2014;5(4):894–900.
94. Marsh V, Davies EJ, Williams GT, Clarke AR. PTEN loss and KRAS activation cooperate in murine biliary tract malignancies. J Pathol. 2013;230(2):165–73.
95. Ando Y, Inada-Inoue M, Mitsuma A, Yoshino T, Ohtsu A, Suenaga N, et al. Phase I dose-escalation

study of buparlisib (BKM120), an oral pan-class I PI3K inhibitor, in Japanese patients with advanced solid tumors. Cancer Sci. 2014;105(3):347–53.
96. Bendell JC, Rodon J, Burris HA, de Jonge M, Verweij J, Birle D, et al. Phase I, dose-escalation study of BKM120, an oral pan-class I PI3K inhibitor, in patients with advanced solid tumors. J Clin Oncol. 2012;30(3):282–90.
97. Rodon J, Braña I, Siu LL, De Jonge MJ, Homji N, Mills D, et al. Phase I dose-escalation and -expansion study of buparlisib (BKM120), an oral pan-class I PI3K inhibitor, in patients with advanced solid tumors. Investig New Drugs. 2014;32(4):670–81.
98. McRee AJ, Sanoff HK, Carlson C, Ivanova A, O'Neil BH. A phase I trial of mFOLFOX6 combined with the oral PI3K inhibitor BKM120 in patients with advanced refractory solid tumors. Investig New Drugs. 2015;33(6):1225–31.
99. Buzzoni R, Pusceddu S, Bajetta E, De Braud F, Platania M, Iannacone C, et al. Activity and safety of RAD001 (everolimus) in patients affected by biliary tract cancer progressing after prior chemotherapy: a phase II ITMO study. Ann Oncol. 2014;25(8):1597–603.
100. Yeung YH, Chionh FJM, Price TJ, Scott AM, Tran H, Fang G, et al. Phase II study of everolimus monotherapy as first-line treatment in advanced biliary tract cancer: RADichol. J Clin Oncol. 2014;32(Suppl; abstr):4101. http://meetinglibrary.asco.org/content/130951-144
101. Kim ST, Lee J, Park SH, Park JO, Park YS, Kang WK, et al. Prospective phase II trial of everolimus in PIK3CA amplification/mutation and/or PTEN loss patients with advanced solid tumors refractory to standard therapy. BMC Cancer. 2017;17:211.
102. Marks EI, Yee NS. Immunotherapeutic approaches in biliary tract carcinoma: current status and emerging strategies. World J Gastrointest Oncol. 2015;7(11):338.
103. Nakakubo Y, Miyamoto M, Cho Y, Hida Y, Oshikiri T, Suzuoki M, et al. Clinical significance of immune cell infiltration within gallbladder cancer. Br J Cancer. 2003;89(9):1736–42.
104. Goeppert B, Frauenschuh L, Zucknick M, Stenzinger A, Andrulis M, Klauschen F, et al. Prognostic impact of tumour-infiltrating immune cells on biliary tract cancer. Br J Cancer. 2013;109(10):2665–74.
105. Takagi S, Miyagawa S-I, Ichikawa E, Soeda J, Miwa S, Miyagawa Y, et al. Dendritic cells, T-cell infiltration, and grp94 expression in cholangiocellular carcinoma. Hum Pathol. 2004;35(7):881–6.
106. Oshikiri T, Miyamoto M, Shichinohe T, Suzuoki M, Hiraoka K, Nakakubo Y, et al. Prognostic value of intratumoral CD8+ T lymphocyte in extrahepatic bile duct carcinoma as essential immune response. J Surg Oncol. 2003;84(4):224–8.
107. Pauff JM, Goff LW. Current progress in immunotherapy for the treatment of biliary cancers. J Gastrointest Cancer. 2016;47(4):351–7.
108. Lepisto AJ, Moser AJ, Zeh H, Lee K, Bartlett D, McKolanis JR, et al. A phase I/II study of a MUC1 peptide pulsed autologous dendritic cell vaccine as adjuvant therapy in patients with resected pancreatic and biliary tumors. Cancer Ther. 2008;6(B):955–64.
109. Kobayashi M, Sakabe T, Abe H, Tanii M, Takahashi H, Chiba A, et al. Dendritic cell-based immunotherapy targeting synthesized peptides for advanced biliary tract cancer. J Gastrointest Surg. 2013;17(9):1609–17.
110. Tran E, Turcotte S, Gros A, Robbins PF, Lu Y-C, Dudley ME, et al. Cancer immunotherapy based on mutation-specific CD4+ T cells in a patient with epithelial cancer. Science. 2014;344(6184):641–5.
111. Shimizu K, Kotera Y, Aruga A, Takeshita N, Takasaki K, Yamamoto M. Clinical utilization of postoperative dendritic cell vaccine plus activated T-cell transfer in patients with intrahepatic cholangiocarcinoma. J Hepatobiliary Pancreat Sci. 2012;19(2):171–8.
112. Bang YJ, Doi T, Braud FD, Piha-Paul S, Hollebecque A, Razak ARA, et al. 525 Safety and efficacy of pembrolizumab (MK-3475) in patients (pts) with advanced biliary tract cancer: interim results of KEYNOTE-028. Eur J Cancer. 2015;51:S112.

Pathological Classification and Surgical Approach to Hepatocellular Adenomas

Safi Dokmak

Risk Factors for HCA

HCA is a benign liver neoplasm that is mainly observed (90%) in young women taking OC [1–5], but it is also rarely observed in men (10%) [6]. In most cases (80–90%), HCA occurs in young women who have been taking OC for many years. Although the exact mechanism of the association between HCA and OC has not been clearly identified, the association is clear because this entity was rarely described before the introduction of OC in the 1970s [1], the incidence of HCA is dose dependent [4, 7] and higher in women taking OC (3–4/100,000) than other women (0.1/100,000) [8, 9], and HCA regresses in some women after OC is withdrawn [10–12]. There are probably many other factors related to the development of HCA. Despite the widespread use of low-content estrogen OC, HCA still exists, but it is more frequent in obese patients and in those with the metabolic syndrome and steatohepatitis [6, 13–18]. Also, genetic alterations may be responsible such as in HNF1A- and β-catenin-mutated HCA [19, 20]. Androgen also plays a role in the pathogenesis of HCA and has been reported in patients with Fanconi anemia treated with androgens, in athletes who have abused steroids, and in patients with high levels of endogenous androgens [21–24]. HCA may also occur in association with certain metabolic diseases such as type 1 glycogen storage disease (GSD) [25–27] and iron overload related to beta-thalassemia or hemochromatosis [28]. In GSD the development of HCA is related to high triglyceride concentrations [27]. Familial cases (HNF1A) have been reported in patients with maturity-onset diabetes type 3 (MODY 3) [29, 30] and the McCune–Albright syndrome [19]. HCA can also occur in patients with hepatic vascular abnormalities such as portosystemic shunts with portal deprivation [31–33], Budd–Chiari syndrome and other vascular diseases [34], and, rarely, cirrhosis [35, 36]. Other rare causes include polycystic ovary syndrome related or not to sodium valproate leading to hyperandrogenemia [37–39], patients with Turner's syndrome receiving growth hormone therapy [40] and Hurler's syndrome with severe immune deficiencies [41], and adults with history of childhood cancer (leukemia) and treated by hematopoietic stem cell transplants with irradiation or estrogen therapy [42].

HCA is rare in men (10%), and androgen use, metabolic syndrome and steatohepatitis, type 1 GSD, and portosystemic shunts with portal deprivation should be systematically searched for.

S. Dokmak
Department of HPB Surgery and Liver Transplantation, Beaujon Hospital, Clichy, France

Assistance Publique Hôpitaux de Paris, Paris, France
e-mail: safi.dokmak@bjn.aphp.fr

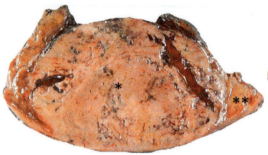 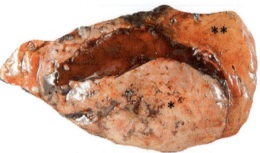

Fig. 12.1 Macroscopic view of a hepatocellular adenoma. Resected specimen showing a non-encapsulated, well-circumscribed tumor (*). Color varies from tan to brown. Congestive and hemorrhagic areas may be seen. The non-tumoral liver (**) appears normal

Clinical Presentation

The mean age at presentation is 37 (16–62), and the mean size is 8.4 cm (±4.2, range: 1–22) [6]. HCA is usually asymptomatic and discovered incidentally during non-related imaging studies, with abnormal liver function tests, or due to nonspecific abdominal pain. Abdominal pain may be present with large or pedunculated HCA. Bleeding usually presents as acute abdominal pain, but hemodynamic instability is rare or is rapidly stabilized with careful treatment. HCA may rarely present with fever, anemia, or pruritus. A single tumor may be present, but multiple tumors (>2 HCA) are more frequently observed [6]. Mild cholestasis or cytolysis is present in two thirds of liver function tests. Alpha-fetoprotein (AFP) should be systematically searched for but is usually normal even when HCA has degenerated. Inflammatory markers (CRP, fibrinogen, and platelets) may be increased with inflammatory HCA [43]. The diagnosis is based on imaging studies including CT scan and MRI [44, 45], and liver biopsy may be necessary in order to confirm the diagnosis or for histological subtyping and management.

Histological Classification

HCA is a soft tumor, and large subcapsular vessels are usually found on macroscopic examination. On cut sections, the tumor is well-delineated, fleshy, and sometimes encapsulated and has a color ranging from white to brown and frequent heterogeneous areas of necrosis and/or hemorrhage (Fig. 12.1). Histologically, HCA consists of a proliferation of benign hepatocytes arranged in a trabecular pattern. However, a normal liver architecture organization is absent. Hepatocytes may have intracellular fat or increased glycogen [46]. However, in the last decade, major progress has been made in the understanding of the histological pathogenesis of the disease, and HCA is no longer considered a single entity. HCA is now classified into at least five histological subtypes with different risks of complication [43, 46, 47].

HNF1A HCA

This subtype is characterized by bi-allelic inactivating mutations of HNF1A (hepatocyte nuclear factor 1 alpha). HNF1A is a key transcription factor that controls several metabolic pathways in the hepatocyte including estrogen metabolism and fatty acid synthesis deregulation with liver fatty acid-binding protein (LFABP), down expression leading to fatty acid accumulation, and steatosis in the tumor hepatocyte. The HNF1A mutation was identified in MODY3 in young patients with a familial context [48] and was later described in some familial cases of adenomatosis and MODY3 [49]. However, adenomatosis is infrequent in MODY3; thus other genetic or environmental factors are probably involved in the development of HCA [47, 50]. The HNF1A subtype is associated with intermediate levels of estrogen exposure [47].

On histology HNF1A is characterized by prominent steatosis associated with an absence of LFABP expression in tumor hepatocytes and high expression in non-tumor hepatocytes [46, 51].

Mutated β-Catenin HCA

This subtype involves mutations of CTNNB1 (protein-coding gene) coding for β-catenin, leading to impaired β-catenin phosphorylation that induces the translocation of β-catenin in the nucleus and expression of Wnt/β-catenin genes such as GLUL (coding for glutamine synthase) and LGR5. These mutations are associated with a higher risk of malignant transformation. These mutations are also observed in colorectal cancer and medulloblastoma. It has recently been shown that mutations on exon 3, but not 7 or 8, are associated with malignancy [47]. These tumors are more related to androgen than estrogen intake, both endogenous and exogenous androgen exposure, and are more frequently observed in men; most HCAs that develop from anabolic steroids are β-catenin mutated [12, 47]. However, women who develop β-catenin HCA have been less exposed to estrogen [47]. Morphologically this subtype is characterized by cellular atypia [52]. Tumor hepatocytes demonstrate strong and homogenous glutamine synthetase positivity (β-catenin target gene) and nuclear expression of β-catenin in some tumor hepatocytes, with high specificity and low sensitivity [52]. These variability and heterogeneity sometimes make the diagnosis difficult by biopsy, and molecular analysis may be needed for an accurate histological diagnosis. For exon 7/exon 8 mutations, glutamine synthetase is less important and heterogeneous, with no β-catenin nuclear staining [53].

Inflammatory HCA

This is the most frequent subtype which is defined by the activation of the IL6/JAK/STAT pathway in tumor hepatocytes with overexpression of acute phase inflammatory proteins such as CRP and SAA. An inflammatory syndrome, anemia and fever, may be observed and is considered to be a paraneoplastic syndrome induced by uncontrolled production of cytokines [43]. Inflammatory HCA can also involve the β-catenin mutation; thus, the Wnt/β-catenin pathway should be searched in the presence of inflammatory HCA. This subgroup is mainly observed in obese patients with extensive exposure to OC [47]. Morphologically these tumors are characterized by the presence of small arteries, inflammatory matrix, and sinusoidal dilatation [54]. Tumor hepatocytes exhibit cytoplasmic expression of SAA and CRP on immunohistochemistry induced by STAT3 activation [46, 51]. They can also contain steatosis and they can be mutated β-catenin [46].

Sonic Hedgehog HCA

The sonic hedgehog mutation (5% of HCA) was recently discovered in the subgroup of unclassified HCA. This mutation results in uncontrolled activation of the sonic hedgehog pathway due to the overexpression of GLI1 [47]. It seems that it is associated with a higher risk of clinical and histological bleeding. It is mainly observed in obese patients with extensive exposure to OC [47].

Unclassified HCA

No genetic alterations can be identified in <10% of HCA.

Radiological Classification

HCAs are usually well-delineated containing fat, vessels, and necrotic or hemorrhagic features. The most marked pathological features are the presence of fat or telangiectatic components; thus, imaging should be fat sensitive (such as MRI) with contrast agents to search for dilated vascular spaces [55]. HCA now includes three subtypes; thus, imaging findings vary depending on the type of HCA.

Steatotic or HNF1A HCA

These HCAs are characterized by the presence of a diffuse and homogeneous signal dropout on chemical shift T1 sequences. This corresponds to fat and is the most marked finding with a high (87–91%) sensitivity and (89–100%) specificity on MRI (Fig. 12.2). These tumors are homogenous and moderately hypervascular and often show washout on portal and/or delayed-phase sequences, while they are hypointense on hepatobiliary phase MRI with hepatospecific contrast agents [56, 57].

Inflammatory HCA

The telangiectatic features of this subtype show a strong, hyperintense signal on T2-weighted sequences, with a diffuse or peripheral (rim-like) image ([58]) and persistent enhancement during the delayed phase that has a high (85–88%) sensitivity and (88–100%) specificity [56, 57]. IHCAs are also markedly hypervascular and heterogeneous (Fig. 12.3). Certain tumors may mimic FNH and be iso- or hyperintense on hepatobiliary phase images with hepatospecific contrast agents [59].

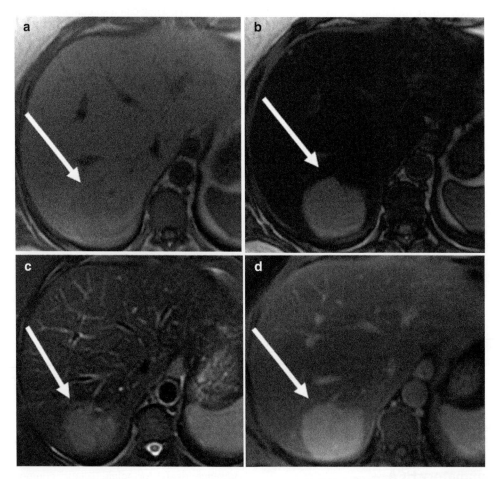

Fig. 12.2 Typical MR imaging appearance of an HNF-1A-inactivated hepatocellular adenoma located in segment 4 in a young female. The lesion appears hyperintense on T1-weighted images (**a**) and shows marked and homogeneous signal dropout on chemical shift images due to the presence of fat (**b**). The fat content is responsible for signal isointensity on T2-weighted images (**c**), mild contrast enhancement on arterial phase images (**d**), and pseudo-washout on delayed-phase images (**e**). The liver parenchyma is normal

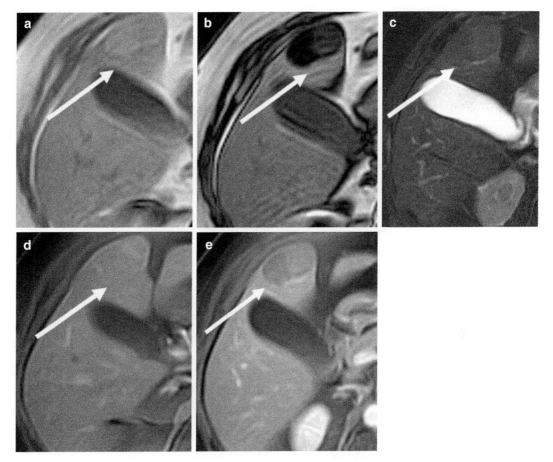

Fig. 12.3 Typical MR imaging appearance of an inflammatory hepatocellular adenoma located in segment 7 in a 37-year-old obese female. The lesion appears isotense on T1-weighted images (arrow in **a**) and does not contain fat (**b**). The lesion shows both signal hyperintensity on T2-weighted images (**c**) and contrast retention on delayed-phase images (**d**). The liver parenchyma is markedly steatotic (**a, b**)

The imaging characteristics of the two other subtypes, β-catenin and unclassified HCA (or classic), are less specific, and the features may be similar to other hepatocellular tumors, mainly arterial enhancement and portal or delayed washout (Fig. 12.4). The content is heterogeneous, but with no features to differentiate them from hepatocellular carcinoma or FNH in relation to β-catenin.

Multiple Adenoma and Adenomatosis

Adenomatosis (>10 HCA) was initially described by Flejou et al. as being more frequent in men with a higher rate of complications [60] and associated with liver steatosis [61]. In fact, multiple HCAs (>2 HCA) are more frequently observed [62] and are not necessarily associated with higher complications. Although we found no clinical difference among the subgroups in a comparison of patients with single or multiple (2–10) [6] HCAs and adenomatosis (>10). Adenomatosis was more frequently associated with microadenomas, obesity, and the steatotic subtype, with a similar risk of complications. The presence of multiple HCAs was not a risk factor for bleeding [6, 63–65]. Thus, management should be based on the size and not the number of tumors [6], limiting the indications for liver transplantation.

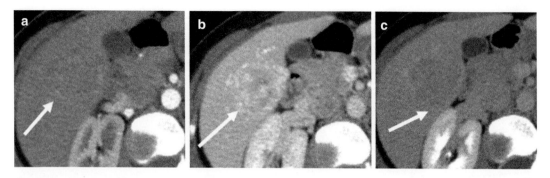

Fig. 12.4 Typical CT appearance of a beta-catenin-activated hepatocellular adenoma in a young female. The lesion shows mild contrast enhancement on arterial phase images (**a**), is heterogeneous on portal venous phase images (**b**), and shows washout on delayed-phase images (**c**). The liver parenchyma is normal. Malignant transformation cannot be excluded. The lesion is indistinguishable from a hepatocellular carcinoma

Risk Factors for Complications

Bleeding

Bleeding is the most frequent complication of HCA, and it may be clinical (acute pain and large zones of bleeding on imaging) or subclinical with small areas of bleeding in HCA discovered on imaging or histology. Although the prevalence of subclinical bleeding is high (30–60%) [6], the clinical impact of this complication is unknown. Clinical bleeding is the most important complication and is observed in 20–25% of cases in surgical series [6, 30, 66]. This may be overestimated because data on prevalence are mainly based on surgical series, which mainly treat complicated HCA. In most cases bleeding HCAs are discovered when the episode of bleeding occurs, and it is less frequent to diagnose bleeding in an observed HCA. The clinical presentation is acute right hypochondrium pain and lower chest pain that can mimic a pulmonary embolism in some patients. Hemodynamic stability must be rapidly obtained following careful reanimation. Bleeding may be intra-tumoral alone with or without parenchymal extension and in 10% of cases associated with intraperitoneal rupture and hemoperitoneum [6]. Biopsy of the viable tissue can be discussed to make certainly the diagnosis of ruptured HCA; however, in patients with complete necrosis at admission, the diagnosis of HCA can be established according to clinical data and prevalence as HCA remains the most frequent cause of liver bleeding in a young female. The main risk factor for bleeding is the presence of inflammatory HCA and tumor size with a 5% risk in HCA < 5 cm and 25% in HCA > 5 cm [6, 63, 66, 67]. Other risk factors are sonic hedgehog HCA [47], exophytic lesions, or lesions located in the left lateral segments and with peripheral arteries visualized on imaging [67], as well as hormone use within the last 6 months [63].

Malignancy

Malignant degeneration is the second complication of HCA. There is no specific clinical or radiological presentation, and in most cases the diagnosis is made following resection. The AFP level is usually normal, and malignant degeneration is suggested in case of rapid growth of an observed or embolized HCA. In clinical practice it may be very difficult to differentiate between malignant HCA and hepatocellular carcinoma (HCC) that develops in a normal liver in young women with or without elevated AFP levels. On histology it can be difficult to differentiate between HCA and well-differentiated HCC, but the presence of both adenomatous tissue and HCC foci is highly suggestive of the diagnosis [68, 69]. The most important risk factors for malignancy are gender and tumor size. The risk of malignant degeneration in men and women is >50% and <5%, respectively [6, 70, 71]. Malignant degeneration is mainly observed in

HCA > 5 cm and has been found in large HCA (>8 cm) [63, 72, 73], but it is rare in HCA < 5 cm [6]. Certain retrospective studies have shown an increased risk of malignancy in β-catenin-mutated HCA [6, 65], but further studies are needed to confirm this, especially because recent results show that only mutations on exon 3 but not those on 7 and 8 are at risk of malignant degeneration [53]. Classic HCAs have an increased risk of malignant degeneration [6].

Risk Factors of Complications by Radiological and Histological Subtypes

Certain retrospective studies have correlated the risk of complications with the new phenotype/genotype classification of HCA [6, 65]. The risk of bleeding is increased in inflammatory HCA, and the risk of malignant degeneration is moderate [6]; steatotic HCAs have a very low risk of bleeding (<10%), and malignant degeneration is rare [6]; β-catenin HCAs with an exon 3 mutation have an estimated risk of malignant degeneration of 20% [6, 65], and the risk of bleeding is increased in sonic hedgehog HCA [47], and the risk of malignant degeneration is also increased in classic HCAs [6]. However, there are no prospective studies on the new subtypes and the risk of complications.

Treatment

When a diagnosis is made, underlying risk factors should be managed in all cases. OC should be stopped [74, 75] and weight loss is suggested because obesity is a risk factor. Encouraging results were recently reported with weight loss alone in obese patients [76]. A period of 6 months was usually needed to observe an effect on tumor size, but it seems that a longer period of OC withdrawal is necessary to obtain a significant reduction. If the tumor does not regress to a size without risk (<5 cm), there are several treatment options including surgical resection, embolization, percutaneous ablation, and, more rarely, liver transplantation.

Non-complicated HCA

In men, HCA should be resected whatever the size due to the high risk of malignant degeneration (>50%). However, in GSD the risk of malignant degeneration is low [26] and has only been reported in case reports [77, 78]. Treatment can be less aggressive, and resection can be limited to large HCA in men with GSD and multiple HCAs. In women, because the risk of complications is mainly observed in HCA > 5 cm, only large HCA (>5 cm) should resected while HCA < 5 cm can be observed.

Indications for Resection Based on the New Classification and the Role of Liver Biopsy

Although the new classification has significantly increased the understanding of the disease, its influence on patient management is still limited because of the absence of valid data. HCA subtyping can be obtained from MRI or liver biopsy, and because the accuracy of MRI for the diagnosis and subtyping of HCA is good [57, 79], the usefulness of biopsy is limited for decision-making; thus, the importance of its role is reduced [80]. Although HNFA1 and inflammatory HCA may be diagnosed on MRI, it is less accurate for the diagnosis of the β-catenin subtype. In men, resection is indicated whatever the subtype, and molecular subtyping can play a role in men with multiple HCAs (such as those with GSD) to prevent unnecessary liver transplantation. In women, HCA >5 cm should be resected whatever the subtype and molecular subtyping should be considered in two cases. First is to diagnose β-catenin mutation in HCA <5 cm. There are no valid data to confirm an increased risk of malignant degeneration in β-catenin-mutated HCA <5 cm, and a preoperative diagnosis may be difficult with liver biopsy because this is made indirectly by measuring glutamine synthetase on immunohistochemistry with a heterogeneity of expression in the nucleus and the cytoplasm [81]. Finally, it was recently demonstrated that only the mutation on exon 3 but not 7 and 8 is associated with malignant degeneration [47]. Thus, in

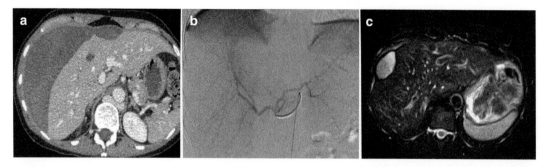

Fig. 12.5 Young female with a long history of oral contraceptive use presented with acute abdominal pain. Bleeding HCA (**a**) with large subcapsular hematoma was diagnosed. After rapid reanimation and stabilization, the patient was treated by embolization. (**b**) A few months later, (**c**) major regression of the hematoma and HCA without any adenomatous tissue. This patient was never operated on and, after a follow-up of 7 years, no recurrence of the disease

our experience management should still be based on gender and size. Second there is a lower risk of complications in steatotic HCA; thus, certain women with large HCA (5–7 cm) may be observed especially if resection is complicated. In these cases, biopsy with molecular subtyping may be needed to confirm the diagnosis of HNF1A [6]. Molecular subtyping may also be systematically performed by biopsy or on the tumor specimen for randomized studies or for the prospective evaluation of liver biopsy.

Bleeding HCA

Stability must be obtained in the presence of hemodynamic instability, and patients should be managed in an intensive care unit [82]. Emergency surgical resection should no longer be performed because this procedure requires a large incision, extended liver resection (resection of HCA and hematoma), and transfusion and is associated with a high morbidity and a long hospital stay [6]. Considerable mortality (12.5%) has been reported following emergency resection [83], and modern management includes stabilization with or without transfusion, arterial embolization, and delayed surgical resection [84–87]. In case of urgent surgery, packing is preferred to liver resection to decrease morbidity and mortality [84]. Delayed resection is performed 3–4 months following embolization once the parenchymal hematoma has disappeared. This is the best surgical strategy because in some cases resection can be performed by laparoscopic approach including minor liver resection, which is associated with less transfusion, reduced morbidity, and a shorter hospital stay. In certain patients with complete necrosis on imaging, simple observation can be an option and bleeding may result in a spontaneous cure of HCA (Fig. 12.5). Observation can also be proposed if bleeding HCAs are not completely necrotic but have downsized to <5 cm because recurrent bleeding in the same HCA is rare.

Indications for Embolization in Bleeding HCA

The indications for arterial embolization are not well known; however, embolization should be systematically performed in unstable patients, in those with severe deglobulization, and if an arterial blush is seen on imaging. Systematic embolization can also be discussed to stop bleeding, to increase the rate of necrosis (to avoid delayed resection), and to downsizing HCA to <5 cm. Repeat embolization to control recurrent bleeding is rare.

Malignant HCA

If a malignant degeneration is suspected preoperatively (rapid growth, slight elevation of AFP, satellites nodules), anatomical liver resection is recommended similar to HCC, especially in a normal liver, making major liver resection safe. If the diagnosis is made postoperatively, there is no need for additional surgery if the resection is performed with free surgical margins because the risk of satellite nodules or vascular invasion is rare [6]. On the other hand, if resection is not satisfactory or is incomplete, we suggest a second intervention for complete resection.

Surgical Resection

When possible the laparoscopic approach should be the standard procedure because HCA is a benign disease in young women with long-term parietal benefits. The advantages of the laparoscopic approach for morbidity and hospital stay were recently reported compared to open surgery in a large French and European multicentric study on 533 resected HCA [88]. Resection with margins of a few millimeters is sufficient, but care should be taken in some patients because it can be difficult to differentiate between adenomatous tissue and the normal liver parenchyma.

Indications for Other Procedures (Ablation and Embolization)

Although embolization is the first choice for bleeding HCA, its role in non-bleeding HCA is a subject of debate. Many retrospective studies have shown a significant decrease in the size of non-bleeding HCA following classic [89, 90] or bland embolization [91]. For some authors this treatment is mainly effective in patients with multiple and small HCA (<3 cm) [72] and in those with adenomatosis [92]. We feel that this treatment is not effective in non-bleeding HCA, and further studies are needed, especially because embolization can result in severe necrosis on the normal liver. Ablation by radiofrequency and more rarely by microwave [93] has already been described with good results [94–99] and a low recurrence rate [96, 97]. However, in most of those studies, ablation was performed on small HCA <5 cm for which general treatment is not needed. However, ablation can be an interesting option for the treatment of limited size HCA (4–5 cm) during pregnancy [100], recurrence after resection [96], difficult intraoperative locations or the need for major liver resection [98], and for small β-catenin-mutated HCA.

Indications for Liver Transplantation

One of the major advantages of the clinical comprehension and genotype phenotype classification (risk factors for complications) of HCA is to limit the indications for liver transplantation, which is therefore rare [62]. In the European Liver Transplant Registry, only 49 liver transplantations were performed between 1986 and 2013 for liver adenomatosis [101]. In women with multiple HCA, only HCA >5 cm should be resected, and remnant HCA <5 cm remains stable in most cases. It should be noted that with the routine and frequent use of modern imaging for abdominal complaints, massive adenomatosis with large HCA involving both liver lobes [102] has become rare. Liver transplantation should only be indicated in symptomatic uncontrolled GSD with multiple HCA [103], men with multiple HCA except GSD (because the risk of malignant degeneration is low), recurrent HCA many years after resection of degenerated HCA, and in patients in which liver resection is a risk due to vascular anomalies [104] (HCA and portacaval shunt) or the presence of underlying liver disease such Budd–Chiari syndrome or other chronic liver diseases.

Pregnancy

Normally pregnancy was contraindicated in patients with HCA due to the risk of disease progression and rupture and reports of maternal and fetal mortality [105]. However, the natural history of HCA from diagnosis to treatment has completely changed in the last 15 years, and

HCA is no longer considered to be a contraindication to pregnancy. We followed 15 pregnancies in 11 women including 9 with residual HCA. HCA did not recur in any of the women without residual HCA (six pregnancies), and two of those with residual HCA ($n = 9$) experienced moderate progression but with no complications. In another study, 17 pregnancies were followed in 12 women with HCA < 5 cm. Progression occurred in four cases, requiring a cesarean in two (>34 weeks) and preventive percutaneous ablation [106]. When the diagnosis of HCA is known before pregnancy (primary diagnosis or residual HCA after resection), it is recommended to treat HCA including those between 3 and 5 cm, and percutaneous ablation could probably play a role in these cases. When the diagnosis is made during pregnancy, the patients with HCA <5 cm can be monitored by ultrasound every 2–3 months and closely observed in HCA >5 cm. In case of disease progression, treatment and indications depend upon the size of HCA and the week of gestation. Surgery should be avoided and replaced by percutaneous ablation or embolization. OC use is not absolutely contraindicated, and low-estrogen content OC or progestative OC can be used once HCA has been managed and the effect of OC withdrawal has been observed on the size of HCA, especially if there are gynecological indications for this treatment.

Follow-Up

After resection of a single HCA, new HCA (<3 cm) may develop in 10–15% of cases, but the patient can be considered cured. After incomplete resection, residual HCA has been shown to progress in 15% and regress in 9% [6, 64, 72, 74]. Follow-up should be mainly radiological, preferable with MRI, but ultrasound can be performed if only the size must be followed. After diagnosis or management, a yearly CT scan or MRI and even ultrasound is sufficient following diagnosis and management. After 5 years and in case of stability, imaging study can be done every 2 years for 5 years, and follow-up may be discontinued after the age of 50 (menopause) because changes are rare after this age. In a recent study, radiological follow-up in 48 women with HCA in the postmenopausal period showed undetectable lesions (44%), stability (33%), or significant regression (19%); thus, follow-up can be discontinued in the postmenopausal period [107]. In all cases, it is very rare to observe complications of residual HCA or newly developed HCA.

Acknowledgments The author would like to thank Dr. Maxime Ronot (Department of Radiology, Beaujon Hospital, Clichy, France) and Dr. Nicolas Pote (Department of Pathology, Beaujon Hospital, Clichy, France) for providing us the radiological (Figs. 12.2, 12.3 and 12.4) and pathological (Fig. 12.1) illustrations and Dr. Roche-Lebrec for her editorial assistance and correction of the article.

References

1. Baum JK, Bookstein JJ, Holtz F, Klein EW. Possible association between benign hepatomas and oral contraceptives. Lancet. 1973;2:926–9.
2. Rooks JB, Ory HW, Ishak KG, Strauss LT, Greenspan JR, Hill AP, Tyler CW Jr. Epidemiology of hepatocellular adenoma. The role of oral contraceptive use. JAMA. 1979;242:644–8.
3. Carrasco D, Barrachina M, Prieto M, Berenguer J. Clomiphene citrate and liver-cell adenoma. N Engl J Med. 1984;310:1120–1.
4. Rosenberg L. The risk of liver neoplasia in relation to combined oral contraceptive use. Contraception. 1991;43:643–52.
5. Heinemann LA, Weimann A, Gerken G, Thiel C, Schlaud M, DoMinh T. Modern oral contraceptive use and benign liver tumors: the German Benign Liver Tumor Case-Control Study. Eur J Contracept Reprod Health Care. 1998;3:194–200.
6. Dokmak S, Paradis V, Vilgrain V, Sauvanet A, Farges O, Valla D, Bedossa P, Belghiti J. A single-center surgical experience of 122 patients with single and multiple hepatocellular adenomas. Gastroenterology. 2009;137:1698–705.
7. Gutiérrez Santiago M, García Ibarbia C, Nan Nan DN, Hernández Hernández JL. Hepatic lesions and prolonged use of oral contraceptive. Rev Clin Esp. 2007;207(5):257–8.
8. Edmondson HA, Henderson B, Benton B. Liver-cell adenomas associated with use of oral contraceptives. N Engl J Med. 1976;294:470–2.
9. Rooks JB, Ory HW, Ishak KG, Strauss LT, Greenspan JR, Tyler CW Jr. The association between oral contraception and hepatocellular ade-

noma—a preliminary report. Int J Gynaecol Obstet. 1977;15:143–4.
10. Bühler H, Pirovino M, Akobiantz A, Altorfer J, Weitzel M, Maranta E, Schmid M. Regression of liver cell adenoma. A follow-up study of three consecutive patients after discontinuation of oral contraceptive use. Gastroenterology. 1982;82(4):775–82.
11. Aseni P, Sansalone CV, Sammartino C, Benedetto FD, Carrafiello G, Giacomoni A, Osio C, Vertemati M, Forti D. Rapid disappearance of hepatic adenoma after contraceptive withdrawal. J Clin Gastroenterol. 2001;33(3):234–6.
12. Svrcek M, Jeannot E, Arrive L, Poupon R, Fromont G, Flejou JF, Zucman-Rossi J, Bouchard P, Wendum D. Regressive liver adenomatosis following androgenic progestin therapy withdrawal: a case report with a 10-year follow-up and a molecular analysis. Eur J Endocrinol. 2007;156:617–21.
13. Brunt EM, Wolverson MK, Di Bisceglie AM. Benign hepatocellular tumors (adenomatosis) in nonalcoholic steatohepatitis: a case report. Semin Liver Dis. 2005;25(2):230–6.
14. Smith BM, Hussain A, Jacobs M, Merrick HW III. Ruptured hepatocellular carcinoma in a patient with nonalcoholic steatohepatitis. Surg Obes Relat Dis. 2009;5(4):510–2.
15. Lefkowitch JH, Antony LV. The evolving role of nonalcoholic fatty liver disease in hepatic neoplasia: inflammatory hepatocellular adenoma in a man with metabolic syndrome. Semin Liver Dis. 2015;35(3):349–54.
16. Bunchorntavakul C, Bahirwani R, Drazek D, Soulen MC, Siegelman ES, Furth EE, Olthoff K, Shaked A, Reddy KR. Clinical features and natural history of hepatocellular adenomas: the impact of obesity. Aliment Pharmacol Ther. 2011;34(6):664–74.
17. Bioulac-Sage P, Taouji S, Possenti L, Balabaud C. Hepatocellular adenoma subtypes: the impact of overweight and obesity. Liver Int. 2012;32(8):1217–21.
18. Chang CY, Hernandez-Prera JC, Roayaie S, Schwartz M, Thung SN. Changing epidemiology of hepatocellular adenoma in the United States: review of the literature. Int J Hepatol. 2013;2013:604860.
19. Nault JC, Bioulac-Sage P, Zucman-Rossi J. Hepatocellular benign tumors-from molecular classification to personalized clinical care. Gastroenterology. 2013;144(5):888–902.
20. Jeannot E, Poussin K, Chiche L, Bacq Y, Sturm N, Scoazec JY, Buffet C, Van Nhieu JT, Bellanné-Chantelot C, de Toma C, Laurent-Puig P, Bioulac-Sage P, Zucman-Rossi J. Association of CYP1B1 germ line mutations with hepatocyte nuclear factor 1alpha-mutated hepatocellular adenoma. Cancer Res. 2007;67(6):2611–6.
21. Bork K, Pitton M, Harten P, Koch P. Hepatocellular adenomas in patients taking danazol for hereditary angio-oedema. Lancet. 1999;353:1066–7.
22. Nakao A, Sakagami K, Nakata Y, Komazawa K, Amimoto T, Nakashima K, Isozaki H, Takakura N, Tanaka N. Multiple hepatic adenomas caused by long-term administration of androgenic steroids for aplastic anemia in association with familial adenomatous polyposis. J Gastroenterol. 2000;35(7):557–62.
23. Velazquez I, Alter BP. Androgens and liver tumors: Fanconi's anemia and non-Fanconi's conditions. Am J Hematol. 2004;77:257–67.
24. Socas L, Zumbado M, Pérez-Luzardo O, Ramos A, Pérez C, Hernández JR, Boada LD. Hepatocellular adenomas associated with anabolic androgenic steroid abuse in bodybuilders: a report of two cases and a review of the literature. Br J Sports Med. 2005;39:e27.
25. Talente GM, Coleman RA, Alter C, Baker L, Brown BI, Cannon RA, Chen YT, Crigler JF Jr, Ferreira P, Haworth JC, Herman GE, Issenman RM, Keating JP, Linde R, Roe TF, Senior B, Wolfsdorf JI. Glycogen storage disease in adults. Ann Intern Med. 1994;120(3):218–26.
26. Reddy SK, Kishnani PS, Sullivan JA, Koeberl DD, Desai DM, Skinner MA, Rice HE, Clary BM. Resection of hepatocellular adenoma in patients with glycogen storage disease type Ia. J Hepatol. 2007;47:658–63.
27. Wang DQ, Fiske LM, Carreras CT, Weinstein DA. Natural history of hepatocellular adenoma formation in glycogen storage disease type I. J Pediatr. 2011;159(3):442–6.
28. Hagiwara S, Takagi H, Kanda D, Sohara N, Kakizaki S, Katakai K, Yoshinaga T, Higuchi T, Nomoto K, Kuwano H, Mori M. Hepatic adenomatosis associated with hormone replacement therapy and hemosiderosis: a case report. World J Gastroenterol. 2006;12(4):652–5.
29. Reznik Y, Dao T, Coutant R, Chiche L, Jeannot E, Clauin S, Rousselot P, Fabre M, Oberti F, Fatome A, Zucman-Rossi J, Bellanne-Chantelot C. Hepatocyte nuclear factor-1 alpha gene inactivation: cosegregation between liver adenomatosis and diabetes phenotypes in two maturity-onset diabetes of the young (MODY)3 families. J Clin Endocrinol Metab. 2004;89(3):1476–80.
30. Barthelmes L, Tait IS. Liver cell adenoma and liver cell adenomatosis. HPB (Oxford). 2005;7(3):186–96.
31. Kawakatsu M, Vilgrain V, Belghiti J, Flejou JF, Nahum H. Association of multiple liver cell adenomas with spontaneous intrahepatic portohepatic shunt. Abdom Imaging. 1994;19(5):438–40.
32. Seyama Y, Sano K, Tang W, Kokudo N, Sakamoto Y, Imamura H, Makuuchi M. Simultaneous resection of liver cell adenomas and an intrahepatic portosystemic venous shunt with elevation of serum PIVKA-II level. J Gastroenterol. 2006;41:909–12.
33. Pupulim LF, Vullierme MP, Paradis V, Valla D, Terraz S, Vilgrain V. Congenital portosystemic shunts associated with liver tumours. Clin Radiol. 2013;68(7):e362–9.

34. Sempoux C, Paradis V, Komuta M, Wee A, Calderaro J, Balabaud C, Quaglia A, Bioulac-Sage P. Hepatocellular nodules expressing markers of hepatocellular adenomas in Budd-Chiari syndrome and other rare hepatic vascular disorders. J Hepatol. 2015;63(5):1173–80.
35. Calderaro J, Nault JC, Balabaud C, Couchy G, Saint-Paul MC, Azoulay D, Mehdaoui D, Luciani A, Zafrani ES, Bioulac-Sage P, Zucman-Rossi J. Inflammatory hepatocellular adenomas developed in the setting of chronic liver disease and cirrhosis. Mod Pathol. 2016;29(1):43–50.
36. Sasaki M, Nakanuma Y. Overview of hepatocellular adenoma in Japan. Int J Hepatol. 2012;2012:648131.
37. Toso C, Rubbia-Brandt L, Negro F, Morel P, Mentha G. Hepatocellular adenoma and polycystic ovary syndrome. Liver Int. 2003;23(1):35–7.
38. Seki A, Inoue T, Maegaki Y, Sugiura C, Toyoshima M, Akaboshi S, Ohno K. Polycystic ovary syndrome and hepatocellular adenoma related to long-term use of sodium valproate in a young woman. No To Hattatsu. 2006;38(3):205–8.
39. Cazorla A, Félix S, Valmary-Degano S, Sailley N, Thévenot T, Heyd B, Bioulac-Sage P. Polycystic ovary syndrome as a rare association with inflammatory hepatocellular adenoma: a case report. Clin Res Hepatol Gastroenterol. 2014;38(6):e107–10.
40. Espat J, Chamberlain RS, Sklar C, Blumgart LH. Hepatic adenoma associated with recombinant human growth hormone therapy in a patient with Turner's syndrome. Dig Surg. 2000;17(6):640–3.
41. Resnick MB, Kozakewich HP, Perez-Atayde AR. Hepatic adenoma in the pediatric age group. Clinicopathological observations and assessment of cell proliferative activity. Am J Surg Pathol. 1995;19(10):1181–90.
42. Tonorezos ES, Barnea D, Abou-Alfa GK, Bromberg J, D'Angelica M, Sklar CA, Shia J, Oeffinger KC. Hepatocellular adenoma among adult survivors of childhood and young adult cancer. Pediatr Blood Cancer. 2017;64(4).
43. Paradis V, Champault A, Ronot M, Deschamps L, Valla DC, Vidaud D, Vilgrain V, Belghiti J, Bedossa P. Telangiectatic adenoma: an entity associated with increased body mass index and inflammation. Hepatology. 2007;46(1):140–6.
44. Brancatelli G, Federle MP, Vullierme MP, Lagalla R, Midiri M, Vilgrain V. CT and MR imaging evaluation of hepatic adenoma. J Comput Assist Tomogr. 2006;30:745–50.
45. Grazioli L, Bondioni MP, Haradome H, Motosugi U, Tinti R, Frittoli B, Gambarini S, Donato F, Colagrande S. Hepatocellular adenoma and focal nodular hyperplasia: value of gadoxetic acid-enhanced MR imaging in differential diagnosis. Radiology. 2012;262:520–9.
46. Bioulac-Sage P, Rebouissou S, Thomas C, Blanc JF, Saric J, Sa Cunha A, Rullier A, Cubel G, Couchy G, Imbeaud S, Balabaud C, Zucman-Rossi J. Hepatocellular adenoma subtype classification using molecular markers and immunohistochemistry. Hepatology. 2007;46:740–8.
47. Nault JC, Couchy G, Balabaud C, Morcrette G, Caruso S, Blanc JF, Bacq Y, Calderaro J, Paradis V, Ramos J, Scoazec JY, Gnemmi V, Sturm N, Guettier C, Fabre M, Savier E, Chiche L, Labrune P, Selves J, Wendum D, Pilati C, Laurent A, De Muret A, Le Bail B, Rebouissou S, Imbeaud S, GENTHEP Investigators, Bioulac-Sage P, Letouzé E, Zucman-Rossi J. Molecular classification of hepatocellular adenoma associates with risk factors, bleeding, and malignant transformation. Gastroenterology. 2017;152(4):880–94.
48. Yamagata K, Oda N, Kaisaki PJ, Menzel S, Furuta H, Vaxillaire M, Southam L, Cox RD, Lathrop GM, Boriraj VV, Chen X, Cox NJ, Oda Y, Yano H, Le Beau MM, Yamada S, Nishigori H, Takeda J, Fajans SS, Hattersley AT, Iwasaki N, Hansen T, Pedersen O, Polonsky KS, Bell GI, et al. Mutations in the hepatocyte nuclear factor-1alpha gene in maturity-onset diabetes of the young (MODY3). Nature. 1996;384:455–8.
49. Bacq Y, Jacquemin E, Balabaud C, Jeannot E, Scotto B, Branchereau S, Laurent C, Bourlier P, Pariente D, de Muret A, Fabre M, Bioulac-Sage P, Zucman-Rossi J. Familial liver adenomatosis associated with hepatocyte nuclear factor 1alpha inactivation. Gastroenterology. 2003;125:1470–5.
50. Iwen KA, Klein J, Hubold C, Lehnert H, Weitzel JM. Maturity-onset diabetes of the young and hepatic adenomatosis—characterisation of a new mutation. Exp Clin Endocrinol Diabetes. 2013;121(6):368–71.
51. Rebouissou S, Imbeaud S, Balabaud C, Boulanger V, Bertrand-Michel J, Tercé F, Auffray C, Bioulac-Sage P, Zucman-Rossi J. HNF1alpha inactivation promotes lipogenesis in human hepatocellular adenoma independently of SREBP-1 and carbohydrate-response element-binding protein (ChREBP) activation. J Biol Chem. 2007;282:14437–46.
52. Zucman-Rossi J, Jeannot E, Nhieu JT, Scoazec JY, Guettier C, Rebouissou S, Bacq Y, Leteurtre E, Paradis V, Michalak S, Wendum D, Chiche L, Fabre M, Mellottee L, Laurent C, Partensky C, Castaing D, Zafrani ES, Laurent-Puig P, Balabaud C, Bioulac-Sage P. Genotype-phenotype correlation in hepatocellular adenoma: new classification and relationship with HCC. Hepatology. 2006;43:515–24.
53. Rebouissou S, Franconi A, Calderaro J, Letouze E, Imbeaud S, Pilati C, Nault JC, Couchy G, Laurent A, Balabaud C, Bioulac-Sage P, Zucman-Rossi J. Genotype-phenotype correlation of CTNNB1 mutations reveals different β-catenin activity associated with liver tumor progression. Hepatology. 2016;64(6):2047–61.
54. Bioulac-Sage P, Rebouissou S, Sa Cunha A, Jeannot E, Lepreux S, Blanc JF, Blanc JF, Blanché H, Le Bail B, Saric J, Laurent-Puig P, Balabaud C, Zucman-Rossi J. Clinical, morphologic, and molec-

54. ular features defining so-called telangiectatic focal nodular hyperplasias of the liver. Gastroenterology. 2005;128:1211–8.
55. Belghiti J, Dokmak S, Vilgrain V, Paradis V. Benign liver lesions, hepatocellular adenoma. Blumgart's surgery of the liver, biliary tract and pancreas, vol. 2. 5th ed. Philadelphia, PA: Elsevier Saunders; 2012.
56. Laumonier H, Bioulac-Sage P, Laurent C, Zucman-Rossi J, Balabaud C, Trillaud H. Hepatocellular adenomas: magnetic resonance imaging features as a function of molecular pathological classification. Hepatology. 2008;48:808–18.
57. Ronot M, Bahrami S, Calderaro J, Valla DC, Bedossa P, Belghiti J, Vilgrain V, Paradis V. Hepatocellular adenomas: accuracy of magnetic resonance imaging and liver biopsy in subtype classification. Hepatology. 2011;53:1182–91.
58. van Aalten SM, Thomeer MG, Terkivatan T, Dwarkasing RS, Verheij J, de Man RA, Ijzermans JN. Hepatocellular adenomas: correlation of MR imaging findings with pathologic subtype classification. Radiology. 2011;261(1):172–81.
59. Bieze M, van den Esschert JW, Nio CY, Verheij J, Reitsma JB, Terpstra V, van Gulik TM, Phoa SS. Diagnostic accuracy of MRI in differentiating hepatocellular adenoma from focal nodular hyperplasia: prospective study of the additional value of gadoxetate disodium. AJR Am J Roentgenol. 2012;199:26–34.
60. Fléjou JF, Barge J, Menu Y, Degott C, Bismuth H, Potet F, Benhamou JP. Liver adenomatosis. An entity distinct from liver adenoma? Gastroenterology. 1985;89:1132–8.
61. Veteläinen R, Erdogan D, de Graaf W, ten Kate F, Jansen PL, Gouma DJ, van Gulik TM. Liver adenomatosis: re-evaluation of aetiology and management. Liver Int. 2008;28:499–508.
62. Dokmak S, Cauchy F, Belghiti J. Resection, transplantation and local regional therapies for liver adenomas. Expert Rev Gastroenterol Hepatol. 2014;8(7):803–10.
63. Deneve JL, Pawlik TM, Cunningham S, Clary B, Reddy S, Scoggins CR, Martin RC, D'Angelica M, Staley CA, Choti MA, Jarnagin WR, Schulick RD, Kooby DA. Liver cell adenoma: a multicenter analysis of risk factors for rupture and malignancy. Ann Surg Oncol. 2009;16:640–8.
64. Toso C, Majno P, Andres A, Rubbia-Brandt L, Berney T, Buhler L, Morel P, Mentha G. Management of hepatocellular adenoma: solitary-uncomplicated, multiple and ruptured tumors. World J Gastroenterol. 2005;11(36):5691–5.
65. Bioulac-Sage P, Laumonier H, Couchy G, Le Bail B, Sa Cunha A, Rullier A, Laurent C, Blanc JF, Cubel G, Trillaud H, Zucman-Rossi J, Balabaud C, Saric J. Hepatocellular adenoma management and phenotypic classification: the Bordeaux experience. Hepatology. 2009;50:481–9.
66. van Aalten SM, de Man RA, IJzermans JN, Terkivatan T. Systematic review of haemorrhage and rupture of hepatocellular adenomas. Br J Surg. 2012;99:911–6.
67. Bieze M, Phoa SS, Verheij J, van Lienden KP, van Gulik TM. Risk factors for bleeding in hepatocellular adenoma. Br J Surg. 2014;101(7):847–55.
68. Farges O, Ferreira N, Dokmak S, Belghiti J, Bedossa P, Paradis V. Changing trends in malignant transformation of hepatocellular adenoma. Gut. 2011;60:85–9.
69. Singhi AD, Jain D, Kakar S, Wu TT, Yeh MM, Torbenson M. Reticulin loss in benign fatty liver: an important diagnostic pitfall when considering a diagnosis of hepatocellular carcinoma. Am J Surg Pathol. 2012;36:710–5.
70. Farges O, Dokmak S. Malignant transformation of liver adenoma: an analysis of the literature. Dig Surg. 2010;27:32–8.
71. Stoot JH, Coelen RJ, De Jong MC, Dejong CH. Malignant transformation of hepatocellular adenomas into hepatocellular carcinomas: a systematic review including more than 1600 adenoma cases. HPB (Oxford). 2010;12:509–22.
72. Karkar AM, Tang LH, Kashikar ND, Gonen M, Solomon SB, Dematteo RP, D'Angelica MI, Correa-Gallego C, Jarnagin WR, Fong Y, Getrajdman GI, Allen P, Kingham TP. Management of hepatocellular adenoma: comparison of resection, embolization and observation. HPB (Oxford). 2013;15(3):235–43.
73. Bossen L, Grønbaek H, Lykke Eriksen P, Jepsen P. Men with biopsy-confirmed hepatocellular adenoma have a high risk of progression to hepatocellular carcinoma: a nationwide population-based study. Liver Int. 2017;37(7):1042–6.
74. van der Windt DJ, Kok NF, Hussain SM, Zondervan PE, Alwayn IP, de Man RA, IJzermans JN. Case-orientated approach to the management of hepatocellular adenoma. Br J Surg. 2006;93:1495–502.
75. Sinclair M, Schelleman A, Sandhu D, Angus PW. Regression of hepatocellular adenomas and systemic inflammatory syndrome after cessation of estrogen therapy. Hepatology. 2017;66(3):989–91.
76. Dokmak S, Belghiti J. Will weight loss become a future treatment of hepatocellular adenoma in obese patients? Liver Int. 2015;35:2228–32.
77. Cassiman D, Libbrecht L, Verslype C, Meersseman W, Troisi R, Zucman-Rossi J, Van Vlierberghe H. An adult male patient with multiple adenomas and a hepatocellular carcinoma: mild glycogen storage disease type Ia. J Hepatol. 2010;53(1):213–7.
78. Iguchi T, Yamagata M, Sonoda T, Yanagita K, Fukahori T, Tsujita E, Aishima S, Oda Y, Maehara Y. Malignant transformation of hepatocellular adenoma with bone marrow metaplasia arising in glycogen storage disease type I: a case report. Mol Clin Oncol. 2016;5(5):599–603.
79. Mounajjed T, Wu TT. Telangiectatic variant of hepatic adenoma: clinicopathologic features and correlation between liver needle biopsy and resection. Am J Surg Pathol. 2011;35:1356–63.

80. Terkivatan T, Ijzermans JN. Hepatocellular adenoma: should phenotypic classification direct management? Nat Rev Gastroenterol Hepatol. 2009;6(12):697–8.
81. Hale G, Liu X, Hu J, Xu Z, Che L, Solomon D, Tsokos C, Shafizadeh N, Chen X, Gill R, Kakar S. Correlation of exon 3 β-catenin mutations with glutamine synthetase staining patterns in hepatocellular adenoma and hepatocellular carcinoma. Mod Pathol. 2016;29(11):1370–80.
82. Marini P, Vilgrain V, Belghiti J. Management of spontaneous rupture of liver tumours. Dig Surg. 2002;19:109–13.
83. Rosales A, Que FG. Spontaneous hepatic hemorrhage: a single institution's 16-year experience. Am Surg. 2016;82(11):1117–20.
84. Terkivatan T, de Wilt JH, de Man RA, van Rijn RR, Tilanus HW, IJzermans JN. Treatment of ruptured hepatocellular adenoma. Br J Surg. 2001;88:207–9.
85. Erdogan D, van Delden OM, Busch OR, Gouma DJ, van Gulik TM. Selective transcatheter arterial embolization for treatment of bleeding complications or reduction of tumor mass of hepatocellular adenomas. Cardiovasc Intervent Radiol. 2007;30:1252–8.
86. Erdogan D, Busch OR, van Delden OM, Ten Kate FJ, Gouma DJ, van Gulik TM. Management of spontaneous haemorrhage and rupture of hepatocellular adenomas. A single centre experience. Liver Int. 2006;26:433–8.
87. Huurman VA, Schaapherder AF. Management of ruptured hepatocellular adenoma. Dig Surg. 2010;27:56–60.
88. Landi F, De' Angelis N, Scatton O, Vidal X, Ayav A, Muscari F, Dokmak S, Torzilli G, Demartines N, Soubrane O, Cherqui D, Hardwigsen J, Laurent A. Short-term outcomes of laparoscopic vs. open liver resection for hepatocellular adenoma: a multicenter propensity score adjustment analysis by the AFC-HCA-2013 study group. Surg Endosc. 2017;31(10):4136–44.
89. Stoot JH, van der Linden E, Terpstra OT, Schaapherder AF. Life-saving therapy for haemorrhaging liver adenomas using selective arterial embolization. Br J Surg. 2007;94:1249–53.
90. van Rosmalen BV, Coelen RJS, Bieze M, van Delden OM, Verheij J, Dejong CHC, van Gulik TM. Systematic review of transarterial embolization for hepatocellular adenomas. Br J Surg. 2017;104(7):823–35.
91. Deodhar A, Brody LA, Covey AM, Brown KT, Getrajdman GI. Bland embolization in the treatment of hepatic adenomas: preliminary experience. J Vasc Interv Radiol. 2011;22(6):795–9.
92. Kobayashi S, Sakaguchi H, Takatsuka M, Suekane T, Iwai S, Morikawa H, Enomoto M, Tamori A, Kawada N. Two cases of hepatocellular adenomatosis treated with transcatheter arterial embolization. Hepatol Int. 2009;3(2):416–20.
93. Smolock AR, Cristescu MM, Potretzke TA, Ziemlewicz TJ, Lubner MG, Hinshaw JL, Brace CL, Lee FT Jr. Microwave ablation for the treatment of hepatic adenomas. J Vasc Interv Radiol. 2016;27(2):244–9.
94. Ahn SY, Park SY, Kweon YO, Tak WY, Bae HI, Cho SH. Successful treatment of multiple hepatocellular adenomas with percutaneous radiofrequency ablation. World J Gastroenterol. 2013;19(42):7480–6.
95. McDaniel JD, Kukreja K, Ristagno RL, Yazigi N, Nathan JD, Tiao G. Radiofrequency ablation of a large hepatic adenoma in a child. J Pediatr Surg. 2013;48(6):E19–22.
96. Rhim H, Lim HK, Kim YS, Choi D. Percutaneous radiofrequency ablation of hepatocellular adenoma: initial experience in 10 patients. J Gastroenterol Hepatol. 2008;23(8 Pt 2):e422–7.
97. Atwell TD, Brandhagen DJ, Charboneau JW, Nagorney DM, Callstrom MR, Farrell MA. Successful treatment of hepatocellular adenoma with percutaneous radiofrequency ablation. AJR Am J Roentgenol. 2005;184(3):828–31.
98. Fujita S, Kushihata F, Herrmann GE, Mergo PJ, Liu C, Nelson D, Fujikawa T, Hemming AW. Combined hepatic resection and radiofrequency ablation for multiple hepatic adenomas. J Gastroenterol Hepatol. 2006;21(8):1351–4.
99. van Vledder MG, van Aalten SM, Terkivatan T, de Man RA, Leertouwer T, Ijzermans JN. Safety and efficacy of radiofrequency ablation for hepatocellular adenoma. J Vasc Interv Radiol. 2011;22:787–93.
100. Scheffer HJ, Melenhorst MC, van Tilborg AA, Nielsen K, van Nieuwkerk KM, de Vries RA, van den Tol PM, Meijerink MR. Percutaneous irreversible electroporation of a large centrally located hepatocellular adenoma in a woman with a pregnancy wish. Cardiovasc Intervent Radiol. 2015;38(4):1031–5.
101. Chiche L, David A1, Adam R, Oliverius MM, Klempnauer J, Vibert E, Colledan M, Lerut J, Mazzafero VV, Di-Sandro S, Laurent C, Scuderi V, Suc B, Troisi R, Bachelier P, Dumortier J, Gugenheim J, Mabrut JY, Gonzalez-Pinto I, Pruvot FR, Le-Treut YP, Navarro F, Ortiz-de-Urbina J, Salamé E, Spada M, Bioulac-Sage P. Liver transplantation for adenomatosis: European experience. Liver Transpl. 2016;22(4):516–26.
102. Chiche L, Dao T, Salamé E, Galais MP, Bouvard N, Schmutz G, Rousselot P, Bioulac-Sage P, Ségol P, Gignoux M. Liver adenomatosis: reappraisal, diagnosis, and surgical management: eight new cases and review of the literature. Ann Surg. 2000;231:74–81.
103. Reddy SK, Austin SL, Spencer-Manzon M, Koeberl DD, Clary BM, Desai DM, Smith AD, Kishnani PS. Liver transplantation for glycogen storage disease type Ia. J Hepatol. 2009;51:483–90.

104. Gordon-Burroughs S, Balogh J, Weiner MA, Monsour HP Jr, Schwartz MR, Gaber AO, Ghobrial RM. Liver transplantation in an adult with adenomatosis and congenital absence of the portal vein: a case report. Transplant Proc. 2014;46(7):2418–21.
105. Cobey FC, Salem RR. A review of liver masses in pregnancy and a proposed algorithm for their diagnosis and management. Am J Surg. 2004;187(2):181–91.
106. Noels JE, van Aalten SM, van der Windt DJ, Kok NF, de Man RA, Terkivatan T, Ijzermans JN. Management of hepatocellular adenoma during pregnancy. J Hepatol. 2011;54(3):553–8.
107. Klompenhouwer AJ, Sprengers D, Willemssen FE, Gaspersz MP, Ijzermans JN, De Man RA. Evidence of good prognosis of hepatocellular adenoma in post-menopausal women. J Hepatol. 2016;65(6):1163–70.

Regional Therapies for Hepatic Adenoma

13

Jack P. Silva and T. Clark Gamblin

Hepatic adenoma (HA) is a rare and benign hepatic tumor classically identified in women exposed to estrogen-based oral contraceptives. Men with anabolic steroid use or glycogen storage disease are also at risk for hepatic adenoma, but prevalence is far lower than in females. Furthermore, obesity and general metabolic disorders have recently been associated with development of HA [1]. In Asian populations, the proportion of men with HA is much higher than in the United States, and concurrent hepatocellular carcinoma is far more prevalent [2]. Patient demographics may influence the course of management, and the treatment modalities available for HA continue to evolve.

Hepatic adenomas in solitude can be an innocuous finding, but can give rise to hemorrhage or malignant conversion. Identifying a patient's risk is essential to the management of hepatic adenoma. As described in the previous chapter, histological subtype is associated with differing outcomes in HA. An inflammatory or telangiectatic adenoma is more likely to hemorrhage or rupture, while tumors with aberrant beta-catenin activation are most likely to harbor malignancy [1]. Despite these predictive variables, the treatment pathway selected is based primarily on tumor size and anatomic location.

J. P. Silva · T. C. Gamblin (✉)
Division of Surgical Oncology, Department of Surgery, Medical College of Wisconsin, Milwaukee, WI, USA
e-mail: jsilva@mcw.edu; tcgamblin@mcw.edu

Imaging and Biopsy

Although some HA patients first present with abdominal pain, an increasing number are identified incidentally on ultrasound or other abdominal imaging. Proper recognition of HA on imaging is important to distinguish it from other processes such as focal nodular hyperplasia (FNH) or hepatocellular carcinoma (HCC). In addition to providing useful information about the size, location, and vascularity of liver lesions, modern cross-sectional imaging can usually distinguish HA from FNH. If necessary, a hepatocyte-specific contrast agent like gadoxetic acid can differentiate between FNH and HA in the hepatobiliary phase [3]. In the rare case where imaging is insufficient and the tumor size necessitates a definitive diagnosis to guide treatment, core needle biopsy may be considered. Alternatively, surgical resection is a diagnostic and therapeutic solution for radiologically ambiguous lesions.

Classical Treatment and Clinical Factors

Following the diagnosis of hepatic adenoma, options for management have historically been either observation or hepatic resection. Most propose that male gender or a tumor size greater than 5 cm should guide resection, given the higher propensity for malignancy in men and increased risk of hemorrhage in larger tumors [4, 5]. If imaging reveals a small (<5 cm) HA, surveillance may be an acceptable course of management. In this pathway, oral contraceptives should be adjusted to minimize estrogen exposure. The presence of symptoms such as pain may also influence the choice to intervene. Surgical resection remains the standard intervention for hepatic adenoma because of the potential risk for hemorrhage and/or malignancy. Orthotopic liver transplantation may also be considered for adenomatosis with suspicion of malignant transformation [6].

Hepatic adenoma carries about a 5–10% risk of malignant transformation. The most widely recognized and easily identified risk factors are patient gender and tumor size. Men have a 6–10× higher malignancy rate than women, and tumors >5 cm are at greater risk of undergoing transformation [5]. Although beta-catenin mutations identified on tumor histology are also known to contribute to the risk of malignancy, diagnostic biopsies are unlikely to guide treatment and thus are rarely performed.

The incidence of hemorrhage associated with HA is 20–40% and also classically correlates with tumor size [1, 4, 5, 7, 8]. Pregnancy and inflammatory/telangiectatic tumor histology have also been described as risk factors for hemorrhage. Tumor number does not appear to be related to malignant transformation or hemorrhage [5]. Most cases of hemorrhage are contained as an intratumoral bleed, but intraperitoneal rupture can occur and lead to hemodynamic instability. The mortality rate for emergency resection in the setting of HA rupture is as high as 10%, so initial stabilization, including embolization, is justified if possible [9].

The surgical management of HA is covered in depth in previous chapter, but the development of new treatment modalities and the improvement of existing ones has provided potential complements and alternatives to HA resection. Arterial embolization has been well-described for the treatment of acute tumoral hemorrhage, and radiofrequency ablation has been proposed as an alternative to resection in select cases. The remainder of this chapter primarily focuses on the expanding role of these regional therapies in the management of hepatic adenoma.

Regional Therapies

The concept of locoregional treatments for liver tumors has evolved significantly over the past 30 years. Continued innovation in the field of ablation and embolization has driven the success in the management of HCC and other hepatic malignancies. These techniques are now being recognized for potential application in the management of hepatic adenoma.

Ablation

Radiofrequency ablation (RFA) is an important tool for small hepatic tumors. In addition to being an intraoperative option (laparoscopically or open), RFA can also be performed percutaneously (Fig. 13.1). The technique places an image-guided

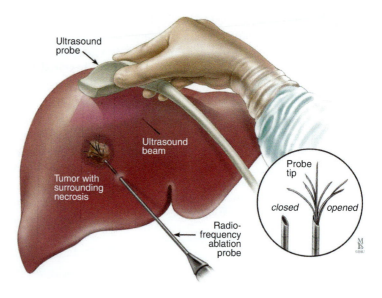

Fig. 13.1 Radiofrequency ablation of a liver mass (http://www.hopkinsmedicine.org/healthlibrary/GetImage.aspx?ImageId=290447)

needle electrode into the tumor, heats the surrounding tissue, and results in cell death necrosis in the ablative zone. The target size of the ablation zone often limits the use of RFA to tumors smaller than 5 cm. A more recent development in the field of ablation is the application of microwaves. Microwave ablation (MWA) utilizes a technique similar to RFA, except the higher frequency achieves tumor necrosis in a shorter amount of time (Fig. 13.2). Both RFA and MWA have been described in small institutional reviews as a possible alternative to resection in select cases of HA. Such studies often report 95–100% local tumor control after one or more treatments [3, 10–13]. Other forms of ablation including high-intensity focused ultrasound (HIFU) ablation, laser ablation, and cryoablation are less established for the treatment of HCC and have not been reported in the management of HA.

Embolization

The other primary locoregional therapy for liver tumors is selective arterial embolization. While the portal system provides most of the blood supply to the liver parenchyma, tumors

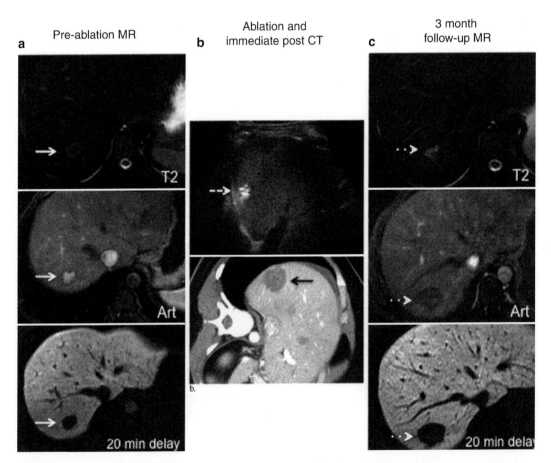

Fig. 13.2 Patient 5 was a 33-year-old woman planning pregnancy. (**a**) MR imaging performed before ablation shows a 2.3 cm T2 hyperintense arterially enhancing lesion (white arrows) in the right hepatic lobe, which is hypointense on the delayed phase image (examination was performed with gadoxetate disodium). (**b**) Gray-scale ultrasound image obtained before and during ablation demonstrate the MW antenna in the tumor and subsequent gas bubble formation (dashed white arrow). Ablation was performed using one gas-cooled MW ablation antenna powered at 65 W for 5 min. Contrast-enhanced CT image obtained immediately after ablation demonstrates complete treatment of the lesion (black arrow). (**c**) MR imaging performed 3 months after ablation demonstrates the nonenhancing ablation zone (dotted white arrows). J Vasc Interv Radiol 2016; 27:244–249, with permission

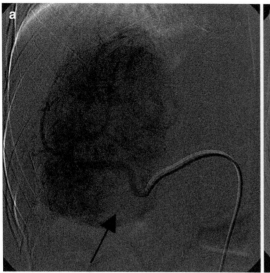 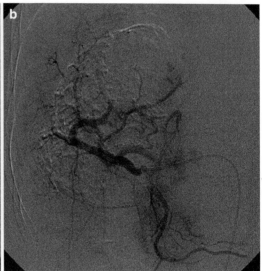

Fig. 13.3 Angiographic images before (**a**) and after (**b**) bland embolization in a 22-year-old patient who was receiving treatment with growth and sex hormones. The patient underwent embolization for abdominal pain and increased risk of bleeding. (**a**) Selective catheterization of a hepatic arterial branch supplying the HA was performed. Note that the posteromedial portion of the tumor is relatively less well perfused by the selected branch (*arrow*). *Journal of Vascular and Interventional Radiology* 2011 22, 795–799 DOI: https://doi.org/10.1016/j.jvir.2011.02.027, with permission

rely primarily on arterial perfusion. Thus, embolization of hepatic arterial supply to a tumor occludes nutrient blood flow while sparing the functional remnant (Fig. 13.3). Hepatic artery embolization (HAE) involves introducing a passing a microcatheter from the femoral artery up to the hepatic artery. The technique has evolved to allow superselective catheter access to maximize targeted isolation. The main indication for HAE in HCC is for unresectable lesions not amenable to ablative therapies or as a bridge to liver transplantation. HAE techniques are often considered palliative in oncologic patients, but bland particle embolization serves a more primarily therapeutic role in HA management.

Arterial Embolization for HA

The majority of literature reporting HA embolization focuses on stabilizing patients presenting with acute tumoral hemorrhage, but limited reports describe it as a bridge or alternative to resection.

Hemorrhage

Hemorrhage and tumor rupture are risks for any hepatic tumor, but the lack of capsule in HA makes it especially susceptible to rupture. Emergency surgery for ruptured HA carries a 5–10% mortality rate, but embolization may provide a first step in management to achieve hemodynamic stability prior to resection. If the HA is under 5 cm and remains stable following embolization, a nonoperative approach involving strict radiological follow-up may be possible [14, 15]. Stoot et al. reported their experience utilizing selective embolization for 11 patients with ruptured HA. Ten of the patients had their hemorrhage controlled by a single embolization, while the one patient required three embolizations. All adenomas decreased in size or were undetectable following treatment, with the median diameter decreasing from 7.0 to 2.5 cm. The first two patients underwent elective resection following embolization, but after histopathological exam revealed complete necrosis, the remaining patients simply received frequent follow-up imaging in lieu of resection [16].

Hypervascular HA with non-emergent intratumoral hemorrhage may be diagnosed on imaging. Embolization may also have a role in this type of patient, followed by interval elective resection. Similarly, elective embolization may also have a role in reducing the size and hemorrhagic potential of large HA prior to surgery [17, 18]. In a report of 17 HA embolizations in eight patients, six patients were asymptomatic, one had abdominal pain, and one had active bleeding. Two of the six asymptomatic patients underwent resection: one received preoperative embolization as a means of decreasing the vascularity of a large adenoma, and the other had an HA resected 3 months after embolization due to persistent peripheral enhancement [19]. With a high rate of technical success, embolization can result in decreased tumor size and a lack of enhancement uniformly. The authors concluded that initial embolization may simplify an eventual surgery, and perhaps resection may be avoided.

Some institutions have also identified malignant potential as an indication for primary HAE in hepatic adenoma patients. Karkar et al. reported 100 HA in 52 patients who underwent resection, embolization, or observation. Multifocal adenomas were more likely to be treated with embolization, while single tumors were more commonly resected. Of the 100 lesions, 37 HAs in 13 patients were treated by 25 embolizations, with suspicion of malignancy being the most common indication (14/25) [20]. Of the 37 embolized tumors, only 3 (8.1%) displayed persistent disease following initial treatment, and all were successfully managed with reintervention. This report is evidence for multifocal HA management with HAE. Although 37 HA in 13 patients is a small sample, a 92% initial effectiveness is noteworthy.

Hepatic arterial embolization has an important role in the management of acute tumoral hemorrhage or rupture and may also provide a benefit in unresectable patients. The role for HAE as an alternative to elective resection remains unclear given the paucity of reports comparing these two methods.

Radiofrequency Ablation for HA

Unlike embolization, ablation is often categorized as a curative treatment, rather than a palliative measure. The success of ablative therapies for hepatic malignancy has led to its possible use for HA, and some have proposed selective ablation as an alternative to surgery.

RFA and other ablation techniques have been well-described for small, unresectable hepatic tumors. Whether as an isolated percutaneous therapy for a single lesion, or as an intraoperative adjunct to a resection, the technique has been proven safe and effective. As with other nontraditional methods for HA treatment, descriptions of RFA are limited to small institutional reviews and case reports, but the results are promising. Ablation has been used in adenomatosis as an addition to surgical resection and also as an option for small unresectable HA [13, 21]. RFA has also been reported as a treatment option to impede HA growth in patients who desire pregnancy or cannot discontinue hormonal therapy. Furthermore, several case reports describe the use of RFA as an alternative to surgery, particularly in patients who might decline resection. As an example, some patients especially concerned about esthetics and invasiveness may prefer RFA if their disease is deemed amenable [22, 23].

To justify replacement of elective surgery, RFA must be able to demonstrate comparable safety and efficacy. Rhim et al. reported their experience with RFA for ten patients with asymptomatic HA as an alternative to surveillance or elective surgery. Tumors ablated were all less than 5 cm, and none showed local tumor progression or new recurrence within a mean follow-up period of 17.5 months (range 2–35) [11]. In a cost analysis, van de Sluis et al. showed that RFA was more effective and cost less than hepatic resection, HAE, or surveillance in the management of small hepatic adenomas [24]. Some current literature supports ablation techniques for tumors under 5 cm [10, 11, 23, 25]. Although reported less frequently, other forms of ablative therapy like microwave ablation (MWA) and irreversible electroporation (IRE) have recently been described as successful treatments for HA. IRE may be an alternative technique for tumors located in an area unsuitable for thermal ablation, and MWA has the advantage of a short ablative time and less potential heat sink [12, 26].

Radiofrequency ablation has a valuable role in unresectable small HA requiring treatment, and its success has led some to consider it as a viable alternative to elective hepatic resection or watchful waiting. However, until RFA can be compared directly to resection, it is unlikely to replace resection in common practice.

Surveillance and Follow-Up

Following ablation or embolization for HA, cross-sectional imaging should be obtained to confirm effective management. Patients with HA under surveillance should minimize estrogen exposure and undergo interval follow-up scans every 3–6 months initially, depending on the planned observation time. Hemorrhagic HA treated initially with HAE should also be imaged and evaluated for subsequent resection. With appropriate surveillance or post-treatment follow-up imaging, management of HA should carry a low risk of complication.

Summary and Conclusion

Hepatic adenomas are a rare and benign disease primarily affecting a young and otherwise healthy patient population, but the risk of hemorrhage and malignant transformation makes identification and treatment crucial. HA may present with abdominal pain but are most often discovered incidentally. Accurate diagnosis of HA is important to properly risk stratify patients. Cross-sectional imaging can often diagnose HA and distinguish it from FNH without the need for core needle biopsy. The most important characteristics guiding treatment of HA are the tumor size, anatomic location, and the patient's gender. Any patient presenting with an HA-associated hemorrhage or rupture should be treated emergently with hepatic artery embolization to stabilize the patient, and resection should be strongly considered.

Asymptomatic patients with HA deemed to be at risk for hemorrhage or malignancy should undergo a treatment of a definitive nature. Unresectable tumors may be treated with HAE or ablation. These regional therapies may result in long-term resolution of the disease or may improve the operative outcomes. Although most HA are currently resected, several institutions and small case series have reported success with HAE or RFA as an alternative.

References

1. Agrawal S, et al. Management of hepatocellular adenoma: recent advances. Clin Gastroenterol Hepatol. 2015;13(7):1221–30.
2. Lin H, et al. Systematic review of hepatocellular adenoma in China and other regions. J Gastroenterol Hepatol. 2011;26(1):28–35.
3. Costa AF, et al. Should fat in the radiofrequency ablation zone of hepatocellular adenomas raise suspicion for residual tumour? Eur Radiol. 2017;27(4):1704–12.
4. Cho SW, et al. Surgical management of hepatocellular adenoma: take it or leave it? Ann Surg Oncol. 2008;15(10):2795–803.
5. Dokmak S, et al. A single-center surgical experience of 122 patients with single and multiple hepatocellular adenomas. Gastroenterology. 2009;137(5):1698–705.
6. Chiche L, et al. Liver transplantation for adenomatosis: European experience. Liver Transpl. 2016;22(4):516–26.
7. Rosales A, Que FG. Spontaneous hepatic hemorrhage: a single institution's 16-year experience. Am Surg. 2016;82(11):1117–20.
8. Deneve JL, et al. Liver cell adenoma: a multicenter analysis of risk factors for rupture and malignancy. Ann Surg Oncol. 2009;16(3):640–8.
9. Nasser F, et al. Minimally invasive treatment of hepatic adenoma in special cases. Einstein (Sao Paulo). 2013;11(4):524–7.
10. Baldwin K, et al. Bipolar radiofrequency ablation of liver tumors: technical experience and interval follow-up in 22 patients with 33 ablations. J Surg Oncol. 2012;106(7):905–10.
11. Rhim H, et al. Percutaneous radiofrequency ablation of hepatocellular adenoma: initial experience in 10 patients. J Gastroenterol Hepatol. 2008;23(8 Pt 2):e422–7.
12. Smolock AR, et al. Microwave ablation for the treatment of hepatic adenomas. J Vasc Interv Radiol. 2016;27(2):244–9.
13. van Vledder MG, et al. Safety and efficacy of radiofrequency ablation for hepatocellular adenoma. J Vasc Interv Radiol. 2011;22(6):787–93.

14. Darnis B, et al. Management of bleeding liver tumors. J Visc Surg. 2014;151(5):365–75.
15. Huurman VA, Schaapherder AF. Management of ruptured hepatocellular adenoma. Dig Surg. 2010;27(1):56–60.
16. Stoot JH, et al. Life-saving therapy for haemorrhaging liver adenomas using selective arterial embolization. Br J Surg. 2007;94(10):1249–53.
17. Erdogan D, et al. Selective transcatheter arterial embolization for treatment of bleeding complications or reduction of tumor mass of hepatocellular adenomas. Cardiovasc Intervent Radiol. 2007;30(6):1252–8.
18. Marini P, Vilgrain V, Belghiti J. Management of spontaneous rupture of liver tumours. Dig Surg. 2002;19(2):109–13.
19. Deodhar A, et al. Bland embolization in the treatment of hepatic adenomas: preliminary experience. J Vasc Interv Radiol. 2011;22(6):795–9. quiz 800
20. Karkar AM, et al. Management of hepatocellular adenoma: comparison of resection, embolization and observation. HPB (Oxford). 2013;15(3):235–43.
21. van Aalten SM, et al. Management of liver adenomatosis by radiofrequency ablation. Dig Surg. 2011;28(3):173–7.
22. Ahn SY, et al. Successful treatment of multiple hepatocellular adenomas with percutaneous radiofrequency ablation. World J Gastroenterol. 2013;19(42):7480–6.
23. Rocourt DV, et al. Contemporary management of benign hepatic adenoma using percutaneous radiofrequency ablation. J Pediatr Surg. 2006;41(6):1149–52.
24. van der Sluis FJ, et al. Hepatocellular adenoma: cost-effectiveness of different treatment strategies. Radiology. 2009;252(3):737–46.
25. Yi B, Somasundar P, Espat NJ. Novel laparoscopic bipolar radiofrequency energy technology for expedited hepatic tumour ablation. HPB (Oxford). 2009;11(2):135–9.
26. Scheffer HJ, et al. Percutaneous irreversible electroporation of a large centrally located hepatocellular adenoma in a woman with a pregnancy wish. Cardiovasc Intervent Radiol. 2015;38(4):1031–5.

Pathologic Classification of Preinvasive Cystic Neoplasms of the Intra- and Extrahepatic Bile Ducts

14

Brian Quigley, Burcin Pehlivanoglu, and Volkan Adsay

Introduction

Preinvasive neoplastic cysts of the liver and extrahepatic bile ducts can be regarded broadly in three groups: (1) those that occur in the bile duct system, i.e., intraductal neoplasms (viz., intraductal papillary neoplasms of the bile ducts [IPNBs], and their close kindreds, intraductal oncocytic papillary neoplasms [IOPNs], and intraductal tubulopapillary neoplasms [ITPNs], (2) mucinous cystic neoplasms (MCNs, with ovarian stroma) which are de novo cystic neoplasms that do not visibly communicate with the native biliary ductal system, and (3) developmental or congenital cysts (including choledochal cysts) that end up developing intraepithelial neoplasia.

Under the 2010 WHO system, regardless of the setting in which they are encountered, dysplastic processes (preinvasive/intraepithelial neoplasia) of the intra- and extrahepatic bile ducts (and gallbladder) are classified similar to their

B. Quigley · B. Pehlivanoglu
Department of Pathology and Laboratory Medicine, Emory University School of Medicine, Atlanta, GA, USA
e-mail: brian.c.quigley@emory.edu; burcin.pehlivanoglu@emory.edu

V. Adsay (✉)
Department of Pathology, Koç University Hospital, Istanbul, Turkey
e-mail: nadsay@mcw.edu

pancreatic counterparts [1] and consist of two generic categories. The first are those that are non-mass-forming (macroscopically appearing as flat lesions and microscopically showing no more than micropapillary formations), which, in the bile ducts, are now classified as biliary intraepithelial neoplasia [BilIN]) [2, 3], which can develop in developmental/congenital cysts as incidental/microscopic lesions [2]. The second group are the clinically and radiologically detectable mass-forming dysplastic (preinvasive) lesions with grossly recognizable papillary/polypoid tumors, classified as tumoral intraepithelial neoplasm, which, as a conceptual category, encompasses the intraductal neoplasms (IPNBs, IOPNs, and ITPNs) [4–14], as well as mucinous cystic neoplasms [1]. In the ensuing sections, the clinicopathologic characteristics of these processes will be discussed.

Biliary Intraepithelial Neoplasia (BilIN) in Congenital/Developmental Cysts

Definition and Terminology

Biliary intraepithelial neoplasia (BilIN) is by definition microscopic flat (non-tumoral) forms of dysplasia [2, 3]. Dysplastic (preinvasive) neoplasms that present as cystic masses (i.e., tumoral intraepithelial neoplasms) are discussed separately below in detail and should not be classified as BilIN. BilINs can develop in and be detected

© Springer Nature Switzerland AG 2018
K. Cardona, S. K. Maithel (eds.), *Primary and Metastatic Liver Tumors*,
https://doi.org/10.1007/978-3-319-91977-5_14

incidentally in congenital or developmental lesions such as choledochal cysts.

A three-tiered grading scheme has been proposed for BilIN in 2007 and was also adopted by the WHO in 2010 (1, 2, and 3, corresponding to low-, intermediate-, and high-grade dysplasia/carcinoma in situ, respectively) [3]; however a two-tiered system (low and high grade), which is more biologically and clinically relevant, is often used instead [15]. In the two-tiered system, BilIN-1 and BilIN-2 correspond to low grade, and BilIN3 is high grade ("carcinoma in situ") [2, 16].

Early BilIN changes (BilIN-1 and BilIN-2, low-grade dysplasia) are rather common incidental findings in biliary resections performed for any cause, and they are believed to be of no clinical significance. BilIN-3 (high-grade dysplasia, CIS), on the other hand, in general is seldom detected outside the setting of invasive adenocarcinoma, while it is commonly observed in the mucosa adjacent to invasive carcinomas of the bile duct [17–19]. However, in congenital or developmental cysts, especially choledochal cyst, high-grade BilIN can be encountered without any invasive carcinoma (see below). The reported incidence of BilIN in different clinical settings varies greatly, possibly owing to the subjectivity in the application of pathologic diagnostic criteria or the well-known challenges in distinguishing dysplasia from its mimickers at the histopathologic level including epithelial ulceration/denudation leading to severe epithelial atypia, or in some cases, to overgrowth by carcinoma, or less extensive sampling [20].

BilINs Arising in Developmental/Congenital Cysts

The main setting that BilIN-3/CIS can be encountered in isolation (without an accompanying invasive carcinoma) and thus becomes a management issue is in choledochal cysts. This is reported to occur in about 10% of the resected choledochal cysts [21, 22]. Some of these cases are associated with pancreatobiliary maljunction (supra-Oddi union of main pancreatic duct and common bile duct that leads to reflux of pancreatic enzymes to the bile duct system). The literature on the clinical outcome of these cases is highly limited, but it is generally believed that such cases require close follow-up. It is also not clear as to what kind of approach is needed if this BilIN-3/CIS also appears at a margin. Thankfully this is a rare occurrence.

We have also seen patients with duplication/congenital cysts occurring in the vicinity of distal biliary tract that contained high-grade dysplasia/CIS. These are technically not designated as BilIN since they often are duplication of GI tract type and contain a muscular coat and respiratory- or intestinal-type epithelium. In some cases, the dysplastic process can form adenomatous masses (tumoral intraepithelial neoplasms) and mimic intraductal papillary neoplasms discussed below.

Histopathologic Diagnosis and Differential of BilIN

Reactive atypia (such as that induced by stones or stents) may closely mimic low- or high-grade dysplasia or even carcinoma on a microscopic level. In fact, it can be impossible to determine whether an atypical lesion is truly neoplastic or merely reactive. Low-grade dysplasia is characterized by cells with pseudostratified nuclei showing slight enlargement and hyperchromasia. That said, some segments of the biliary epithelium are pseudostratified even in the normal state; for this reason, low-grade dysplasia can show considerable morphologic overlap with non-dysplastic epithelium, particularly when it is either thickly sectioned or hyperplastic. Reactive epithelial cells maintain smooth nuclear membranes and homogenous pale chromatin. Fine chromatin stippling of reactive biliary epithelial cells sometimes mimics neuroendocrine cell nuclei. In contrast, dysplastic epithelium shows large nuclei and coarse chromatin. True high-grade dysplasia often (but not always) shows loss of nuclear polarity and nuclear hyperchromasia, enlargement, and pleomorphism (variation in size and shape).

Dysplasia extending into and involving peribiliary mucous glands can mimic invasive carcinoma. The most helpful distinguishing feature is retained lobular architecture of the peribiliary mucous glands, which are also uniform and small with narrow lumens in contrast to the irregular distribution, variable sizes, and irregular shapes of true invasive carcinoma glands.

Probably the most challenging aspect of high-grade dysplasia (CIS; BilIN-3), problematic both clinically and for researchers, is how to distinguish it from the "colonization/cancerization" phenomenon. It is now well established that invasive carcinoma cells can retrogradely invade into the mucosa and colonize the surface epithelium, in which case it becomes indistinguishable from "in situ" carcinoma although it is actually composed of cells that have proven the ability to invade. The importance of recognition of this phenomenon comes from the fact that any time a BilIN of high-grade is discovered in a cystic lesion, this cyst (and this patient) needs to be investigated very thoroughly in order to exclude the presence of invasive carcinoma associated with it (or perhaps colonizing the surface and mimicking dysplasia).

In terms of pathologic diagnosis and molecular investigation of BilINs, there is a variety of markers that have been shown to be overexpressed in these lesions. Among the more routinely used diagnostic immunohistochemical markers, BilIN expresses CEA immunohistochemically. MUC1 is also expressed, with degrees of expression roughly correlating with the grade of dysplasia [23–26]. BilIN does not express MUC2 [23–26], which is mostly confined to intestinal-type IPNBs (see below). Some high-grade BilINs express IMP3 (insulin-like growth factor II mRNA binding protein 3) [27]. Invasive adenocarcinomas that arise from BilIN3 are of tubular type and incite stromal desmoplasia [15]. Similar to IPNBs, low-grade BilIN may harbor KRAS mutations, but this is at a far less frequency than in the pancreas, and it becomes more common as the lesion progresses [28–31]. Additionally, the frequency of KRAS mutation goes down with the distance from the pancreas (higher in distal CBD lesions and far less common in proximal tumors). Loss of SMAD4, nuclear TP53 expression, p16 inactivation, and altered p21 and cyclin D1 expression occur late [28–31].

Tumoral Intraepithelial Neoplasms Presenting as Cyst

Tumor types that are by nature preinvasive (dysplastic) and cystic are regarded as tumoral forms of intraepithelial neoplasia. In essence, these are adenoma-carcinoma sequence. It is believed that whatever leads to these neoplastic cells to grow intraluminally/intraductally (before they become invasive carcinomas) impart a distinctive biology to these tumors. These entities (discussed below in detail) often present as cystic lesions. The criteria for their grading are very similar to the grading described above for BilINs.

Intraductal Papillary Neoplasms of the Bile Duct (IPNB)

Intraductal papillary neoplasms of bile duct (IPNBs) [3, 12, 32–36] are intraepithelial (preinvasive) neoplasms with papillary architecture (Fig. 14.1), and they often lead to cystic dilatation of the ductal system and present as cystic masses. By definition, IPNBs are distinguished from BilIN by the formation of grossly detectable papillary/polypoid (and/or cystic) tumors measuring at least 1 centimeter. They are essentially the biliary counterpart of pancreatic intraductal papillary mucinous neoplasms (IPMNs) [36–43] although mucin production is relatively less in IPNBs. Intraductal papillary neoplasms of bile ducts can result in extensive cystic distension of the bile ducts (similar to pancreatic IPMNs) [44], explaining why some cases had previously been referred to as cystadenocarcinoma. Ampullary or duodenal adenomas may grow into the bile ducts and mimic IPNBs; the distinction is made through careful gross examination and correlation with imaging studies.

Patients with IPNBs present at a mean age in the early 60s [3, 12, 32–35]. The presenting symptoms (abdominal pain, jaundice, and cholangitis) tend to be related to biliary obstruction, and, consequently, cases that are disseminated or multifocal (the so-called papillomatosis) tend to present at a slightly younger age [45–47]. Stones can be present at any level of the biliary

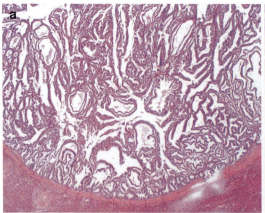 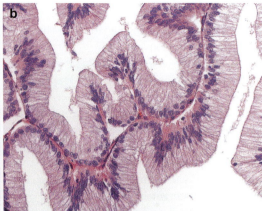

Fig. 14.1 Intraductal papillary neoplasm of the bile duct, low grade. The tumor is composed of compact papillary and glandular elements filling and markedly dilating the ductal system. The background liver is also seen and is unremarkable. The tumor itself is composed of innocuous cells with abundant apical mucinous cytoplasm showing the texture and color characteristic of gastric foveolar epithelium and thus qualifies the lesion as gastric-type IPNB. Despite the prolific nature of the lesion and architectural complexity, the cytologic atypia is minimal. The nuclei are very well polarized and have very mature appearance (virtually indistinguishable from gastric mucosa) showing abundant apical mucin. There is no atypia to qualify the lesion as "high-grade dysplastic" by cytology. However, these low-grade cases may prove to be associated with (or progress into) invasive carcinoma

tract in IPNB cases. Parasites (especially *Clonorchis sinensis*) may also be found. Twenty percent of cases had a history of prior cholecystectomy. Approximately 10% of intra-or extrahepatic bile ducts resected for biliary neoplasia contain an IPNB component. About three-fourths of IPNBs have an invasive component at the time of diagnosis [12, 35]; therefore, if an example is discovered in a biopsy, it should be regarded highly to suspect to harbor invasion, even if the invasive carcinoma may not be present in the biopsy sample itself. At the time of diagnosis, most IPNBs have high-grade dysplasia, although any grade of dysplasia may be observed. For the grading of dysplasia, the criteria discussed above for BilINs are employed.

IPNBs display different types of epithelium that have been well described for their pancreatic counterparts, IPMNs. Some are intestinal type, resembling adenomas of the colon. These may lead to mucinous colloid-type invasive carcinoma. They typically show diffuse expression of intestinal lineage markers such as CDX2 and MUC2 [23]. A significant proportion of IPNBs, however, have gastric or gastro-pancreatobiliary lineage (and show MUC1 and/or MUC6 expression), and these appear to be more aggressive. Oncocytic-type lesions have distinctive clinicopathologic characteristics and seem to warrant a separate classification [4, 48] (see below). The immunoprofile matches the epithelial phenotype [36, 49].

In the absence of invasion, IPNBs behave in an indolent fashion; the recurrence and metastasis that occasionally ensue may either be secondary to a small focus of invasion that was missed or to multifocality [3, 12, 32–36]. The cases with extensive papillary nodules and multifocality ("papillomatosis") often occur in younger patients but more prone to have invasion. Invasive carcinomas arising in IPNBs are aggressive, although their prognosis is better than that of conventional cholangiocarcinoma. Colloid-type invasive carcinoma that is well described to develop in the pancreatic counterparts of these tumors (i.e., IPMNs), and which have more protracted clinical course, appears to have a more benevolent course in the bile ducts as well, but this impression needs to be confirmed in larger studies. Cases with minimal invasion seem to have an intermediate prognosis [45], highlighting the necessity for detailed and proper pathologic reporting of cases with invasion. There is some evidence that invasive carcinomas arising from IPNBs, which are morphologically indistinguishable from conventional cholangiocarcinomas, may be less aggressive than ordinary cholangiocarcinomas (arising de novo or from BilINs) even when stage matched, which goes along with the impression that they represent a distinct pathway of carcinogenesis with a different biology.

Intraductal Oncocytic Papillary Neoplasms ("Oncocytic Papillary Cystadenocarcinomas")

Cystic tumors with complex papillary nodules lined by oncocytic cells are relatively rare but increasingly being recognized as a distinct category also in the bile ducts [4, 48]. These tend to present as complex heterogeneous cystic masses and are often also multifocal and thus typically misdiagnosed as ordinary cholangiocarcinomas (with metastasis). In fact, some cases are diagnosed only after the surprisingly protracted clinical course (which would be unexpected from an ordinary cholangiocarcinoma of this complexity and size). Their morphology is highly distinctive. The papillae are unusually complex and arborizing and show either delicate cores that may acquire edematous change. In addition to the oncocytic cytology, these tumors also show the characteristic intraepithelial lumen formation described for their pancreatic counterpart [48]. Despite their complexity (that leads to the impression of an aggressive "cystadenocarcinoma"), these tumors are proving to have a shockingly benevolent behavior. In fact, they are often cured with complete removal. And even when they are not resected, their growth and progression rate seem to be surprisingly slow.

Intraductal Tubulopapillary Neoplasm of the Bile Ducts (ITPNs)

Intraductal tubulopapillary neoplasms of the bile ducts (ITPNs) are very similar to IPNBs clinically and grossly [50, 51]. They can present with cystic dilatation of the ducts, although they are more commonly detected as multinodular tumors with focal cystic changes [51]. They are distinguished from IPNBs by their predominantly tubular architecture and minimal papilla formation and non-mucinous cells [51]. ITPNs are now regarded to be a distinct category. Some examples were published under the title of intraductal tubular neoplasms [50] although the term intraductal tubulopapillary neoplasm (ITPN) is becoming the norm [51]. Having said that, it should be noted here that papilla formation is very limited, if any, in these tumors; they are typically composed of florid compact nodules of back-to-back tubular units. Over half are intrahepatic [3, 12, 32–36, 50, 51]. Some solid examples have comedo-type (central) necrosis. They have other distinctive histomorphologic findings including intratubular acidophilic secretions, psammoma bodies, and calcifications that can impart a thyroid-like follicular appearance. Immunohistochemically, they usually express MUC1 and MUC6 [51]. They usually do not stain for MUC2 or CDX2, and in contrast to IPNBs many of which are of intestinal lineage. ITPNs do not express MUC5AC. Their molecular makeup also appears to be different than IPNBs and ordinary cholangiocarcinomas. ITPNs present clinically in a similar fashion as IPNBs. Approximately 80% have associated invasive carcinomas. Nevertheless, true to their predominantly preinvasive nature, these seem to have a relatively protracted clinical course based on the currently available limited data [51].

Mucinous Cystic Neoplasms (with Ovarian Stroma)

Mucinous cystic neoplasms (MCNs) are neoplastic cysts defined by the presence of mural ovarian stroma according to the 2010 WHO criteria (Fig. 14.2) [1, 52–57]. This ovarian stroma has all the characteristics of the ovarian cortical cells, including progesterone receptor expression and the presence of scattered luteal-type cells. The requirement of ovarian stroma for the diagnosis of mucinous cystic neoplasm is based on the recognition that these neoplasms are clinically and

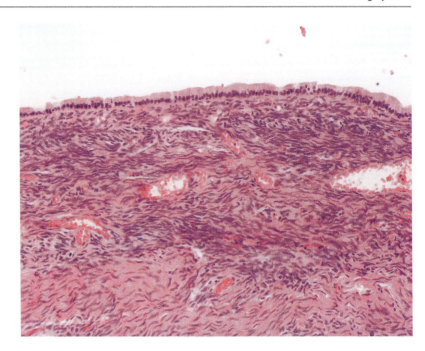

Fig. 14.2 Mucinous cystic neoplasm. The spindle cell stroma underlying the epithelium has all the characteristics of ovarian cortex, and as such it is diagnostic (and pathognomonic) for mucinous cystic neoplasm. The epithelium is tall columnar mucinous in this area; however, often in MCNs the cyst lining is composed of non-mucinous biliary-type cells which is the predominant pattern in some cases

biologically distinct from other hepatobiliary cysts and mirrors classification of mucinous cystic neoplasm of the pancreas [1, 57]. The antiquated term "hepatobiliary cystadenoma" is best avoided, as this term was previously used to refer to a variety of cystic liver lesions including those that did not all have the ovarian stroma that is a requirement for the diagnosis of mucinous cystic neoplasm according to the 2010 WHO criteria. Since the relatively recent definitional changes, the clinicopathologic characteristics of true hepatobiliary MCNs with ovarian stroma are just beginning to be elucidated in more recent literature with studies that stringently apply the requirement for ovarian stroma [57]. The vast majority occur in adult women. They may involve the liver or the extrahepatic bile ducts; some involve the liver and prolapse into an extrahepatic bile duct [57–59]. Curiously, the majority of intrahepatic MCNs (72–75%) involve the left hepatic lobe, despite its smaller size [57]. The ovarian stroma may be diffusely present throughout the lesion, or it may be focal. The cysts are epithelial-lined although in many examples the lining is at least focally denuded and in some cases epithelial denudation is extensive. The lining may be low cuboidal biliary-type or tall columnar mucinous. Given the occasional focal nature of the ovarian stroma, the frequent epithelial denudation, and the frequent occurrence of at least focal non-mucinous cuboidal epithelial lining, it is important to bear in mind that mucinous cystic neoplasm cannot be excluded on a limited sampling of a cyst wall that happens not to have ovarian stroma, even if there is a non-mucinous cuboidal lining or no epithelium at all.

By definition, all mucinous cystic neoplasms are neoplastic and harbor at least low-grade dysplasia although cytologically the cells are typically very "normal-appearing," closely resembling normal endocervical or gastric surface epithelial cells. Recent studies have shown that many MCNs that are defined by 2010 WHO criteria (with ovarian-type stroma) actually have a substantial non-mucinous biliary-type epithelial lining, and, in fact, this non-mucinous cytology may predominate the picture in many cases [60].

Grading of dysplasia follows the criteria discussed above for BilINs and, following the trend in the pancreas, now uses a two-tiered system (low and high grade). Recent studies have shown that, defined by the presence of the ovarian-type stroma (as in the pancreas), high-grade dysplasia and invasive carcinoma are in fact relatively uncommon in hepatobiliary mucinous cystic neoplasms (reported combined frequency ranging from 2 to 10%) [35, 57, 58] compared to their pancreatic counterparts (combined prevalence, 24%; invasive, 17%) [61]. Prior to the requirement of ovarian stroma for diagnosis, the term mucinous cystadenocarcinoma had been applied to lesions that would currently be called intraductal neoplasms of the bile ducts (IPNBs, IOPNs, and ITPNs discussed above). Even cholangiocarcinomas with cystic degeneration have been classified as "hepatobiliary cystadenocarcinoma." A recent study suggests that high-grade dysplasia was not identified in any case that did not have tall columnar mucinous epithelium, suggesting that transition from non-mucinous cuboidal biliary epithelium to tall columnar mucinous epithelium may be a step in the progression toward higher-grade neoplasia [62]. As most hepatobiliary MCNs are low-grade, the lining is usually flat. When there are polypoid intraluminal projections comprising epithelium (tumoral intraepithelial neoplasia), these often harbor high-grade dysplasia/CIS; papillary/polypoid epithelial proliferation is uncommon in low-grade MCNs. That said, not all high-grade dysplasia or carcinoma will be grossly recognizable, and consequently, extensive (if not complete) sampling is often necessary for accurate pathologic assessment to exclude carcinoma. Conversely, not all mural nodules necessarily represent tumoral epithelial proliferation [57] (i.e., not all signify high-grade dysplasia or carcinoma). Polypoid intraluminal projections/mural nodules may also comprise various combinations of protruding ovarian stroma with or without mural daughter cysts, fibrosis, hemorrhage, or inflammation; mural nodules of these types (sometimes measuring over 1 cm) occasionally occur in low-grade MCNs [57].

True to their neoplastic nature, MCNs tend to persist/recur when they are not completely excised. Therefore, procedures such as aspiration, fenestration, or unroofing are not curative; complete resection is necessary to minimize the chances of recurrence and/or progression [57, 58, 60]. We have seen examples to recur many years after the original incomplete removal [57].

In summary, there is a spectrum of cystic lesions that can harbor preinvasive neoplasia and thus progress into invasive cancer. Their biologic behavior can vary greatly by type, and their clinical associations also differ depending on the entity. Therefore, it is important to make every attempt to classify such cases as accurately as possible.

References

1. Bosman FT, World Health Organization., International Agency for Research on Cancer. WHO classification of tumours of the digestive system. 4th ed. Lyon: International Agency for Research on Cancer; 2010. 417 p.
2. Zen Y, Adsay NV, Bardadin K, Colombari R, Ferrell L, Haga H, et al. Biliary intraepithelial neoplasia: an international interobserver agreement study and proposal for diagnostic criteria. Mod Pathol. 2007;20(6):701–9.
3. Albores-Saavedra J, Adsay NV, Crawford JM, Klimstra DS, Klöppel G, Sripa B, et al. Carcinoma of the gallbladder and extrahepatic bile ducts. In: Bosman FT, Carneiro F, Hruban R, Theise ND, editors. World health organization classification of tumors tumors of digestive system. 4th ed. Lyon: IARC Press; 2010. p. 266–74.
4. Adsay NV, Adair CF, Heffess CS, Klimstra DS. Intraductal oncocytic papillary neoplasms of the pancreas. Am J Surg Pathol. 1996;20(8):980–94.
5. Adsay NV, Kloeppel G, Fukushima N, Offerhaus GJ, Furukawa N. Intraductal neoplasms of the pancreas. In: Bosman FT, Carneiro F, Hruban RH, Theise ND, editors. WHO classification of tumors. Lyon: WHO Press; 2010. p. 304–13.
6. Adsay V, Mino-Kenudson M, Furukawa T, Basturk O, Zamboni G, Marchegiani G, et al. Pathologic evaluation and reporting of intraductal papillary mucinous neoplasms of the pancreas and other tumoral intraepithelial neoplasms of pancreatobiliary tract: recommendations of Verona consensus meeting. Ann Surg. 2016;263(1):162–77.
7. Basturk O, Hong SM, Wood LD, Adsay NV, Albores-Saavedra J, Biankin AV, et al. A revised classification system and recommendations from the Baltimore consensus meeting for neoplastic precursor lesions in the pancreas. Am J Surg Pathol. 2015;39(12):1730–41.
8. Furukawa T, Kloppel G, Volkan Adsay N, Albores-Saavedra J, Fukushima N, Horii A, et al. Classification of types of intraductal papillary-mucinous neoplasm of the pancreas: a consensus study. Virchows Arch. 2005;447(5):794–9.
9. Hruban RH, Takaori K, Klimstra DS, Adsay NV, Albores-Saavedra J, Biankin AV, et al. An illustrated consensus on the classification of pancreatic intraepithelial neoplasia and intraductal papillary mucinous neoplasms. Am J Surg Pathol. 2004;28(8):977–87.

10. Kloppel G, Basturk O, Schlitter AM, Konukiewitz B, Esposito I. Intraductal neoplasms of the pancreas. Semin Diagn Pathol. 2014;31(6):452–66.
11. Ohhashi KMY, Maruyama M. Four cases of mucous secreting pancreatic cancer. Prog Digest Endosc. 1982;20:348–51.
12. Rocha FG, Lee H, Katabi N, DeMatteo RP, Fong Y, D'Angelica MI, et al. Intraductal papillary neoplasm of the bile duct: a biliary equivalent to intraductal papillary mucinous neoplasm of the pancreas? Hepatology. 2012;56(4):1352–60.
13. Hruban R, Pitman MB, Klimstra DS. Tumors of the pancreas. Washington, DC: American Registry of Pathology; 2007.
14. Basturk O, Adsay V, Askan G, Dhall D, Zamboni G, Shimizu M, et al. Intraductal tubulopapillary neoplasm of the pancreas: a clinicopathologic and immunohistochemical analysis of 33 cases. Am J Surg Pathol. 2017;41(3):313–25.
15. Kloppel G, Adsay V, Konukiewitz B, Kleeff J, Schlitter AM, Esposito I. Precancerous lesions of the biliary tree. Best Pract Res Clin Gastroenterol. 2013;27(2):285–97.
16. Zen Y, Aishima S, Ajioka Y, Haratake J, Kage M, Kondo F, et al. Proposal of histological criteria for intraepithelial atypical/proliferative biliary epithelial lesions of the bile duct in hepatolithiasis with respect to cholangiocarcinoma: preliminary report based on interobserver agreement. Pathol Int. 2005;55(4):180–8.
17. Laitio M. Carcinoma of extrahepatic bile ducts. A histopathologic study. Pathol Res Pract. 1983;178(1):67–72.
18. Suzuki M, Takahashi T, Ouchi K, Matsuno S. The development and extension of hepatohilar bile duct carcinoma. A three-dimensional tumor mapping in the intrahepatic biliary tree visualized with the aid of a graphics computer system. Cancer. 1989;64(3):658–66.
19. Davis RI, Sloan JM, Hood JM, Maxwell P. Carcinoma of the extrahepatic biliary tract: a clinicopathological and immunohistochemical study. Histopathology. 1988;12(6):623–31.
20. Albores-Saavedra J, Henson DE, Klimstra DS. Tumors of the gallbladder, extrahepatic bile ducts, and ampulla of vater. Atlas of tumor pathology, 3rd ed. 27. Washington, DC: Armed Forces Institute of Pathology; 2000. p. 21–113.
21. Hacihasanoglu E, Reid M, Muraki T, Memis B, Mittal P, Polito H, Zarrabi N, Saka B, Krasinskas A, Quigley B, Adsay V. Choledochal cysts in the west: clinicopathologic analysis of 84 cases. (abstract). Modern Pathol. 2016;29:441A.
22. Katabi NPV, DeMatteo R, Klimstra DS. Choledochal cysts: a clinicopathologic study of 36 cases with emphasis on the morphologic and the immunohistochemical features of premalignant and malignant alterations. Hum Pathol. 2014;45(10):2107–14.
23. Shibahara H, Tamada S, Goto M, Oda K, Nagino M, Nagasaka T, et al. Pathologic features of mucin-producing bile duct tumors: two histopathologic categories as counterparts of pancreatic intraductal papillary-mucinous neoplasms. Am J Surg Pathol. 2004;28(3):327–38.
24. Moschovis D, Bamias G, Delladetsima I. Mucins in neoplasms of pancreas, ampulla of Vater and biliary system. World J Gastrointest Oncol. 2016;8(10):725–34.
25. Nagata K, Horinouchi M, Saitou M, Higashi M, Nomoto M, Goto M, et al. Mucin expression profile in pancreatic cancer and the precursor lesions. J Hepato-Biliary-Pancreat Surg. 2007;14(3):243–54.
26. Yonezawa S, Taira M, Osako M, Kubo M, Tanaka S, Sakoda K, et al. MUC-1 mucin expression in invasive areas of intraductal papillary mucinous tumors of the pancreas. Pathol Int. 1998;48(4):319–22.
27. Riener MO, Fritzsche FR, Clavien PA, Pestalozzi BC, Probst-Hensch N, Jochum W, et al. IMP3 expression in lesions of the biliary tract: a marker for high-grade dysplasia and an independent prognostic factor in bile duct carcinomas. Hum Pathol. 2009;40(10):1377–83.
28. Wu J, Matthaei H, Maitra A, Dal Molin M, Wood LD, Eshleman JR, et al. Recurrent GNAS mutations define an unexpected pathway for pancreatic cyst development. Sci Transl Med. 2011;3(92):92ra66.
29. Matthaei H, Wu J, Dal Molin M, Debeljak M, Lingohr P, Katabi N, et al. GNAS codon 201 mutations are uncommon in intraductal papillary neoplasms of the bile duct. HPB (Oxford). 2012;14(10):677–83.
30. Furukawa T, Kuboki Y, Tanji E, Yoshida S, Hatori T, Yamamoto M, et al. Whole-exome sequencing uncovers frequent GNAS mutations in intraductal papillary mucinous neoplasms of the pancreas. Sci Rep. 2011;1:161.
31. Kanda M, Knight S, Topazian M, Syngal S, Farrell J, Lee J, et al. Mutant GNAS detected in duodenal collections of secretin-stimulated pancreatic juice indicates the presence or emergence of pancreatic cysts. Gut. 2013;62(7):1024–33.
32. Schlitter AM, Kloppel G, Esposito I. Intraductal papillary neoplasms of the bile duct (IPNB). Diagnostic criteria, carcinogenesis and differential diagnostics. Pathologe. 2013;34(Suppl 2):235–40.
33. Sasaki M, Matsubara T, Nitta T, Sato Y, Nakanuma Y. GNAS and KRAS mutations are common in intraductal papillary neoplasms of the bile duct. PLoS One. 2013;8(12):e81706.
34. Kim KM, Lee JK, Shin JU, Lee KH, Lee KT, Sung JY, et al. Clinicopathologic features of intraductal papillary neoplasm of the bile duct according to histologic subtype. Am J Gastroenterol. 2012;107(1):118–25.
35. Zen Y, Jang KT, Ahn S, Kim DH, Choi DW, Choi SH, et al. Intraductal papillary neoplasms and mucinous cystic neoplasms of the hepatobiliary system: demographic differences between Asian and western populations, and comparison with pancreatic counterparts. Histopathology. 2014;65(2):164–73.
36. Sclabas GM, Barton JG, Smyrk TC, Barrett DA, Khan S, Kendrick ML, et al. Frequency of subtypes of biliary intraductal papillary mucinous neoplasm and their MUC1, MUC2, and DPC4 expression patterns differ

37. from pancreatic intraductal papillary mucinous neoplasm. J Am Coll Surg. 2012;214(1):27–32.
37. Zen Y, Fujii T, Itatsu K, Nakamura K, Minato H, Kasashima S, et al. Biliary papillary tumors share pathological features with intraductal papillary mucinous neoplasm of the pancreas. Hepatology. 2006;44(5):1333–43.
38. Chen TC, Nakanuma Y, Zen Y, Chen MF, Jan YY, Yeh TS, et al. Intraductal papillary neoplasia of the liver associated with hepatolithiasis. Hepatology. 2001;34(4 Pt 1):651–8.
39. Abraham SC, Lee JH, Boitnott JK, Argani P, Furth EE, Wu TT. Microsatellite instability in intraductal papillary neoplasms of the biliary tract. Mod Pathol. 2002;15(12):1309–17.
40. Kim HJ, Kim MH, Lee SK, Yoo KS, Park ET, Lim BC, et al. Mucin-hypersecreting bile duct tumor characterized by a striking homology with an intraductal papillary mucinous tumor (IPMT) of the pancreas. Endoscopy. 2000;32(5):389–93.
41. Abraham SC, Lee JH, Hruban RH, Argani P, Furth EE, Wu TT. Molecular and immunohistochemical analysis of intraductal papillary neoplasms of the biliary tract. Hum Pathol. 2003;34(9):902–10.
42. Kloppel G, Kosmahl M. Is the intraductal papillary mucinous neoplasia of the biliary tract a counterpart of pancreatic papillary mucinous neoplasm? J Hepatol. 2006;44(2):249–50.
43. Nakanuma Y, Harada K, Sasaki M, Sato Y. Proposal of a new disease concept "biliary diseases with pancreatic counterparts". Anatomical and pathological bases. Histol Histopathol. 2014;29(1):1–10.
44. Zen Y, Fujii T, Itatsu K, Nakamura K, Konishi F, Masuda S, et al. Biliary cystic tumors with bile duct communication: a cystic variant of intraductal papillary neoplasm of the bile duct. Mod Pathol. 2006;19(9):1243–54.
45. Albores-Saavedra J, Murakata L, Krueger JE, Henson DE. Noninvasive and minimally invasive papillary carcinomas of the extrahepatic bile ducts. Cancer. 2000;89(3):508–15.
46. Madden JJ Jr, Smith GW. Multiple biliary papillomatosis. Cancer. 1974;34(4):1316–20.
47. Taguchi J, Yasunaga M, Kojiro M, Arita T, Nakayama T, Simokobe T. Intrahepatic and extrahepatic biliary papillomatosis. Arch Pathol Lab Med. 1993;117(9):944–7.
48. Rouzbahman M, Serra S, Adsay NV, Bejarano PA, Nakanuma Y, Chetty R. Oncocytic papillary neoplasms of the biliary tract: a clinicopathological, mucin core and Wnt pathway protein analysis of four cases. Pathology. 2007;39(4):413–8.
49. Zen Y, Sasaki M, Fujii T, Chen TC, Chen MF, Yeh TS, et al. Different expression patterns of mucin core proteins and cytokeratins during intrahepatic cholangiocarcinogenesis from biliary intraepithelial neoplasia and intraductal papillary neoplasm of the bile duct--an immunohistochemical study of 110 cases of hepatolithiasis. J Hepatol. 2006;44(2):350–8.
50. Katabi N, Torres J, Klimstra DS. Intraductal tubular neoplasms of the bile ducts. Am J Surg Pathol. 2012;36(11):1647–55.
51. Schlitter AM, Jang KT, Kloppel G, Saka B, Hong SM, Choi H, et al. Intraductal tubulopapillary neoplasms of the bile ducts: clinicopathologic, immunohistochemical, and molecular analysis of 20 cases. Mod Pathol. 2016;29(1):93.
52. Devaney K, Goodman ZD, Ishak KG. Hepatobiliary cystadenoma and cystadenocarcinoma. A light microscopic and immunohistochemical study of 70 patients. Am J Surg Pathol. 1994;18(11):1078–91.
53. Ishak KG, Willis GW, Cummins SD, Bullock AA. Biliary cystadenoma and cystadenocarcinoma: report of 14 cases and review of the literature. Cancer. 1977;39(1):322–38.
54. O'Shea JS, Shah D, Cooperman AM. Biliary cystadenocarcinoma of extrahepatic duct origin arising in previously benign cystadenoma. Am J Gastroenterol. 1987;82:1307–10.
55. Subramony C, Herrera GA, Turbat-Herrera EA. Hepatobiliary cystadenoma. A study of five cases with reference to histogenesis. Arch Pathol Lab Med. 1993;117(10):1036–42.
56. Wheeler DA, Edmondson HA. Cystadenoma with mesenchymal stroma (CMS) in the liver and bile ducts. A clinicopathologic study of 17 cases, 4 with malignant change. Cancer. 1985;56(6):1434–45.
57. Quigley B, Reid MD, Squires MH, Maithel S, Xue Y, Hyejong C, Akkas G, Muraki T, Pehlivanoglu B, Kooby DA, Sarmiento JM, Cardona K, Sekhar AK, Krasinskas A, Adsay V. Hepatobiliary mucinous cystic neoplasms with ovarian type stroma (so-called "hepatobiliary cystadenoma/cystadenocarcinoma"): clinicopathologic analysis of 36 cases illustrates rarity of carcinomatous change. Am J Surg Pathol. 2018;42(1):95–102.
58. Albores-Saavedra J, Cordova-Ramon JC, Chable-Montero F, Dorantes-Heredia R, Henson DE. Cystadenomas of the liver and extrahepatic bile ducts: morphologic and immunohistochemical characterization of the biliary and intestinal variants. Ann Diagn Pathol. 2015;19(3):124–9.
59. Takano Y, Nagahama M, Yamamura E, Maruoka N, Mizukami H, Tanaka J, et al. Prolapse into the bile duct and expansive growth is characteristic behavior of mucinous cystic neoplasm of the liver: report of two cases and review of the literature. Clin J Gastroenterol. 2015;8(3):148–55.
60. Lee CW, Tsai HI, Lin YS, Wu TH, Yu MC, Chen MF. Intrahepatic biliary mucinous cystic neoplasms: clinicoradiological characteristics and surgical results. BMC Gastroenterol. 2015;15:67.
61. Jang KT, Park SM, Basturk O, Bagci P, Bandyopadhyay S, Stelow EB, et al. Clinicopathologic characteristics of 29 invasive carcinomas arising in 178 pancreatic mucinous cystic neoplasms with ovarian-type stroma: implications for management and prognosis. Am J Surg Pathol. 2015;39(2):179–87.
62. Zhelnin K, Xue Y, Quigley B, Reid MD, Choi H, Memis B, et al. Nonmucinous biliary epithelium is a frequent finding and is often the predominant epithelial type in mucinous cystic neoplasms of the pancreas and liver. Am J Surg Pathol. 2017;41(1):116–20.

Indications for Resection of Preinvasive Cystic Neoplasms of the Intra- and Extrahepatic Bile Ducts

15

Jad Abou-Khalil and Flavio G. Rocha

Introduction

A variety of liver lesions are cystic in nature, with the majority being of benign or parasitic etiology. Simple cysts are extremely common and have no malignant potential, with surgical indications focusing on relief of symptoms related to mass effect or hemorrhage. Cystic hamartomas are also described, usually small and with a universally benign course. In certain regions, parasitic cysts due to echinococcal infection are prevalent, and high suspicion is important to rule out this entity in patients from endemic areas presenting for the workup of a cystic liver lesion, as the unplanned entry into a parasitic cyst can be associated with intraperitoneal parasitic recurrence or anaphylactic reactions. Metastasis of certain neoplasms, namely, those with cystic components such as mucinous carcinomas of the colon, cystadenocarcinomas of the pancreas, and ovarian cancer, presents as cystic liver masses, whereas solid liver tumors, whether primary or metastatic, that display central necrosis or degeneration can have a cystic appearance without being true hepatic cysts.

J. Abou-Khalil
Department of Surgery, The Ottawa Hospital, Ottawa, ON, Canada

F. G. Rocha (✉)
Section of General, Thoracic and Vascular Surgery, Virginia Mason Medical Center, Seattle, WA, USA
e-mail: Flavio.Rocha@virginiamason.org

Primary cystic neoplasms of the liver are much rarer than the aforementioned lesions and constitute a minority of premalignant and malignant liver lesions. These rare tumors will be the focus of this chapter. The different clinical and pathological entities will be reviewed with a focus on indications for surgical resection.

Mucinous Cystic Neoplasms of the Liver

Mucinous cystic neoplasms of the liver [1] are rare cystic hepatic lesions affecting predominantly women in the fourth and fifth decade of life. Previously known as biliary cystadenomas, they have been reclassified by the World Health Organization (WHO) in 2010 to mirror similar entities found in the pancreas [2]. Histologically they are characterized by a biliary epithelial lining with mucin-containing and mucin-secreting cells, occasional islands of atypia and micropapillary projections, and universally an ovarian-like stroma. The presence of this ovarian stroma is the defining characteristic of this pathologic entity, similar to its corollary in the pancreas [3]. A key feature of MCN-L is their lack of communication with the biliary tree. The pathogenesis of MCN-L is unknown, with both intrahepatic peri-biliary glandular epithelium or endodermal remnants of embryonic biliary epithelium proposed as the likely origin [4].

These tumors are generally asymptomatic and are increasingly identified incidentally. When associated with symptoms, these are often non-specific and associated with stretch of the Glisson's capsule or compression of adjacent organs. Very uncommonly, MCN-L can present with biliary obstructive symptoms such as jaundice. Less than 10% of lesions historically characterized as biliary adenomas arise in the extrahepatic bile ducts, and some have been documented to grow as a tumor embolus along the bile duct and obstruct the biliary confluence. However it is possible that such tumors would not be classified as MCN-L today after the WHO reclassification [5] and that many series reporting on MCN-L associated intimately or growing into the biliary tree in fact represent intraductal papillary neoplasms of the bile duct (IPNB).

Radiographically, MCN-L are multilocular, usually with thin or thick septations sometimes described as a "cyst-on-cyst" appearance. Only a third of MCN-L have mural nodules. Although upstream biliary tree dilatation can be present, it is much more commonly associated with IPNB [6] as MCN-L are not associated with downstream biliary dilatation.

MCN-L are mostly benign and have an indolent course, but progression to their malignant counterpart, mucinous cystic carcinomas of the liver (previously known as biliary cystadenocarcinomas), is documented. The exact natural history of this progression, its risk factors, and its associated radiologic, pathologic, and biochemical associations are not well defined but appear to be less frequent than in pancreatic MCN [7]. The proportion of MCN-L progressing to carcinoma, estimated at 20% in early series, is likely overestimated due to misclassification of other tumors with higher malignant potential such as intraductal papillary neoplasms of the bile ducts and in series restricted to tumors with ovarian stroma is closer to 2%. In a series of 29 patients with true MCN-L with ovarian stroma, only 1 (3%) had malignancy at postoperative pathologic examination [3]. In older series of patients diagnosed with biliary cystadenocarcinomas, the absence of an ovarian stroma and the equal proportion of men and women in this population suggest these tumors were in fact misclassified IPNB [8].

Every attempt should be made to excise these tumors completely with a negative margin [9]. Aspiration, fenestration, and sclerosant application are associated with an unacceptable recurrence rate and may leave behind a potential malignancy. When MCN-L are diagnosed after cyst unroofing of lesions thought to represent simple cysts, a completion resection of the remaining lesion is prudent. Even though the risk of the remaining cyst wall harboring invasive carcinoma is low, the malignant potential means that all, but patients with the most prohibitive surgical risk, should undergo complete excision [10]. This approach is supported by a meta-analysis of reported MCN-L in the literature which demonstrates a slight decrease in survival in patients undergoing incomplete resections—71% at 2 years and 36% at 5 years, compared to 100% survival with complete resection [11].

However, occasionally these can be quite large and located either deep within the liver or adjacent to the hepatic vein or biliary confluence. In cases where the potential for significant morbidity is present, we recommend a partial cyst excision with frozen section analysis to determine the need for complete resection. If benign, we have performed marsupialization with ablation of the retained interior of the cyst (see Fig. 15.1).

Intraductal Papillary Mucinous Neoplasms of the Bile Duct

Intraductal papillary neoplasm of the bile duct (IPNB) is a newly defined clinical entity sharing many pathological and clinical characteristics of pancreatic IPMN. Both pancreatic and IPNB are thought to represent similar processes in different parts of the biliopancreatic system and share many histologic and biochemical characteristics [12]. Like pancreatic IPMNs, IPNB are classified into four histologic types: pancreaticobiliary, intestinal, oncocytic, and gastric [13]. Unlike MCN-L, they communicate with the biliary tree, contain papillary projections and mural nodules, have no ovarian-like stroma, and are not more common in women. Significant geographic variation exists in the proportion of IPNB and MCN-L, with IPNB constituting the majority of mucinous liver cysts in

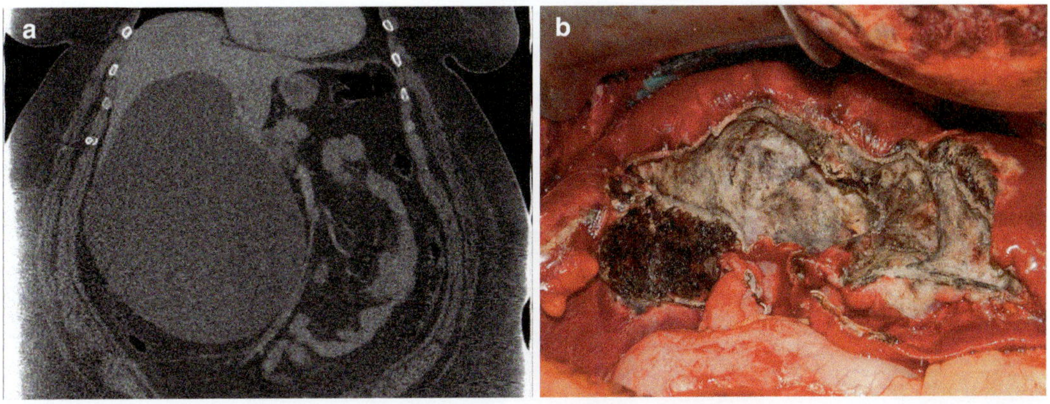

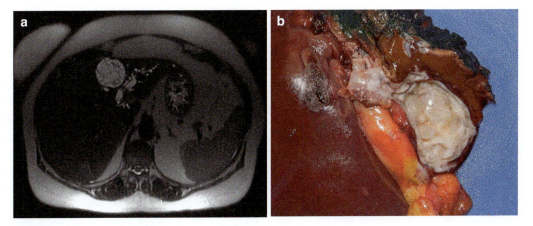

Fig. 15.1 A 58-year-old female with a large, symptomatic MCN-L that was partially excised and cyst epithelium ablated given the extent of liver involvement

Fig. 15.2 A 62-year-old female who presented with abnormal liver function tests and was noted to have a cystic mass causing biliary obstruction. A left hepatectomy with bile duct reconstruction was required given the presence of IPNB

Asia, whereas western Europe and North America report a predominance of MCN-L [7].

Radiographically, IPNB tend to have more central septations and are more often associated with mural nodules than MCN-L. Upstream biliary dilatation is present in two thirds of IPNB but can also be seen in MCN-L, whereas downstream biliary dilatation is only seen with IPNB (Fig. 15.2) [6]. They tend to be located more frequently in the left liver for unclear reasons but perhaps due to the longer course of the left extrahepatic bile duct.

A high proportion (40–80%) [14] of IPNB have a component of invasive carcinoma. No clinical, radiological, or biochemical markers can adequately predict the presence of carcinoma, but this may be due to most published series combining MCN-L and IPNB [15]. The prognosis of cholangiocarcinoma in this setting is better than that of cholangiocarcinoma arising in flat dysplasia [13]. However, the depth of invasion is also predictive of survival. Given the significant malignant potential, complete surgical excision with a negative bile duct margin is indicated, as patients with residual dysplasia are at higher risk of recurrence [16].

Intraductal Tubulopapillary Neoplasms of the Bile Duct

Intraductal tubulopapillary neoplasm of the bile duct (ITPN) is a newly described unique pathologic entity closely paralleling its homologous

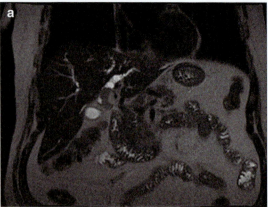 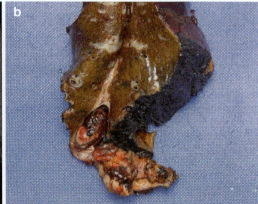

Fig. 15.3 A 66-year-old male with obstructive jaundice found to have an intrabiliary tumor at the confluence. Final pathology demonstrated a poorly differentiated intrahepatic cholangiocarcinoma arising in a background of ITPN extending into the hilum

entity in the pancreas. Unlike IPNB which have a mostly papillary intraductal growth pattern, ITPNs show glands with a predominantly tubular growth pattern and minimal papillary architecture [17, 18]. Often the intraductal tumor grows as a solid, compact polypoid mass preserving the ductal epithelium except where an invasive component is found. In the largest series of 20 patients from multiple institutions, 80% of resected ITPNs contained invasive carcinoma [19]. Despite this, the 5-year survival was 90%, indicating the possibly indolent nature of these tumors even in the presence of invasive carcinoma. These unique tumors are unlikely to be distinguished preoperatively from other cholangiocarcinomas (Fig. 15.3). They should therefore be excised in their entirety with negative margins. The rarity of these tumors makes it difficult to posit on the ways in which their treatment should differ from the management of other cholangiocarcinomas.

Choledochal Cysts

This cluster of entities present as cystic dilatation of the extrahepatic, the intrahepatic bile ducts, or both. The original Alonso-Lej classification [20], which only included cysts of the common bile duct, was then expanded to include intrahepatic cysts by Todani [21], who rapidly pointed out the association of these cysts with malignant transformation of the abnormally dilated bile ducts and the necessity of excising the abnormal ducts. We will focus our discussion on the management of choledochal cyst types associated with the development of cholangiocarcinoma.

Type 1 choledochal cysts consist of cystic (1A) or fusiform (1C) dilatation of the entire extrahepatic portions of the biliary tree associated with an abnormal pancreaticobiliary junction (APBJ) or of focal segments thereof (1B and 1D) without an association with APBJ. Type 2 and 3 choledochal cysts represent, respectively, true diverticuli of the extrahepatic bile ducts and choledochocele. Type 4 cysts consist of intra- and extrahepatic cystic dilatation of the bile ducts (4A) or multiple cystic dilatations of the extrahepatic ducts (4B) without associated APBJ. Type 5 choledochal cysts, also known as Caroli's disease, represent multiple cystic dilatations of the intrahepatic biliary tree.

Types 1 and 4 are the classes of choledochal cysts thought to be most at risk for malignant transformation (Fig. 15.4), whereas types 2 and 3 are at a much lower risk. The exact risk conferred by such lesion is difficult to estimate. Early series appeared to describe a high lifetime risk of cholangiocarcinoma, with the risk increasing with age from 0.7% in the pediatric population to over

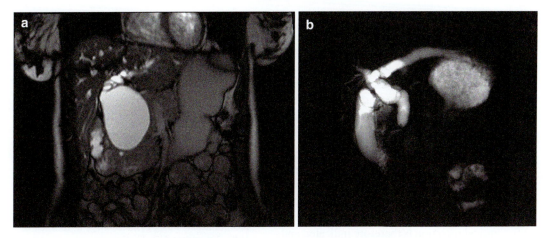

Fig. 15.4 Characteristic MRI/MRCP images of type I and type IV choledochal cysts

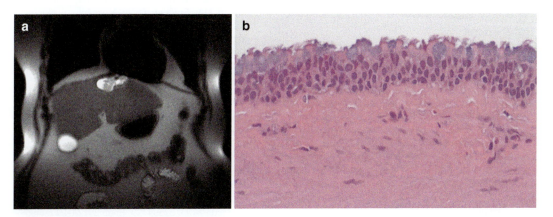

Fig. 15.5 Ciliated hepatic foregut cyst found in the typical location of segment 4 along the falciform ligament. Pathologic examination reveals pseudostratified respiratory epithelium with fimbria and goblet cells

14% in by the third decade of life [22]. Some series calculate an even higher proportion of carcinoma—up to 30% [23], but it is likely that these estimates are biased and inaccurate due to the inability to capture the experience of all patients with clinically occult choledochal cysts.

In patients that are surgical candidates, a complete resection of the extrahepatic biliary tree in its entirety, between the pancreaticobiliary junction and the confluence of the left and right hepatic ducts, is indicated. This is done to decrease the risk of developing cholangiocarcinoma. However, surgeons must remain vigilant while following such patients. Despite an adequate resection, the risk of cholangiocarcinoma in the remnant biliary tree remains high, estimated at 5% [24]. This may be due to a "field defect" within the remaining biliary epithelium, or possibly to the chronic low-grade inflammation that accompanies the hepaticoenterostomy itself.

Ciliated Hepatic Foregut Cysts

This rare congenital cyst, equivalent to bronchogenic cysts in its embryonic origin and its histologic structure, presents in children and young adults. Generally asymptomatic and identified incidentally on imaging performed for other reasons, they can also present with a variety of nonspecific symptoms such as abdominal pain, early satiety, and occasionally jaundice [25]. The cysts are usually well circumscribed and mostly unilocular, although rare reported cases have multilocular cysts or solid components. Most are located in segment 4, but they have also been described in the porta hepatis and the falciform ligament. The cyst fluid can contain CA19-9 and CEA [26]. Histologically, they contain a classic four-layered structure of an inner lining of ciliated columnar epithelium overlying a smooth muscle and loose connective tissue layers, surrounded by a fibrous capsule (Fig. 15.5). These cysts have the potential of developing squamous metaplasia as well as squamous cell carcinoma [27]. Surgical resection is therefore indicated and preferred over ablative or sclerosing techniques.

References

1. Takano Y, Nagahama M, Yamamura E, Maruoka N, Mizukami H, Tanaka J-I, et al. Prolapse into the bile duct and expansive growth is characteristic behavior of mucinous cystic neoplasm of the liver: report of two cases and review of the literature. Clin J Gastroenterol. 2015;8(3):148–55. 05/0801/09/received 04/16/accepted. PubMed PMID: PMC4481294.
2. Nakanuma Y. A novel approach to biliary tract pathology based on similarities to pancreatic counterparts: is the biliary tract an incomplete pancreas? Pathol Int. 2010;60(6):419–29. PubMed PMID: 20518896. Epub 2010/06/04. eng.
3. Zen Y, Pedica F, Patcha VR, Capelli P, Zamboni G, Casaril A, et al. Mucinous cystic neoplasms of the liver: a clinicopathological study and comparison with intraductal papillary neoplasms of the bile duct. Mod Pathol. 2011;24(8):1079–89. PubMed PMID: 21516077. Epub 2011/04/26. eng.
4. Erdogan D, Lamers WH, Offerhaus GJ, Busch OR, Gouma DJ, van Gulik TM. Cystadenomas with ovarian stroma in liver and pancreas: an evolving concept. Dig Surg. 2006;23(3):186–91. PubMed PMID: 16837797. Epub 2006/07/14. eng.
5. Yi B, Cheng Q-B, Jiang X-Q, Liu C, Luo X-J, Dong H, et al. A special growth manner of intrahepatic biliary cystadenoma. World J Gastroenterol. 2009;15(48):6134–6. 12/2810/22/received 11/18/revised 11/25/accepted. PubMed PMID: PMC2797675.
6. Kim HJ, Yu ES, Byun JH, Hong S-M, Kim KW, Lee JS, et al. CT differentiation of mucin-producing cystic neoplasms of the liver from solitary bile duct cysts. Am J Roentgenol. 2013;202(1):83–91. 2014/01/01.
7. Zen Y, Jang KT, Ahn S, Kim DH, Choi DW, Choi SH, et al. Intraductal papillary neoplasms and mucinous cystic neoplasms of the hepatobiliary system: demographic differences between Asian and western populations, and comparison with pancreatic counterparts. Histopathology. 2014;65(2):164–73. PubMed PMID: 24456415. Epub 2014/01/25. eng.
8. Ishak KG, Willis GW, Cummins SD, Bullock AA. Biliary cystadenoma and cystadenocarcinoma: report of 14 cases and review of the literature. Cancer. 1977;39(1):322–38. PubMed PMID: 318915. Epub 1977/01/01. eng.
9. Ahanatha Pillai S, Velayutham V, Perumal S, Ulagendra Perumal S, Lakshmanan A, Ramaswami S, et al. Biliary cystadenomas: a case for complete resection. HPB Surg. 2012;2012:501705. 06/2003/14/received04/30/revised 05/08/accepted. PubMed PMID: PMC3388282.
10. Martel G, Alsharif J, Aubin J-M, Marginean C, Mimeault R, Fairfull-Smith RJ, et al. The management of hepatobiliary cystadenomas: lessons learned. HPB. 2013;15(8):617–22. 12/0608/21/received10/28/accepted. PubMed PMID: PMC3731583.
11. Simo KA, McKillop IH, Ahrens WA, Martinie JB, Iannitti DA, Sindram D. Invasive biliary mucinous cystic neoplasm: a review. HPB. 2012;14(11):725–40. 01/20/received 06/08/accepted. PubMed PMID: PMC3482668.
12. Wang M, Deng BY, Wen TF, Peng W, Li C, Trishul NM. An observational and comparative study on intraductal papillary mucinous neoplasm of the biliary tract and the pancreas from a Chinese cohort. Clin Res Hepatol Gastroenterol. 2016;40(2):161–8. PubMed PMID: 26823040. Epub 2016/01/30. eng.
13. Rocha FG, Lee H, Katabi N, DeMatteo RP, Fong Y, D'Angelica MI, et al. Intraductal papillary neoplasm of the bile duct: a biliary equivalent to intraductal papillary mucinous neoplasm of the pancreas? Hepatology (Baltimore, Md). 2012;56(4):1352–60. PubMed PMID: 22504729. Epub 2012/04/17. eng.
14. Wan XS, Xu YY, Qian JY, Yang XB, Wang AQ, He L, et al. Intraductal papillary neoplasm of the bile duct. World J Gastroenterol. 2013;19(46):8595–604. PubMed PMID: 24379576. Pubmed Central PMCID: PMC3870504. Epub 2014/01/01. eng.
15. Arnaoutakis DJ, Kim Y, Pulitano C, Zaydfudim V, Squires MH, Kooby D, et al. Management of biliary cystic tumors: a multi-institutional analysis of a rare liver tumor. Ann Surg. 2015;261(2):361–7. PubMed PMID: 24509187. Pubmed Central PMCID: PMC4655107. Epub 2014/02/11. eng.
16. Jung G, Park KM, Lee SS, Yu E, Hong SM, Kim J. Long-term clinical outcome of the surgically resected intraductal papillary neoplasm of the bile duct. J Hepatol. 2012;57(4):787–93. PubMed PMID: 22634127. Epub 2012/05/29. eng.
17. Katabi N, Torres J, Klimstra DS. Intraductal tubular neoplasms of the bile ducts. Am J Surg Pathol. 2012;36(11):1647–55. PubMed PMID: 23073323. Epub 2012/10/18. eng.
18. Sato Y, Osaka H, Harada K, Sasaki M, Nakanuma Y. Intraductal tubular neoplasm of the common bile duct. Pathol Int. 2010;60(7):516–9. PubMed PMID: 20594273. Epub 2010/07/03. eng.

19. Schlitter AM, Jang KT, Kloppel G, Saka B, Hong SM, Choi H, et al. Intraductal tubulopapillary neoplasms of the bile ducts: clinicopathologic, immunohistochemical, and molecular analysis of 20 cases. Mod Pathol. 2015;28(9):1249–64. PubMed PMID: 26111977. Epub 2015/06/27. eng.
20. Alonso-Lej F, Rever WB Jr, Pessagno DJ. Congenital choledochal cyst, with a report of 2, and an analysis of 94, cases. Int Abstr Surg. 1959;108(1):1–30. PubMed PMID: 13625059. Epub 1959/01/01. eng.
21. Todani T, Watanabe Y, Narusue M, Tabuchi K, Okajima K. Congenital bile duct cysts: classification, operative procedures, and review of thirty-seven cases including cancer arising from choledochal cyst. Am J Surg. 1977;134(2):263–9. PubMed PMID: 889044. Epub 1977/08/01. eng.
22. Voyles CR, Smadja C, Shands WC, Blumgart LH. Carcinoma in choledochal cysts. Age-related incidence. Arch Surg (Chicago, IL: 1960). 1983;118(8):986–8. PubMed PMID: 6870530. Epub 1983/08/01. eng.
23. Soreide K, Soreide JA. Bile duct cyst as precursor to biliary tract cancer. Ann Surg Oncol. 2007;14(3):1200–11. PubMed PMID: 17187167. Epub 2006/12/26. eng.
24. Ohashi T, Wakai T, Kubota M, Matsuda Y, Arai Y, Ohyama T, et al. Risk of subsequent biliary malignancy in patients undergoing cyst excision for congenital choledochal cysts. J Gastroenterol Hepatol. 2013;28(2):243–7. PubMed PMID: 22989043. Pubmed Central PMCID: PMC3816325. Epub 2012/09/20. eng.
25. Bishop KC, Perrino CM, Ruzinova MB, Brunt EM. Ciliated hepatic foregut cyst: a report of 6 cases and a review of the English literature. Diagn Pathol. 2015;10:81. 06/3001/22/received 06/10/accepted. PubMed PMID: PMC4486693.
26. Ben Ari Z, Cohen-Ezra O, Weidenfeld J, Bradichevsky T, Weitzman E, Rimon U, et al. Ciliated hepatic foregut cyst with high intra-cystic carbohydrate antigen 19-9 level. World J Gastroenterol. 2014;20(43):16355–8. 11/2103/28/received 05/25/revised 07/16/accepted. PubMed PMID: PMC4239529.
27. Zhang X, Wang Z, Dong Y. Squamous cell carcinoma arising in a ciliated hepatic foregut cyst: case report and literature review. Pathol Res Pract. 2009;205(7):498–501. PubMed PMID: 19410383. Epub 2009/05/05. eng.

Part III

Metastatic Liver Tumors

Patient Selection and Surgical Approach to Colorectal Cancer Liver Metastases

16

Jordan M. Cloyd and Thomas A. Aloia

Introduction

Colorectal cancer (CRC) is the second leading cause of cancer-related mortality in the United States [1]. Although more than 50% of patients will develop liver metastases during the course of their disease, as few as 25% of patients with colorectal cancer liver metastases (CRLM) are thought to be resectable at initial presentation. On the other hand, response rates to contemporary systemic chemotherapy have increased considerably resulting in longer survival durations for many patients. In fact, multimodality therapy with margin-negative resection can be associated with 5-year survival rates as high as 50% at experienced centers, even in patients with complex bilobar CRLM [2, 3].

Over the past two decades, there has been exponential growth in the knowledge of and experience in the management of CRLM. While surgical options have expanded, so have nonoperative therapies. At the same time, advances in diagnostic imaging, future liver remnant (FLR) augmentation, perioperative anesthesia and medicine, and patient selection have made liver surgery safer, enabling more complex liver resections without associated increases in morbidity and mortality [4, 5]. Finally, a better understanding of the tumor biology and the underlying molecular mechanisms have provided important prognostic information and soon should lead to more targeted therapeutic options.

This chapter provides an overview of the management of complex CRLM with a particular emphasis on patient selection and surgical approaches.

Patient Selection

Although the number of liver resections performed for CRLM has increased over the past several decades, a critical concept in patient selection for surgery is acknowledging that, by definition, all patients have stage IV disease. Therefore, identifying which patients are "resectable" and most likely to benefit from surgical resection is imperative. In general, resectability of CRLM should be defined along three separate domains and in a particular sequence: (1) physiologic, (2) oncologic, and (3) technical.

Physiologic Assessment

Physiologic resectability refers to the patient's ability to safely undergo one or more major abdominal operations. Although perioperative medicine, pre-

J. M. Cloyd
Division of Surgical Oncology, The Ohio State University Wexner Medical Center, Columbus, OH, USA
e-mail: jmcloyd@mdanderson.org

T. A. Aloia (✉)
Department of Surgical Oncology, University of Texas MD Anderson Cancer Center, Houston, TX, USA
e-mail: taaloia@mdanderson.org

© Springer Nature Switzerland AG 2018
K. Cardona, S. K. Maithel (eds.), *Primary and Metastatic Liver Tumors*,
https://doi.org/10.1007/978-3-319-91977-5_16

habilitation, the application of minimally invasive surgery, and enhanced recovery after surgery protocols have helped foster safer surgery, patient selection remains paramount. Multiple risk calculators [6], frailty indices [7], and other tools [8] have been developed to identify patients with adequate performance status to undergo major surgery with acceptably low risks of perioperative adverse events. If performance status is inadequate to tolerate hepatectomy, non-operative liver-directed therapies can be considered.

Oncologic Resectability

After a patient meets physiologic resectability criteria, a multidisciplinary assessment of oncologic resectability ensues. This concept refers to the selection of patients most likely to benefit from major surgery based on their underlying tumor biology. Patients considered candidates for resection of bilateral liver metastases should have minimal extrahepatic disease, stable or responding disease during preoperative systemic chemotherapy, and normal or improved CEA levels in response to chemotherapy. Although low-volume extrahepatic disease is not a contraindication to liver resection, these patients are at higher risk of recurrence and should demonstrate disease stability and favorable tumor biology prior to proceeding with hepatectomy [3, 9]. Emerging evidence regarding the poor prognosis of some tumor mutational profiles (e.g., KRAS or BRAF mutations) may also influence surgical decision-making in the near future [10].

Technical Resectability

After patients have met physiologic and oncologic resectability criteria, the ability to surgically resect all metastases with negative microscopic margins while leaving an adequate FLR must be critically assessed. In general, technical resectability requires the retention of two contiguous liver segments with adequate vascular inflow, outflow, and biliary drainage. FLR volume serves as a surrogate for function, and an FLR $\geq 20\%$ of standardized total liver volume (TLV) in chemotherapy-naïve patients and $\geq 30\%$ in chemotherapy-treated patients is considered necessary [11, 12]. In cases where predicted FLR is inadequate based on liver volumetry, PVE may be used to stimulate hypertrophy of the FLR [13, 14].

Technical Aspects

Perioperative Chemotherapy

Although still controversial, there is a growing consensus that patients with CRLM should receive preoperative chemotherapy prior to resection. The EORTC 40983 trial randomized patients with ≤ 4 CRLM to perioperative FOLFOX (5-FU, leucovorin, oxaliplatin) and surgical resection versus resection alone and found an absolute increase in progression-free survival (PFS) of 7 months in the perioperative chemotherapy plus surgery group [15]. While this modest increase in PFS is noteworthy, several other advantages to perioperative chemotherapy exist. First, a strategy of preoperative chemotherapy affords an opportunity to select out patients who develop progressive disease and select in those with favorable tumor biology and adequate personal physiology to undergo major hepatectomy. In fact, in the EORTC trial, 11% of patients in the surgery alone group underwent non-therapeutic laparotomy compared to 5% in the chemotherapy plus surgery group. Second, the mean reduction in tumor size among patients who received chemotherapy prior to surgery in EORTC 40983 was 26%, and therefore preoperative chemotherapy may enable sufficient downstaging to convert unresectable disease to resectable in a subset of patients.

We routinely administer 4–6 cycles of FOLFOX to patients with CRLM as we have previously shown that rates of chemotherapy-associated liver injury and postoperative hepatic insufficiency (PHI) increase with longer durations of chemotherapy [16]. The antiangiogenesis agent bevacizumab is added to the first 3–5 cycles as it is associated with an improved response rate and partially protects against oxaliplatin-associated sinusoidal injury [17]. Importantly, the response to preoperative chemotherapy provides useful prognostic information. Patients who experience a significant radiographic response [18], marked by homogenization of the tumor with a sharp tumor-liver interface, and/or a major pathologic response [19], defined as <50% of viable tumor cells, have significantly improved overall survival. The concept of disappearing liver metastases is important but in practice rarely occurs during short-interval chemotherapy. In exceptional circumstances, placement of fiducial markers prior to the administration of chemotherapy may help localize metastases that are small and/or located deeper than the subcapsular area [20].

Margin Status

The goal of resection is complete removal of all known disease, as seen on pretreatment imaging, with microscopically negative margins. However, in the era of modern chemotherapy, the importance of negative margins and the optimal margin width continues to be controversial. Several studies have suggested worse survival in patients with an R1 resection margin [21, 22], and some have even demonstrated a stepwise increase in survival as the margin width increases [23]. These observations likely reflect biological phenomena as opposed to technical consequences. In fact, when stratified by response to preoperative chemotherapy, the impact of R1 resection margin status is no longer significant in patients who experienced either a radiographic or pathologic response to induction systemic therapy [21]. Importantly, RAS mutations are associated with higher rates of margin positivity and narrower resection margins [24] as well as suboptimal responses to preoperative chemotherapy [25]. In practice, we aim for a 1 cm resection margin in KRAS wild type and 1.5 cm resection margin in KRAS-mutant metastases at the time of parenchymal transection in order to achieve optimal microscopic pathologic margins.

FLR Augmentation

The need for extended hepatectomy (i.e., trisegmentectomy) occurs relatively frequently among patients with advanced CRLM. An FLR volume <20% of the standardized TLV is directly linked to postoperative hepatic insufficiency, and therefore attempts at increasing the size of the liver remnant preoperatively are justified. First described by Kinoshita and later refined by Makuuchi, PVE diverts portal flow away from the hemiliver to be resected and toward the liver remnant thereby leading to compensatory hyperplasia of hepatocytes and organ hypertrophy [26, 27]. Utilized both prior to extended right hepatectomy [12] and part of a two-stage hepatectomy (TSH) strategy [2], PVE is associated with reductions in PHI as well as overall perioperative morbidity and mortality. Various techniques have been described, but we recommend an ipsilateral percutaneous approach, which may be extended to segment 4 when applicable, using embolic microspheres and coils as the best strategy to maximize the FLR [28]. In patients who demonstrate inadequate hypertrophy, hepatic vein embolization may be considered to further optimize the FLR [29].

Liver augmentation strategies also allow the opportunity to evaluate hepatic growth capacity. CT-based volumetry should be calculated 3–4 weeks following PVE with particular attention to the degree of hypertrophy (DH) and kinetic growth rate (KGR). The DH, defined as the change in FLR percentage based on CT volumetry before and after PVE, is independently associated with postoperative outcomes [30]. The KGR, defined as the DH divided by the length of time between PVE and first post-PVE volumetry, has been shown to be the most accurate predictor of postoperative morbidity and mortality secondary to liver insufficiency [31]. Confirming the importance of measuring hepatic regenerative capacity, patients with a KGR > 2%, in our experience, rarely develop PHI, and there have been no perioperative mortalities in this high-risk major hepatectomy group.

Non-resectional Therapies

For patients who are not optimal surgical candidates, either because of poor performance status, prohibitive comorbidities, significant previous surgical history, or inadequate hepatic reserve, non-resectional therapies offer alternatives. Ablative techniques are probably the most frequently utilized non-resectional therapy for CRLM. Ablation can be performed either percutaneously (guided by US, CT, or MRI) or via laparotomy or laparoscopy (guided by intraoperative ultrasound). Ablation should be reserved for lesions <3 cm in size, as recurrence rates rise for larger tumors [32]. Most lesions are accessible via a percutaneous approach although optimal targets are non-peripheral, distant from the diaphragm, and separate from major vessels [33, 34]. While cryotherapy has been used in the past, most centers utilize radiofrequency ablation (RFA, for which the most data is available) or the emerging technology of microwave ablation [35].

In addition to ablation, there has been a growing experience with transarterial chemoembolization (TACE) for CLRM [36]. Selective targeting of the tumor-supplying vessels allows for the direct delivery of chemotherapy, while concomitant embolization aids in decreased chemotherapy clearance and tumor perfusion. Various techniques are available including traditional chemoembolization using cytotoxic chemotherapy (e.g., 5-fluorouracil, mitomycin C, doxorubicin, irinotecan) with an embolic agent (e.g., iodized oil, polyvinyl alcohol particles, gelatin sponge, or microspheres). More recently, drug eluting-bead (DEB)-TACE which permits controlled drug release of either doxorubicin or irinotecan has become popularized.

Finally, growing evidence suggests a role for external beam radiation therapy for CRLM. This may be especially helpful in unresectable disease and/or when previous hepatotoxicity prevents the use of additional systemic chemotherapy. Ongoing experience with newer forms of radiotherapy, including proton beam radiation, may help spare normal liver parenchyma and expand the indications for radiation [37]. Nevertheless, traditional liver-directed radiation poses distinct challenges and limitations. An alternative is hepatic artery-based radioembolization, also known as selective internal radiation therapy (SIRT), typically using yttrium-90 (y90) resin microspheres. Most frequently, SIRT is used in unresectable patients after failure of first- or second-line chemotherapy [36]. The SIRFLOX trial randomized treatment-naïve patients with unresectable CRLM to FOLFOX chemotherapy with or without SIRT using y90 and found no difference in overall progression-free survival, though liver-specific progression was delayed in the group receiving radioembolization [38].

Minimally Invasive Approaches

While the adoption of minimally invasive approaches to liver resection has been slower than in other fields, laparoscopic hepatectomy still affords the same benefits of minimally invasive surgery: less postoperative pain, shorter length of hospital stay, and earlier return to activity [39]. Furthermore, despite the absence of level I evidence, oncologic outcomes appear to be similar to traditional open hepatectomy. In addition, hand-assisted approaches share the same recovery benefits as totally laparoscopic plus extraction incision approaches, with the added benefit of liver palpation for detection of radiographically occult lesions [40]. A steep learning curve persists especially in the performance of major hepatectomy, hilar dissection, parenchymal transection, and the use of intraoperative ultrasound [41]. However, in experienced centers, laparoscopic ultrasound appears to be similar to open ultrasound with regard to sensitivity and specificity of identifying small CRLM [42].

Surgical Approach

Extent and Distribution

The number of surgical approaches for patients with CRLM, especially those with bilateral disease, has significantly increased in recent years. Surgical options for CRLM now include anatomic hepatectomy, parenchymal sparing hepatectomy (PSH), traditional TSH with or without PVE, associated liver partition and portal vein ligation for staged hepatectomy (ALPPS), local ablative techniques, and hepatic arterial infusion

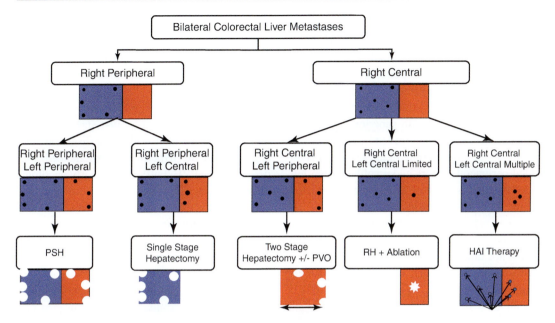

Fig. 16.1 A systematic algorithm for assessing the distribution and extent of bilateral colorectal liver metastases that informs surgical treatment strategy. Each scenario is modeled with the right liver in blue (representing approximately 65% of total liver volume) and the left liver in red (representing approximately 35% of total liver volume). Tumors are represented as closed circles, parenchymal-sparing resections as open circles, and ablations as open stars. *PSH* parenchymal-sparing hepatectomy, *PVO* portal vein occlusion, *RH* right hepatectomy, *HAI* hepatic arterial infusion. Used with permission from: Cloyd JM, Aloia TA. Hammer vs Swiss Army Knife: Developing a Strategy for the Management of Bilobar Colorectal Liver Metastases. Surgery. 2017 doi: https://doi.org/10.1016/j.surg.2016.11.035

(HAI) therapy. However, comparative studies demonstrating superiority of one approach over another are lacking. Rather than championing a single strategy, we recommend a *tailored approach* that takes advantage of all available surgical tools and individually applies them based on an algorithmic assessment of the extent and distribution of metastatic disease. In the case of bilateral disease, this conceptual framework is best understood by classifying the burden of intrahepatic disease in two dimensions, with assessment of the right versus left hemilivers and the peripheral versus central distribution of disease (Fig. 16.1).

Parenchymal-Sparing Hepatectomy

While anatomic hepatectomy is often required based on the number and location of CRLMs, it is not necessarily associated with oncologic benefits over non-anatomic hepatectomy. The advantage of the latter is preservation of uninvolved liver tissue. Although initial concerns had been raised regarding higher rates of local (because of closer margins) and intrahepatic (because of greater "at-risk" residual liver) recurrence, studies have shown similar rates of recurrence and survival in parenchymal-sparing hepatectomy (PSH) compared to a strategy of anatomic hepatectomy [43, 44]. In fact, through preservation of uninvolved liver tissue at the initial operation, PSH is associated with greater salvageability and survival in the case of subsequent liver-only recurrences [3]. For patients with bilobar CRLM that are all peripheral in nature, a one-stage PSH may be most appropriate.

Resection + Ablation

Local ablation techniques can also be used in conjunction with surgical resection especially in patients with bilobar CRLM. In this strategy, the majority of metastases are resected (either via hemihepatectomy or multiple non-anatomic resections), and the residual small, deeply located lesion(s) are treated with percutaneous or operative ablation. Although inferior to surgical resection of all disease, a strategy of resection and ablation is associated with superior results compared to nonsurgical therapies [45]. This approach might be most appropriate in the setting of right-sided peripheral tumors and a solitary deep left-sided metastasis in which a single-stage resection of the right-sided lesions and RFA of the left lesion is performed. In addition, while patients with bilobar centrally located metastases are typically not amenable to surgical resection of all disease, when left-sided metastases are limited (e.g., solitary lesion), a right hepatectomy may be combined with left-sided ablation.

Two-Stage Hepatectomy

In its initial description, TSH was performed without PVE and was associated with high postoperative mortality rates, most commonly due to liver insufficiency [46]. The addition of PVE between the two stages induced hypertrophy of the FLR and lowered postoperative morbidity and mortality after the second-stage procedure [14]. In the first stage, often performed with minimally invasive techniques, the FLR is cleared of metastatic disease, either via parenchymal-sparing resections or ablation. One to four weeks after surgery, percutaneous ipsilateral transhepatic PVE is performed to induce hypertrophy of the FLR. In patients who demonstrate adequate hypertrophy on CT volumetry 3–4 weeks after PVE, a second-stage operation, typically a right hepatectomy that may be extended to include all or part of segment 4, is performed.

In 2012, the novel approach to two-stage hepatectomy known as ALPPS was introduced by Schnitzbauer et al. [47]. In the first stage of ALPPS, a right PVL is combined with parenchymal transection and clearance of the FLR of metastatic disease. The second stage is performed during the same hospital admission 1–2 weeks after the first stage and involves complete hemihepatectomy. While ALPPS is associated with rapid and significant hypertrophy of the FLR, as well as high completion rates of both stages of surgery, perioperative morbidity and mortality rates are significantly higher than in a traditional TSH approach [48, 49]. It also appears that the rapid hypertrophy seen after first-stage ALPPS is less reliably linked to adequate liver function compared to the hypertrophy experienced after percutaneous PVE. Furthermore, early oncologic outcomes suggest lower recurrence-free and overall survival rates compared to other approaches, with long-term data not yet available [50, 51]. For these reasons, the current standard of care for this distribution of disease remains TSH with PVE, which has consistently demonstrated high completion rates, low perioperative morbidity and mortality, and good survival outcomes [2, 52].

A TSH is most commonly required in the setting of dominant right liver metastases and peripherally located metastases in the left liver. However, the need to perform a formal right hepatectomy and additional left-sided resections places this subset of patients with bilobar disease at the highest risk of PHI. This risk is reduced with careful patient selection via assurance of adequate FLR and calculation of the DH and KGR following PVE.

Unresectable Bilateral Metastases

The presence of multiple, bilobar, centrally located metastases likely represents true unresectable disease and an indication for HAI therapy. HAI allows for a higher concentration of cytotoxic drugs and/or radiation to be delivered directly to metastases while decreasing the potential systemic toxicities. When used in the first-line setting, chemotherapy administered via a HAI pump results in tumor response rates of 40–50% [53], with rates even higher when combined with systemic chemotherapy [54] or when used after failure of first-line systemic chemotherapy [55, 56]. The use of HAI therapy in initially unresectable patients may also result in downsizing that permits subsequent resection in a limited subset of patients [57]. Importantly, consensus guidelines recommend that HAI therapy should be delivered as part of a multidisciplinary program at experienced centers only [58]. Other hepatic artery-based therapies, such as radioembolization and transcatheter arterial chemoembolization, as well as ongoing systemic chemotherapy should also be considered [59].

Conclusions

The management of complex CRLM continues to evolve as improvements in systemic chemotherapy, liver augmentation strategies, non-resectional therapies, surgical technologies, and perioperative care occur. Critical to optimizing patient outcomes is an orderly and consistent approach to patient selection. Namely, resectability should be defined along three domains, physiologic, then oncologic, and then technical, in order to identify patients best suited to benefit from liver-directed therapies. It is important that surgeons not constrain themselves to a single treatment strategy, but rather, rely on a multidisciplinary approach and utilization of all surgical tools available, permitting the extension of curative-intent treatments to the largest number of patients. Further advances in systemic therapy, as well as a better understanding of the genetic correlates to tumor biology, should only continue to expand the opportunities to help patients with CRLM.

References

1. American Cancer Society. Cancer facts & figures [internet]. Atlanta: American Cancer Society; 2016. http://www.cancer.org/acs/groups/content/@research/documents/document/acspc-047079.pdf
2. Brouquet A, Abdalla EK, Kopetz S, Garrett CR, Overman MJ, Eng C, et al. High survival rate after two-stage resection of advanced colorectal liver metastases: response-based selection and complete resection define outcome. J Clin Oncol. 2011;29(8):1083–90.
3. Mise Y, Aloia TA, Brudvik KW, Schwarz L, Vauthey J-N, Conrad C. Parenchymal-sparing hepatectomy in colorectal liver metastasis improves salvageability and survival. Ann Surg. 2016;263(1):146–52.
4. Passot G, Chun YS, Kopetz SE, Zorzi D, Brudvik KW, Kim BJ, et al. Predictors of safety and efficacy of 2-stage hepatectomy for bilateral colorectal liver metastases. J Am Coll Surg. 2016;223(1):99–108.
5. Chun YS, Vauthey J-N, Ribero D, Donadon M, Mullen JT, Eng C, et al. Systemic chemotherapy and two-stage hepatectomy for extensive bilateral colorectal liver metastases: perioperative safety and survival. J Gastrointest Surg. 2007;11(11):1498–504; discussion 1504–1505.
6. Bilimoria KY, Liu Y, Paruch JL, Zhou L, Kmiecik TE, Ko CY, et al. Development and evaluation of the universal ACS NSQIP surgical risk calculator: a decision aid and informed consent tool for patients and surgeons. J Am Coll Surg. 2013;217(5):833–842.e1-3.
7. Wagner D, Büttner S, Kim Y, Gani F, Xu L, Margonis GA, et al. Clinical and morphometric parameters of frailty for prediction of mortality following hepatopancreaticobiliary surgery in the elderly. Br J Surg. 2016;103(2):e83–92.
8. Reddy S, Contreras CM, Singletary B, Bradford TM, Waldrop MG, Mims AH, et al. Timed stair climbing is the single strongest predictor of perioperative complications in patients undergoing abdominal surgery. J Am Coll Surg. 2016;222(4):559–66.
9. Hadden WJ, de Reuver PR, Brown K, Mittal A, Samra JS, Hugh TJ. Resection of colorectal liver metastases and extra-hepatic disease: a systematic review and proportional meta-analysis of survival outcomes. HPB. 2016;18(3):209–20.
10. Karagkounis G, Torbenson MS, Daniel HD, Azad NS, Diaz LA, Donehower RC, et al. Incidence and prognostic impact of KRAS and BRAF mutation in patients undergoing liver surgery for colorectal metastases. Cancer. 2013;119(23):4137–44.
11. Vauthey JN, Chaoui A, Do KA, Bilimoria MM, Fenstermacher MJ, Charnsangavej C, et al. Standardized measurement of the future liver remnant prior to extended liver resection: methodology and clinical associations. Surgery. 2000;127(5):512–9.
12. Kishi Y, Abdalla EK, Chun YS, Zorzi D, Madoff DC, Wallace MJ, et al. Three hundred and one consecutive extended right hepatectomies: evaluation of outcome based on systematic liver volumetry. Ann Surg. 2009;250(4):540–8.
13. Azoulay D, Castaing D, Smail A, Adam R, Cailliez V, Laurent A, et al. Resection of nonresectable liver metastases from colorectal cancer after percutaneous portal vein embolization. Ann Surg. 2000;231(4):480–6.
14. Jaeck D, Oussoultzoglou E, Rosso E, Greget M, Weber J-C, Bachellier P. A two-stage hepatectomy procedure combined with portal vein embolization to achieve curative resection for initially unresectable multiple and bilobar colorectal liver metastases. Ann Surg. 2004;240(6):1037–49; discussion 1049–1051.
15. Nordlinger B, Sorbye H, Glimelius B, Poston GJ, Schlag PM, Rougier P, et al. Perioperative chemotherapy with FOLFOX4 and surgery versus surgery alone for resectable liver metastases from colorectal cancer (EORTC Intergroup trial 40983): a randomised controlled trial. Lancet. 2008;371(9617):1007–16.

16. Kishi Y, Zorzi D, Contreras CM, Maru DM, Kopetz S, Ribero D, et al. Extended preoperative chemotherapy does not improve pathologic response and increases postoperative liver insufficiency after hepatic resection for colorectal liver metastases. Ann Surg Oncol. 2010;17(11):2870–6.
17. Ribero D, Wang H, Donadon M, Zorzi D, Thomas MB, Eng C, et al. Bevacizumab improves pathologic response and protects against hepatic injury in patients treated with oxaliplatin-based chemotherapy for colorectal liver metastases. Cancer. 2007;110(12):2761–7.
18. Chun YS, Vauthey J-N, Boonsirikamchai P, Maru DM, Kopetz S, Palavecino M, et al. Association of computed tomography morphologic criteria with pathologic response and survival in patients treated with bevacizumab for colorectal liver metastases. JAMA. 2009;302(21):2338–44.
19. Blazer DG, Kishi Y, Maru DM, Kopetz S, Chun YS, Overman MJ, et al. Pathologic response to preoperative chemotherapy: a new outcome end point after resection of hepatic colorectal metastases. J Clin Oncol. 2008;26(33):5344–51.
20. Passot G, Odisio BC, Zorzi D, Mahvash A, Gupta S, Wallace MJ, et al. Eradication of missing liver metastases after fiducial placement. J Gastrointest Surg. 2016;20(6):1173–8.
21. Andreou A, Aloia TA, Brouquet A, Dickson PV, Zimmitti G, Maru DM, et al. Margin status remains an important determinant of survival after surgical resection of colorectal liver metastases in the era of modern chemotherapy. Ann Surg. 2013;257(6):1079–88.
22. Pawlik TM, Scoggins CR, Zorzi D, Abdalla EK, Andres A, Eng C, et al. Effect of surgical margin status on survival and site of recurrence after hepatic resection for colorectal metastases. Ann Surg. 2005;241(5):715–22; discussion 722–724.
23. Sadot E, Groot Koerkamp B, Leal JN, Shia J, Gonen M, Allen PJ, et al. Resection margin and survival in 2368 patients undergoing hepatic resection for metastatic colorectal cancer: surgical technique or biologic surrogate? Ann Surg. 2015;262(3):476–85; discussion 483–485.
24. Brudvik KW, Mise Y, Chung MH, Chun YS, Kopetz SE, Passot G, et al. RAS mutation predicts positive resection margins and narrower resection margins in patients undergoing resection of colorectal liver metastases. Ann Surg Oncol. 2016;23(8):2635–43.
25. Mise Y, Zimmitti G, Shindoh J, Kopetz S, Loyer EM, Andreou A, et al. RAS mutations predict radiologic and pathologic response in patients treated with chemotherapy before resection of colorectal liver metastases. Ann Surg Oncol. 2015;22(3):834–42.
26. Kinoshita H, Sakai K, Hirohashi K, Igawa S, Yamasaki O, Kubo S. Preoperative portal vein embolization for hepatocellular carcinoma. World J Surg. 1986;10(5):803–8.
27. Makuuchi M, Thai BL, Takayasu K, Takayama T, Kosuge T, Gunvén P, et al. Preoperative portal embolization to increase safety of major hepatectomy for hilar bile duct carcinoma: a preliminary report. Surgery. 1990;107(5):521–7.
28. Madoff DC, Abdalla EK, Gupta S, Wu T-T, Morris JS, Denys A, et al. Transhepatic ipsilateral right portal vein embolization extended to segment IV: improving hypertrophy and resection outcomes with spherical particles and coils. J Vasc Interv Radiol JVIR. 2005;16(2 Pt 1):215–25.
29. Hwang S, Lee S-G, Ko G-Y, Kim B-S, Sung K-B, Kim M-H, et al. Sequential preoperative ipsilateral hepatic vein embolization after portal vein embolization to induce further liver regeneration in patients with hepatobiliary malignancy. Ann Surg. 2009;249(4):608–16.
30. Ribero D, Abdalla EK, Madoff DC, Donadon M, Loyer EM, Vauthey J-N. Portal vein embolization before major hepatectomy and its effects on regeneration, resectability and outcome. Br J Surg. 2007;94(11):1386–94.
31. Shindoh J, Truty MJ, Aloia TA, Curley SA, Zimmitti G, Huang SY, et al. Kinetic growth rate after portal vein embolization predicts posthepatectomy outcomes: toward zero liver-related mortality in patients with colorectal liver metastases and small future liver remnant. J Am Coll Surg. 2013;216(2):201–9.
32. Bleicher RJ, Allegra DP, Nora DT, Wood TF, Foshag LJ, Bilchik AJ. Radiofrequency ablation in 447 complex unresectable liver tumors: lessons learned. Ann Surg Oncol. 2003;10(1):52–8.
33. Kennedy TJ, Cassera MA, Khajanchee YS, Diwan TS, Hammill CW, Hansen PD. Laparoscopic radiofrequency ablation for the management of colorectal liver metastases: 10-year experience. J Surg Oncol. 2013;107(4):324–8.
34. Berber E, Pelley R, Siperstein AE. Predictors of survival after radiofrequency thermal ablation of colorectal cancer metastases to the liver: a prospective study. J Clin Oncol. 2005;23(7):1358–64.
35. Stang A, Fischbach R, Teichmann W, Bokemeyer C, Braumann D. A systematic review on the clinical benefit and role of radiofrequency ablation as treatment of colorectal liver metastases. Eur J Cancer. 2009;45(10):1748–56.
36. Xing M, Kooby DA, El-Rayes BF, Kokabi N, Camacho JC, Kim HS. Locoregional therapies for metastatic colorectal carcinoma to the liver—an evidence-based review. J Surg Oncol. 2014;110(2):182–96.
37. Colbert LE, Cloyd JM, Koay EJ, Crane CH, Vauthey J-N. Proton beam radiation as salvage therapy for bilateral colorectal liver metastases not amenable to second-stage hepatectomy. Surgery. 2017;161(6):1543–8.
38. van Hazel GA, Heinemann V, Sharma NK, Findlay MPN, Ricke J, Peeters M, et al. SIRFLOX: randomized phase III trial comparing first-line mFOLFOX6 (plus or minus bevacizumab) versus mFOLFOX6 (plus or minus bevacizumab) plus selective internal radiation therapy in patients with metastatic colorectal cancer. J Clin Oncol. 2016;34(15):1723–31.
39. Wei M, He Y, Wang J, Chen N, Zhou Z, Wang Z. Laparoscopic versus open hepatectomy with

or without synchronous colectomy for colorectal liver metastasis: a meta-analysis. PLoS One. 2014;9(1):e87461.
40. Cardinal JS, Reddy SK, Tsung A, Marsh JW, Geller DA. Laparoscopic major hepatectomy: pure laparoscopic approach versus hand-assisted technique. J Hepatobiliary Pancreat Sci. 2013;20(2):114–9.
41. Komatsu S, Scatton O, Goumard C, Sepulveda A, Brustia R, Perdigao F, et al. Development process and technical aspects of laparoscopic hepatectomy: learning curve based on 15 years of experience. J Am Coll Surg. 2017;224(5):841–50.
42. Viganò L, Ferrero A, Amisano M, Russolillo N, Capussotti L. Comparison of laparoscopic and open intraoperative ultrasonography for staging liver tumours. Br J Surg. 2013;100(4):535–42.
43. Torzilli G, Procopio F, Botea F, Marconi M, Del Fabbro D, Donadon M, et al. One-stage ultrasonographically guided hepatectomy for multiple bilobar colorectal metastases: a feasible and effective alternative to the 2-stage approach. Surgery. 2009;146(1):60–71.
44. Gold JS, Are C, Kornprat P, Jarnagin WR, Gönen M, Fong Y, et al. Increased use of parenchymal-sparing surgery for bilateral liver metastases from colorectal cancer is associated with improved mortality without change in oncologic outcome: trends in treatment over time in 440 patients. Ann Surg. 2008;247(1):109–17.
45. Abdalla EK, Vauthey J-N, Ellis LM, Ellis V, Pollock R, Broglio KR, et al. Recurrence and outcomes following hepatic resection, radiofrequency ablation, and combined resection/ablation for colorectal liver metastases. Ann Surg. 2004;239(6):818–25; discussion 825–827.
46. Adam R, Laurent A, Azoulay D, Castaing D, Bismuth H. Two-stage hepatectomy: a planned strategy to treat irresectable liver tumors. Ann Surg. 2000;232(6):777–85.
47. Schnitzbauer AA, Lang SA, Goessmann H, Nadalin S, Baumgart J, Farkas SA, et al. Right portal vein ligation combined with in situ splitting induces rapid left lateral liver lobe hypertrophy enabling 2-staged extended right hepatic resection in small-for-size settings. Ann Surg. 2012;255(3):405–14.
48. Ratti F, Schadde E, Masetti M, Massani M, Zanello M, Serenari M, et al. Strategies to increase the resectability of patients with colorectal liver metastases: a multi-center case-match analysis of ALPPS and conventional two-stage hepatectomy. Ann Surg Oncol. 2015;22(6):1933–42.
49. Schadde E, Ardiles V, Robles-Campos R, Malago M, Machado M, Hernandez-Alejandro R, et al. Early survival and safety of ALPPS: first report of the international ALPPS registry. Ann Surg. 2014;260(5):829–36; discussion 836–838.
50. Alvarez FA, Ardiles V, de Santibañes M, Pekolj J, de Santibañes E. Associating liver partition and portal vein ligation for staged hepatectomy offers high oncological feasibility with adequate patient safety: a prospective study at a single center. Ann Surg. 2015;261(4):723–32.
51. Oldhafer KJ, Donati M, Jenner RM, Stang A, Stavrou GA. ALPPS for patients with colorectal liver metastases: effective liver hypertrophy, but early tumor recurrence. World J Surg. 2014;38(6):1504–9.
52. Wicherts DA, Miller R, de Haas RJ, Bitsakou G, Vibert E, Veilhan L-A, et al. Long-term results of two-stage hepatectomy for irresectable colorectal cancer liver metastases. Ann Surg. 2008;248(6):994–1005.
53. Kemeny N, Daly J, Reichman B, Geller N, Botet J, Oderman P. Intrahepatic or systemic infusion of fluorodeoxyuridine in patients with liver metastases from colorectal carcinoma. A randomized trial. Ann Intern Med. 1987;107(4):459–65.
54. Ducreux M, Ychou M, Laplanche A, Gamelin E, Lasser P, Husseini F, et al. Hepatic arterial oxaliplatin infusion plus intravenous chemotherapy in colorectal cancer with inoperable hepatic metastases: a trial of the gastrointestinal group of the Federation Nationale des Centres de Lutte Contre le Cancer. J Clin Oncol. 2005;23(22):4881–7.
55. Boige V, Malka D, Elias D, Castaing M, De Baere T, Goere D, et al. Hepatic arterial infusion of oxaliplatin and intravenous LV5FU2 in unresectable liver metastases from colorectal cancer after systemic chemotherapy failure. Ann Surg Oncol. 2008;15(1):219–26.
56. Kemeny N, Gonen M, Sullivan D, Schwartz L, Benedetti F, Saltz L, et al. Phase I study of hepatic arterial infusion of floxuridine and dexamethasone with systemic irinotecan for unresectable hepatic metastases from colorectal cancer. J Clin Oncol. 2001;19(10):2687–95.
57. Kemeny NE, Melendez FDH, Capanu M, Paty PB, Fong Y, Schwartz LH, et al. Conversion to resectability using hepatic artery infusion plus systemic chemotherapy for the treatment of unresectable liver metastases from colorectal carcinoma. J Clin Oncol. 2009;27(21):3465–71.
58. Karanicolas PJ, Metrakos P, Chan K, Asmis T, Chen E, Kingham TP, et al. Hepatic arterial infusion pump chemotherapy in the management of colorectal liver metastases: expert consensus statement. Curr Oncol. 2014;21(1):e129–36.
59. Zacharias AJ, Jayakrishnan TT, Rajeev R, Rilling WS, Thomas JP, George B, et al. Comparative effectiveness of hepatic artery based therapies for unresectable colorectal liver metastases: a meta-analysis. PLoS One. 2015;10(10):e0139940.

Ablative Techniques for Colorectal Cancer Liver Metastases

17

Camilo Correa-Gallego and T. Peter Kingham

Introduction

The use of extreme temperatures to treat tumors dates back over a century [1]. However, in parallel with the dramatic evolution of liver surgery, the last three decades have seen an accelerated expansion of techniques and indications for liver tumor ablation, and they are currently considered complementary strategies in the treatment of primary and secondary liver malignancies. Moreover, ablation has become an accepted alternative to hepatic resection in a select group of patients with both primary and metastatic liver neoplasms. Indications for ablative therapies include patients considered unfit for surgery due to either location of the lesion or poor health, those with smaller lesions, or those in whom a small amount of remnant liver parenchyma precludes resection [2, 3]. These techniques have also been advocated as a bridge to transplantation in patients facing a long waiting list for a liver allograft [4, 5].

It is thus important for any practitioner involved in the treatment of liver malignancies to understand the basic principles, indications, operative techniques, as well as procedural and oncologic outcomes of patients treated in this fashion. This chapter discusses basic principles of radiofrequency ablation (RFA), microwave ablation (MWA), cryoablation (Cryo), and irreversible electroporation (IRE), which are the most commonly used ablation methods. Their indications in the management of colorectal cancer liver metastases (CRLM) and general technical approaches are outlined, and the outcomes in the different settings (i.e., solitary peripheral lesions, tumor recurrence, combined resection/ablation, etc.) are analyzed. Furthermore, while there is scarce level I data directly comparing these techniques, important nuances that justify the use of one method over the others are reviewed.

Techniques

Ablative techniques in liver surgery aim at the destruction of malignant cells within a tumor while preserving the surrounding liver parenchyma and protecting the adjacent structures. The generation of extreme temperatures that cause cell death is the principle behind RFA, MWA, and Cryo. While the former two techniques generate heat that reliably induces coagulative necrosis after temperatures reach 60 °C, the latter achieves cell death by consecutive

C. Correa-Gallego (✉)
Department of Surgery, Memorial Sloan Kettering Cancer Center, New York, NY, USA
e-mail: correagj@mskcc.org

T. P. Kingham
Division of Hepatopancreatobiliary Surgery, Memorial Sloan Kettering Cancer Center, New York, NY, USA

freeze-thawing cycles. IRE induces apoptosis-mediated cell death in a nonthermal manner by disrupting the cell membrane potential and creating pores that allow the flow of micro- and macromolecules that ultimately disrupt cellular homeostasis. These effects are limited to the target tissue while preserving blood vessels and bile ducts [6, 7]. In this chapter, we will review the basic mechanisms of action of these different techniques, as well as their applications and potential pitfalls.

Approach

Liver ablation can be approached through the percutaneous route, laparoscopically, and via a laparotomy. While percutaneous ablations have a comparatively low morbidity compared to the other two approaches [8, 9], it can be challenging for radiologists to target lesions that are not easily seen on computed tomography or ultrasound and those in which a direct in-line plane for probe placement is not safely attainable percutaneously. Furthermore, not uncommonly, lesions are located in close proximity to vital structures such as the diaphragm, the heart, major blood vessels, or other abdominal viscera. While hydrodissection with saline is sometimes possible to create a safe ablation zone, all of these situations increase the procedural risk of percutaneous ablations [9]. Given these limitations, the percutaneous approach traditionally has the highest local recurrence rate. Laparoscopy provides the ability to isolate and expose the liver, to directly visualize the ablation probe placement, and has the ability to identify smaller tumors that would otherwise remain untreated with percutaneous ablation. Furthermore, it also allows for additional procedures to be performed during the same intervention (e.g., limited liver resection, cholecystectomy, etc.) and for immediate management of procedural complications [9]. On the other end of the spectrum, ablation performed during laparotomy, albeit most invasive, has the lowest recurrence rates of the three approaches.

Image guidance is a key component of ablative procedures ensuring precise ablation of the tissue of interest while avoiding injury to adjacent biliary and vascular structures. Ultrasound has become the gold standard modality for image-guided ablations in the operating room given its ease of use and availability. In addition, its ability to provide real-time feedback to the practitioner performing the procedure is valuable [3]. It is limited by lack of reproducibility, operator dependence, and the sonographic artifact produced by the ablation itself which limits ablation monitoring [10–19]. However, when systematically applied, ultrasound monitoring of ablations allows for the creation of an adequate ablation margin. Analogous to the concept of surgical margins, liver RFA aims to generate an ablation zone that includes a rim of normal tissue along the perimeter of the target tumor, to ensure complete destruction and minimize the incidence of local recurrence.

Indications

Colorectal cancer remains the third most common cancer in both men and women with a projected incidence of 130,000 new cases in 2017 [20]. Approximately half of patients with colorectal cancer either present with or will develop liver metastases during their disease course [21]. Complete resection remains the standard of care for the management of CRLM, and despite elevated recurrence rates, it achieves 5-year survival rates close to 50% and cure rates that approximate 20% [22, 23]. Unfortunately, the vast majority of patients (80–90%) present with unresectable disease [21]. Liver ablation is widely practiced in patients with CRLM who have unresectable disease, those with single or limited recurrence sites, and in patients who are otherwise unfit to tolerate a major liver resection due to comorbid diseases.

Radiofrequency Ablation

Medical application of radiofrequency waves dates back to the early twentieth century. In 1910 Dr. Edwin Beer reported on the use of radiofrequency energy to successfully ablate unresectable papillary growths of the urinary bladder in two patients with significant hematuria [24]. Around the same time, yet independently, Dr. William Clark in Philadelphia popularized the use of high-frequency desiccation and coagulation for the treatment of neoplasms of the skin, head, neck, oral cavity, breast, and cervix [25]. Furthermore, it was the modulated application of radiofrequency waves that allowed Bovie and Cushing to device the electrocautery as we know it today and successfully apply it in surgical procedures [26]. However, it would take several decades until the first preliminary description of the use of RFA of liver neoplasms in the early 1990s [27, 28]. These early ablation probes were essentially modified Bovie electrocauteries with long insulated shafts that allowed guided placement of the uninsulated tip into the tumor of interest mainly with the use of ultrasound [29].

Radiofrequency (RF) refers to the part of the electromagnetic spectrum bounded by the frequencies of 3 Hz and 300 GHz. RF application causes thermal damage and induces coagulative necrosis of a defined volume of tissue. This stems from high temperatures generated by the rapid vibration of water molecules in contact with the RF electrode tip, which is induced by the application of alternating current [29]. This technique relies on tissue conductivity to spread the heat generated by the tissue immediately adjacent to the probe; hence as the distance from the probe increases, the temperature decreases in an exponential fashion. It is important to note that if temperature rises too quickly with the application of RF energy, resultant tissue charring will act as an insulator which prevents the propagation of heat and likely limits the effectiveness of ablation. Thus, RFA is a methodical process which aims to gradually increase the temperature to a goal between 60 and 100 °C over a period of approximately 5 min. The reliance on tissue conductivity explains another important limitation of RFA: heat sink effect. Blood flow in vessels that are in close proximity with the target ablation dissipates heat, thereby preventing tissue from reaching lethal temperatures. This effect should be taken into consideration while planning and executing liver tumor ablation as incomplete ablation along blood vessels may cause residual tumor and potentially lead to increased risk of local recurrence [30]. Given these limitations, as a general rule, RFA is considered most effective for lesions ≤3 cm in diameter.

Microwave Ablation

Similar to RFA, tissue heating in MWA is generated via the continuous realignment of polar molecules in the tissue (mainly water molecules) forced by the alternating current applied by the microwave probe. Thus, the efficiency of this ablation modality is directly proportional to the water content of the target tissue. One of the key differences between MWA and RFA is the ability of microwaves to radiate from the antenna and affect a surrounding volume of tissue. As opposed to RFA which is only able to heat tissue in direct contact with the electrode and thus relies on tissue conductivity to create and ablation zone, MWA induces heat generation by excitation of water molecules in a volume of tissue beyond the immediate vicinity of the probe [31]. This ability overcomes the limitation effected by the charring effect which hampers RFA. Furthermore, MWA has been shown to be much less susceptible to heat sink effect which is of particular importance in ablation of CRLM given the highly vascular nature of the liver parenchyma [32]. In comparison with RFA, MWA achieves higher temperatures with significantly shorter ablation times (Fig. 17.1).

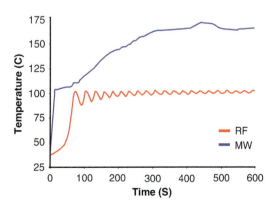

Fig. 17.1 Microwave versus RF temperatures in porcine kidney in vivo. Data collected with a fiber-optic sensor 5 mm away from an RF electrode or microwave antenna in normal porcine kidney in vivo show higher temperatures (well greater than 100 °C) over time around the microwave antenna. Used with permission from Lubner 2010

While RFA is a well-established technique and the most commonly used method for ablation of lesions ≤3 cm, the ability to achieve larger ablations with shorter procedure times, less susceptibility to heat sinking, and the ability to design overlapping ablation zones make MWA an attractive alternative for the treatment of lesions up to 6.5 cm [31, 33]. There are limited randomized studies directly comparing these two methods for treatment of CRLM; however, retrospective series support the use of either modality as an effective treatment particularly for small lesions [34, 35]. In a single institution-matched cohort analysis evaluating 254 matched tumors treated with either RFA or MWA at a 1:1 ratio, the authors identified a lower ablation site recurrence rate in tumors treated with MWA (6% vs 20%; $P < 0.01$), while the follow-up time was significantly shorter for the MWA-treated patients, actuarial local failure estimations corroborated these findings [36].

Cryoablation

Cryoablation was one of the earliest established methods of ablation. However, over the last several decades, it has been slowly abandoned and replaced by RFA and MWA for ablation of tumors due to suboptimal oncologic outcomes and increased morbidity. The general mechanism of action will be discussed for historical interest only. Cryoablation probes induce tissue freezing temperatures by reliance on the Joule-Thompson effect, whereby rapid expansion of a compressed gas changes its temperature [37]. Current cryoablation systems rely mostly on two different compressed gases, argon and helium, which decrease and increase their temperature in response to rapid expansion, respectively. The change in temperature is transmitted to the tissue of interest via the cryo-probe thus allowing for repetitive cycles of freeze-thawing. Three distinct mechanisms of cell injury and death are depicted in Fig. 17.2. Cell death occurs during the initial freezing when extracellular ice formation leads to relative extracellular hypertonicity and cellular dehydration. Furthermore cellular freezing results in protein and membrane malfunction that lead to cell death. During thawing, the reverse process occurs: extracellular ice melts before intracellular ice crystals, and the resultant intracellular hypertonicity leads to osmotic fluid shift that induces cellular edema and death. Lastly delayed cellular death occurs as a result of could-induced cellular injury which activates caspases and leads to apoptosis [37].

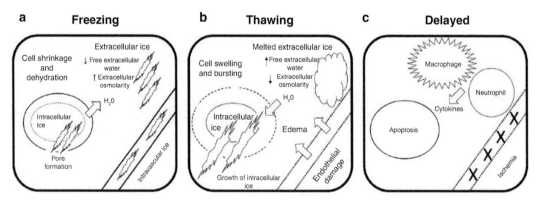

Fig. 17.2 Cryoablation-induced injury. (**a**) During freezing, extracellular ice formation results in sequestration of free extracellular water, increasing the osmolarity of the extracellular space. This leads to cellular dehydration and cell shrinkage. Intracellular ice formation results in disruption of organelle and plasma membranes, impairing cellular function. (**b**) During thawing, extracellular ice melts before intracellular ice, creating an osmotic fluid shift of water into damaged cells, causing swelling and bursting. Growth of intracellular ice crystals can continue during thawing, exacerbating cellular damage. (**c**) Damage to the vascular endothelium results in tissue edema. Delayed cellular damage occurs because of the initiation of apoptosis by the cold-induced cellular injury. Thrombosis of blood vessels causes tissue ischemia, hindering repair. Inflammatory cells, including macrophages and neutrophils, remove damaged cells and clear cellular debris Used with permission from Erinjeri et al. [37]

Complication rates following liver cryoablation range between 30 and 40% which are exceedingly high when compared with rates in the single digits for RFA and MWA. Additionally, series comparing cryoablation with other thermal ablation techniques show that local recurrence rates are generally higher with cryoablation [38–40].

Outcomes of Thermal Ablation

Even though there are no large randomized studies comparing complete resection and ablation for CRLM, a recent meta-analysis pooled data from 13 studies and compared oncologic outcomes between the two approaches [41]. In this study, liver resection proved to be superior to RFA in every relevant metric. Namely, complete resection was significantly superior to RFA in 3- and 5-year OS (RR 1.4 and 1.5, respectively) and 3- and 5-year DFS (RR 1.7 and 2.2, respectively). As could be anticipated, liver resection resulted in higher operative morbidity rates (18% vs 4%; $P < 0.001$—RR 2.5) and longer hospital stay. However, there was no significant difference in mortality. Subgroup analyses were performed for small tumors (<3 cm) and solitary tumors as well as different analyses for patients undergoing open or laparoscopic ablations; in all cases liver resection exhibited superior oncologic outcomes than ablation.

An adequately powered randomized trial comparing thermal ablation and complete resection is unlikely to be performed due to lack of equipoise and the overwhelming evidence in favor of complete resection. The main role of thermal ablation in CRLM remains as an adjunct to surgical resection in patients with extensive bilobar disease, in the treatment of recurrent disease, or as local control for patients who are otherwise considered unfit for surgery. In these appropriately selected scenarios, thermal ablation provides valuable opportunities for tumor control. To this end, it is imperative that surgeons, medical oncologists, and interventional radiologists caring for patients with CRLM reach multidisciplinary consensus as to who are the ideal patients to receive this treatment. Recently a panel of experts published a set of guidelines derived from the critical appraisal of published studies reporting on the treatment of at least 100 CRLM and providing at least 3 years of follow-up [42]. This consensus statement based on the best available evidence and expert opinion provided recommendations regarding tumor size, number of tumors, overall liver tumor volume, relationship to central bile ducts and major blood vessels, and presence of extrahepatic disease.

As previously stated, lesion size is closely related to the effectiveness of ablation. Thermal ablation is optimal for lesions ≤1 cm. While some studies report on lesions of up to 5 cm that are adequately treated if they are located favorably within the liver parenchyma and properly planned and monitored ablations are carried out, the most commonly cited threshold for complete ablation is 3 cm [40]. Local recurrence rates are reported around 3–15% for lesions ≤3 cm, while for lesions >5 cm local recurrence rates range between 30 and 45% [42]. Based on these unacceptable failure rates, the authors recommend ablation for small lesions (<3 cm) or lesions up to 5 cm in size as long as they can be readily accessible, such that efficient ablation with clear margins can be achieved avoiding such limitations as heat sinking.

Beyond size itself which determines the technical feasibility of ablation, it is important to consider the total number of lesions as the other determinant of total liver tumor volume. It has been well documented that the tumor burden has a direct correlation with survival after ablation of unresectable CRLM. A prospective study from the UK which analyzed the outcomes of 309 patients with unresectable disease treated with RFA found size and number of lesions to be these two variables to be independently correlated with overall survival on multivariate analysis. The only other significant variable in this model was the presence of extrahepatic disease [43]. Based on these findings, patients with five or fewer lesions are considered ideal candidates for thermal ablation in the setting of unresectable disease. In certain scenarios, particularly in patients with small lesions, ablation of a greater number of tumors might be considered.

Location of the target lesion has important implications both for the effectiveness of ablation and for the safety profile of the procedure. Thermal treatment of lesions that are within 1 cm of a major bile duct increases the risk of injury to the ductal system. Potential complications include development of biloma, cholangitis, intrahepatic abscess, and biliary fistulization. Ablation is thus not recommended in the vicinity of the common bile duct, common hepatic duct, or right and left hepatic ducts. Irreversible electroporation (see later) is a potential strategy that allows ablation of lesions in these locations while protecting biliary structures. Moreover, the location of the lesion in relationship to major blood vessels is an important determinant of the success and completeness of ablation. As previously discussed, the heat sink effect from vessels >3 mm significantly impairs the ability of RFA (and MWA albeit to a lesser degree) to consistently generate and sustain tissue temperatures in the lethal range. Given the highly vascular nature of the liver parenchyma, it is important to keep these considerations in mind while planning liver ablation of CRLM and for post-ablation monitoring, as lesions in the vicinity of blood vessels have a higher likelihood of local recurrence. Lastly, in terms of location, it is paramount to assess proximity to vulnerable extrahepatic structures (e.g., gallbladder, colon, diaphragm, stomach, right atrium, etc.) as these too can be injured by the heat generated resulting in significant complications. Ablation of liver surface lesions is particularly prone to this type of complication, and precise probe positioning often precludes the percutaneous route.

Additional recommendations aimed at maximizing local control are outlined in the consensus document. These include obtaining adequate ablation margins of at least 1 cm, precisely defining the extent of tumor by the use of contrast-enhanced imaging, performing ablations by experienced operators, liberally using general anesthesia to allow for appropriate patient positioning and duration of ablation, planning ablations based on updated scans, and using real-time contrast-enhanced imaging to monitor ablation.

A particularly advantageous application of liver ablation is in the treatment of patients who present with otherwise unresectable disease. Historically, these patients were treated with systemic chemotherapy alone which is associated with a median survival of 20 months and does not allow the possibility of cure unless tumors are downstaged and become resectable which occurs in 25–30% of patients [44, 45]. However, with the advent and reliable application of ablation techniques, lesions that were considered unresectable due to location are now potentially targetable. Furthermore, patients with unresectable disease due to extensive bilobar involvement who are not amenable to resection due to insufficient future liver remnant can now be treated with combined resection and ablation. In an attempt to prove the oncologic legitimacy of this approach, a recent study reports the long-term outcomes of patients with newly diagnosed CRLM who were treated with resection and ablation and compares them to those patients who underwent liver resection without the need for ablation. The cohorts were analyzed using propensity score matching [46]. Overall and disease-free survival among patients in the resection and ablation group were no different from those for patients who had liver resection alone (5-year OS, 57 vs. 61%; $P = 0.6$; 5-year DFS: 19 vs 17%; $P = 0.9$). There was no difference in intrahepatic disease-free survival despite higher overall local recurrence rate in the resection + ablation group (29 vs 12%; P, 0.03). This study supports the notion that patients with extensive disease that is nonetheless amenable to local control with aggressive combined modality that includes thermal ablation might experience similar oncologic outcomes as those patients who are considered resectable at presentation. Furthermore, such a combined approach for patients presenting with unresectable disease has proven to provide superior oncologic outcomes compared with chemotherapy alone. The CLOCC trial randomized patients with initially unresectable disease to systemic chemotherapy vs systemic chemotherapy plus RFA (+/− resection) [47]. In the recently published long-term outcomes at a median follow-up of nearly 10 years, the CLOCC investigators report a statistically significant difference in overall survival favoring patients treated with combined modality with systemic chemotherapy and RFA +/− resection compared to those treated with chemotherapy alone (HR 0.58 95%CI, 0.38–0.88; P, 0.01) [47, 48].

Of note, half of the patients randomized to combined modality (30/60) underwent radiofrequency ablation alone (without liver resection). This is one of the few randomized studies to demonstrate a survival benefit for patients with unresectable disease treated with such an aggressive approach and underscores the utility of ablation techniques in carefully selected patients.

Irreversible Electroporation

Irreversible electroporation has emerged as a safe ablative technique for liver lesions that are not amenable to RFA or MWA due to close proximity to bilio-vascular structures. IRE does not depend on thermal energy and thus is not limited by the heat sink effect and has a safer profile for ablation near sensitive structures. As the name indicates, this technique creates permanent nano-pores in cell membranes of the target tissue by delivery of electrical pulses of very short duration. Membrane physiology disruption leads to loss of homeostasis and ultimately cell death [6]. This targeted cellular injury explains the ability of IRE to achieve a complete ablation in the immediate vicinity of sensitive vascular or biliary structures without causing undue damage; structures mostly formed by proteins and connective tissue are not susceptible to injury by IRE. In our early experience, over half of 65 tumors treated with IRE were within a centimeter of either a major hepatic vein (n, 25) or a portal pedicle (n, 16). In this series, the overall morbidity was 3%, and there were no ablation-related deaths. Complete ablation was achieved in 98% of tumors [49].

In a recent single-institution experience, patients with liver tumors not amenable to RFA or MWA due to location, IRE ablation was associated with a local recurrence rate of 13% at median follow-up 26 months [50]. This recurrence rate is promising particularly taking into consideration that these patients are by definition not amenable to resection or other ablation modalities. There are scarce data regarding long-term outcomes of patients undergoing IRE for CRLM. There is an ongoing Phase II single-arm clinical trial aiming to accrue 29 patients with unresectable, centrally located CRLM. The primary endpoint of this study is treatment efficacy defined as percentage of tumors eradicated at 12 months after IRE [51]. Results of trials of these kinds with carefully selected prospectively followed patients will be instrumental in furthering our understanding of this modality and identifying patients who can best benefit from this novel technique.

Summary and Conclusions

Different ablative techniques are available for the treatment of patients with colorectal cancer liver metastases. While complete resection remains the standard of care for this patient, these techniques provide good alternatives for local disease control in patients that are not eligible for surgery because of physiologic restrictions or unresectable disease. While thermal ablations (i.e., RFA and MWA) have different mechanisms of action, both methods induce necrosis by generating extreme heat within the tumor and immediate surrounding tissue. They are both limited by heat sink effect and the risk of injuring neighboring structures. While there are no large randomized studies directly comparing these two modalities, data suggest that MWA may be more effective and result in lower local recurrence rates than RFA. IRE has been recently applied to the treatment of CRLM; while there is limited data on this technique and short follow-up, its ability to overcome some of the major limitations faced by thermal ablative techniques makes it a very promising technique worthy of further study.

Practitioners involved in the care of patients with CRLM should be familiar with ablative techniques, their ideal applications, limitations, and outcomes, as they constitute an excellent complement to surgical resection and are thus an essential tool in the therapeutic armamentarium.

References

1. Beer E. Landmark article May 28, 1910: removal of neoplasms of the urinary bladder. By Edwin Beer. JAMA. 1983;250(10):1324–5.
2. Rocha FG, D'Angelica M. Treatment of liver colorectal metastases: role of laparoscopy, radiofrequency

ablation, and microwave coagulation. J Surg Oncol. 2010;102(8):968–74.
3. Livraghi T. Radiofrequency ablation of hepatocellular carcinoma. Surg Oncol Clin N Am. 2011;20(2):281–99, viii.
4. DuBay DA, Sandroussi C, Kachura JR, Ho CS, Beecroft JR, Vollmer CM, et al. Radiofrequency ablation of hepatocellular carcinoma as a bridge to liver transplantation. HPB (Oxford). 2011;13(1):24–32.
5. Panaro F, Piardi T, Audet M, Gheza F, Woehl-Jaegle ML, Portolani N, et al. Laparoscopic ultrasound-guided radiofrequency ablation as a bridge to liver transplantation for hepatocellular carcinoma: preliminary results. Transplant Proc. 2010;42(4):1179–81.
6. Lee EW, Thai S, Kee ST. Irreversible electroporation: a novel image-guided cancer therapy. Gut Liver. 2010;4(Suppl 1):S99–S104.
7. Lee EW, Chen C, Prieto VE, Dry SM, Loh CT, Kee ST. Advanced hepatic ablation technique for creating complete cell death: irreversible electroporation. Radiology. 2010;255(2):426–33.
8. Topal B, Aerts R, Penninckx F. Laparoscopic radiofrequency ablation of unresectable liver malignancies: feasibility and clinical outcome. Surg Laparosc Endosc Percutan Tech. 2003;13(1):11–5.
9. Asahina Y, Nakanishi H, Izumi N. Laparoscopic radiofrequency ablation for hepatocellular carcinoma. Dig Endosc. 2009;21(2):67–72.
10. Vogl TJ, Mack MG, Straub R, Roggan A, Felix R. Magnetic resonance imaging--guided abdominal interventional radiology: laser-induced thermotherapy of liver metastases. Endoscopy. 1997;29(6):577–83.
11. Boaz TL, Lewin JS, Chung YC, Duerk JL, Clampitt ME, Haaga JR. MR monitoring of MR-guided radiofrequency thermal ablation of normal liver in an animal model. J Magn Reson Imaging. 1998;8(1):64–9.
12. Lewin JS, Connell CF, Duerk JL, Chung YC, Clampitt ME, Spisak J, et al. Interactive MRI-guided radiofrequency interstitial thermal ablation of abdominal tumors: clinical trial for evaluation of safety and feasibility. J Magn Reson Imaging. 1998;8(1):40–7.
13. Aschoff AJ, Rafie N, Jesberger JA, Duerk JL, Lewin JS. Thermal lesion conspicuity following interstitial radiofrequency thermal tumor ablation in humans: a comparison of STIR, turbo spin-echo T2-weighted, and contrast-enhanced T1-weighted MR images at 0.2 T. J Magn Reson Imaging. 2000;12(4):584–9.
14. Breen MS, Lazebnik RS, Fitzmaurice M, Nour SG, Lewin JS, Wilson DL. Radiofrequency thermal ablation: correlation of hyperacute MR lesion images with tissue response. J Magn Reson Imaging. 2004;20(3):475–86.
15. Breen MS, Lazebnik RS, Nour SG, Lewin JS, Wilson DL. Three-dimensional comparison of interventional MR radiofrequency ablation images with tissue response. Comput Aided Surg. 2004;9(5):185–91.
16. Mahnken AH, Buecker A, Spuentrup E, Krombach GA, Henzler D, Gunther RW, et al. MR-guided radiofrequency ablation of hepatic malignancies at 1.5 T: initial results. J Magn Reson Imaging. 2004;19(3):342–8.
17. Cernicanu A, Lepetit-Coiffe M, Viallon M, Terraz S, Becker CD. New horizons in MR-controlled and monitored radiofrequency ablation of liver tumours. Cancer Imaging. 2007;7:160–6.
18. Boss A, Rempp H, Martirosian P, Clasen S, Schraml C, Stenzl A, et al. Wide-bore 1.5 Tesla MR imagers for guidance and monitoring of radiofrequency ablation of renal cell carcinoma: initial experience on feasibility. Eur Radiol. 2008;18(7):1449–55.
19. Chopra SS, Schmidt SC, Wiltberger G, Denecke T, Streitparth F, Seebauer C, et al. Laparoscopic radiofrequency ablation of liver tumors: comparison of MR guidance versus conventional laparoscopic ultrasound for needle positioning in a phantom model. Minim Invasive Ther Allied Technol. 2011;20(4):212–7.
20. Siegel RL, Miller KD, Fedewa SA, Ahnen DJ, Meester RGS, Barzi A, et al. Colorectal cancer statistics, 2017. CA Cancer J Clin. 2017;67(3):177–93.
21. D'Angelica MI, Correa-Gallego C, Paty PB, Cercek A, Gewirtz AN, Chou JF, et al. Phase II trial of hepatic artery infusional and systemic chemotherapy for patients with unresectable hepatic metastases from colorectal cancer: conversion to resection and long-term outcomes. Ann Surg. 2015;261(2):353–60.
22. D'Angelica M, Brennan MF, Fortner JG, Cohen AM, Blumgart LH, Fong Y. Ninety-six five-year survivors after liver resection for metastatic colorectal cancer. J Am Coll Surg. 1997;185(6):554–9.
23. Tomlinson JS, Jarnagin WR, DeMatteo RP, Fong Y, Kornprat P, Gonen M, et al. Actual 10-year survival after resection of colorectal liver metastases defines cure. J Clin Oncol. 2007;25(29):4575–80.
24. Beer E. Removal of neoplasms of the urinary bladder; a new method, employing high-frequency (oudin) currents through a catheterizing cystoscope. Am J Med. 1952;13(5):542–3.
25. Clark WL. Indications for the use of electrosurgical methods. N Engl J Med. 1931;204(3):110–5.
26. Goldwyn RM. Bovie: the man and the machine. Ann Plast Surg. 1979;2(2):135–53.
27. McGahan JP, Browning PD, Brock JM, Tesluk H. Hepatic ablation using radiofrequency electrocautery. Investig Radiol. 1990;25(3):267–70.
28. McGahan JP, Gu WZ, Brock JM, Tesluk H, Jones CD. Hepatic ablation using bipolar radiofrequency electrocautery. Acad Radiol. 1996;3(5):418–22.
29. Hong K, Georgiades C. Radiofrequency ablation: mechanism of action and devices. J Vasc Interv Radiol. 2010;21(8 Suppl):S179–86.
30. Lu DS, Raman SS, Limanond P, Aziz D, Economou J, Busuttil R, et al. Influence of large peritumoral vessels on outcome of radiofrequency ablation of liver tumors. J Vasc Interv Radiol. 2003;14(10):1267–74.
31. Lubner MG, Brace CL, Hinshaw JL, Lee FT Jr. Microwave tumor ablation: mechanism of action, clinical results, and devices. J Vasc Interv Radiol. 2010;21(8 Suppl):S192–203.

32. Yu NC, Raman SS, Kim YJ, Lassman C, Chang X, Lu DS. Microwave liver ablation: influence of hepatic vein size on heat-sink effect in a porcine model. J Vasc Interv Radiol. 2008;19(7):1087–92.
33. Brace CL, Laeseke PF, Sampson LA, Frey TM, van der Weide DW, Lee FT Jr. Microwave ablation with multiple simultaneously powered small-gauge triaxial antennas: results from an in vivo swine liver model. Radiology. 2007;244(1):151–6.
34. Leung U, Kuk D, D'Angelica MI, Kingham TP, Allen PJ, DeMatteo RP, et al. Long-term outcomes following microwave ablation for liver malignancies. Br J Surg. 2015;102(1):85–91.
35. van Tilborg AA, Scheffer HJ, de Jong MC, Vroomen LG, Nielsen K, van Kuijk C, et al. MWA versus RFA for perivascular and peribiliary CRLM: a retrospective patient- and lesion-based analysis of two historical cohorts. Cardiovasc Intervent Radiol. 2016;39(10):1438–46.
36. Correa-Gallego C, Fong Y, Gonen M, D'Angelica MI, Allen PJ, DeMatteo RP, et al. A retrospective comparison of microwave ablation vs. radiofrequency ablation for colorectal cancer hepatic metastases. Ann Surg Oncol. 2014;21(13):4278–83.
37. Erinjeri JP, Clark TW. Cryoablation: mechanism of action and devices. J Vasc Interv Radiol. 2010;21(8 Suppl):S187–91.
38. Pearson AS, Izzo F, Fleming RY, Ellis LM, Delrio P, Roh MS, et al. Intraoperative radiofrequency ablation or cryoablation for hepatic malignancies. Am J Surg. 1999;178(6):592–9.
39. Adam R, Akpinar E, Johann M, Kunstlinger F, Majno P, Bismuth H. Place of cryosurgery in the treatment of malignant liver tumors. Ann Surg. 1997;225(1):39–8; discussion 48–50.
40. Kingham TP, Tanoue M, Eaton A, Rocha FG, Do R, Allen P, et al. Patterns of recurrence after ablation of colorectal cancer liver metastases. Ann Surg Oncol. 2012;19(3):834–41.
41. Weng M, Zhang Y, Zhou D, Yang Y, Tang Z, Zhao M, et al. Radiofrequency ablation versus resection for colorectal cancer liver metastases: a meta-analysis. PLoS One. 2012;7(9):e45493.
42. Gillams A, Goldberg N, Ahmed M, Bale R, Breen D, Callstrom M, et al. Thermal ablation of colorectal liver metastases: a position paper by an international panel of ablation experts, the interventional oncology sans frontieres meeting 2013. Eur Radiol. 2015;25(12):3438–54.
43. Gillams AR, Lees WR. Five-year survival in 309 patients with colorectal liver metastases treated with radiofrequency ablation. Eur Radiol. 2009;19(5):1206–13.
44. Folprecht G, Gruenberger T, Bechstein WO, Raab HR, Lordick F, Hartmann JT, et al. Tumour response and secondary resectability of colorectal liver metastases following neoadjuvant chemotherapy with cetuximab: the CELIM randomised phase 2 trial. Lancet Oncol. 2010;11(1):38–47.
45. Pozzo C, Basso M, Cassano A, Quirino M, Schinzari G, Trigila N, et al. Neoadjuvant treatment of unresectable liver disease with irinotecan and 5-fluorouracil plus folinic acid in colorectal cancer patients. Ann Oncol. 2004;15(6):933–9.
46. Imai K, Allard MA, Castro Benitez C, Vibert E, Sa Cunha A, Cherqui D, et al. Long-term outcomes of radiofrequency ablation combined with hepatectomy compared with hepatectomy alone for colorectal liver metastases. Br J Surg. 2017;104(5):570–9.
47. Ruers T, Punt C, Van Coevorden F, Pierie JP, Borel-Rinkes I, Ledermann JA, et al. Radiofrequency ablation combined with systemic treatment versus systemic treatment alone in patients with non-resectable colorectal liver metastases: a randomized EORTC Intergroup phase II study (EORTC 40004). Ann Oncol. 2012;23(10):2619–26.
48. Ruers T, Van Coevorden F, Punt CJ, Pierie JE, Borel-Rinkes I, Ledermann JA, et al. Local treatment of unresectable colorectal liver metastases: results of a randomized phase II trial. J Natl Cancer Inst. 2017;109(9).
49. Kingham TP, Karkar AM, D'Angelica MI, Allen PJ, Dematteo RP, Getrajdman GI, et al. Ablation of perivascular hepatic malignant tumors with irreversible electroporation. J Am Coll Surg. 2012;215(3):379–87.
50. Langan RC, Goldman DA, D'Angelica MI, DeMatteo RP, Allen PJ, Balachandran VP, et al. Recurrence patterns following irreversible electroporation for hepatic malignancies. J Surg Oncol. 2017;115(6):704–10.
51. Scheffer HJ, Vroomen LG, Nielsen K, van Tilborg AA, Comans EF, van Kuijk C, et al. Colorectal liver metastatic disease: efficacy of irreversible electroporation—a single-arm phase II clinical trial (COLDFIRE-2 trial). BMC Cancer. 2015;15:772.

Hepatic Arterial Therapy for Colorectal Cancer Liver Metastases

18

Neal Bhutiani and Robert C. G. Martin II

Background

The presence and extent of colorectal cancer liver metastases (CLM) are major prognostic factors with respect to overall survival. A large percentage (25–50%) of patients exhibit liver metastases at the time of diagnosis with colon cancer, while approximately 80% of patients diagnosed with colorectal cancer will develop liver metastases on follow-up evaluation. A variety of therapies exist for the treatment of for CLM—surgical resection, systemic chemotherapy, molecular therapy, and local ablative treatments. Optimal treatment for a given patient depends on the biology of the disease, which is defined by tumor stage (IVa vs. IVb), timing, extent of, and pattern of metastases. Additional patient factors also play a role in relation to performance status and patient preference [1, 2].

Hepatic resection currently constitutes the optimal first-line treatment and is discussed in detail in a previous chapter. At the time of diagnosis, fewer than 20% of patients have resectable CLM [3, 4], with 60–80% of those undergoing resection developing recurrence of their CLM on distant follow-up, of which half have an intrahepatic recurrence [5, 6].

The greater than 80% of patients who are not candidates for CLM resection at the time of initial diagnosis receive systemic chemo- and/or biologic therapy according to current guidelines [1]. Currently, 5-fluorouracil (5-FU)-based regimens consisting of 5-FU, irinotecan, and/or oxaliplatin (e.g., FOLFOX, FOLFIRI, and FOLFOXIRI) result in response rates and median overall survival of 40–57% and 15–20 months, respectively. Still, reported 5-year overall survival rates are close to 0% [1, 2, 7–12]. The introduction of molecular-targeted therapies such as anti-epidermal growth factor receptor (EGFR) and anti-vascular endothelial growth factor (VEGF) antibodies have further improved outcomes with or after the administration of systemic therapies, with randomized control trials showing that the addition of a monoclonal antibody to systemic chemotherapy regimens increased overall survival to more than 24 months [1, 13].

Current evidence suggests that systemic chemotherapy with or without the use of biologic agents followed by liver resection is safe and effective for selected patients with initially unresectable CLM [14–18]. The use of hepatic arterial therapy to augment the response rates of systemic chemotherapy is an enticing concept, as it allows

N. Bhutiani
Department of Surgery, Division of Surgical Oncology, University of Louisville, Louisville, KY, USA

Department of Microbiology and Immunology, University of Louisville, Louisville, KY, USA
e-mail: neal.bhutiani@louisville.edu

R. C. G. Martin II (✉)
Division of Surgical Oncology, Upper Gastrointestinal and Hepato-Pancreatico-Biliary Clinic, Louisville, KY, USA
e-mail: Robert.Martin@louisville.edu

for higher concentration of drugs or radiation therapy within a target liver area while decreasing toxicity and adverse effects associated with systemic chemotherapy or external beam radiation therapy [19].

Transarterial Hepatic Embolization

Rationale

While normal liver parenchyma draws >85% of its blood supply from the portal vein, malignant liver tumors primarily derive their blood supply from hepatic arterial branches [20]. Thus, transarterial drug-eluting beads (chemotherapy or radiation therapy) deliver substantially greater concentrations of chemotherapy/radiation to the liver compared with systemic chemotherapy/external beam radiation therapy while sparing normal liver parenchyma and minimizing both hepatic and systemic toxicity [19].

Chemotherapy-associated liver injury (CALI)—e.g., sinusoidal obstruction syndrome (SOS) and nonalcoholic steato-hepatitis (NASH)—limits the duration of cytotoxic therapy and impacts preoperative treatment plans. For example, SOS may occur with oxaliplatin treatment, with increased severity associated with prolonged treatments (>6 cycles). Bevacizumab, meanwhile, can be used safely in the preoperative setting when discontinued at least 4–6 weeks before liver resection and seems to decrease the incidence of oxaliplatin-induced sinusoidal injury [21].

Since angiogenesis is integral to hematogenous spread of primary tumors as well as growth of distant metastases, EGF, VEGF, angiopoietin, and cyclooxygenase all represent potential targets to modulate the arterial blood supply of CLM. The exact role of these pathways and targeted biologic therapies with respect to treatment of colorectal cancer remains nebulous. While cetuximab and bevacizumab have been used in the treatment of ependymoma and glioblastoma, respectively, no groups have reported transarterial use of biologic agents in treatment of CLM [22, 23].

Reported Techniques

Due to the lack of an evidence-based treatment standard, multiple chemotherapeutics and embolic agents are used in different combinations and doses [24–26]. Historically, transarterial therapies have been classified as (1) conventional transarterial chemoembolization (cTACE), (2) degradable starch microscophere chemoembolization (DSM-TACE), and (3) hepatic arterial drug-eluting bead (HAT-DEB) therapy. Today, DSM-TACE and HAT-DEB comprise the majority of transarterial treatments for CLM.

cTACE involves direct injection of chemotherapeutics into the hepatic arterial system followed by infusion of a vascular occlusive agent (e.g., Gelfoam) to induce embolization. In the case of DSM-TACE, one or more chemotherapeutics (e.g., mitomycin C, gemcitabine, and/or irinotecan) are infused concurrently with DSM (as an admixture) or immediately prior to infusion of DSM [27, 28]. In both cases, solutions are injected directly into the right and left hepatic arteries over a period of approximately 10 min after gaining access to the arterial circulation via the femoral artery. Pre-infusion embolization of gastric or duodenal arterial branches is performed in situations where there is concern for infusion overflow into these vessels. In cTACE, infusion of a solution containing a vascular occlusive agent is then performed; in DSM-TACE, that agent is DSM. cTACE results in permanent arterial embolization, while DSM-TACE causes only temporary vascular occlusion since human serum amylase dissolves the DSMs. In Europe, available DSMs (EmboCept S; PharmaCept, Berlin, Germany) have a mean microsphere diameter of 50 μm and a recanalization time of about 60 min. Table 18.1 lists various published studies assessing the safety and efficacy of various cTACE and DSM-TACE regimens.

With respect to tumor response, the specific combination of drug and embolic agent that yields an optimal treatment result remains unclear and requires assessment with randomized controlled studies. The predefined calibration of microsphere size allows precise control of embolization depth,

Table 18.1 Original studies of safety and efficacy of cTACE and DSM for CLM

Study/year/reference	Patients (n)	Therapy stage (first line, second line, third line, beyond third line)	Chemoembolics (embolic agents + chemotherapeutics)	Median follow-up (months)	Progression-free survival (months)	Median OS (months)
Ceelen et al./1996/[31]	14 9	NR	Lipiodol and Gelfoam + cisplatin + surgery Surgery alone	15.5 17.5	NR	NR
Tellez et al./1998/[75]	30	NR	Bovine collagen material + cisplatin, doxorubicin, and mitomycin C	NR	NR	8.6
Leichman, et al./1999/[76]	31	NR	Collagen suspension + doxorubicin, mitomycin C, and cisplatin	NR	8	14
Müller et al./2001/[77]	103	Beyond second line	Group (A) HAI 5-FUx4d; HAI GM-CSFx2d; cTACE Lipiodol, Gelfoam, melphalan × 1 day Group (B) HAI 5-FU/leucovorin/GM-CSF × 2 days; cTACE Lipiodol, Gelfoam, melphalan × 1 day	42	7 8	17 28
Salman et al./2002/[78]	26 24	Second line	PVA PVA AND 5-FU + IFN	NR	4 3	10 15
Tsuchiya et al./2007/[28]	27	NR	DSMs + irinotecan and mitomycin C	NR	NR	NR
Vogl et al./2009/[79]	463	Second line	Lipiodol and DSMs + mitomycin C alone (52.5%), mitomycin C and gemcitabine (33.0%), or mitomycin C and irinotecan (14.5%)	NR	NR	14
Albert, et al./2011/[80]	121	Beyond second line	Lipiodol and PVA + mitomycin C, doxorubicin, cisplatin	NR	3	9
Nishiofuku et al./2013/[27]	24	Beyond second line	DSMs + cisplatin powder	17.4	8.8	21.1
Gruber-Roth et al./2014/[81]	564	NR	Lipiodol and mitomycin C or mitomycin C + irinotecan or mitomycin C + irinotecan + cisplatin	NR	NR	14.3

No statistically significant difference between chemonaive patients and patients pretreated with any kind of systemic therapy
TACE versus systemic therapy
TACE + capecitabine versus TACE only

as the occluded vessel diameters correspond to the nominal diameter of the microsphere. Furthermore, in contrast to permanent embolic agents, DSMs result in reduced ischemic effects and, therefore, less neoangiogenesis. Should future randomized trials demonstrate efficacy of angiogenesis inhibitors such as bevacizumab in the setting of HAT, inclusion of these biologics in cTACE or DSM-TACE regimens could further address the issue of neoangiogenesis.

Hepatic Arterial Drug-Eluting Bead (HAT-DEB) Embolization

Rationale

Recently, HAT-DEB has emerged as an increasingly popular embolization-drug delivery technique. The concept is based on loading permanent microspheres with a cytotoxic chemotherapy such as irinotecan and doxorubicin. After intra-arterial injection of DEBs, the drug is released in a controlled manner over a period of hours to days within the target tissue [29]. Since the type and dose of the chemotherapeutic can be modulated and combined with a particular microsphere size and volume, HAT-DEB is gaining significant popularity among HAT techniques in the treatment of CLM.

After lobar, selective, or superselective injection of one or more chemotherapeutic drugs and one or more embolic agents into the blood supply to liver metastases, chemotoxic and ischemic tumor effects are observed. The combination of intra-arterial chemotherapy and hemostasis in embolized vessels can, however, lead to great toxicity and worse adverse effects [19, 30]. Some authors believe that halting the progression of metastatic colorectal disease can lead to improved outcomes, though this has not proven to reliably improve overall survival [4, 30–34]. According to the current guidelines, and in contrast to hepatocellular carcinoma, HAT-DEB is still not recommended as a standard therapy for CLM. Nevertheless, use of this technology for treatment of CLM is increasing. Recent studies have demonstrated the efficacy of repetitive HAT-DEB, placing greater emphasis on drug delivery and less on inducing stasis/anoxia in patients with liver-dominant CLM after failure of surgical, ablative, and/or systemic therapies or as an induction therapy to induce downsizing of disease for resection.

Technique

HAT-DEB is indicated for patients with a life expectancy >3 months and an appropriate performance status (e.g., Eastern Cooperative Oncology Group (ECOG) status ≤2) [20, 24]. Patients must have adequate liver function, generally defined as bilirubin <3 mg/dL, albumin >3 g/dL, and international normalized ratio (INR) <1.6. Pre-interventional staging within 1 month of treatment with high-quality, thin-slice, triphasic contrast-enhanced CT or dynamic magnetic resonance imaging (MRI) before conventional catheter angiography is required to adequately assess the intra- and extrahepatic extent of disease.

During the peri-HAT period, analgesics and antiemetics can help prophylax against and/or treat common therapy-related side effects (pain and nausea). In case of large-volume tumors, intravenous corticosteroids (e.g., dexamethasone 250 mg) can effectively treat the tumor edema often occurring after HAT-DEB. Prophylactic antibiotics to prevent bloodstream and/or intrahepatic infections are recommended only in high-risk patients [35].

The correct choice of the catheter position for drug delivery and the DEB end point are key factors for safe and effective treatments. One must also consider both the nature and amount of drug to be delivered (i.e., number of vials of beads) as well as the size, location, and vascularization of the liver metastases. Treatment via the right or left hepatic artery is used for selective targeting of either the right or left lobe of the liver [33, 34, 36]. Diagnostic angiography and intra-procedural cone-beam computed tomography (CT) can help delineate the anatomy of all tumor-feeding arteries and allow operators to navigate the microcatheter accordingly. Catheter location is confirmed intra-procedurally using fluoroscopy.

After HAT-DEB, patients are monitored for treatment effect and disease recurrence through use of clinical examination, blood tests, and contrast-enhanced imaging. Subsequent HAT-DEB treatments are commonly required and should be scheduled in conjunction with the off week of the patient's systemic therapy, usually within 4–6 weeks of initial HAT-DEB, with exact timing based on patient tolerance of combined therapy. Oftentimes, the right lobe is treated twice and the left lobe once over a 10–12-week time interval before repeat imaging is obtained to assess for radiographic response. Official recommendations such as the Standards of Practice Guidelines of the Cardiovascular and Interventional Radiological Society of Europe (CIRSE) can help to further standardize HAT-DEB for colorectal liver metastases [37].

Technical Success, Complications, and Adverse Effects

In key studies of HAT-DEB for colorectal liver metastases, technical success—successful catheterization with subsequent selective/superselective deposition of chemoembolic agents within the target region—is close to 100%. Dissection or thrombosis of the hepatic artery is extremely rare [20]. Temporary vasospasm during catheterization is common but can be effectively treated with vasodilators (i.e., repetitive transarterial bolus injections of 0.25 mg nitroglycerin). Arterioportal and arteriovenous shunts should be occluded to avoid the risk for nontarget embolization. After one or more HAT-DEB cycles, the chemoembolics can alter the larger tumor-feeding arteries. Very small microspheres (e.g., irinotecan-loaded microspheres with a diameter of 40 ± 10 μm) can then be employed to embolize the diffuse tumor vasculature, with concomitant use of DSMs as need to provide temporary protective embolization of nontarget liver tissue [38].

The "post-embolization syndrome" was a relatively frequent side effect of HAT-DEB and comprised one or more of the following: fatigue, nausea, vomiting, mild fever, and laboratory values indicative of tumor necrosis. Commonly, this phenomenon was associated with over-embolization (i.e., going to hard stasis), selective HAT-DEB, and irinotecan-based therapy [30]. A recent review compared relevant toxicities of HAT-DEB, cTACE, systemic chemotherapy (CTx), and hepatic arterial infusion (HAI) [20]. For HAT-DEB, cited toxicities were nausea/vomiting (2–55%), hypertension (4–80%), liver dysfunction/failure (6%), cholecystitis (1%), gastritis (1%), anorexia (3%), abdominal pain (0–57%), hematologic toxicity (9–90%), fatigue (60%), and alopecia (5–35%). For cTACE, toxicities included nausea/vomiting (18–83%), fever (13–83%), fatigue (24–60%), abdominal pain (82–100%), liver dysfunction/failure (13–33%), gastritis (17%), neurotoxicity (45%), diarrhea (9–31%), hematologic toxicity (13–33%), and renal failure (4%). Finally, for CTx and HAI, cited toxicities were chemical hepatitis (7–15% and 4–79%, respectively), biliary sclerosis (not reported (NR) and 4–21%, respectively), peptic/duodenal ulceration (0–3% and 0–17%, respectively), gastritis/duodenitis (1–7% and 1–21%, respectively), diarrhea (16–70% and 1–44%, respectively), nausea/vomitus (35–46% and 21–61%, respectively), and stomatitis (14–87% and 0–76%, respectively). Recent reports have outlined appropriate use of HAT-DEB in metastatic colorectal cancer, which can significantly reduce any and all side effects [30, 39].

As previously mentioned, complications of HAT-DEB—such as liver abscess and tumor rupture—are rare, particularly in experienced centers [25–27, 31]. Results of nontarget embolization (e.g., pancreatitis or cholecystitis) can be avoided by sufficient evaluation of the arterial anatomy through the use of high-resolution angiography or intra-procedural cone-beam CT and by using accepted hepatic embolization techniques such as flow-mediated embolization or balloon protection [24, 30]. In general, the procedure can be regarded as safe and well-tolerated provided that standard catheterization

Oncologic Outcomes

In summary, HAT-DEB for CLM is usually performed after failure of at least one systemic and/or surgical therapy. Elsewise, it is performed in conjunction with systemic therapy or in the period after hepatic resection. HAT-DEB regimens can produce a tumor response rate of 89%, a progression-free survival (PFS) rate of 13.6 months, and an overall survival (OS) of >28 months. Original studies assessing efficacy along with their relevant characteristics and disease-free and overall survival figures are detailed in Table 18.2.

Since 2011, a number of review articles addressing HAT-DEB for CLM have been published [13, 20, 25, 26, 40–43]. Some authors emphasize an increased survival benefit and conclude that HAT-DEB should be implemented earlier in treatment algorithms for CLM, specifically after patients fail first- and second-line systemic therapy [13]. Others, meanwhile, state that HAT-DEB cannot be definitively recommended for unresectable CLM because of the lack of prospective, randomized trials that would allow for appropriate comparison with systemic regimens [25]. Regardless of their recommendations, all authors acknowledge the appeal of evolving HAT-DEB techniques but recognize the lack of prospective clinical data from randomized trials [4, 10, 26–31]. They also agree that the safety and toxicity profile of HAT-DEB are comparable to or better than that of salvage systemic chemotherapy.

In terms of oncologic long-term goals, the optimal timing and utilization of HAT-DEB are based on the current disease biology and the short- and long-term plan for the patient (e.g., downstage to resection, control of chemorefractory disease, need for a systematic chemotherapy holiday). Thus, the patient's multidisciplinary team of physicians should work together at the *initial* diagnosis of disease to establish these goals.

HAT in Combination with Systemic Chemotherapy and/or Surgery

Few studies have reported outcomes of patients with CLM after HAT-DEB in combination with surgical resection. HAT, including HAT-DEB, does not confer additional risk in patients undergoing hepatectomy, with a retrospective study showing no differences in postoperative overall or liver-specific complication rate or grade [44]. Two prospective trials have been performed assessing outcomes following HAT-DEB and cTACE, respectively, prior to resection [31, 45]. In the HAT-DEB study, 55 patients with CLM underwent HAI as initial therapy, with 20% of patients demonstrating either downstaging or stability of their disease, thus enabling resection. In the cTACE study, 14 patients underwent preoperative cTACE, while 9 patients were treated with partial hepatectomy alone. Reported OS and tumor recurrence rates were 93 and 8% (mean follow-up 15.5 months) versus 67 and 67% (mean follow-up 17.5 months), respectively. In this context, cTACE was not associated with increased operating time, transfusion requirement, or perioperative complication rates. The authors concluded that preoperative cTACE reduces a 12-month recurrence rate after curative liver resection and may improve overall survival.

Two recent studies have assessed the radiologic-pathologic correlation of resection specimens in patients who underwent HAT-DEB prior to surgical resection. The first, a case-control series, involved three patients who were treated with HAT-DEB (DEBIRI; 200 mg irinotecan loaded in a particle volume of 2 mL (particle size of 100–300 μm) (DC Bead; BTG, London, Great Britain)) [46]. Pathologic analysis of the surgical specimen demonstrated 0% tumor viability for all targeted liver metastases. Nontargeted liver metastases as well as those detected at the time of operation also showed a response: two in the non-treated contralateral liver lobe (30% and 45% tumor viability, respectively) as well as three in the ipsilateral liver lobe (0%, 0%, and 60% tumor viability, respectively). Such data support the hypothesis that HAT-DEB has the potential to treat nontargeted liver metastases as well as micrometastases. In the second study,

Table 18.2 Original studies of safety and efficacy of HAT-DEB for CLM

Study/year/reference	Patients (n)	Therapy stage (first line, second line, third line, beyond third line)	Chemoembolics (embolic agents + chemotherapeutics)	Median follow-up (months)	Progression-free survival (months)	Median OS (months)
Aliberti et al./2006/[82]	10	NR	DEBIRI (100 mg irinotecan) every 3 weeks	NR	NR	NR
Martin, et al./2009/[33]	30	Second line	DEBs (100–700 μm)	9	NR	NR
Martin, et al./2009/[34]	55	Second line	DEBs (100–900 μm)	18	6.5	11.3
Martin, et al./2010/[30]	84	Second line	DEBs (100–700 μm)	NR	NR	NR
Martin, et al./2011/[83]	55	Second line	DEBs (100–700 μm)	18	11	19
Aliberti et al./2011/[84]	82	Second line	DEBIRI	29	8	25
Fiorentini et al./2012/[85]	36 38	NR	DEBIRI FOLFIRI	NR	7 4	22 15
Martin, et al./2012/[86]	10	During the off week of FOLFOX	DEBIRI (100 mg irinotecan, 100–300 μm)	NR	NR	15.2
Jones et al./2013/[46]	22	Easily resectable colorectal liver metastases were treated with TACE 4 weeks prior to resection	DEBIRI	22	13.6	NR
Eichler et al./2012/[87]	11	Second line	DEBIRI(100–500 μm)	2.7	5.1	NR
Jones et al./2013/[88]	10	NR	DEBIRI (200 mg irinotecan) as part of PARAGON II	NR	NR	NR
Narayanan et al./2013/[89]	28	NR	DEBIRI	6.9	4	13.3
Huppert et al./2014/[90]	29	Beyond second line	DEBIRI (35–400 mg irinotecan)	8	5	8
Akinwande et al./2014/[49]	22 149	NR	DEBIRI + capecitabine DEBIRI only	10	7 9	22 13
Martin et al./2015/[50]	70	First line	FOLFOX + DEBIRI FOLFOX alone	NR	17 15	13.7 16

NR not reported, *DEBIRI* drug-eluting beads loaded with irinotecan

22 patients were treated with HAT-DEB for 4 weeks prior to liver resection [46, 47]. Disease-free survival was 13.6 months. However, the authors noted that the Response Evaluation Criteria in Solid Tumors (RECIST) failed to accurately predict either pathologic response or clinical outcome. Thus, clinicians have discussed the use of different modalities for response assessment, including cone-beam CT, angio-CT, hybrid imaging, and biomarkers.

Recent work has demonstrated the therapeutic potential of combining transarterial and systemic therapies [48]. Fifty-three patients with primarily unresectable CLM (defined as at least one of the following: >5 liver metastases, bilobar disease, ≥6 involved segments) were treated with transarterial 5-fluoro-deoxyuridine and dexamethasone as HAI along with systemic oxaliplatin and irinotecan. Tumor response rate was 92%, with 47% converting to resectability. Analogously, HAT-DEB plus Xeloda may confer a survival advantage without additional toxicity compared with patients undergoing HAT-DEB only (22 versus 13 months) [49].

A recent randomized controlled trial assessed the safety and efficacy of DEBIRI with FOLFOX and bevacizumab vs. FOLFOX and bevacizumab alone [50]. They demonstrated no difference in toxicity between the FOLFOX-DEBIRI and FOLFOX/bevacizumab treatment arms, a 6-month ORR of 76 vs. 60% ($p = 0.05$), a conversion to resectability of 35% vs. 16% ($0 = 0.05$), and a median progression-free survival of 15.3 vs. 7.6 months. These findings suggest that DEBIRI represents a powerful adjunct to first-line systemic chemotherapy in patients with unresectable CLM, and further studies should be undertaken to assess the effects of combining HAT-DEB with various combinations of oral and systemic agents for the treatment of CLM.

Yttrium-90 (Y-90) Radioembolization

Rationale and Patient Selection

Initially described in the 1980s, radioembolization represents another locoregional modality for the treatment of CLM [51]. Targeted arterial injection of Y-90 microspheres results in embolization and stasis of tumor blood supply as well as localized radiation delivery to hepatic tumors. As with patients being considered for HAT-DEB, candidates for Y-90 therapy should have metastatic colorectal cancer with liver-predominant tumor burden and >3 months life expectancy. Absolute contraindications include the potential delivery of >30 Gy of radiation to the lung or the gastrointestinal tract as a result of the embolization procedure. A pretreatment macroaggregated albumin (MAA) scan can help determine the likelihood of either of these occurrences. Relative contraindications include poor baseline liver function, persistently elevated serum bilirubin, portal venous compromise, and prior hepatic radiation therapy. As with HAT-DEB, pretreatment planning should also include contrasted CT or MRI, tumor markers, and serum chemistries. Furthermore, hepatic arterial flow characteristics should be carefully delineated using both pre-procedural hepatic angiogram and intra-procedural fluoroscopy via percutaneously inserted intra-arterial catheters. Protective embolization of feeding blood vessels to the gastrointestinal tract should be performed prior to radioembolization of the target hepatic lesions to protect the gastrointestinal tract from inadvertent delivery of Y-90 [52, 53].

Treatment and Toxicity

Y-90 treatments can be performed in one of three ways: whole liver, sequential (treating one hepatic lobe followed by the other), and lobar (treating only a single lobe of the liver). The optimal treatment varies based on disease burden and distribution, baseline hepatic function, and the patient's overall performance status. Projecting Y-90 microsphere activity is generally performed using the body surface area (BSA) method. Dosing can be reduced by as much as 30% to account for impaired hepatic function or marginal hepatic reserve [52, 53].

Toxicity and complications of Y-90 treatment, much like DEBIRI, arise from the treatment itself, destruction of normal hepatocytes, and aberrant delivery of Y-90 microspheres. Post-radioembolization syndrome, an analogue of post-embolization syndrome, consists of fatigue, nausea/vomiting, cachexia, and/or abdominal pain. Incidence ranges from 20 to 70%, though symptoms are rarely severe enough to warrant hospitalization [54, 55]. Additionally, while hepatic dysfunction occurs with 40–60% of Y-90 treatments, the vast majority is mild (Grade I or II) and resolves within 30 days of treatment. Factors associated with persistent hepatic dysfunction are repeated radioembolization, prior external beam radiation therapy to the liver, and elevated pretreatment serum bilirubin and/or transaminases [54, 56]. Other sequelae include biliary complications such as cholecystitis and cholangitis, pancreatitis, and gastroenteritis [57–59]. These occur in fewer than 5–10% of patients and result from aberrant deposition of microspheres into arterial communications with biliary, pancreatic, and/or enteric structures. They can be prevented through careful pre-procedural assessment of each patient's arterial anatomy and prudent utilization of protective embolization prior to deposition of Y-90 beads [54].

Efficacy and Response Evaluation

The safety and efficacy of Y-90 embolization for treatment of chemotherapy–refractory CLM have been demonstrated by several groups (Table 18.3) [60–67]. Median overall survival ranged from 6.1 to 14.5 months with an adverse event rate of approximately 8% [65]. An increased survival benefit was shown in patients experiencing decrease in carcinoembryonic antigen (CEA) level as well as a response on posttreatment imaging [12]. When stratifying by hepatic burden of disease (HBD) and number of prior chemotherapy regimens, patients with less than 25% HBD have significantly greater median OS compared to those with greater than 25% HBD (19.6 months vs. 3.4 months, $p < 0.001$) [66]. On multivariate analysis, factors associated with decreased OS were age, three or more lines of prior chemotherapy, HBD >25%, and higher CEA level.

Several groups have investigated the optimal means of assessing response to Y-90. A 2007 study found that use of combined necrosis and RECIST criteria resulted in the highest response rate and also detected responses earlier than size criteria alone [68]. PET also allowed for greater detection of treatment response than CT using RECIST or combined criteria. PET in conjunction with CT imaging has been shown to detect recurrence earlier after treatment and should be considered a useful tool in posttreatment follow-up of patients treated with Y-90 embolization for CLM [69].

Currently, Y-90 beads exist in two forms: glass (TheraSphere; MDS Nordion) and biocompatible resin (selective internal radiation, SIR-Spheres, SIRTeX). Given that SIR-Spheres were developed after their glass counterparts, most early studies report efficacy using TheraSpheres, while more recent studies largely employ SIR-Spheres. Given that little data exists to help guide physician selection of one type of Y-90 bead over the other, a recent study compared safety and efficacy in patients treated with TheraSpheres and SIR-Spheres. For patients with CLM, treatment with SIR-Spheres was associated with a longer mean survival compared to treatment with TheraSpheres (26.8 vs. 16.3 months, log-rank = 0097). However, it was also associated with a higher incidence of Grade III side effects (16.3% vs. 0%). These results highlight the need for future prospective trials directly comparing these Y-90 embolization vehicles in treating patients with CLM.

Concomitant Use with Systemic Chemotherapy, Surgery

As with HAT-DEB, several investigators have recently examined the use of Y-90 with systemic chemotherapy [70–73]. Combined Y-90 therapy with systemic FOLFOX4 in patients with CLM resulted in median progression-free survival of 9.3 months and hepatic-specific progression of 12.3 months. Rate of conversion to hepatic resection was approximately 9% [71]. Two groups are currently conducting randomized controlled trials assessing Y-90 therapy combined with FOLFOX6 ± bevacizumab vs.

Table 18.3 Original studies of safety and efficacy of Y-90 Radioembolization for CLM

Study/year/reference	Patients (n)	Therapy stage (first line, second line, third line, >third line)	Radioembolic agent	Median follow-up (months)	Median PFS (months)	Median OS (months)
Mantravadi et al./1982/[51]	15	NR	TheraSpheres	NR	NR	NR
Herba et al./2002/[64]	37	Second line or beyond	TheraSpheres	8	NR	NR
Murthy et al./2007/[91]	10	Third line or beyond	SIR-Spheres	5	NR	5.8
Sharma et al./2007/[71]	22	First line	SIR-Spheres (+FOLFOX4)	NR	9.3	NR
Jakobs et al./2008/[65]	36	Second line or beyond	SIR-Spheres	7.9	NR	10.5
Mulcahy et al./2009/[67]	72	Second line or beyond	TheraSpheres	26.2	15.4	14.5
Nace et al./2011/[92]	51	Third line	SIR-Spheres	NR	NR	10.2
Lam et al./2013/[56]	8	First line or beyond	TheraSpheres SIR-Spheres	24.7	NR	3.1
Gunduz et al./2014/[93]	78	NR	SIR-Spheres	NR	4.4	10.1
Kalva et al./2017/[62]	45	Second line or beyond	SIR-Spheres	4.9	NR	6.1
Abbott et al./2015/[66]	68	First line or beyond	TheraSpheres	NR	NR	11.6

FOLFOX6 ± bevacizumab alone and OxMdG with or without Y-90 therapy for treatment of unresectable CLM, with a projected increase in PFS from 9.4 to 12.5 months [70, 73].

Finally, with respect to the safety of hepatic resection after administration of Y-90, a recent series of four patients who underwent Y-90 therapy with good response and subsequently underwent hepatic resection with or without concomitant hepatic ablation reported no hepatic dysfunction or hepatic-specific recurrence after hepatectomy. Median survival was 2 years [74]. As noted by the authors of this study, the utility of preoperative Y-90 therapy lies not only in downstaging patients but also in assessing tumor biology, informing prognosis, and guiding therapy.

Conclusion

Recent years have seen a marked increase in the use of HAT-DEB in patients with therapy-refractory colorectal liver metastases. The emergence of calibrated microspheres, together with improvements in DEB technology, has enabled physicians to perform both HAT-DEB and Y-90 embolization in a highly standardized and effective manner. Preoperatively, HAT may be used for tumor downsizing and conversion to resectability of CLM with minimal toxicity and fewer adverse effects compared with systemic therapy. In the postoperative setting, it may prevent recurrence and improve overall survival. However, to date, most published studies describe HAT-DEB and Y-90 use either in the setting of controlled trials with patients who had failed first- or second-line chemotherapy or as a salvage intervention for patients who had failed multiple previous surgical, ablative, and/or systemic therapies. Though the results of a randomized trial demonstrating the benefit of adding HAT-DEB to first-line systemic chemotherapy for unresectable CLM have recently been published and two similarly oriented trials for Y-90 are currently underway, future prospective trials are needed to optimally characterize the efficacy of HAT as first-, second-, or third-line and palliative therapy in patients with CLM.

Disclosures Neither author has any relevant disclosures or conflicts of interest.

References

1. Zhao Z, Pelletier E, Barber B, Bhosle M, Wang S, Gao S, et al. Patterns of treatment with chemotherapy and monoclonal antibodies for metastatic colorectal cancer in Western Europe. Curr Med Res Opin. 2012;28(2):221–9. https://doi.org/10.1185/03007995.2011.650503.
2. Schwarz RE, Berlin JD, Lenz HJ, Nordlinger B, Rubbia-Brandt L, Choti MA. Systemic cytotoxic and biological therapies of colorectal liver metastases: expert consensus statement. HPB. 2013;15(2):106–15. https://doi.org/10.1111/j.1477-2574.2012.00558.x.
3. Bentrem DJ, Dematteo RP, Blumgart LH. Surgical therapy for metastatic disease to the liver. Ann Rev Med. 2005;56:139–56. https://doi.org/10.1146/annurev.med.56.082103.104630.
4. Folprecht G. Treatment of colorectal liver metastases. Deutsche medizinische Wochenschrift (1946). 2013;138(41):2098–103. https://doi.org/10.1055/s-0033-1349610.
5. Goere D, Benhaim L, Bonnet S, Malka D, Faron M, Elias D, et al. Adjuvant chemotherapy after resection of colorectal liver metastases in patients at high risk of hepatic recurrence: a comparative study between hepatic arterial infusion of oxaliplatin and modern systemic chemotherapy. Ann Surg. 2013;257(1):114–20. https://doi.org/10.1097/SLA.0b013e31827b9005.
6. Bozzetti F, Doci R, Bignami P, Morabito A, Gennari L. Patterns of failure following surgical resection of colorectal cancer liver metastases. Rationale for a multimodal approach. Ann Surg. 1987;205(3):264–70.
7. Hind D, Tappenden P, Tumur I, Eggington S, Sutcliffe P, Ryan A. The use of irinotecan, oxaliplatin and raltitrexed for the treatment of advanced colorectal cancer: systematic review and economic evaluation. Health Technol Assess. 2008;12(15):iii–x, xi–162.
8. Hochster HS, Hart LL, Ramanathan RK, Childs BH, Hainsworth JD, Cohn AL, et al. Safety and efficacy of oxaliplatin and fluoropyrimidine regimens with or without bevacizumab as first-line treatment of metastatic colorectal cancer: results of the TREE study. J Clin Oncol. 2008;26(21):3523–9. https://doi.org/10.1200/jco.2007.15.4138.
9. Thirion P, Michiels S, Pignon JP, Buyse M, Braud AC, Carlson RW, et al. Modulation of fluorouracil by leucovorin in patients with advanced colorectal cancer: an updated meta-analysis. J Clin Oncol. 2004;22(18):3766–75. https://doi.org/10.1200/jco.2004.03.104.
10. Tournigand C, Andre T, Achille E, Lledo G, Flesh M, Mery-Mignard D, et al. FOLFIRI followed by FOLFOX6 or the reverse sequence in advanced colorectal cancer: a randomized GERCOR study. J Clin Oncol. 2004;22(2):229–37. https://doi.org/10.1200/jco.2004.05.113.
11. Van Cutsem E, Kohne CH, Hitre E, Zaluski J, Chang Chien CR, Makhson A, et al. Cetuximab and chemotherapy as initial treatment for metastatic colorectal cancer. N Engl J Med. 2009;360(14):1408–17. https://doi.org/10.1056/NEJMoa0805019.
12. Ychou M, Viret F, Kramar A, Desseigne F, Mitry E, Guimbaud R, et al. Tritherapy with fluorouracil/leucovorin, irinotecan and oxaliplatin (FOLFIRINOX): a phase II study in colorectal cancer patients with non-resectable liver metastases. Cancer Chemother Pharmacol. 2008;62(2):195–201. https://doi.org/10.1007/s00280-007-0588-3.
13. Foubert F, Matysiak-Budnik T, Touchefeu Y. Options for metastatic colorectal cancer beyond the second line of treatment. Dig Liver Dis. 2014;46(2):105–12. https://doi.org/10.1016/j.dld.2013.07.002.
14. Alberts SR, Horvath WL, Sternfeld WC, Goldberg RM, Mahoney MR, Dakhil SR, et al. Oxaliplatin, fluorouracil, and leucovorin for patients with unresectable liver-only metastases from colorectal cancer: a North Central Cancer Treatment Group phase II study. J Clin Oncol. 2005;23(36):9243–9. https://doi.org/10.1200/jco.2005.07.740.
15. Nordlinger B, Sorbye H, Glimelius B, Poston GJ, Schlag PM, Rougier P, et al. Perioperative chemotherapy with FOLFOX4 and surgery versus surgery alone for resectable liver metastases from colorectal cancer (EORTC Intergroup trial 40983): a randomised controlled trial. Lancet. 2008;371(9617):1007–16. https://doi.org/10.1016/s0140-6736(08)60455-9.
16. Haraldsdottir S, Wu C, Bloomston M, Goldberg RM. What is the optimal neo-adjuvant treatment for liver metastasis? Ther Adv Med Oncol. 2013;5(4):221–34. https://doi.org/10.1177/1758834013485111.
17. Lam VW, Spiro C, Laurence JM, Johnston E, Hollands MJ, Pleass HC, et al. A systematic review of clinical response and survival outcomes of downsizing systemic chemotherapy and rescue liver surgery in patients with initially unresectable colorectal liver metastases. Ann Surg Oncol. 2012;19(4):1292–301. https://doi.org/10.1245/s10434-011-2061-0.
18. Malik H, Khan AZ, Berry DP, Cameron IC, Pope I, Sherlock D, et al. Liver resection rate following downsizing chemotherapy with cetuximab in metastatic colorectal cancer: UK retrospective observational study. Eur J Surg Oncol. 2015;41(4):499–505. https://doi.org/10.1016/j.ejso.2015.01.032.
19. Collins JM. Pharmacologic rationale for regional drug delivery. J Clin Oncol. 1984;2(5):498–504.
20. Lewandowski RJ, Geschwind JF, Liapi E, Salem R. Transcatheter intraarterial therapies: rationale and overview. Radiology. 2011;259(3):641–57. https://doi.org/10.1148/radiol.11081489.
21. Abdalla EK, Vauthey JN. Chemotherapy prior to hepatic resection for colorectal liver metastases: helpful until harmful? Dig Surg. 2008;25(6):421–9. https://doi.org/10.1159/000184733.
22. Rajappa P, Krass J, Riina HA, Boockvar JA, Greenfield JP. Super-selective basilar artery infusion of bevacizumab and cetuximab for multiply recur-

rent pediatric ependymoma. Interv Neuroradiol. 2011;17(4):459–65.
23. Burkhardt JK, Riina H, Shin BJ, Christos P, Kesavabhotla K, Hofstetter CP, et al. Intra-arterial delivery of bevacizumab after blood-brain barrier disruption for the treatment of recurrent glioblastoma: progression-free survival and overall survival. World Neurosurg. 2012;77(1):130–4. https://doi.org/10.1016/j.wneu.2011.05.056.
24. Pellerin O, Geschwind JF. Intra-arterial treatment of liver metastases from colorectal carcinoma. J Radiol. 2011;92(9):835–41. https://doi.org/10.1016/j.jradio.2011.07.008.
25. Xing M, Kooby DA, El-Rayes BF, Kokabi N, Camacho JC, Kim HS. Locoregional therapies for metastatic colorectal carcinoma to the liver—an evidence-based review. J Surg Oncol. 2014;110(2):182–96. https://doi.org/10.1002/jso.23619.
26. Alberts SR. Update on the optimal management of patients with colorectal liver metastases. Crit Rev Oncol Hematol. 2012;84(1):59–70. https://doi.org/10.1016/j.critrevonc.2012.02.007.
27. Nishiofuku H, Tanaka T, Matsuoka M, Otsuji T, Anai H, Sueyoshi S, et al. Transcatheter arterial chemoembolization using cisplatin powder mixed with degradable starch microspheres for colorectal liver metastases after FOLFOX failure: results of a phase I/II study. J Vasc Interv Radiol. 2013;24(1):56–65. https://doi.org/10.1016/j.jvir.2012.09.010.
28. Tsuchiya M, Watanabe M, Otsuka Y, Yamazaki K, Tamura A, Ishii J, et al. Transarterial chemoembolization with irinotecan (CPT-11) and degradable starch microspheres (DSM) in patients with liver metastases from colorectal cancer. Gan To Kagaku Ryoho. 2007;34(12):2038–40.
29. Gnutzmann DM, Mechel J, Schmitz A, Kohler K, Krone D, Bellemann N, et al. Evaluation of the plasmatic and parenchymal elution kinetics of two different irinotecan-loaded drug-eluting embolics in a pig model. J Vasc Interv Radiol. 2015;26(5):746–54. https://doi.org/10.1016/j.jvir.2014.12.016.
30. Martin RC, Howard J, Tomalty D, Robbins K, Padr R, Bosnjakovic PM, et al. Toxicity of irinotecan-eluting beads in the treatment of hepatic malignancies: results of a multi-institutional registry. Cardiovasc Interv Radiol. 2010;33(5):960–6. https://doi.org/10.1007/s00270-010-9937-4.
31. Ceelen W, Praet M, Villeirs G, Defreyne L, Pattijn P, Hesse U, et al. Initial experience with the use of preoperative transarterial chemoembolization in the treatment of liver metastasis. Acta Chir Belg. 1996;96(1):37–40.
32. Cohen AD, Kemeny NE. An update on hepatic arterial infusion chemotherapy for colorectal cancer. Oncologist. 2003;8(6):553–66.
33. Martin RC, Joshi J, Robbins K, Tomalty D, O'Hara R, Tatum C. Transarterial chemoembolization of metastatic colorectal carcinoma with drug-eluting beads, irinotecan (DEBIRI): multi-institutional registry. J Oncol. 2009;2009:539795. https://doi.org/10.1155/2009/539795.
34. Martin RC, Robbins K, Tomalty D, O'Hara R, Bosnjakovic P, Padr R, et al. Transarterial chemoembolisation (TACE) using irinotecan-loaded beads for the treatment of unresectable metastases to the liver in patients with colorectal cancer: an interim report. World J Surg Oncol. 2009;7:80. https://doi.org/10.1186/1477-7819-7-80.
35. Geschwind JF, Kaushik S, Ramsey DE, Choti MA, Fishman EK, Kobeiter H. Influence of a new prophylactic antibiotic therapy on the incidence of liver abscesses after chemoembolization treatment of liver tumors. J Vasc Interv Radiol. 2002;13(11):1163–6.
36. Liu DM, Thakor AS, Baerlocher M, Alshammari MT, Lim H, Kos S, et al. A review of conventional and drug-eluting chemoembolization in the treatment of colorectal liver metastases: principles and proof. Future Oncol. 2015;11(9):1421–8. https://doi.org/10.2217/fon.15.3.
37. Basile A, Carrafiello G, Ierardi AM, Tsetis D, Brountzos E. Quality-improvement guidelines for hepatic transarterial chemoembolization. Cardiovasc Interv Radiol. 2012;35(4):765–74. https://doi.org/10.1007/s00270-012-0423-z.
38. Meyer C, Pieper CC, Ezziddin S, Wilhelm KE, Schild HH, Ahmadzadehfar H. Feasibility of temporary protective embolization of normal liver tissue using degradable starch microspheres during radioembolization of liver tumours. Eur J Nucl Med Mol Imaging. 2014;41(2):231–7. https://doi.org/10.1007/s00259-013-2550-4.
39. Lencioni R, Aliberti C, de Baere T, Garcia-Monaco R, Narayanan G, O'Grady E, et al. Transarterial treatment of colorectal cancer liver metastases with irinotecan-loaded drug-eluting beads: technical recommendations. J Vasc Interv Radiol. 2014;25(3):365–9. https://doi.org/10.1016/j.jvir.2013.11.027.
40. Chan DL, Alzahrani NA, Morris DL, Chua TC. Systematic review and meta-analysis of hepatic arterial infusion chemotherapy as bridging therapy for colorectal liver metastases. Surg Oncol. 2015;24(3):162–71. https://doi.org/10.1016/j.suronc.2015.06.014.
41. Fiorentini G, Aliberti C, Mulazzani L, Coschiera P, Catalano V, Rossi D, et al. Chemoembolization in colorectal liver metastases: the rebirth. Anticancer Res. 2014;34(2):575–84.
42. Richardson AJ, Laurence JM, Lam VW. Transarterial chemoembolization with irinotecan beads in the treatment of colorectal liver metastases: systematic review. J Vasc Interv Radiol. 2013;24(8):1209–17. https://doi.org/10.1016/j.jvir.2013.05.055.
43. Cai GX, Cai SJ. Multi-modality treatment of colorectal liver metastases. World J Gastroenterol. 2012;18(1):16–24. https://doi.org/10.3748/wjg.v18.i1.16.
44. Brown RE, Bower MR, Metzger TL, Scoggins CR, McMasters KM, Hahl MJ, et al. Hepatectomy after hepatic arterial therapy with either yttrium-90 or drug-eluting bead chemotherapy: is it safe? HPB. 2011;13(2):91–5. https://doi.org/10.1111/j.1477-2574.2010.00246.x.

45. Bower M, Metzger T, Robbins K, Tomalty D, Valek V, Boudny J, et al. Surgical downstaging and neo-adjuvant therapy in metastatic colorectal carcinoma with irinotecan drug-eluting beads: a multi-institutional study. HPB. 2010;12(1):31–6. https://doi.org/10.1111/j.1477-2574.2009.00117.x.
46. Jones RP, Dunne D, Sutton P, Malik HZ, Fenwick SW, Terlizzo M, et al. Segmental and lobar administration of drug-eluting beads delivering irinotecan leads to tumour destruction: a case-control series. HPB. 2013;15(1):71–7. https://doi.org/10.1111/j.1477-2574.2012.00587.x.
47. Jones RP, Stattner S, Dunne DF, O'Grady E, Smethurst A, Terlizzo M, et al. Radiological assessment of response to neoadjuvant transcatheter hepatic therapy with irinotecan-eluting beads (DEBIRI((R))) for colorectal liver metastases does not predict tumour destruction or long-term outcome. Eur J Surg Oncol. 2013;39(10):1122–8. https://doi.org/10.1016/j.ejso.2013.07.087.
48. Kemeny NE, Melendez FD, Capanu M, Paty PB, Fong Y, Schwartz LH, et al. Conversion to resectability using hepatic artery infusion plus systemic chemotherapy for the treatment of unresectable liver metastases from colorectal carcinoma. J Clin Oncol. 2009;27(21):3465–71. https://doi.org/10.1200/jco.2008.20.1301.
49. Akinwande O, Miller A, Hayes D, O'Hara R, Tomalty D, Martin RC. Concomitant capecitabine with hepatic delivery of drug eluting beads in metastatic colorectal cancer. Anticancer Res. 2014;34(12):7239–45.
50. Martin RC II, Scoggins CR, Schreeder M, Rilling WS, Laing CJ, Tatum CM, et al. Randomized controlled trial of irinotecan drug-eluting beads with simultaneous FOLFOX and bevacizumab for patients with unresectable colorectal liver-limited metastasis. Cancer. 2015;121(20):3649–58. https://doi.org/10.1002/cncr.29534.
51. Mantravadi RV, Spigos DG, Tan WS, Felix EL. Intraarterial yttrium 90 in the treatment of hepatic malignancy. Radiology. 1982;142(3):783–6. https://doi.org/10.1148/radiology.142.3.7063703.
52. Kennedy A, Nag S, Salem R, Murthy R, McEwan AJ, Nutting C, et al. Recommendations for radioembolization of hepatic malignancies using yttrium-90 microsphere brachytherapy: a consensus panel report from the radioembolization brachytherapy oncology consortium. Int J Radiat Oncol Biol Phys. 2007;68(1):13–23. https://doi.org/10.1016/j.ijrobp.2006.11.060.
53. Lau WY, Kennedy AS, Kim YH, Lai HK, Lee RC, Leung TW, et al. Patient selection and activity planning guide for selective internal radiotherapy with yttrium-90 resin microspheres. Int J Radiat Oncol Biol Phys. 2012;82(1):401–7. https://doi.org/10.1016/j.ijrobp.2010.08.015.
54. Riaz A, Awais R, Salem R. Side effects of yttrium-90 radioembolization. Front Oncol. 2014;4:198. https://doi.org/10.3389/fonc.2014.00198.
55. Peterson JL, Vallow LA, Johnson DW, Heckman MG, Diehl NN, Smith AA, et al. Complications after 90Y microsphere radioembolization for unresectable hepatic tumors: an evaluation of 112 patients. Brachytherapy. 2013;12(6):573–9. https://doi.org/10.1016/j.brachy.2013.05.008.
56. Lam MG, Louie JD, Iagaru AH, Goris ML, Sze DY. Safety of repeated yttrium-90 radioembolization. Cardiovasc Interv Radiol. 2013;36(5):1320–8. https://doi.org/10.1007/s00270-013-0547-9.
57. Atassi B, Bangash AK, Lewandowski RJ, Ibrahim S, Kulik L, Mulcahy MF, et al. Biliary sequelae following radioembolization with Yttrium-90 microspheres. J Vasc Interv Radiol. 2008;19(5):691–7. https://doi.org/10.1016/j.jvir.2008.01.003.
58. Murthy R, Brown DB, Salem R, Meranze SG, Coldwell DM, Krishnan S, et al. Gastrointestinal complications associated with hepatic arterial Yttrium-90 microsphere therapy. J Vasc Interv Radiol. 2007;18(4):553–61. https://doi.org/10.1016/j.jvir.2007.02.002. quiz 62.
59. Hoffmann RT, Jakobs TF, Kubisch CH, Stemmler HJ, Trumm C, Tatsch K, et al. Radiofrequency ablation after selective internal radiation therapy with Yttrium90 microspheres in metastatic liver disease—is it feasible? Eur J Radiol. 2010;74(1):199–205. https://doi.org/10.1016/j.ejrad.2009.02.001.
60. Gulec SA, Mesoloras G, Dezarn WA, McNeillie P, Kennedy AS. Safety and efficacy of Y-90 microsphere treatment in patients with primary and metastatic liver cancer: the tumor selectivity of the treatment as a function of tumor to liver flow ratio. J Transl Med. 2007;5:15. https://doi.org/10.1186/1479-5876-5-15.
61. Padia SA, Kwan SW, Roudsari B, Monsky WL, Coveler A, Harris WP. Superselective yttrium-90 radioembolization for hepatocellular carcinoma yields high response rates with minimal toxicity. J Vasc Interv Radiol. 2014;25(7):1067–73. https://doi.org/10.1016/j.jvir.2014.03.030.
62. Kalva SP, Rana RS, Liu R, Rachamreddy N, Dave B, Sharma A, et al. Yttrium-90 radioembolization as salvage therapy for liver metastases from colorectal cancer. Am J Clin Oncol. 2017;40(3):288–93. https://doi.org/10.1097/coc.0000000000000151.
63. Deleporte A, Flamen P, Hendlisz A. State of the art: radiolabeled microspheres treatment for liver malignancies. Expert Opin Pharmacother. 2010;11(4):579–86. https://doi.org/10.1517/14656560903520916.
64. Herba MJ, Thirlwell MP. Radioembolization for hepatic metastases. Semin Oncol. 2002;29(2):152–9.
65. Jakobs TF, Hoffmann RT, Dehm K, Trumm C, Stemmler HJ, Tatsch K, et al. Hepatic yttrium-90 radioembolization of chemotherapy-refractory colorectal cancer liver metastases. J Vasc Interv Radiol. 2008;19(8):1187–95. https://doi.org/10.1016/j.jvir.2008.05.013.
66. Abbott AM, Kim R, Hoffe SE, Arslan B, Biebel B, Choi J, et al. Outcomes of therasphere radioembolization for colorectal metastases. Clin Colorectal Cancer. 2015;14(3):146–53. https://doi.org/10.1016/j.clcc.2015.02.002.

67. Mulcahy MF, Lewandowski RJ, Ibrahim SM, Sato KT, Ryu RK, Atassi B, et al. Radioembolization of colorectal hepatic metastases using yttrium-90 microspheres. Cancer. 2009;115(9):1849–58. https://doi.org/10.1002/cncr.24224.
68. Miller FH, Keppke AL, Reddy D, Huang J, Jin J, Mulcahy MF, et al. Response of liver metastases after treatment with yttrium-90 microspheres: role of size, necrosis, and PET. AJR Am J Roentgenol. 2007;188(3):776–83. https://doi.org/10.2214/ajr.06.0707.
69. Annunziata S, Treglia G, Caldarella C. The role of 18F-FDG-PET and PET/CT in patients with colorectal liver metastases undergoing selective internal radiation therapy with yttrium-90: a first evidence-based review. Sci World J. 2014;2014:879469. https://doi.org/10.1155/2014/879469.
70. Gibbs P, Gebski V, Van Buskirk M, Thurston K, Cade DN, Van Hazel GA. Selective internal radiation therapy (SIRT) with yttrium-90 resin microspheres plus standard systemic chemotherapy regimen of FOLFOX versus FOLFOX alone as first-line treatment of non-resectable liver metastases from colorectal cancer: the SIRFLOX study. BMC Cancer. 2014;14:897. https://doi.org/10.1186/1471-2407-14-897.
71. Sharma RA, Van Hazel GA, Morgan B, Berry DP, Blanshard K, Price D, et al. Radioembolization of liver metastases from colorectal cancer using yttrium-90 microspheres with concomitant systemic oxaliplatin, fluorouracil, and leucovorin chemotherapy. J Clin Oncol. 2007;25(9):1099–106. https://doi.org/10.1200/jco.2006.08.7916.
72. De Souza A, Daly KP. Safety and efficacy of combined yttrium 90 resin radioembolization with aflibercept and FOLFIRI in a patient with metastatic colorectal cancer. Case Rep Oncol Med. 2015;2015:461823. https://doi.org/10.1155/2015/461823.
73. Dutton SJ, Kenealy N, Love SB, Wasan HS, Sharma RA. FOXFIRE protocol: an open-label, randomised, phase III trial of 5-fluorouracil, oxaliplatin and folinic acid (OxMdG) with or without interventional Selective Internal Radiation Therapy (SIRT) as first-line treatment for patients with unresectable liver-only or liver-dominant metastatic colorectal cancer. BMC Cancer. 2014;14:497. https://doi.org/10.1186/1471-2407-14-497.
74. Whitney R, Tatum C, Hahl M, Ellis S, Scoggins CR, McMasters K, et al. Safety of hepatic resection in metastatic disease to the liver after yttrium-90 therapy. J Surg Res. 2011;166(2):236–40. https://doi.org/10.1016/j.jss.2009.05.021.
75. Tellez C, Benson AB III, Lyster MT, Talamonti M, Shaw J, Braun MA, et al. Phase II trial of chemoembolization for the treatment of metastatic colorectal carcinoma to the liver and review of the literature. Cancer. 1998;82(7):1250–9.
76. Leichman CG, Jacobson JR, Modiano M, Daniels JR, Zalupski MM, Doroshow JH, et al. Hepatic chemoembolization combined with systemic infusion of 5-fluorouracil and bolus leucovorin for patients with metastatic colorectal carcinoma: a Southwest Oncology Group pilot trial. Cancer. 1999;86(5):775–81.
77. Muller H, Nakchbandi W, Chatzissavvidis I, Valek V. Intra-arterial infusion of 5-fluorouracil plus granulocyte-macrophage colony-stimulating factor (GM-CSF) and chemoembolization with melphalan in the treatment of disseminated colorectal liver metastases. Eur J Surg Oncol. 2001;27(7):652–61. https://doi.org/10.1053/ejso.2001.1193.
78. Salman HS, Cynamon J, Jagust M, Bakal C, Rozenblit A, Kaleya R, et al. Randomized phase II trial of embolization therapy versus chemoembolization therapy in previously treated patients with colorectal carcinoma metastatic to the liver. Clin Colorectal Cancer. 2002;2(3):173–9. https://doi.org/10.3816/CCC.2002.n.022.
79. Vogl TJ, Gruber T, Balzer JO, Eichler K, Hammerstingl R, Zangos S. Repeated transarterial chemoembolization in the treatment of liver metastases of colorectal cancer: prospective study. Radiology. 2009;250(1):281–9. https://doi.org/10.1148/radiol.2501080295.
80. Albert M, Kiefer MV, Sun W, Haller D, Fraker DL, Tuite CM, et al. Chemoembolization of colorectal liver metastases with cisplatin, doxorubicin, mitomycin C, ethiodol, and polyvinyl alcohol. Cancer. 2011;117(2):343–52. https://doi.org/10.1002/cncr.25387.
81. Gruber-Rouh T, Naguib NN, Eichler K, Ackermann H, Zangos S, Trojan J, et al. Transarterial chemoembolization of unresectable systemic chemotherapy-refractory liver metastases from colorectal cancer: long-term results over a 10-year period. Int J Cancer. 2014;134(5):1225–31. https://doi.org/10.1002/ijc.28443.
82. Aliberti C, Tilli M, Benea G, Fiorentini G. Transarterial chemoembolization (TACE) of liver metastases from colorectal cancer using irinotecan-eluting beads: preliminary results. Anticancer Res. 2006;26(5b):3793–5.
83. Martin RC, Joshi J, Robbins K, Tomalty D, Bosnjakovik P, Derner M, et al. Hepatic intra-arterial injection of drug-eluting bead, irinotecan (DEBIRI) in unresectable colorectal liver metastases refractory to systemic chemotherapy: results of multi-institutional study. Ann Surg Oncol. 2011;18(1):192–8. https://doi.org/10.1245/s10434-010-1288-5.
84. Aliberti C, Fiorentini G, Muzzio PC, Pomerri F, Tilli M, Dallara S, et al. Trans-arterial chemoembolization of metastatic colorectal carcinoma to the liver adopting DC Bead(R), drug-eluting bead loaded with irinotecan: results of a phase II clinical study. Anticancer Res. 2011;31(12):4581–7.
85. Fiorentini G, Aliberti C, Tilli M, Mulazzani L, Graziano F, Giordani P, et al. Intra-arterial infusion of irinotecan-loaded drug-eluting beads (DEBIRI) versus intravenous therapy (FOLFIRI) for hepatic metastases from colorectal cancer: final results of a phase III study. Anticancer Res. 2012;32(4):1387–95.

86. Martin RC II, Scoggins CR, Tomalty D, Schreeder M, Metzger T, Tatum C, et al. Irinotecan drug-eluting beads in the treatment of chemo-naive unresectable colorectal liver metastasis with concomitant systemic fluorouracil and oxaliplatin: results of pharmacokinetics and phase I trial. J Gastrointest Surg. 2012;16(8):1531–8. https://doi.org/10.1007/s11605-012-1892-8.
87. Eichler K, Zangos S, Mack MG, Hammerstingl R, Gruber-Rouh T, Gallus C, et al. First human study in treatment of unresectable liver metastases from colorectal cancer with irinotecan-loaded beads (DEBIRI). Int J Oncol. 2012;41(4):1213–20. https://doi.org/10.3892/ijo.2012.1572.
88. Jones RP, Sutton P, Greensmith RM, Santoyo-Castelazo A, Carr DF, Jenkins R, et al. Hepatic activation of irinotecan predicts tumour response in patients with colorectal liver metastases treated with DEBIRI: exploratory findings from a phase II study. Cancer Chemother Pharmacol. 2013;72(2):359–68. https://doi.org/10.1007/s00280-013-2199-5.
89. Narayanan G, Barbery K, Suthar R, Guerrero G, Arora G. Transarterial chemoembolization using DEBIRI for treatment of hepatic metastases from colorectal cancer. Anticancer Res. 2013;33(5):2077–83.
90. Huppert P, Wenzel T, Wietholtz H. Transcatheter arterial chemoembolization (TACE) of colorectal cancer liver metastases by irinotecan-eluting microspheres in a salvage patient population. Cardiovasc Interv Radiol. 2014;37(1):154–64. https://doi.org/10.1007/s00270-013-0632-0.
91. Murthy R, Eng C, Krishnan S, Madoff DC, Habbu A, Canet S, et al. Hepatic yttrium-90 radioembolotherapy in metastatic colorectal cancer treated with cetuximab or bevacizumab. J Vasc Interv Radiol. 2007;18(12):1588–91. https://doi.org/10.1016/j.jvir.2007.08.015.
92. Nace GW, Steel JL, Amesur N, Zajko A, Nastasi BE, Joyce J, et al. Yttrium-90 radioembolization for colorectal cancer liver metastases: a single institution experience. Int J Surg Oncol. 2011;2011:571261. https://doi.org/10.1155/2011/571261.
93. Gunduz S, Ozgur O, Bozcuk H, Coskun HS, Ozdogan M, Erkilic M, et al. Yttrium-90 radioembolization in patients with unresectable liver metastases: determining the factors that lead to treatment efficacy. Hepato-Gastroenterol. 2014;61(134):1529–34.

Hepatic Artery Infusion Therapy for Colorectal Cancer Liver Metastases

Camilo Correa-Gallego and Michael I. D'Angelica

Introduction

Colorectal cancer (CRC) is a leading cause of cancer death [1]. Approximately 50% of patients with CRC will develop liver metastases (colorectal cancer liver metastases—CRLM) during their disease course, and about one-third of these patients have disease that is confined to the liver. Historically, CRLM were associated with high mortality rates due the lack of effective treatments. With the evolution of liver surgery, resection has come to the forefront and is now routinely used in the treatment of these patients. Complete resection is the most effective treatment for CRLM and is associated with a 5-year disease-specific survival of approximately 50% [2]. However, only a minority of patients (~20%) present with resectable disease. In the remaining patients, standard treatment involves cytotoxic chemotherapy and targeted therapy which are employed with the goal of response and disease control aiming at prolonged survival and potentially conversion to resectable

disease. Furthermore, chemotherapy has been employed in the adjuvant setting after complete resection for CRLM with the aim of improving survival and cure rates.

Despite significant improvements, systemic chemotherapy has limited efficacy in this advanced setting. Modern combination regimens yield response rates (RR) around 50% in the first-line setting, but this drops to approximately 20% or less in the second-line setting. For patients with unresectable disease, systemic treatment is associated with a time to progression of under 10 months and a median survival of roughly 20 months [3]. Hepatic artery infusion (HAI) chemotherapy is an attractive alternative for regional treatment of liver malignancies that is currently used in combination with systemic chemotherapy and has been demonstrated to have significantly higher response rates (RR) than systemic chemotherapy alone. This has resulted in an associated substantial improvement in disease-specific survival (DSS), as well as rates of conversion to complete resection [4, 5].

HAI is predicated on the fact that metastatic liver tumors derive their blood supply from the hepatic arterial circulation [6], whereas the normal liver has a dual blood supply from both the hepatic artery and portal vein. Furthermore, HAI therapy takes advantage of the high hepatic extraction rate of floxuridine (FUDR) which when directly infused into the hepatic artery minimizes systemic exposure and toxicity even when

C. Correa-Gallego
Department of Surgery, Memorial Sloan Kettering Cancer Center, New York, NY, USA
e-mail: correagj@mskcc.org

M. I. D'Angelica (✉)
Division of Hepatopancreatobiliary Surgery, Department of Surgery, Memorial Sloan Kettering Cancer Center, New York, NY, USA
e-mail: dangelim@mskcc.org

administering high doses [7]. This chapter reviews the technical aspects of hepatic arterial infusion pump (HAIP) placement, as well as the outcomes in the adjuvant and unresectable settings.

Technical Aspects

Totally implantable infusion pumps for administration of intrahepatic chemotherapy have been safely used for many decades [7–10]. The outcomes of our current placement technique have been previously published and shown to have an adequate safety profile [11, 12]. In essence, a mechanical reservoir with the ability to provide continuous or bolus infusion is implanted in the abdominal wall. This pump is connected transperitoneally to the hepatic arterial circulation via a catheter that is most commonly (see below) placed in the gastroduodenal artery (GDA), thus allowing direct and exclusive drug delivery to the liver via the proper hepatic artery (PHA).

Placement

After exclusion of extrahepatic disease, the most important consideration is each patient's individual hepatic vascular anatomy. Approximately one-third of patients have anatomical variations that impact the placement of the catheter. It is thus imperative to obtain and carefully study angiographic images (now readily available from cross-sectional imaging reconstruction) in every patient being considered for HAIP placement. A variety of incisions, including right subcostal and upper midline, which provide adequate access to the porta hepatis, have been used for pump placement. It is important to keep in mind the potential for future liver and/or colorectal resections when deciding which incision to use.

Once access to the hepatoduodenal ligament is gained, a standard cholecystectomy is performed. Since the cystic artery originates from the hepatic artery branches, it is imperative to perform a cholecystectomy to prevent chemical cholecystitis. Next, the hepatic artery and its branches are circumferentially dissected. In the normal arterial configuration, the common hepatic artery (CHA) is palpated running anteriorly and to the right, parallel to the body of the pancreas. As it approaches the hepatoduodenal ligament, the CHA bifurcates into the GDA and PHA, which are found running parallel and immediately to the left of the common bile duct (CBD). The right gastric artery, which has a variable origin, is identified, ligated, and divided. The CHA, PHA, as well as the right and left hepatic arterial branches are circumferentially dissected, dividing all minor branches, and freed for at least 2 cm. It has been shown that the majority of post-HAIP placement extrahepatic perfusion originates from the right hepatic artery and is within 2 cm of the origin of the GDA [13]. The GDA is dissected for a maximal distance to help with catheter placement. A limited Kocher maneuver, division of any small vessels along the supraduodenal area, as well as resection of lymph nodes in the portacaval space and along the hepatic artery facilitates the dissection and minimizes the risk of extrahepatic perfusion. Vascular control is obtained with rubber vessel loops or vascular clamps. It is important to assess competency of the celiac axis by clamping the GDA and palpating pulses in the PHA to rule out critical stenosis at the origin of the celiac artery and retrograde flow through the GDA (Fig. 19.1).

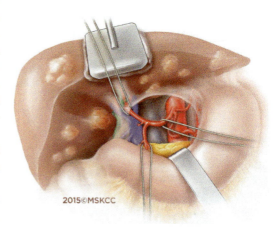

Fig. 19.1 Common hepatic artery (CHA) and its branches are completely dissected in preparation for catheter placement. Modified from Qadan [14], with permission

The GDA is then ligated at its most distal aspect, and either the proximal GDA or PHA/CHA is clamped for vascular control. A transverse arteriotomy is made in the distal GDA with an 11-blade scalpel. The previously flushed arterial catheter is inserted into the GDA up to, but not beyond, the junction with the hepatic artery. It is important to avoid protrusion of the catheter into the CHA or PHA, as turbulent flow in this location can lead to thrombosis and malfunction. Bilobar liver perfusion is assessed by injection of diluted methylene blue into the pump which should show uniform discoloration of the liver surface. This can also be achieved by using fluorescein and a Wood's lamp. At this point any extrahepatic perfusion should be ruled out by careful inspection of the duodenum, pancreas, and stomach for any sign of discoloration. If extrahepatic perfusion is detected, this mandates a search for the culprit vessel with further dissection, ligation, and retesting.

Our experience has shown that the GDA is the ideal location for catheter placement regardless of the presence of aberrant hepatic arterial anatomy. Abnormal anatomy was seen in 37% of patients analyzed in our series and was not associated with catheter-related complications or inadequate pump function or survival. In patients with accessory or replaced hepatic vessels, ligation of the aberrant vessel with catheter placement in the GDA universally resulted in complete liver perfusion via cross-perfusion from the contralateral hepatic artery. Cannulation of any vessel other than the GDA was associated with increased pump-related complications and decreased pump survival [11, 12]. Therefore, our general rule is to place the pump catheter in the GDA and to ligate all replaced/accessory vessels in nearly all cases. On rare occasions, one has to consider using other conduits for the catheter. This includes the right or left hepatic artery or in rare situations an anastomosed vein graft to an aberrant vessel. In the case where a relevant celiac stenosis is found, an attempt at lysing the arcuate ligament should be considered. Alternatively, the catheter can be placed in the CHA up to the level of the GDA and rely on flow through the GDA.

One major hurdle for widespread adoption of HAI chemotherapy is the need for a laparotomy for HAIP placement. The development of minimally invasive techniques for pump placement may overcome this barrier. Laparoscopic pump placement is feasible but technically challenging even in experienced hands and often results in conversion to laparotomy given the fine motion required for vascular dissection and precise placement of the catheter. The use of the robotic platform has the potential to overcome some of these issues with articulated wrist motion and elimination of fine tremor. In a single-center, early experience, Qadan et al. reported on 24 robotically placed HAIP and compared their outcomes to patients undergoing open pump placement by the same surgeon and laparoscopic placement by another single surgeon at the same institution. Technical outcomes and complications were comparable between the three groups, and the conversion to open surgery was lower in the robotic than the laparoscopic group (17% vs 67%) [14]. The authors conclude that robotic placement of HAIP is feasible and safe, and this report provides support for continued study and analysis of this minimally invasive approach.

Complications

The technical outcomes of HAIP placement were evaluated by Allen et al. [12]. The overall pump-related complication rate in this report was 22%. These were divided between early and late complications which had implications for the likelihood of HAIP salvage. Overall, in nearly half of all complications, the HAIP was salvaged, but early complications were more likely to be salvaged than late complications (30% vs 70%, respectively). Early complications were most commonly misperfusions that were correctable by angiographic or surgical intervention, while late complications were most commonly catheter dislodgement or occlusions, or arterial thrombosis for which effective interventions were not available. Overall, 12% of patients experienced a pump-related complication that deemed the pump not usable. In some cases, these occurred after the patient had received therapy. HAI chemotherapy was discontinued because of a pump-related complication in 9% of patients.

Biliary sclerosis (BS) is a well-documented late complication of HAI chemotherapy and deserves special mention. First described by Kemeny et al. in the 1980s, this complication is currently estimated to occur in approximately 5% of patients treated with FUDR and dexamethasone. It is more common in the adjuvant setting when a liver resection has been performed and is quite uncommon in the unresectable setting. The development of postoperative infectious complications, as well as the as the type and dose of intra-arterial chemotherapy, may contribute to the development of BS [15, 16]. Since it is adequately salvaged by stenting or dilation, this complication is not associated with worse oncologic outcomes. Biliary sclerosis is often suspected by sustained elevation of liver function tests, which underscores the importance of frequent close monitoring of laboratory values in these patients. It is critical that dose reduction algorithms are carefully followed during the administration of HAI chemotherapy. Of note, in several prospective studies, the addition of bevacizumab to systemic therapy and HAI FUDR resulted in unacceptable rates of biliary toxicity, and its use is thus not recommended in this setting [5].

Postoperative Assessment

Once the patient has recovered from surgery and before the initiation of chemotherapy, it is crucial to document adequate perfusion of the liver through the pump and rule out any extrahepatic perfusion. This is achieved by comparison of an intravenous technetium-99m sulfur colloid scan which defines the liver contour to the same scan obtained after injection of 99mTc-labeled macroaggregated albumin (MAA) through the bolus port of the pump. Incomplete hepatic perfusion or extrahepatic perfusion is readily identified with this method and should be investigated and corrected before initiation of pump therapy (Fig. 19.2) [17].

Hepatic Arterial Infusion Chemotherapy in the Adjuvant Setting

While complete resection of CRLM is associated with long-term survival and cure, at least two-thirds of patients experience disease recurrence during follow-up. The most common pattern of recurrence is liver-only disease (31%), followed by lung-only disease (27%). Approximately 30% of patients present with multiple sites of recurrence, and less commonly, patients recur in other

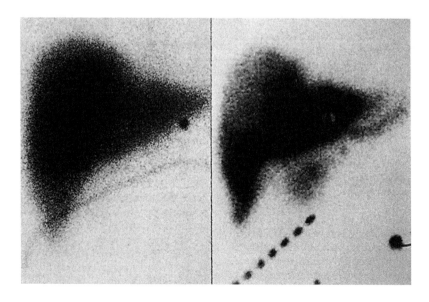

Fig. 19.2 The liver-spleen technetium-99m sulfur colloid scan on the left shows the normal liver. The macroaggregated albumin scan on the right shows extrahepatic perfusion to the duodenum and head of the pancreas. From Motaz Qadan; Nancy E. Kemeny in Blumgart's Surgery of the Liver, Biliary Tract, and Pancreas (Chapter 99—Regional Chemotherapy for Liver Tumors), with permission

single sites (12%). These various patterns of recurrence, as well as the timing at which they occur after resection, are associated with differing survival rates [18]. The high recurrence rates seen after resection highlight the need for effective adjuvant therapy in this setting.

Randomized prospective studies evaluating systemic chemotherapy regimens in this setting have failed to demonstrate improvement in overall survival. Mitry et al. pooled data from two prospective phase III trials in an attempt to evaluate the impact of adjuvant 5-fluorouracil chemotherapy on survival [19]. This study demonstrated marginal improvements in PFS (28 vs 19 months; P, 0.058) and overall survival (62 vs 47 months; P, 0.095) which did not reach statistical significance. In a large randomized controlled trial, Nordlinger et al. reported a marginal improvement of 7% in 3-year PFS for patients who received perioperative 5-FU + leucovorin + oxaliplatin (FOLFOX4) compared with surgery alone; this difference did not reach statistical significance [20]. Long-term follow-up of this cohort and assessment of overall survival revealed no difference at a median follow-up of 8.5 years. The estimated 5-year overall survival rates were 51% and 48% for patients treated with perioperative FOLFOX4 and surgery alone, respectively (P, 0.34) [21]. Furthermore, adjuvant modern chemotherapy regimens do not appear to improve survival as compared to standard regimens. In a randomized trial of adjuvant FOLFIRI versus 5FU, there was no difference in outcome [22]. In a trial comparing adjuvant chemotherapy with and without cetuximab, there was also no difference in outcomes [23].

Four randomized controlled trials have evaluated the impact of HAI chemotherapy after complete resection of hepatic arterial metastases; their outcomes are summarized in Table 19.1 [24–28]. In a multicenter study conducted in Germany, patients were randomized to resection alone vs resection + HAI with 5-FU + leucovorin. This trial was halted before complete accrual due to an interim analysis that determined futility. Hepatic disease-free survival and disease-free survival favored patients receiving HAI; however, the difference did not reach statistical significance. Notably, patients in this trial received 5-FU HAI which has a low hepatic extraction rate and lower efficacy compared with FUDR which is generally used in North American trials [26]. Lygidakis et al. reported on 122 patients that were randomized to receive mitomycin C, 5-FU, and interleukin-2 by both HAI and the systemic route versus systemic alone. This trial showed improved overall survival at 2 years (92% versus 75%) and 5 years (73% versus 60%) for the HAI + systemic group compared to the systemic-alone group. Similarly, DFS and hepatic DFS were significantly better for the combined treatment group [27]. The intergroup study (ECOG and Southwest Oncology Group) randomized patients with up to three resectable liver metastases and adequate

Table 19.1 Randomized controlled trials of adjuvant HAI chemotherapy for colorectal liver metastases

Author (year)		Hepatic disease-free survival				Disease-free survival				
		% 2-year		% 5-year		% 2-year		% 5-year		
	No. of patients	HAI	Control	HAI	Control	P value	HAI	Control	HAI	Control	P value
Lorenz (1998)[a] [26]	186	Median (mo)		43	27	NS	Median (mo)		20	12.6	NS
Lygidakis (2001) [27]	122	90	60	85	50	0.0001	66	48	60	35	0.0002
Kemeny (2002)[a] [24]	75	75	50	70	40[a]	0.0001	60	40	40	20[a]	0.03
Kemeny (2005) [25]	156	90	60	75	40	0.0001	55	45	40	30	0.02

Modified from Zervoudakis et al. [41]
HAI hepatic arterial infusion, *mo* months
[a]Control did not receive adjuvant systemic therapy

functional status to resection plus adjuvant HAI FUDR + systemic 5-FU + leucovorin versus resection alone. At 4 years, recurrence-free survival (46 vs 25%; P, 0.04) and liver recurrence-free survival rates (67 vs 43%; P, 0.03) were significantly improved for patients receiving HAI chemotherapy [24]. Lastly, in a single-institution randomized trial, Kemeny et al. randomized 156 patients with resected CRLM to treatment with systemic 5-FU + leucovorin vs systemic 5-FU + leucovorin + HAI with FUDR. Primary end points were overall survival and progression-free survival at 2 years. Patients in the HAI arm experienced better survival at the prespecified 2-year time point (86% vs 72%; P, 0.03). Furthermore, in a subsequent analysis at a median follow-up time of 10 years, overall PFS was significantly greater in the HAI group (31 vs 17 months; P, 0.02), as was hepatic RFS (not reached vs 32 months; $P < 0.01$). This trial also demonstrated a large difference in median overall survival that did not reach statistical significance (68 vs 59 months; P, 0.10) [25, 28].

One common argument cited against HAI chemotherapy is that the randomized studies that justify its use were largely performed in 1990s and thus did not included patients treated with "modern" systemic chemotherapy. The term "modern" chemotherapy refers to regimens including oxaliplatin and/or irinotecan (i.e., FOLFOX, FOLFIRI, etc.), which were introduced in the early 2000s. In this context it is important to recall that adjuvant FOLFOX and FOLFIRI were not proven to improve outcomes as compared to surgery alone and adjuvant 5-FU, respectively (see above) [21, 22]. The use of adjuvant HAI in combination with modern systemic chemotherapy has been studied at our institution in two early phase studies with favorable results [29, 30]. In a phase I/II study, 96 patients were treated with HAI FUDR/dexamethasone plus escalating doses of irinotecan in the adjuvant setting. The 2-year survival rate was 89% at a median follow-up of 26 months [30]. In a separate phase I trial, 35 patients were treated with HAI FUDR/dexamethasone with escalating doses of oxaliplatin and 5-FU. With a median follow-up of 43 months, the 4-year survival and progression-free survival were 88% and 50%, respectively [29]. While these studies were not designed to detect survival differences, they showed promising outcomes and adequate safety profile for combined HAI/FUDR and modern systemic chemotherapy. Recently, the long-term survival of all patients included in four consecutive adjuvant protocols of combined HAI and systemic chemotherapy between 1991 and 2009 was evaluated by Kemeny et al. [31]. Patients treated before 2003 had a median follow-up of 15 years; 5- and 10-year survivals of 56% and 40%, respectively; and median survival of 71 months. Patients treated after 2003 had a median follow-up of 9 years and 5- and 10-year survivals of 78% and 61%, respectively; median survival has not been reached in these patients.

Further evidence supporting the use of HAI chemotherapy after complete resection in patients with CRLM in the modern era is derived from large nonrandomized institutional series that evaluate long-term outcomes and factors associated with survival on these patients. In a retrospective analysis, House et al. analyzed patients who received HAI FUDR/dexamethasone and concurrent modern systemic therapy between 2000 and 2005 ($n = 125$) and compared their outcomes with the latest consecutive cohort of patients ($n = 125$) undergoing complete resection of CRLM and receiving only systemic chemotherapy including oxaliplatin or irinotecan [32]. The cohorts were well-balanced in terms of extent of disease and other known prognostic factors. At a median follow-up of 43 months, adjuvant HAI FUDR was associated with an improved overall and liver RFS, as well as DSS. The favorable effect of adjuvant HAI FUDR remained on multivariate analysis for all oncologic outcomes (liver RFS HR = 0.34; RFS HR = 0.65; DSS HR = 0.39; all $P < 0.01$) [32]. The largest institutional experience with HAI for CRLM was recently published by our group [33]. In this large study spanning 20 years, the impact of adjuvant HAI chemotherapy on overall survival was evaluated. This study included a propensity score analysis matching patients for known prognostic factors. A total of 2368 patients were included in this analysis (HAI $n = 785$; no HAI = 1583). At a median follow-up of 55 months, patients treated with HAI FUDR had a significantly better OS compared with patients without HAI treatment (67 vs 44 months; $P < 0.001$). This difference was nearly identical when only patients receiving modern systemic chemotherapy were analyzed ($n = 1442$ - 67 vs 47; $P < 0.001$). The propensity score (adjusting for sex, age, year of resection, presence of extrahepatic disease, number of treated tumors, size of largest resected tumor, and margin status) demonstrated longer OS with HAI, 0.67 (95% CI, 0.59–0.76; $P < 0.001$). Interestingly, a very pronounced difference in median OS was found for patients with node-negative colorectal cancer (129 vs 51 months; $P < 0.001$) and those with low clinical risk score (89 vs 53 months; $P < 0.001$). Altogether, these data provide strong evidence supporting the use of adjuvant HAI FUDR in patients with completely resected CRLM. It is clear that a randomized trial evaluating the role of adjuvant HAI/FUDR is justified.

HAI Chemotherapy in the Treatment of Unresectable Colorectal Liver Metastases

While complete resection is associated with favorable outcomes in CRLM, the majority of patients present with unresectable disease. In this setting, chemotherapy is administered aiming to achieve disease control and improved survival. Furthermore, a subgroup of these patients will have enough volumetric response to be converted to a resectable state. Patients who achieve complete resection after downstaging with chemotherapy are expected to have oncologic outcomes that mimic those of patients with extensive but resectable disease at presentation [34]. Conversion to resectability is thus an important goal of chemotherapy for patients with unresectable CRLM.

Historically, studies evaluating systemic chemotherapy report conversion to resection rates ranging between 12 and 60% [5, 34]. Such a wide range is explained by multiple different trial designs with highly variable inclusion criteria, definitions of resectability, and what needs to be achieved to become resectable. In fact, many trials do not explicitly provide such definitions. Furthermore, the true denominator of unresectable patients is often not reported, and there is heterogeneity in terms of previous treatment lines. In a systematic review of prospective studies published between 1998 and 2013, Jones et al. performed a pooled analysis of phase II and III trials of systemic chemotherapy for unresectable CRLM that reported RR and conversion to resectability [35]. A total of 25 studies were identified (15 single arm and 10 randomized trials). Only 20 studies explicitly defined criteria for resectability, and only 11 of these mentioned the involvement of a liver surgeon in this assessment. Furthermore, less than half (4/10) of the RCTs included resectability criteria upfront. Of note, they found that phase II trials were more likely to report high conversion rates (10–59%) than phase III trials (4–36%). Response rates in this systematic review ranged between 39 and 80% in single-arm studies and 33 and 76% in RCTs. For all included series, response rate demonstrated a strong correlation with rates of conversion to resectability ($R^2 = 0.44$, P, 0.008) [35].

We have published several trials of combination HAI + systemic therapy in the treatment of unresectable CRLM [5, 36, 37]. Most recently, a phase II prospective trial was specifically designed to evaluate conversion to resectability as the primary outcome measure. This study provided strict definitions of irresectability and what is needed to be achieved to be considered resectable which was determined by consensus between two experienced liver surgeons and a radiologist with experience in hepatobiliary imaging. The initial cohort included 49 patients with a median of 14 tumors. Two-thirds of patients were previously treated. Overall RR was 76% (86% for chemotherapy-naïve patients and 67% for previously treated patients), and 47% of patients achieved conversion to complete resection [5]. Conversion was the only factor associated with prolonged OS and PFS in multivariate analysis. This cohort was expanded, and the long-term outcomes were analyzed [38]. The expansion cohort included an additional 15 patients (total n,

64), of which 10 achieved conversion to resection for an overall rate of 52% (33/64). At a median follow-up among survivors of 81 months, median PFS and OS were 12 and 37 months; 5-year-OS in the entire cohort was 36%. At last follow-up, 21 patients were alive and 9 were free of disease. However, when only chemotherapy-naïve patients were analyzed, the 5-year-OS was 51%. Conversion to resection was the only independent factor prognostic of improved PFS and OS. Furthermore, in a recent analysis of patients refractory to at least three standard chemotherapy regimens (oxaliplatin, irinotecan, and 5-FU), HAI chemotherapy achieved an objective response rate of 33% in those with liver only and 36% in those with liver and low-volume extrahepatic disease [39].

A recent meta-analysis evaluated the impact of KRAS status and treatment with targeted monoclonal antibodies on response and conversion rates. In a pooled analysis of 13 randomized controlled trials included in that study, KRAS WT (wild type) and treatment with either bevacizumab or cetuximab were associated with RR and conversion in patients with unresectable CRLM [40]. In our recent experience, patients with KRAS WT tumors had improved RR compared to KRAS mutant (68 vs 56%; P, 0.009). However, mutational status was not associated with a difference in conversion to resection, PFS, HPFS, or 5-year OS (41 vs 35%; $P > 0.05$) [38]. This robust data support the use of HAI in selected patients who present with unresectable CRLM. Using this proactive treatment strategy combining HAI, systemic therapy, and aggressive resection, long-term survival (and potentially cure) can be achieved in this setting.

Conclusion

Hepatic arterial infusion chemotherapy in combination with systemic chemotherapy is an extensively studied treatment strategy for patients with colorectal cancer liver metastases. It is based on sound anatomical and pharmacological principles, and it has been proven to be safe. Over the last several decades, multiple studies have demonstrated improved oncologic outcomes in the adjuvant setting when compared to surgery alone or systemic therapy alone. Furthermore, in patients who present with unresectable disease, HAI achieves very high response rates (even as second or third line), and conversion to resection occurs roughly 50% of the time. These patients have outcomes that are comparable to those of patients who are resectable at presentation and have a true chance of cure.

References

1. Siegel RL, Miller KD, Jemal A. Cancer statistics, 2017. CA Cancer J Clin. 2017;67(1):7–30.
2. House MG, Ito H, Gonen M, Fong Y, Allen PJ, DeMatteo RP, et al. Survival after hepatic resection for metastatic colorectal cancer: trends in outcomes for 1,600 patients during two decades at a single institution. J Am Coll Surg. 2010;210(5):744–52, 52–5.
3. Sanoff HK, Sargent DJ, Campbell ME, Morton RF, Fuchs CS, Ramanathan RK, et al. Five-year data and prognostic factor analysis of oxaliplatin and irinotecan combinations for advanced colorectal cancer: N9741. J Clin Oncol. 2008;26(35):5721–7.
4. Kemeny NE, Niedzwiecki D, Hollis DR, Lenz HJ, Warren RS, Naughton MJ, et al. Hepatic arterial infusion versus systemic therapy for hepatic metastases from colorectal cancer: a randomized trial of efficacy, quality of life, and molecular markers (CALGB 9481). J Clin Oncol. 2006;24(9):1395–403.
5. D'Angelica MI, Correa-Gallego C, Paty PB, Cercek A, Gewirtz AN, Chou JF, et al. Phase II trial of hepatic artery infusional and systemic chemotherapy for patients with unresectable hepatic metastases from colorectal cancer: conversion to resection and long-term outcomes. Ann Surg. 2015;261(2):353–60.
6. Breedis C, Young G. The blood supply of neoplasms in the liver. Am J Pathol. 1954;30(5):969–77.
7. Ensminger WD, Gyves JW. Clinical pharmacology of hepatic arterial chemotherapy. Semin Oncol. 1983;10(2):176–82.
8. Ramming KP, Sparks FC, Eilber FR, Holmes EC, Morton DL. Hepatic artery ligation and 5-fluorouracil infusion for metastatic colon carcinoma and primary hepatoma. Am J Surg. 1976;132(2):236–42.
9. Daly JM, Kemeny N, Oderman P, Botet J. Long-term hepatic arterial infusion chemotherapy. Anatomic considerations, operative technique, and treatment morbidity. Arch Surg. 1984;119(8):936–41.
10. Kemeny N, Daly J, Oderman P, Shike M, Chun H, Petroni G, et al. Hepatic artery pump infusion: toxicity and results in patients with metastatic colorectal carcinoma. J Clin Oncol. 1984;2(6):595–600.
11. Allen PJ, Stojadinovic A, Ben-Porat L, Gonen M, Kooby D, Blumgart L, et al. The management of variant

arterial anatomy during hepatic arterial infusion pump placement. Ann Surg Oncol. 2002;9(9):875–80.
12. Allen PJ, Nissan A, Picon AI, Kemeny N, Dudrick P, Ben-Porat L, et al. Technical complications and durability of hepatic artery infusion pumps for unresectable colorectal liver metastases: an institutional experience of 544 consecutive cases. J Am Coll Surg. 2005;201(1):57–65.
13. Perez DR, Kemeny NE, Brown KT, Gewirtz AN, Paty PB, Jarnagin WR, et al. Angiographic identification of extrahepatic perfusion after hepatic arterial pump placement: implications for surgical prevention. HPB (Oxford). 2014;16(8):744–8.
14. Qadan M, D'Angelica MI, Kemeny NE, Cercek A, Kingham TP. Robotic hepatic arterial infusion pump placement. HPB (Oxford). 2017;19(5):429–35.
15. Ito K, Ito H, Kemeny NE, Gonen M, Allen PJ, Paty PB, et al. Biliary sclerosis after hepatic arterial infusion pump chemotherapy for patients with colorectal cancer liver metastasis: incidence, clinical features, and risk factors. Ann Surg Oncol. 2012;19(5):1609–17.
16. Kemeny MM, Battifora H, Blayney DW, Cecchi G, Goldberg DA, Leong LA, et al. Sclerosing cholangitis after continuous hepatic artery infusion of FUDR. Ann Surg. 1985;202(2):176–81.
17. Sofocleous CT, Schubert J, Kemeny N, Covey AM, Brody LA, Getrajdman GI, et al. Arterial embolization for salvage of hepatic artery infusion pumps. J Vasc Interv Radiol. 2006;17(5):801–6.
18. D'Angelica M, Kornprat P, Gonen M, DeMatteo RP, Fong Y, Blumgart LH, et al. Effect on outcome of recurrence patterns after hepatectomy for colorectal metastases. Ann Surg Oncol. 2011;18(4):1096–103.
19. Mitry E, Fields AL, Bleiberg H, Labianca R, Portier G, Tu D, et al. Adjuvant chemotherapy after potentially curative resection of metastases from colorectal cancer: a pooled analysis of two randomized trials. J Clin Oncol. 2008;26(30):4906–11.
20. Nordlinger B, Sorbye H, Glimelius B, Poston GJ, Schlag PM, Rougier P, et al. Perioperative chemotherapy with FOLFOX4 and surgery versus surgery alone for resectable liver metastases from colorectal cancer (EORTC Intergroup trial 40983): a randomised controlled trial. Lancet. 2008;371(9617):1007–16.
21. Nordlinger B, Sorbye H, Glimelius B, Poston GJ, Schlag PM, Rougier P, et al. Perioperative FOLFOX4 chemotherapy and surgery versus surgery alone for resectable liver metastases from colorectal cancer (EORTC 40983): long-term results of a randomised, controlled, phase 3 trial. Lancet Oncol. 2013;14(12):1208–15.
22. Ychou M, Hohenberger W, Thezenas S, Navarro M, Maurel J, Bokemeyer C, et al. A randomized phase III study comparing adjuvant 5-fluorouracil/folinic acid with FOLFIRI in patients following complete resection of liver metastases from colorectal cancer. Ann Oncol. 2009;20(12):1964–70.
23. Primrose J, Falk S, Finch-Jones M, Valle J, O'Reilly D, Siriwardena A, et al. Systemic chemotherapy with or without cetuximab in patients with resectable colorectal liver metastasis: the New EPOC randomised controlled trial. Lancet Oncol. 2014;15(6):601–11.
24. Kemeny MM, Adak S, Gray B, Macdonald JS, Smith T, Lipsitz S, et al. Combined-modality treatment for resectable metastatic colorectal carcinoma to the liver: surgical resection of hepatic metastases in combination with continuous infusion of chemotherapy—an intergroup study. J Clin Oncol. 2002;20(6):1499–505.
25. Kemeny NE, Gonen M. Hepatic arterial infusion after liver resection. N Engl J Med. 2005;352(7):734–5.
26. Lorenz M, Muller HH, Schramm H, Gassel HJ, Rau HG, Ridwelski K, et al. Randomized trial of surgery versus surgery followed by adjuvant hepatic arterial infusion with 5-fluorouracil and folinic acid for liver metastases of colorectal cancer. German Cooperative on Liver Metastases (Arbeitsgruppe Lebermetastasen). Ann Surg. 1998;228(6):756–62.
27. Lygidakis NJ, Sgourakis G, Vlachos L, Raptis S, Safioleas M, Boura P, et al. Metastatic liver disease of colorectal origin: the value of locoregional immunochemotherapy combined with systemic chemotherapy following liver resection. Results of a prospective randomized study. Hepatogastroenterology. 2001;48(42):1685–91.
28. Kemeny N, Huang Y, Cohen AM, Shi W, Conti JA, Brennan MF, et al. Hepatic arterial infusion of chemotherapy after resection of hepatic metastases from colorectal cancer. N Engl J Med. 1999;341(27):2039–48.
29. Kemeny N, Capanu M, D'Angelica M, Jarnagin W, Haviland D, Dematteo R, et al. Phase I trial of adjuvant hepatic arterial infusion (HAI) with floxuridine (FUDR) and dexamethasone plus systemic oxaliplatin, 5-fluorouracil and leucovorin in patients with resected liver metastases from colorectal cancer. Ann Oncol. 2009;20(7):1236–41.
30. Kemeny N, Jarnagin W, Gonen M, Stockman J, Blumgart L, Sperber D, et al. Phase I/II study of hepatic arterial therapy with floxuridine and dexamethasone in combination with intravenous irinotecan as adjuvant treatment after resection of hepatic metastases from colorectal cancer. J Clin Oncol. 2003;21(17):3303–9.
31. Kemeny NE, Chou JF, Boucher TM, Capanu M, DeMatteo RP, Jarnagin WR, et al. Updated long-term survival for patients with metastatic colorectal cancer treated with liver resection followed by hepatic arterial infusion and systemic chemotherapy. J Surg Oncol. 2016;113(5):477–84.
32. House MG, Kemeny NE, Gonen M, Fong Y, Allen PJ, Paty PB, et al. Comparison of adjuvant systemic chemotherapy with or without hepatic arterial infusional chemotherapy after hepatic resection for metastatic colorectal cancer. Ann Surg. 2011;254(6):851–6.
33. Groot Koerkamp B, Sadot E, Kemeny NE, Gonen M, Leal JN, Allen PJ, et al. Perioperative hepatic arterial infusion pump chemotherapy is associated with longer survival after resection of colorectal liver metastases: a propensity score analysis. J Clin Oncol. 2017;35(17):1938–44.

34. Adam R, Delvart V, Pascal G, Valeanu A, Castaing D, Azoulay D, et al. Rescue surgery for unresectable colorectal liver metastases downstaged by chemotherapy: a model to predict long-term survival. Ann Surg. 2004;240(4):644–57; discussion 57–8.
35. Jones RP, Hamann S, Malik HZ, Fenwick SW, Poston GJ, Folprecht G. Defined criteria for resectability improves rates of secondary resection after systemic therapy for liver limited metastatic colorectal cancer. Eur J Cancer. 2014;50(9):1590–601.
36. Kemeny N, Jarnagin W, Paty P, Gonen M, Schwartz L, Morse M, et al. Phase I trial of systemic oxaliplatin combination chemotherapy with hepatic arterial infusion in patients with unresectable liver metastases from colorectal cancer. J Clin Oncol. 2005;23(22):4888–96.
37. Kemeny NE, Melendez FD, Capanu M, Paty PB, Fong Y, Schwartz LH, et al. Conversion to resectability using hepatic artery infusion plus systemic chemotherapy for the treatment of unresectable liver metastases from colorectal carcinoma. J Clin Oncol. 2009;27(21):3465–71.
38. Ma LW, Kemeny NE, Capanu M, Chou J, Cercek A, Kingham TP, et al. Prospective phase II trial of combination hepatic artery and systemic chemotherapy for unresectable colorectal liver metastases: long-term results and curative potential. J Am Coll Surg. 2016;223(4):S78–S9.
39. Cercek A, Boucher TM, Gluskin JS, Aguilo A, Chou JF, Connell LC, et al. Response rates of hepatic arterial infusion pump therapy in patients with metastatic colorectal cancer liver metastases refractory to all standard chemotherapies. J Surg Oncol. 2016;114(6):655–63.
40. Wang L, Sun Y, Zhao B, Zhang H, Yu Q, Yuan X. Chemotherapy plus targeted drugs in conversion therapy for potentially resectable colorectal liver metastases: a meta-analysis. Oncotarget. 2016;7(34):55732–40.
41. Zervoudakis A, Boucher T, Kemeny NE. Treatment options in colorectal liver metastases: hepatic arterial infusion. Visc Med. 2017;33(1):47–53.

Patient Selection and Surgical Approach to Neuroendocrine Tumor Liver Metastases

20

Kendall J. Keck and James R. Howe

Introduction

Neuroendocrine tumors (NETs) are slow-growing neoplasms of the thymus, lungs, stomach, pancreas, small bowel, colon, and rectum that have been increasing in incidence, recently reported to affect 6.98 persons per 100,000 [1]. Many patients with these tumors will present with metastases at the time of diagnosis. For those diagnosed with gastroenteropancreatic NETs (GEPNETs), 50–60% of patients will be found to have metastases [2]. GEPNETs are the most common source of NETLMs, and up to 95% of distant metastases in GEPNET patients are found in the liver [3].

NETLMs may present as large solitary lesions, but most patients have diffuse, bilobar disease (Fig. 20.1). Frilling et al. divided 119 patients with NETLMs into three categories: (1) those with solitary metastases, which was made up 19% of their patients; (2) those with isolated bulky disease as well as smaller bilobar metastases, which was 15% of their cohort; and (3) patients with disseminated bilobar disease, which accounted for the majority (66%) [4]. This study provided insight into the type and extent of disease seen in NET patients and illustrates the important fact that a large proportion of patients have bilobar NETLMs. These findings were similar to those of Glazer et al. and Mayo et al., who reported bilobar disease in 84 of 172 (49%) and 183 of 309 (60%) of patients, respectively [5, 6]. The multiplicity of lesions and the generally long survival of these patients dictate that any surgical approach be carefully planned. Several options exist regarding the surgical resection of NETLMs, including major hepatectomies, segmentectomy, as well as the parenchymal-sparing procedures (PSPs) of wedge resection and enucleation. Ablative techniques are also effective for cytoreduction, which include radio-frequency ablation (RFA), microwave ablation, and irreversible electroporation. The goal of these interventions for NETLMs is to improve symptom control and survival, while minimizing morbidity. These procedures will often require the use of multiple, complimentary techniques. Studies have demonstrated that use of these strategies results in symptom improvement in up to 96% of patients [7] and 5-year survival rates ranging from 60 to 90% [6, 8–10]. These survival rates represent a substantial improvement over the 5-year survival noted for historical controls, which range from

K. J. Keck
Department of General Surgery, University of Iowa Hospitals and Clinics, Iowa City, IA, USA
e-mail: kendall-keck@uiowa.edu

J. R. Howe (✉)
Department of General Surgery, University of Iowa Hospitals and Clinics, Iowa City, IA, USA

University of Iowa College of Medicine, Iowa City, IA, USA
e-mail: james-howe@uiowa.edu

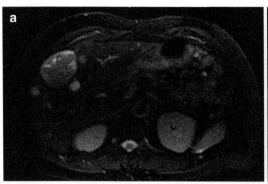 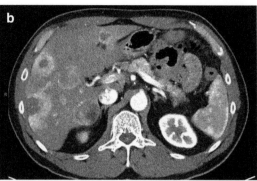

Fig. 20.1 (a) T2 MRI sequence in a 53 years old with over 20 SBNET metastases to the liver, with this single image showing 5 of these lesions. (b) CT with contrast showing multiple liver lesions in a patient with a metastatic SBNET diagnosed 5 years earlier, treated nonoperatively with somatostatin analogues, everolimus, and three hepatic embolizations 1.5 year earlier. Note the central necrosis of several lesions but peripheral enhancement, indicating viable tumors

10 to 51% for patients with metastatic NETs, depending on the primary site [2, 11, 12].

Patient Selection

As with any surgical procedure, surgical resection of NETLMs should only take place after careful patient evaluation, with the type and extent of surgical intervention tailored to each patient. Similar to surgical resection for other liver tumors, comorbidities such as cirrhosis, atherosclerotic disease, pulmonary disease, and functional status should be thoroughly assessed prior to any surgery. Liver function should also be assessed, and the guidelines used for patients undergoing resection for hepatocellular carcinoma provide a good framework for this evaluation, requiring patients to lack significant portal hypertension, be Child-Pugh class A or have a MELD <9, and have serum bilirubin <1 mg/dL [13]. Special attention should be given to patients who have previously undergone PRRT or hepatic artery embolization, and particularly radioembolization, to ensure that they have not developed cirrhosis or liver dysfunction secondary to these therapies.

In 2014, the working group on neuroendocrine tumor liver metastases utilized the available data to develop criteria that should be met in order for patients to be considered for NETLM resection, in addition to the more general functional assessments mentioned above. They recommended that patients selected for NETLM resection meet the following five criteria: (1) WHO tumor grade of 1 or 2, (2) absence of unresectable extrahepatic disease, (3) type 1 or 2 NETLMs amenable to R0 or R1 resection while maintaining a viable liver remnant of >30%, (4) no advanced carcinoid heart disease, (5) and that resections should be carried out at tertiary referral centers [14]. This collaborative only considered the evidence with regard to formal hepatic resections and did not specifically consider PSPs or ablation. Thus, while these recommendations provide a good basis for judging patient suitability for resection, failure to meet all of these criteria is not an absolute contraindication to resection.

Aside from the above criteria, other studies have indicated that the percent of liver replacement, number of NETLMs, size of NETLMs, and number of NETLMs treated affect prognosis, and these factors should also be considered. A 2003 study by Elias et al. of 47 patients who underwent hepatic resection for NETLMs showed a trend toward increased survival when the percent of liver replacement was <25%, with 5-year survival rates of 68% for <25% replacement and 40% for >25% replacement ($p = 0.10$) [15]. Maxwell et al. expanded on this finding and demonstrated that having more than five or ten lesions preoperatively as well as liver replacement >25% (as determined by radiologic assessment) was both significantly associated with worse prognosis. Their study included 108 patients with GEPNETs who underwent resection of NETLMs utilizing primarily PSPs [9]. Touzios et al. found similar results in 60 patients with NETLMs. Using a liver replacement cutoff of 50%, they noted that patients with greater than 50% replacement had a 5-year survival of 8%, versus 67% for those patients with <50% replacement [16]. In a larger study, Ruzzenente and colleagues reviewed 133 patients undergoing NETLM resection and found that the number of NETLMs, grade as determined by Ki-67%, and NETLM size <3 cm were all independently associated with survival, and they used these parameters to construct a nomogram to predict prognosis [17]. Frilling et al. excluded patients with >70% liver replacement from resection, while Chamberlain et al. reported very poor prognoses for the subset of their 85 patients who had >75% replacement and noted that they rarely performed surgical resections on these individuals [4, 18]. Thus, patients with >25–50% replacement generally will have a worse prognosis, and those with greater than 50–75% liver replacement need to be even more carefully assessed and potentially not be offered surgery due to the increased risk of severe liver dysfunction and/or death after resection.

Summarizing this information, patients selected to undergo NETLM resection should be good surgical candidates (ECOG performance status of 0 or 1) with low-grade lesions (G1 or G2), lack signs of liver dysfunction, have >30% uninvolved remnant liver parenchyma, and a tumor distribution amenable to significant cytoreduction. Other patient factors to be considered preoperatively should be the number of tumors to be treated, their distribution, amenability to significant cytoreduction (70–90%), and the total percentage of hepatic replacement. Once a patient is deemed to be a surgical candidate, then the surgeon must plan the extent and type of cytoreduction to be performed.

Extent of Resection

Unlike many other malignancies, the inability to completely remove all liver metastases is not a contraindication to resection in NET patients. Several studies have shown that complete resection of NETLMs does not confer a survival benefit over incomplete resection [5, 6, 9, 15, 19]. In a study of 172 patients undergoing operations for NETLMs, Glazer et al. noted no significant difference in survival between patients who had an R0 resection when compared to patients with R1/R2 resections [5]. This was confirmed by Graff-Baker et al., who noted similar survival rates in 52 patients and statistically similar rates of liver progression between those having R0 resections and those having R2 resections [8]. A large, multi-institutional study of 339 patients came to the same conclusion, where they found that patients with nonfunctional tumors who underwent R2 resections had a similar survival as patients undergoing R0/R1 resections ($p = 0.64$) [6]. Since R1/R2 resections give comparable rates of liver progression and survival, another important question is how much cytoreduction is needed to provide a survival benefit for patients.

The first mention of a threshold for adequate debulking of NETLMs was introduced by McEntee et al. in 1990, where in 37 patients, they observed that those with <90% debulking were less likely to have symptom improvement [20]. This was in a time prior to the common use of somatostatin analogues, and they were unable to identify any factors (including debulking threshold) associated with survival, and these resections were performed for symptom relief only. Subsequent studies from the Mayo Clinic used this 90% threshold for patient selection, including publications by Que et al. in 1995 ($n = 74$) and Sarmiento et al. in 2003 ($n = 170$) [7, 19]. Que et al. noted that there was no survival benefit for R0 resections but suggested that there was an overall survival benefit with resection, while Sarmiento et al. found an improved 5-year survival of 60% relative to historical controls using the same strategy. The Sarmiento study was one of the first studies to include asymptomatic patients, and the increase in survival reported was statistically similar for both those with and without symptoms.

One of the issues with utilizing a threshold for cytoreduction that requires 90% of the metastases to be amenable to resection is that 67–90% of patients will not be considered for a debulking procedure [18]. Subsequently, several centers have published results showing improved 5-year survival for NET patients undergoing liver resection without using any specific threshold for debulking [6, 21–24]. Therefore, this previously held threshold of 90% has been called into question, and it is possible that lower levels of cytoreduction may still provide benefit. One of the first studies that sought to address the use of a decreased debulking threshold was Graff-Baker et al., who found similar recurrence rates in patients having cytoreduction percentages of 70–90%, 90–99%, and 100%, using primarily PSPs. They reported 5-year disease-specific survival of 90% in their 52 patients, with no differences between these three levels of cytoreduction [8]. The 70% threshold was more thoroughly examined by Maxwell et al. in their analysis of 108 patients undergoing NETLM resection whose extent of cytoreduction ranged from <50 to 100%. Utilizing primarily PSPs, they demonstrated that patients who had >70% of their NETLMs debulked (64% of all patients) had significantly improved progression-free survival (PFS, median 3.2 vs. 1.3 years; $p < 0.01$) and overall survival (OS, median not reached vs. 6.5 years; $p < 0.01$) versus those with <70% cytoreduction. Those with >90% cytoreduction (39% of patients) had a PFS of 4.4 years vs. 1.3 years for those with <90% ($p = 0.05$), but the OS difference was not significant (not reached vs. 6.1 years; $p = 0.14$). Lowering of the cytoreduction threshold allowed 102 of 142 patients (76%) to undergo debulking procedures in this study [9]. Therefore, if one believes that cytoreduction prolongs survival in patients with NETLMs, then reducing the target for cytoreduction from 90 to >70% will increase the number of patients who might benefit from these procedures.

In this pursuit of improved survival, it is important to recognize that many patients with NETLMs can have relatively long survival on medical therapy and minimizing morbidity and mortality is paramount in these patients. One also needs to recognize that recurrence rates are extremely high, 94% at 5 years in the report of Mayo et al. [6], and therefore these procedures are not curative. Proper patient selection and minimization of operative risk are very important in providing benefit to patients with NETLMs.

Anatomic Liver Resections

In order to achieve the 90% resection threshold that was believed to be necessary for NETLM management, many surgeons performed large resections such as hemihepatectomies in their attempt to accomplish adequate cytoreduction. While formal hepatic resections can be performed laparoscopically by some, most surgeons prefer an open approach given the extent of disease in most patients. The open approach is preferred in order to gain better access to all tumors, as well as to allow for concurrent resection of the primary tumor(s) and nodal metastases (Fig. 20.2). Use of formal hepatic resections in the treatment of NETLMs can result in high levels of debulking, but it also often results in higher rates of complications and/or mortality.

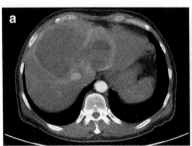
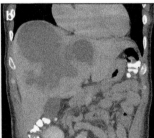
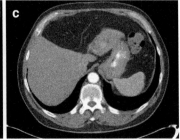

Fig. 20.2 (a) Transverse view of central liver lesion in a patient with NET of unknown primary. (b) Coronal view of the central liver lesion. (c) Transverse CT 30 months postcentral liver resection with no evidence of liver recurrence. The patient was found to have a small bowel primary at exploration, which was removed at the time of liver resection

In their retrospective review of 47 patients undergoing formal hepatic resection for NETLMs, in which they found no survival difference based on resection status (R0 vs. R1 vs. R2), Elias et al. reported a complication rate of 45% and a 5% mortality rate [15]. They also demonstrated an improved 5-year overall survival of 71%. This was in a group of patients where 31 of 47 (66%) of patients underwent resection of >3 segments, while the remainder underwent resection of 3 or fewer segments, and 5 of 47 (11%) patients also had RFA performed. These complication and mortality rates were concerning, raising the question of whether less extensive, parenchymal-sparing techniques could also provide benefit.

In Sarmiento and colleagues larger cohort of 170 patients, 91 (54%) underwent resection of 4 or more segments, and the remainder had resections of <4 segments or underwent wedge resection [7]. They were able to demonstrate symptom control in 96% of their patients and a 5-year overall survival rate of 61%. The complication rate in this series was 21.1%, and the mortality was 1.2%. They also found that despite these large resections, the majority of patients (143 of 170; 84%) had disease recurrence within 5 years. In the multi-institutional series of Mayo et al., the mortality rate was 0.4% for patients with functional tumors and 1.1% for patients with nonfunctional tumors [6]. While the majority (329 of 339; 97%) had resection of 2 or more liver segments, 66 (19%) of those patients also had ablation performed, and 10 patients (3%) had ablation only. The 5-year PFS for all patients was 5.9%, while the PFS for those patients only having ablation was 4.5%. The high rate of recurrence and the preservation of survival benefit with R1 and R2 resections invited the question of whether extensive resections are necessary and whether PSPs, including ablation, may be equally effective. In order to address this question, several studies sought to determine the efficacy of PSPs.

Parenchymal-Sparing Procedures

Parenchymal-sparing procedures provide a means of cytoreduction that address the liver lesions while preserving normal liver. Since most patients with metastatic disease will die of liver failure, it makes sense to try and preserve as much normal liver as possible. Since the distribution of lesions in most patients is bilobar and multifocal, one often needs to combine several techniques in the treatment of patients with NETLMs, including PSPs, which include wedge resection, enucleation, and ablation. Similar to formal liver resections, laparoscopic approaches can be performed, but the majority of cases are done in an open fashion because of the presence of multiple of lesions and concurrent resection of the primary tumor.

Wedge Resection

Wedge resections utilize nonanatomic margins in order to resect tumors, with the advantage being that just the lesion and a small amount of normal liver are resected. The borders of resection are commonly marked on the liver capsule using electrocautery, and dissection is carried out using any number of devices, such as Aquamantys, Cavitron Ultrasonic Surgical Aspirator (CUSA), water dissection, and other methods to reduce blood loss (Fig. 20.3).

In a study of 52 patients undergoing resection of NETLMs, Graff-Baker et al. described the efficacy of wedge resection [8]. They utilized the technique in 51 of 52 (98%) patients in their study with 15 of those 51 patients also undergoing an anatomic hepatic resection. They found that they could achieve 90% disease-specific survival at 5 years with the type of resection having no effect on survival and younger age being the only factor independently associated with worse survival. Another technique, which removes even less normal liver parenchyma and can also be applied to individual lesions, especially those near the surface of the liver, is enucleation.

Enucleation

Enucleation is a useful method for NETLM removal due to the fact that most tumors are firm

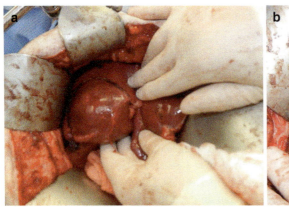
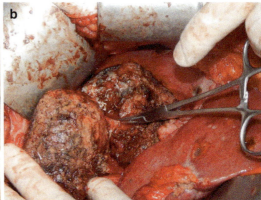

Fig. 20.3 (a) Wedge resection of liver lesion; scoring of the liver capsule around the lesion. This is the larger lesion seen on the MRI in Fig. 20.1a. (b) Final stage of excision with ligation of a hepatic vein branch after dissection of liver tissue with Aquamantys device

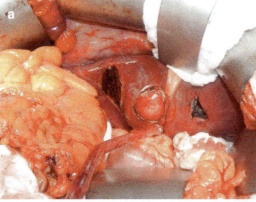
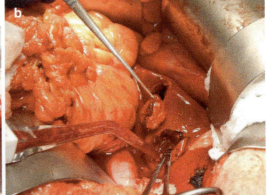

Fig. 20.4 (a) Surface NETLM amenable to enucleation. The liver capsule around the lesion has been scored with electrocautery. The gallbladder fossa after cholecystectomy is at the left, and a previous enucleation site is seen on the right. (b) NETLM completely enucleated. Note the white edge of the tumor and color (and texture) difference relative to the normal liver parenchyma

and push normal liver tissue away rather than infiltrate the adjacent liver. This allows one to remove these lesions at the tumor-liver interface with minimal normal liver tissue resected. With this technique, recurrence of NETLMs is rare even though the resection margins are always positive. This method is most readily accomplished in tumors located on or near the liver surface. Enucleation is usually performed using cautery to essentially carve out lesions at the edge of the lesion-liver junction with hemostasis being achieved by argon beam and/or sutures (Fig. 20.4).

A 2016 study by Maxwell et al. presented their results in 80 small bowel and 28 pancreatic NET patients undergoing treatment of NETLMs, with the majority undergoing wedge resection, enucleation, and/or ablation (97 of 108; 90%) [9]. They also included radio-frequency or microwave ablation in their parenchymal-sparing approaches, with 70 of the 97 patients also having some ablative technique used. They were able to demonstrate increased median progression-free (3.2 years) and overall survival (not reached) for patients undergoing >70% cytoreduction. This study reported a major complication rate of only 13%, which was lower than the complication rates of 21, 23, and 26% previously described by Sarmiento, Landry, and Chambers, respectively [7, 9, 22, 23]. This study showed that PSPs could be done with good results in terms of survival and postoperative complication rates, which are generally higher for major resections. Furthermore, there were no mortalities reported in the Maxwell, Landry, or Chambers studies, which are important for patients with NETs, as they can still live a long time even without intervention.

Ablative Techniques

Radio-frequency ablation (RFA) utilizes alternating current passed through a probe to create heat. This heat is produced at the edges of the tines of the probe. The probe is inserted into the center of the tumors and the tines gradually advanced outward as the target temperature is reached. The goal is to induce cell death and coagulative necrosis within the tumor while sparing the surrounding normal parenchyma. This technique is commonly used as an adjunct to other techniques and can be used to treat multiple lesions throughout the liver. It is vulnerable to the heat-sink effect, where the edge of tumors along the major blood vessels remains cooler than the rest of the tumor and may not achieve the temperature required for inducing cell death.

Akyildiz et al. investigated the long-term outcomes for the use of RFA in the treatment of NETLMs, which they performed laparoscopically in a cohort of 89 patients [25]. The majority of patients (65 of 89; 73%) underwent a single RFA treatment, while 19 patients (21%) underwent 2 RFA treatments, 4 underwent 3 treatments, and 1 patient underwent 4 RFA procedures. They were able to improve symptoms in 97% of these patients having RFA, which is similar to studies of surgical resection. The 5-year overall survival after the first RFA procedure was 57%, and the complication rate was 5.6%, with one mortality. Roughly 60% of these patients demonstrated new hepatic lesions or extrahepatic disease during follow-up, and the 5-year recurrence rate was 84%, which the authors argue and demonstrate the need for extrahepatic disease control.

Fairweather and colleagues performed a retrospective review of 649 patients with NETLM, of whom 58 underwent NETLM resection and 28 underwent RFA. They found that while the 5-year overall survival for patients undergoing RFA (84%) was better than that for patients who underwent chemoembolization (55%, $n = 130$) and systemic therapy (58%, $n = 316$), it still fell short of the 5-year survival for those patients who underwent surgical resection (90%, $p < 0.001$) [10]. These findings, along with observations of Akyildiz, indicate that while RFA may improve survival, it may have the most impact when used in conjunction with surgical resections as reported in other studies. A summary of the studies and their use of ablative techniques and resections can be found in Table 20.1.

Ablation can also be performed utilizing probes that generate microwaves (Fig. 20.5). Microwave ablation (MWA) functions similar to RFA in that it creates heat, which in turn destroys tumor cells. Although both methods induce thermal destruction, MWA has several advantages over RFA, including increased intratumoral temperatures, faster ablation time, and decreased heat-sink effect [26]. Groeschl et al. reported a multi-institutional experience of 473 MWA procedures, of which 61 were for NETLMs. In the subset of patients with NETLMs, there was a local recurrence rate of 3%, a median recurrence-free survival of 33 months, and a median OS of 92 months [27]. For most surgeons, the decreased ablation time, reduction of heat-sink effect, and effectiveness of therapy have made MWA the preferred ablative therapy for NETLMs at this time.

Irreversible electroporation (IRE) is a more recently developed method of ablation. This technique utilizes high-voltage electrical fields in order to induce cell membrane damage in the tumor cell and subsequent cell death. This is performed using a single needle (bipolar electrode) or multiple (at least two) unipolar electrode needles. The advantage of this technique is the ability to treat tumors adjacent to blood vessels or

Table 20.1 Summary of studies addressing the surgical management of NETLMs [5–10, 15, 21–25, 35–40]

	N	Surgical procedures	Survival	Postoperative morbidity*	Postoperative mortality
Elias, 2003	47	Minor resection: 34% Major resection: 66% Ablation: 10.6%	5-year OS: 71%	Major and minor: 45%	5%
Sarmiento, 2003	170	Major resection: 54%	5-year OS: 61%	Major and minor: 21.1%	1.2%
Boudreaux, 2005	82	Resection +/− ablation: 100%	*4-year OS*: No NETLM or unilateral disease: 89% Bilobar hepatic disease: 52%	Major and minor: 56%	2.4%
Osborne, 2006	Surgical: 61 Embolization: 59	NR	*Median survival*: Curative: 50 months Palliative: 3 months Embolization: 24 months	Surgical: 3.3%	Surgical: 1.7%
Hibi, 2007	21	Resection: 100%	5-year OS: 41%	Major only: 19%	0%
Landry, 2008	Surgical: 23 Nonsurgical: 31	Major resection: 70% Wedge resection: 17% Major + wedge: 13% Ablation: 17%	*5-year OS*: Surgery: 75% No surgery: 62%	Major only: 26%	0%
Chambers, 2008	Surgical: 30 Nonsurgical: 33	Major resection: 23% Wedge resection: 57% Ablation: 53%	5-year OS: 74%	Major only: 23%	0%
Elias, 2009	16	Major resection: 56% Minor resection: 44% Ablation: 100%	3-year OS: 84%	Major only: 47%	0%
Glazer, 2010	172	Resection: 73.3% Ablation alone: 10.5%	5-year OS: 77.4%	Major and minor: 22.1%	0%
Akyildiz, 2010	89	1 Ablative procedure: 73% 2 Ablative procedures: 21% 3 Ablative procedures: 4.5% 4 Ablative procedures: 1.1%	5-year OS: 57% (after 1st procedure)	5.6%	1.1%
Mayo, 2010	339	Resection: 77.6% Ablation: 2.9% Resection + ablation: 19.5%	*Median OS* 1st operation: 125 months 2nd operation: 141 months from 1st operation 89 months from 2nd operation	NR	NR
Norlen, 2012	162	Resection: 35.2% Ablation: 42%	*5-year OS*: Resection: 86% RFA: 94% No debulking: 53%	Major only: 1.9%	Resection: 1.8% Ablation: 2.9%
Taner, 2013	94	Minor resection: 81% Major resection: 19% Ablation: 100%	5-year OS: 80%	Local complication in 1 patient	0%
Boudreaux, 2014	189	Resection: 72% Ablation: 31%	5-year OS: 87%	Major only: 13%	7%

Table 20.1 (continued)

	N	Surgical procedures	Survival	Postoperative morbidity*	Postoperative mortality
Graff-Baker, 2014	52	Formal resection: 31% Wedge resection: 98%	5-year PFS: 64%	NR	NR
Maxwell, 2016	108	PSP only: 95% PSP + major resection: 4% Major only: 1%	5-year OS: 72%	Major only: 13%	0%
Fairweather, 2017	86	Resection: 67% Ablation: 33%	5-year OS: Resection: 90% RFA: 84%	NR	NR

*The calculation of the morbidity rate was calculated as the total number of complications divided by the total number of patients. Major morbidity included complications that would fall into the Level III and IV classifications in the Clavien-Dindo classification system

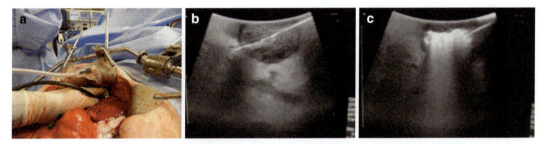

Fig. 20.5 (**a**) Microwave ablation device within a needle guide attached to an intraoperative ultrasound probe. (**b**) Microwave ablation probe traversing the NETLM; yellow dotted lines indicate different potential paths within the ultrasound needle guide. (**c**) Microwave ablation proceeding at 100 W after 1 min. Note that white (hyperechoic) area reflects boiling within the ablation zone

major bile ducts with less risk of injury. Implementation has been limited by the high initial cost of equipment, cardiac side effects (arrhythmias), and the inability to treat larger tumors. Early results of IRE treatment of several types of liver metastases in 44 patients (including 3 NETLMs) reported by Cannon et al. demonstrated a 12-month local recurrence-free survival (LRFS) of 59.5% and trend toward higher recurrence with tumors >4 cm and use of a percutaneous approach [28]. Niessen et al. published a series of 65 tumors (3 NETLMs) treated with IRE and demonstrated an increased 12-month LRFS of 75% [29]. Of note, Niessen excluded those patients with resectable tumors, multifocal hepatic lesions, and cardiac disease. Niessen et al. performed all IRE treatments percutaneously, while Cannon and colleagues performed 76% of their cases percutaneously. This is in contrast to the studies of the other ablative modalities where the majority of procedures were performed in an open fashion with a small proportion performed laparoscopically. Percutaneous approaches are possible with all of the mentioned ablative techniques, but given that most patients with NETLMs have multiple lesions and possibly synchronous primary tumors, open approaches are usually preferred (or laparoscopic in selected cases). Percutaneous ablative techniques are discussed in more detail in a subsequent chapter.

Liver Transplantation

In patients with diffuse hepatic disease who are not candidates for effective surgical cytoreduction, there remains another option: liver transplantation. The Milan criteria and ENETs guidelines provide a framework for the selection of NETLM patients for liver transplantation.

These require that patients are <55 years old, have had their primary tumor removed, have no extrahepatic disease on advanced imaging (DOTATOC/DOTATATE, SPECT/CT-SRS, PET/CT), have Ki-67 <10% (ENETS), have <50% liver involvement (Milan), and have had stable disease for 6 months [30, 31].

In 2015 Fan et al. performed a review of the available studies reporting results of liver transplantation for NETLMs. They identified a total of 706 patients, 514 of which came from 3 large series. These studies combined demonstrated a 5-year disease-free survival rate of 30% and overall survival of 50% [32]. Mazzaferro et al. sought to determine if there was a survival advantage in 88 consecutive patients who were candidates for transplant as determined by the Milan criteria [33]. A total of 42 patients underwent transplant, while the other 46 were treated with other modalities. After propensity matching patients in both groups, they identified that patients undergoing transplant had significantly better survival and that the transplant-related survival benefits at 5 and 10 years were 6.82 and 38.4 months, respectively. They found a 5-year survival rate of 97.2% for transplanted patients versus 50.9% for non-transplanted patients. Norlen et al. examined their patients under 65 who had small bowel primary tumors and NETLMs and who underwent multimodality treatment ($n = 78$) and observed that those patients who met the Milan criteria ($n = 33$) had a 5-year OS of 97%, which is similar or better than the survival for patients undergoing liver transplant [34]. Thus, the use of liver transplantation for patients with NETLMs is an option, but allocation of organs to a population of patients who have long survival with other treatments and the possibility that immunosuppression will activate occult extrahepatic disease are factors which have limited its use.

Conclusion

Patients with NETs often present with NETLMs upon initial evaluation. Resection of NETLMs in appropriately selected patients (those who do not have high-grade tumors, extensively replaced livers, or severe comorbidities) results in improved symptoms and prolonged survival in the majority of patients. The required extent of resection to provide benefit is still a matter of debate, but recent studies suggest that at least 70% cytoreduction should be performed in order to achieve a survival advantage. This can be achieved by formal anatomic hepatic resections or parenchymal-sparing procedures such as wedge resection, enucleation, and ablations. Parenchymal-sparing procedures should be considered when possible given the decreased risk of these procedures, preservation of normal liver parenchyma, and nearly universal recurrence rates regardless of the method used for cytoreduction. Liver transplantation is an option for a small subset of patients with low-grade tumors and diffuse hepatic disease who are not otherwise candidates for resection and who meet several very specific criteria.

References

1. Dasari A, Shen C, Halperin D, Zhao B, Zhou S, Xu Y, et al. Trends in the incidence, prevalence, and survival outcomes in patients with neuroendocrine tumors in the United States. JAMA Oncol. 2017;3(10):1335–42.
2. Yao JC, Hassan M, Phan A, Dagohoy C, Leary C, Mares JE, et al. One hundred years after "carcinoid": epidemiology of and prognostic factors for neuroendocrine tumors in 35,825 cases in the United States. J Clin Oncol. 2008;26(18):3063–72.
3. Pape UF, Berndt U, Muller-Nordhorn J, Bohmig M, Roll S, Koch M, et al. Prognostic factors of long-term outcome in gastroenteropancreatic neuroendocrine tumours. Endocr Relat Cancer. 2008;15(4):1083–97.
4. Frilling A, Li J, Malamutmann E, Schmid KW, Bockisch A, Broelsch CE. Treatment of liver metastases from neuroendocrine tumours in relation to the extent of hepatic disease. Br J Surg. 2009;96(2):175–84.
5. Glazer ES, Tseng JF, Al-Refaie W, Solorzano CC, Liu P, Willborn KA, et al. Long-term survival after surgical management of neuroendocrine hepatic metastases. HPB (Oxford). 2010;12(6):427–33.
6. Mayo SC, de Jong MC, Pulitano C, Clary BM, Reddy SK, Gamblin TC, et al. Surgical management of hepatic neuroendocrine tumor metastasis: results from an international multi-institutional analysis. Ann Surg Oncol. 2010;17(12):3129–36.
7. Sarmiento JM, Heywood G, Rubin J, Ilstrup DM, Nagorney DM, Que FG. Surgical treatment of neuroendocrine metastases to the liver: a plea for

resection to increase survival. J Am Coll Surg. 2003;197(1):29–37.
8. Graff-Baker AN, Sauer DA, Pommier SJ, Pommier RF. Expanded criteria for carcinoid liver debulking: maintaining survival and increasing the number of eligible patients. Surgery. 2014;156(6):1369–76; discussion 76-7.
9. Maxwell JE, Sherman SK, O'Dorisio TM, Bellizzi AM, Howe JR. Liver-directed surgery of neuroendocrine metastases: what is the optimal strategy? Surgery. 2016;159(1):320–35.
10. Fairweather M, Swanson R, Wang J, Brais LK, Dutton T, Kulke MH, et al. Management of neuroendocrine tumor liver metastases: long-term outcomes and prognostic factors from a large prospective database. Ann Surg Oncol. 2017;24(8):2319–25.
11. Maggard MA, O'Connell JB, Ko CY. Updated population-based review of carcinoid tumors. Ann Surg. 2004;240(1):117–22.
12. Modlin IM, Sandor A. An analysis of 8305 cases of carcinoid tumors. Cancer. 1997;79(4):813–29.
13. Ribero D, Curley SA, Imamura H, Madoff DC, Nagorney DM, Ng KK, et al. Selection for resection of hepatocellular carcinoma and surgical strategy: indications for resection, evaluation of liver function, portal vein embolization, and resection. Ann Surg Oncol. 2008;15(4):986–92.
14. Frilling A, Modlin IM, Kidd M, Russell C, Breitenstein S, Salem R, et al. Recommendations for management of patients with neuroendocrine liver metastases. Lancet Oncol. 2014;15(1):e8–21.
15. Elias D, Lasser P, Ducreux M, Duvillard P, Ouellet JF, Dromain C, et al. Liver resection (and associated extrahepatic resections) for metastatic well-differentiated endocrine tumors: a 15-year single center prospective study. Surgery. 2003;133(4):375–82.
16. Touzios JG, Kiely JM, Pitt SC, Rilling WS, Quebbeman EJ, Wilson SD, et al. Neuroendocrine hepatic metastases: does aggressive management improve survival? Ann Surg. 2005;241(5):776–83; discussion 83–5.
17. Ruzzenente A, Bagante F, Bertuzzo F, Aldrighetti L, Ercolani G, Giuliante F, et al. A novel nomogram to predict the prognosis of patients undergoing liver resection for neuroendocrine liver metastasis: an analysis of the Italian neuroendocrine liver metastasis database. J Gastrointest Surg. 2017;21(1):41–8.
18. Chamberlain RS, Canes D, Brown KT, Saltz L, Jarnagin W, Fong Y, et al. Hepatic neuroendocrine metastases: does intervention alter outcomes? J Am Coll Surg. 2000;190(4):432–45.
19. Que FG, Nagorney DM, Batts KP, Linz LJ, Kvols LK. Hepatic resection for metastatic neuroendocrine carcinomas. Am J Surg. 1995;169(1):36–42; discussion 42–3.
20. McEntee GP, Nagorney DM, Kvols LK, Moertel CG, Grant CS. Cytoreductive hepatic surgery for neuroendocrine tumors. Surgery. 1990;108(6):1091–6.
21. Boudreaux JP, Wang YZ, Diebold AE, Frey DJ, Anthony L, Uhlhorn AP, et al. A single institution's experience with surgical cytoreduction of stage IV, well-differentiated, small bowel neuroendocrine tumors. J Am Coll Surg. 2014;218(4):837–44.
22. Chambers AJ, Pasieka JL, Dixon E, Rorstad O. The palliative benefit of aggressive surgical intervention for both hepatic and mesenteric metastases from neuroendocrine tumors. Surgery. 2008;144(4):645–51; discussion 51–3.
23. Landry CS, Scoggins CR, McMasters KM, Martin RC II. Management of hepatic metastasis of gastrointestinal carcinoid tumors. J Surg Oncol. 2008;97(3):253–8.
24. Norlen O, Stalberg P, Zedenius J, Hellman P. Outcome after resection and radiofrequency ablation of liver metastases from small intestinal neuroendocrine tumours. Br J Surg. 2013;100(11):1505–14.
25. Akyildiz HY, Mitchell J, Milas M, Siperstein A, Berber E. Laparoscopic radiofrequency thermal ablation of neuroendocrine hepatic metastases: long-term follow-up. Surgery. 2010;148(6):1288–93; discussion 93.
26. Simon CJ, Dupuy DE, Mayo-Smith WW. Microwave ablation: principles and applications. Radiographics. 2005;25(Suppl 1):S69–83.
27. Groeschl RT, Pilgrim CH, Hanna EM, Simo KA, Swan RZ, Sindram D, et al. Microwave ablation for hepatic malignancies: a multiinstitutional analysis. Ann Surg. 2014;259(6):1195–200.
28. Cannon R, Ellis S, Hayes D, Narayanan G, Martin RC II. Safety and early efficacy of irreversible electroporation for hepatic tumors in proximity to vital structures. J Surg Oncol. 2013;107(5):544–9.
29. Niessen C, Beyer LP, Pregler B, Dollinger M, Trabold B, Schlitt HJ, et al. Percutaneous ablation of hepatic tumors using irreversible electroporation: a prospective safety and midterm efficacy study in 34 patients. J Vasc Interv Radiol. 2016;27(4):480–6.
30. Pavel M, Baudin E, Couvelard A, Krenning E, Oberg K, Steinmuller T, et al. ENETS Consensus Guidelines for the management of patients with liver and other distant metastases from neuroendocrine neoplasms of foregut, midgut, hindgut, and unknown primary. Neuroendocrinology. 2012;95(2):157–76.
31. Mazzaferro V, Pulvirenti A, Coppa J. Neuroendocrine tumors metastatic to the liver: how to select patients for liver transplantation? J Hepatol. 2007;47(4):460–6.
32. Fan ST, Le Treut YP, Mazzaferro V, Burroughs AK, Olausson M, Breitenstein S, et al. Liver transplantation for neuroendocrine tumour liver metastases. HPB (Oxford). 2015;17(1):23–8.
33. Mazzaferro V, Sposito C, Coppa J, Miceli R, Bhoori S, Bongini M, et al. The long-term benefit of liver transplantation for hepatic metastases from neuroendocrine tumors. Am J Transplant. 2016;16(10):2892–902.
34. Norlen O, Daskalakis K, Oberg K, Akerstrom G, Stalberg P, Hellman P. Indication for liver transplantation in young patients with small intestinal NETs is rare? World J Surg. 2014;38(3):742–7.
35. Osborne DA, Zervos EE, Strosberg J, Boe BA, Malafa M, Rosemurgy AS, et al. Improved outcome with cytoreduction versus embolization for symptomatic

hepatic metastases of carcinoid and neuroendocrine tumors. Ann Surg Oncol. 2006;13(4):572–81.
36. Hibi T, Sano T, Sakamoto Y, Takahashi Y, Uemura N, Ojima H, et al. Surgery for hepatic neuroendocrine tumors: a single institutional experience in Japan. Jpn J Clin Oncol. 2007;37(2):102–7.
37. Elias D, Goere D, Leroux G, Dromain C, Leboulleux S, de Baere T, et al. Combined liver surgery and RFA for patients with gastroenteropancreatic endocrine tumors presenting with more than 15 metastases to the liver. Eur J Surg Oncol. 2009;35(10):1092–7.
38. Taner T, Atwell TD, Zhang L, Oberg TN, Harmsen WS, Slettedahl SW, et al. Adjunctive radiofrequency ablation of metastatic neuroendocrine cancer to the liver complements surgical resection. HPB (Oxford). 2013;15(3):190–5.
39. Boudreaux JP, Putty B, Frey DJ, et al. Surgical treatment of advanced-stage carcinoid tumors: lessons learned. Ann Surg. 2005;241(6):839–45; discussion 45–6.
40. Norlen O, Stalberg P, Oberg K, et al. Long-term results of surgery for small intestinal neuroendocrine tumors at a tertiary referral center. World J Surg. 2012;36(6):1419–31.

Liver-Directed Therapies for Neuroendocrine Metastases

Erica S. Alexander and Michael C. Soulen

Neuroendocrine tumors (NET) have historically been considered rare tumors, comprising about 0.5% of all malignancies [1]. In spite of the relative rarity of NET, the incidence of diagnosis has been rising, which is thought to be secondary to increased detection [2]. According to Surveillance, Epidemiology, and End Results data, the incidence of NET rose from 1.9 to 5.25 cases per 100,000 people between 1973 and 2004 [3]. NET comprise a heterogeneous group of malignancies that arise from neuroendocrine cells throughout the body and are characterized by their ability to synthesize and secrete hormonally active polypeptides [4]. The clinical course of NET is variable, with some tumors having an indolent course and others exhibiting aggressive behavior.

At the time of diagnosis, 46–93% of patients with NET have synchronous hepatic metastases [5]. The presence of hepatic metastases is the single most important prognostic indicator of survival in patients with NET, with an associated 5-year survival rate of 0–40% [4, 6, 7]. Although no study has compared therapies for liver metastases to natural history alone, local therapies such as resection and embolization appear to increase the 5-year survival rates as compared to historical controls [8–10]. Choice among the various liver-directed therapies is largely dictated by localization and the degree of tumor burden [8, 11]. When metastases are confined to a single hepatic lobe or two adjacent segments, surgery is considered the treatment of choice [11–13]. However, complete excision of NET liver metastases is only feasible in about 10–20% of patients presenting with metastatic disease [5, 14]. For patients with diffuse and/or multifocal disease, treatment options have included liver transplantation, non-curative surgical debulking, medical therapy, ablation, hepatic artery (chemo)embolization, and radioembolization [15–19]. This chapter discusses minimally invasive therapies, including tumor ablation and transarterial therapies, utilized by interventional radiologists to treat NET liver metastases.

Tumor Ablation

Tumor ablation involves the percutaneous, laparoscopic, or open surgical placement of an ablation applicator into a tumor. Ablation utilizes thermal energy to create controlled coagulation necrosis of malignant cells. For the purpose of this chapter, we will discuss the percutaneous, image-guided approach to tumor ablation, which

E. S. Alexander
Department of Diagnostic Radiology, Hospital of the University of Pennsylvania, Philadelphia, PA, USA
e-mail: Erica.alexander@uphs.upenn.edu

M. C. Soulen (✉)
Department of Radiology, Abramson Cancer Center, University of Pennsylvania, Philadelphia, PA, USA
e-mail: michael.soulen@uphs.upenn.edu

utilizes either ultrasound, computed tomographic (CT), or magnetic resonance (MR) guidance. The three mainstays of ablation therapy are radiofrequency ablation (RFA), microwave ablation (MWA), and cryoablation (CA). Ablation is primarily utilized for palliation of carcinoid symptoms and management of recurrent disease in patients with a limited tumor burden.

Ablation Modalities

Radiofrequency Ablation

RFA is the most researched ablation modality for the treatment of NET metastases to the liver. It utilizes high-frequency alternating current that passes from an electrode into surrounding tissues to create frictional heating of tissues to temperatures between 60 and 100 °C. The goal of RFA is to produce instantaneous protein coagulation with irreversible damage to mitochondria and cytosolic cell enzymes [20, 21].

The largest study to date evaluating RFA for NET metastases to the liver evaluated 34 patients with a total of 234 metastases. Relief of symptoms was achieved in 95% of patients, and 41% of patients showed no evidence of progression [22]. Several other retrospective studies have observed symptom relief in patients treated with RFA for NET liver metastases [23–25]. Wessels et al. evaluated a small series of patients with unresectable NET liver metastases treated with RFA and noted that one of the three patients was able to discontinue octreotide therapy and the other two patients were able to decrease their dosages [24]. A recent study, evaluating multiple modalities in the treatment of liver metastases related to NETs, noted a median overall survival of 160 months in patients treated with surgical resection compared to 123 months for those treated with RFA [26].

Microwave Ablation

MWA utilizes alternative electromagnetic microwaves to produce rapid oscillation of water molecules. The molecules flip several billion times per second, which produces frictional, cytotoxic heating [27]. MWA may be superior to RFA in treating larger tumors, as it has broader energy deposition, a larger zone of active heating, achieves higher intratumoral temperatures, larger ablation volumes, faster ablation times, and is less susceptible to cooling from surrounding vessels [28–30]. There are no dedicated publications evaluating MWA in the treatment of NET metastases; however, several papers have shown promising safety and efficacy of MWA in the treatment of metastatic liver lesions [29, 31–36].

Cryoablation

Cryoablation relies on alternating freeze-thaw cycles to create osmotic shifts that result in cellular membrane rupture and cell death. Advantages of cryoablation include the creation of an ice ball, which can be visualized intraprocedurally and is a surrogate for ablation zone size. Cryoablation preserves the collagenous structures within the parenchyma, making it safe to use near major vessels and bile ducts.

There are several small studies in the surgical literature evaluating cryoablation in the treatment of NET metastases to the liver [37–39]. The largest series to date by Seifert et al. evaluated the use of intraoperative cryotherapy in 13 patients with NETS. Twelve of the treated patients were alive and mostly asymptomatic at 13.5 months, and all patients with elevated preoperative tumor markers saw a fall of >85% posttreatment [38].

Patient Selection

Percutaneous image-guided ablation is generally considered best suited for nonsurgical patients with metastases less than 3 cm [40, 41]. Local failure rates increase as tumor size increases; however, several studies have shown that combination therapy with transarterial therapy can prove beneficial in the treatment of larger liver lesions [42–47]. Additionally, larger tumors can be adequately treated with the use of altered ablation parameters, including increasing the number of ablation antennae or applicators, increasing the treatment time, or utilizing MWA to achieve larger treatment sizes [48, 49].

There is no absolute upper limit for the number of hepatic tumors that can be ablated; however, for patients presenting with more than four tumors, there is a high probability of occult malignancy [50]. Contraindications to ablation include uncorrectable coagulopathy, liver failure, uncorrectable proximity to critical structures, or widely metastatic disease [41]. Caution should be used when treating patients with bilioenteric anastomoses, as studies have demonstrated an increased risk of developing liver abscesses and sepsis [51–54].

Prior to treatment, an interventional oncologist should assess patient's health and treatment history. Laboratory tests, including a complete blood count, creatinine level, coagulation profile, liver function panel, and relevant tumor markers, should be obtained [50]. Additionally, recent cross-sectional imaging should be reviewed for treatment planning and as a baseline to assess posttreatment response.

Procedure

To reduce the risk of sedation-related aspiration, all patients are instructed to fast overnight, prior to the procedure. Patients who take cardiac or hypertension medications are instructed to take their medications as directed. Those patients with diabetes should take half of their morning insulin dose. Patients should stop anticoagulant medications 2–7 days prior to ablation. Given that patients with NET can exhibit the release of vasoactive hormones during ablation, patients should be premedicated with somatostatin analogs prior to ablation to avoid a carcinoid crisis [55]. Preoperative administration of octreotide can reduce the incidence of carcinoid crisis and should be used in patients with a history of carcinoid crisis. If a carcinoid crisis occurs intra-procedurally, the blood pressure should be supported with infusion of plasma and octreotide [11, 56–58].

Percutaneous ablation is generally performed as an outpatient procedure with the use of intravenous moderate sedation or monitored anesthesia care. Heat-based ablation therapies, such as RFA and MWA, are associated with greater pain and may require deeper sedation with general anesthesia. Vital signs, including pulse oximetry and electrocardiogram, are monitored throughout the procedure.

Ultrasound is an efficient modality for ablation guidance for those tumors that can be sonographically visualized. Of note, the echogenic steam generated during the procedure can obscure the tumor and liver parenchyma, making targeting of subsequent activations difficult. CT generally provides the best depiction of the target tumor and the antenna or applicator, but the CT gantry can make probe positioning difficult and the procedures generally take more time. MR guidance can be used at institutions with MRI-compatible ablation equipment. Regardless of modality, dynamic contrast-enhanced imaging is helpful to guide ablation and provide immediate assessment of efficacy.

Prior to the procedure, the skin is prepped and draped in a sterile fashion, and lidocaine is injected at the skin. For tumors adjacent to critical structures, such as adjacent organs, the body wall, or diaphragm, hydrodissection can be performed. This involves direct infusion of dextrose solution or saline into the peritoneum, to create artificial ascites, which protects structures from thermal injury and is also associated with decreased post-procedure pain [59, 60].

The ablation parameters, including the number of probes and number of activations, are intended to achieve a total ablation zone that extends 5–10 mm beyond the periphery of the tumor. A consideration for treatment is the proximity of the tumor to surrounding veins, as blood vessels near or within the treatment zone can create perfusion-mediated cooling, also referred to as the "heat sink effect," which can hinder complete tumor eradication [61–63].

After treatment, the probe(s) are removed, and post-procedure imaging can be obtained to evaluate for hemorrhage or complications and to determine if the targeted tumor was treated. Typical

CT features of a successful ablation on immediate posttreatment imaging include an area of low attenuation completely covering the tumor, as well as a 5–10 mm rim of ablated hepatic parenchyma around the treated tumor [64–66]. It is important to note that the immediate inflammatory response associated with ablation can result in significant perilesional enhancement. For patients with persistent pain or post-procedural complications, inpatient admission can be considered.

Treatment Follow-Up

In the immediate post-procedure period, patients should be monitored for possible complications. In general, ablation is very well tolerated, with major complication rates of 5–12% in several large studies evaluating RFA in the treatment of liver metastases [23, 67]. Complications can include carcinoid crisis, liver abscesses, biliopleural fistulas, bile leakage, pleural effusion, postablation syndrome, and liver failure.

Clinical and laboratory assessment and triple-phase enhanced imaging should be performed 1 month after treatment to monitor for complications and to determine if the treatment was technically successful. Subsequent imaging follow-up should be performed at 3-month intervals for 12 months thereafter. A complete lack of enhancement in the ablation zone and evidence of the postablation coagulation volume covering the index lesion are indicative of a technically successful ablation. Residual or recurrent disease most often occurs in the periphery of the ablation zone and generally presents as distortion and/or enhancement of the otherwise smooth interface with the liver parenchyma [64, 68, 69].

Transarterial Therapy

Transarterial therapies, including transarterial embolization (TAE), transarterial chemoembolization (TACE), and radioembolization (TARE), exploit the vascular nature of NET. Liver metastases are fed primarily by the hepatic artery, while healthy liver parenchyma is predominantly supplied by the portal venous system [70]. Current NANETS, ENETS, and NCCN guidelines recommend transarterial therapies in patients with unresectable NET metastases with symptoms related to tumor bulk, excess hormone production, and/or progression of disease [71].

Transarterial Embolization

TAE therapy delivers targeted embolic agents to tumor microvasculature, resulting in blood vessel occlusion, which promotes tissue infarction and necrosis. TAE has been shown to improve biophysical markers, palliate symptoms, and reduce radiographic tumor burden [72, 73]. Embolic agents used include cyanoacrylate, gel foam particles, polyvinyl alcohol, and microspheres. It remains debatable if the addition of cytotoxic drugs to embolics is superior to bland embolization alone [74–77]. A multicenter, retrospective review of 100 patients treated with TAE versus TACE, revealed no difference in overall survival, symptom improvement, morbidity, or mortality between treatment groups [76].

Transarterial Chemoembolization

TACE delivers high doses of targeted chemotherapy and embolic agents to intrahepatic tumors, while sparing healthy surrounding parenchyma. Most NET metastases are treated using doxorubicin or streptozotocin, although the latter regimen requires general anesthesia due to significant pain during hepatic intra-arterial injection [78–80]. Some reports have suggested that drug-eluting beads (DEBs) are associated with increased complications, including bilomas and liver abscesses [81–83]. The drug(s) selected for TACE are combined with Lipiodol, an ethyl ester of iodized fatty acids of poppy seed oil, to form an emulsion. Embolic agents are injected after the Lipiodol TACE mixture. Embolics slow drug efflux from the hepatic circulation, which increases the delivered drug concentration, duration of delivery, and rate of tumor necrosis [84, 85]. In general, patients undergo two sequential TACE procedures, performed 2–8 weeks apart.

For localized disease demonstrating incomplete necrosis on posttreatment imaging, the second session targets the same lobe or subsegmental location. For patients with bilobar disease, each lobe is targeted in two separate sessions.

Chemoembolization using Lipiodol has been used for over 30 years and has shown significant efficacy in treating NET metastases and associated carcinoid syndrome [75, 86–90]. Bloomston et al. conducted one of the largest single-center studies, evaluating TACE in 122 patients with metastatic carcinoid tumors.

Median follow-up was 21.5 months, and 94% of patients showed either no evidence of tumor progression or stabilization of disease on posttreatment imaging. TACE was associated with a significant reduction in pancreastatin levels, and symptom improvement was reported in 92% of patients. A lack of symptom improvement correlated with a lack of radiographic evidence of tumor regression. The median progression-free survival after TACE was 10.0 months and the median overall survival was 33.3 months. Complications occurred in 23% of patients, and there were six periprocedural deaths, which were related to multisystem organ failure, gangrenous cholecystitis, myocardial infarction, and carcinoid crisis [89]. The MD Anderson group evaluated prognostic factors for progression-free survival in patients with NET liver metastases who underwent bland embolization or transarterial chemoembolization and concluded that those patients with carcinoid tumors, compared to pancreatic NET, had a longer cumulative survival, better radiologic response rate, and a longer median progression-free survival. The only independent risk factor for mortality in carcinoid patients was male gender. Poor predictors for survival in patients with pancreatic NET included a persistent primary tumor, $\geq 75\%$ tumor liver involvement, and the presence of bone metastases [87].

Transarterial Radioembolization

TARE is a catheter-directed, targeted cancer treatment that uses high-dose radiation selectively delivered to the tumor microvasculature. The technology utilizes ^{90}Yttrium (^{90}Y) microspheres, which are pure beta emitters that deliver high doses of targeted radiation therapy in a short radius around each microsphere.

Several studies evaluating SIRT in the treatment of NET liver metastases have shown that the therapy has a substantial and durable biologic and morphologic response rate [91–95]. Kennedy et al. conducted a multi-institution retrospective study that evaluated 148 patients with unresectable NET metastases treated with ^{90}Y. Complete or partial response to treatment was demonstrated in 63.2% of patients, and the median survival was 70 months [95]. In another study evaluating 34 patients with liver metastases related to NET treated with SIRT, the mean overall survival was 29.4 months, and chromogranin A levels decreased to 50%, with a sustained response lasting 30 months [94].

Patient Selection

Patients should be evaluated by an interventional oncologist prior to treatment. All patients should undergo evaluation of cross-sectional abdominal imaging, thoracic imaging, complete blood counts, hepatic function panels, coagulation profile, creatinine levels, and tumor markers.

Patients receiving transarterial therapies must have sufficient portal vein inflow to allow for hepatic artery occlusion. Relative contraindications include greater than 50% of liver volume being replaced by tumor, lactate dehydrogenase greater than 425 IU/L, aspartate aminotransferase greater than 100 IU/L, and total bilirubin greater than 2.0 IU/L [96, 97]. Absolute contraindications to embolization include hepatic encephalopathy and jaundice [84]. Presence of a bilioenteric anastomosis or stent increases the risk of postembolization liver abscess or cholangitis.

Prior to TARE, patients are required to have a celiac angiogram to map the vascular supply to the liver and identify any aberrant vasculature to the gastrointestinal tract that may need to be avoided or embolized. ^{99}Technitium macroalbumin is infused intra-arterially into the selected hepatic artery, and the patient then has a single photon emission computed tomography

(SPECT) scan to evaluate for shunting to the lungs or gastrointestinal tract. The ^{99}Technitium imaging is intended to avoid unintentional infusion of radioactive materials outside of the targeted treatment zone, as radiation pneumonitis or enteritis are highly morbid complications. Several recent studies have indicated that a high lung shunt function (>10%) is associated with lower overall survival [98, 99].

Procedure

All patients are instructed to fast overnight prior to the procedure. Preoperative medication instructions are identical to those provided to ablation patients. At our institution, patients are admitted to the hospital the morning of the procedure. An intravenous (IV) line is placed and IV hydration is initiated, along with prophylactic antibiotics (cefazolin, 1 g; metronidazole, 500 mg) and antiemetics (ondansetron, 24 mg; dexamethasone, 10 mg; diphenhydramine, 50 mg). Prophylactic use of somatostatin analogs is recommended to avoid a carcinoid crisis.

Embolization procedures start with visceral arteriography for treatment planning. This is designed to identify the hepatic vasculature, patency of the portal vein, and location of tumors [84]. For TAE and TACE, the embolic regimen is injected into the selected artery until near complete stasis of flow is achieved. For TARE, radioembolics are not infused until stasis of blood flow is achieved, as cell death through radiation requires normal oxygen tension [100].

Embolotherapy is performed as selectively as possible, particularly for patients with a single or localized tumors. A microcatheter is placed into segmental or subsegmental tumor-feeding arteries. For patients with widespread disease involving an entire lobe, lobar treatment is required. Many institutions administer intra-arterial lidocaine between each aliquot of drug and/or embolic to help alleviate pain.

Immediately after the procedure, patients receive vigorous intravenous hydration, antibiotics, and antiemetic and pain medications as needed. Patients receiving TAE/TACE at our institution are admitted to an observation unit and are discharged the next morning if they have adequate oral intake and pain is controlled. TARE is performed on an outpatient basis due to the low rate of postembolization syndrome.

Treatment Follow-Up

The most frequent complication association with embolization is postembolization syndrome, which is marked by fever, abdominal pain, leukocytosis, transaminitis, and hyperbilirubinemia. Postembolization syndrome is generally self-limited; the risk may be minimized by treating a single lobe per session over several sessions [101, 102]. Major treatment complications include gallbladder necrosis, liver infarction or insufficiency, hepatorenal syndrome, pancreatitis, liver abscess, biloma, gastrointestinal ulceration or hemorrhage, and aneurysm formation [8, 103]. Complications unique to TARE can result from nontargeted delivery of radioactive materials to other organs and include pneumonitis, cholecystitis, gastrointestinal ulcer, pancreatitis, and biliary injury [104, 105]. In the literature the incidence of nontarget embolization ranges from 0 to 24%; these complications can be incredibly morbid for patients [95, 106–110]. Scrupulous evaluation of the vascular anatomy on pretreatment angiography is essential to help minimize these risks.

Patients should be followed up post-procedure with clinical, laboratory, and radiologic exams, to assess tumor response and to identify any complications. Cross-sectional imaging should be performed 1 month after treatment and then every 3 months subsequently. There is no clear consensus by which to evaluate the response of transarterial treatments for metastatic lesions to the liver; however, most institutions use a combination of World Health Organization (WHO), Response Evaluation Criteria in Solid Tumors (RECIST), modified RECIST (mRECIST), and/or European Association for the Study of the Liver (EASL) guidelines [111–113]. Assessment of tumor response should take into account target index lesion size and the presence of necrosis [114, 115].

An early imaging feature of TARE is the presence of a fibrotic, enhancing capsule around the lesion; this should not be mistaken for residual tumor [115]. In the 8–12 weeks after TARE, completely treated tumors should undergo shrinkage. Also, the surrounding parenchyma undergoes atrophy as a result of hepatic fibrosis and capsular retraction of the treated lesion; this atrophy, particularly after lobar treatments, results in a compensatory hypertrophy of the contralateral lobe. Other common imaging features after TARE include perfusion abnormalities in the treated lesion and hypoattenuating perivascular edema near the hepatic and portal veins [116].

Conclusion

The high incidence of patients with NET presenting with inoperable hepatic metastases necessitates a broad range of treatment approaches to help improve patient outcomes. Minimally invasive interventional oncology procedures have been used for several decades and have shown promising efficacy in the treatment of carcinoid-related symptoms and in the overall survival of treated patients. Thermal ablation and transarterial therapies are important tools in the armamentarium of NET treatment and should be integrated with other surgical, systemic, and supportive therapies.

References

1. Buchanan KD, Johnston CF, O'Hare MM, Ardill JE, Shaw C, Collins JS, et al. Neuroendocrine tumors. A European view. Am J Med. 1986;81(6B):14–22.
2. Hallet J, Law CH, Cukier M, Saskin R, Liu N, Singh S. Exploring the rising incidence of neuroendocrine tumors: a population-based analysis of epidemiology, metastatic presentation, and outcomes. Cancer. 2015;121(4):589–97.
3. Yao JC, Hassan M, Phan A, Dagohoy C, Leary C, Mares JE, et al. One hundred years after "carcinoid": epidemiology of and prognostic factors for neuroendocrine tumors in 35,825 cases in the United States. J Clin Oncol. 2008;26(18):3063–72.
4. Modlin IM, Lye KD, Kidd M. A 5-decade analysis of 13,715 carcinoid tumors. Cancer. 2003;97(4):934–59.
5. Chamberlain RS, Canes D, Brown KT, Saltz L, Jarnagin W, Fong Y, et al. Hepatic neuroendocrine metastases: does intervention alter outcomes? J Am Coll Surg. 2000;190(4):432–45.
6. Rindi G, D'Adda T, Froio E, Fellegara G, Bordi C. Prognostic factors in gastrointestinal endocrine tumors. Endocr Pathol. 2007;18(3):145–9.
7. Modlin IM, Sandor A. An analysis of 8305 cases of carcinoid tumors. Cancer. 1997;79(4):813–29.
8. Steinmuller T, Kianmanesh R, Falconi M, Scarpa A, Taal B, Kwekkeboom DJ, et al. Consensus guidelines for the management of patients with liver metastases from digestive (neuro)endocrine tumors: foregut, midgut, hindgut, and unknown primary. Neuroendocrinology. 2008;87(1):47–62.
9. Chen H, Hardacre JM, Uzar A, Cameron JL, Choti MA. Isolated liver metastases from neuroendocrine tumors: does resection prolong survival? J Am Coll Surg. 1998;187(1):88–92; discussion 92–3.
10. Elias D, Lasser P, Ducreux M, Duvillard P, Ouellet JF, Dromain C, et al. Liver resection (and associated extrahepatic resections) for metastatic well-differentiated endocrine tumors: a 15-year single center prospective study. Surgery. 2003;133(4):375–82.
11. Macedo D, Amaral T, Fernandes I, Sousa AR, Costa AL, Tavora I, et al. The treatment of liver metastases in patients with neuroendocrine tumors in 2012. ISRN Hepatol. 2013;2013:702167.
12. Ramage JK, Ahmed A, Ardill J, Bax N, Breen DJ, Caplin ME, et al. Guidelines for the management of gastroenteropancreatic neuroendocrine (including carcinoid) tumours (NETs). Gut. 2012;61(1):6–32.
13. Frilling A, Sotiropoulos GC, Li J, Kornasiewicz O, Plockinger U. Multimodal management of neuroendocrine liver metastases. HPB (Oxford). 2010;12(6):361–79.
14. Jagannath P, Chhabra D, Shrikhande S, Shah R. Surgical treatment of liver metastases in neuroendocrine neoplasms. Int J Hepatol. 2012;2012:782672.
15. Lehnert T. Liver transplantation for metastatic neuroendocrine carcinoma: an analysis of 103 patients. Transplantation. 1998;66(10):1307–12.
16. Le Treut YP, Gregoire E, Belghiti J, Boillot O, Soubrane O, Mantion G, et al. Predictors of long-term survival after liver transplantation for metastatic endocrine tumors: an 85-case French multicentric report. Am J Transplant. 2008;8(6):1205–13.
17. Mathe Z, Tagkalos E, Paul A, Molmenti EP, Kobori L, Fouzas I, et al. Liver transplantation for hepatic metastases of neuroendocrine pancreatic tumors: a survival-based analysis. Transplantation. 2011;91(5):575–82.
18. Harring TR, Nguyen NT, Goss JA, O'Mahony CA. Treatment of liver metastases in patients with neuroendocrine tumors: a comprehensive review. Int J Hepatol. 2011;2011:154541.
19. Modlin IM, Latich I, Kidd M, Zikusoka M, Eick G. Therapeutic options for gastrointestinal carcinoids. Clin Gastroenterol Hepatol. 2006;4(5):526–47.

20. Goldberg SN, Gazelle GS, Mueller PR. Thermal ablation therapy for focal malignancy: a unified approach to underlying principles, techniques, and diagnostic imaging guidance. AJR Am J Roentgenol. 2000;174(2):323–31.
21. Goldberg SN, Gazelle GS, Halpern EF, Rittman WJ, Mueller PR, Rosenthal DI. Radiofrequency tissue ablation: importance of local temperature along the electrode tip exposure in determining lesion shape and size. Acad Radiol. 1996;3(3):212–8.
22. Gillams A, Cassoni A, Conway G, Lees W. Radiofrequency ablation of neuroendocrine liver metastases: the Middlesex experience. Abdom Imaging. 2005;30(4):435–41.
23. Akyildiz HY, Mitchell J, Milas M, Siperstein A, Berber E. Laparoscopic radiofrequency thermal ablation of neuroendocrine hepatic metastases: long-term follow-up. Surgery. 2010;148(6):1288–93; discussion 93.
24. Wessels FJ, Schell SR. Radiofrequency ablation treatment of refractory carcinoid hepatic metastases. J Surg Res. 2001;95(1):8–12.
25. Henn AR, Levine EA, McNulty W, Zagoria RJ. Percutaneous radiofrequency ablation of hepatic metastases for symptomatic relief of neuroendocrine syndromes. AJR Am J Roentgenol. 2003;181(4):1005–10.
26. Fairweather M, Swanson R, Wang J, Brais LK, Dutton T, Kulke MH, et al. Management of neuroendocrine tumor liver metastases: long-term outcomes and prognostic factors from a large prospective database. Ann Surg Oncol. 2017;24(8):2319–25.
27. Simon CJ, Dupuy DE, Mayo-Smith WW. Microwave ablation: principles and applications. Radiographics. 2005;25(Suppl 1):S69–83.
28. Dodd GD III, Dodd NA, Lanctot AC, Glueck DA. Effect of variation of portal venous blood flow on radiofrequency and microwave ablations in a blood-perfused bovine liver model. Radiology. 2013;267(1):129–36.
29. Martin RC, Scoggins CR, McMasters KM. Safety and efficacy of microwave ablation of hepatic tumors: a prospective review of a 5-year experience. Ann Surg Oncol. 2010;17(1):171–8.
30. Wright AS, Sampson LA, Warner TF, Mahvi DM, Lee FT Jr. Radiofrequency versus microwave ablation in a hepatic porcine model. Radiology. 2005;236(1):132–9.
31. Zaidi N, Okoh A, Yigitbas H, Yazici P, Ali N, Berber E. Laparoscopic microwave thermosphere ablation of malignant liver tumors: an analysis of 53 cases. J Surg Oncol. 2016;113(2):130–4.
32. Martin RC, Scoggins CR, McMasters KM. Microwave hepatic ablation: initial experience of safety and efficacy. J Surg Oncol. 2007;96(6):481–6.
33. Liang P, Wang Y, Yu X, Dong B. Malignant liver tumors: treatment with percutaneous microwave ablation—complications among cohort of 1136 patients. Radiology. 2009;251(3):933–40.
34. Groeschl RT, Pilgrim CH, Hanna EM, Simo KA, Swan RZ, Sindram D, et al. Microwave ablation for hepatic malignancies: a multiinstitutional analysis. Ann Surg. 2014;259(6):1195–200.
35. Livraghi T, Meloni F, Solbiati L, Zanus G, Collaborative Italian Group Using AMICA System. Complications of microwave ablation for liver tumors: results of a multicenter study. Cardiovasc Intervent Radiol. 2012;35(4):868–74.
36. Liang P, Dong B, Yu X, Yang Y, Yu D, Su L, et al. Prognostic factors for percutaneous microwave coagulation therapy of hepatic metastases. AJR Am J Roentgenol. 2003;181(5):1319–25.
37. Cozzi PJ, Englund R, Morris DL. Cryotherapy treatment of patients with hepatic metastases from neuroendocrine tumors. Cancer. 1995;76(3):501–9.
38. Seifert JK, Cozzi PJ, Morris DL. Cryotherapy for neuroendocrine liver metastases. Semin Surg Oncol. 1998;14(2):175–83.
39. Duperier T, Ali A, Pereira S, Davies RJ, Ballantyne GH. Laparoscopic cryoablation of a metastatic carcinoid tumor. J Laparoendosc Adv Surg Tech A. 2001;11(2):105–9.
40. Solbiati L, Livraghi T, Goldberg SN, Ierace T, Meloni F, Dellanoce M, et al. Percutaneous radiofrequency ablation of hepatic metastases from colorectal cancer: long-term results in 117 patients. Radiology. 2001;221(1):159–66.
41. Lencioni R, Crocetti L, Della Pina C, Cioni D. Image-guided ablation of hepatocellular carcinoma. In: Geschwind JH, Soulen MC, editors. Interventional oncology: principles and practice. 1st ed. Cambridge: Cambridge University Press; 2008. p. 145–59.
42. Veltri A, Moretto P, Doriguzzi A, Pagano E, Carrara G, Gandini G. Radiofrequency thermal ablation (RFA) after transarterial chemoembolization (TACE) as a combined therapy for unresectable non-early hepatocellular carcinoma (HCC). Eur Radiol. 2006;16(3):661–9.
43. Peng ZW, Zhang YJ, Chen MS, Xu L, Liang HH, Lin XJ, et al. Radiofrequency ablation with or without transcatheter arterial chemoembolization in the treatment of hepatocellular carcinoma: a prospective randomized trial. J Clin Oncol. 2013;31(4):426–32.
44. Kim JH, Won HJ, Shin YM, Kim SH, Yoon HK, Sung KB, et al. Medium-sized (3.1-5.0 cm) hepatocellular carcinoma: transarterial chemoembolization plus radiofrequency ablation versus radiofrequency ablation alone. Ann Surg Oncol. 2011;18(6):1624–9.
45. Morimoto M, Numata K, Kondou M, Nozaki A, Morita S, Tanaka K. Midterm outcomes in patients with intermediate-sized hepatocellular carcinoma: a randomized controlled trial for determining the efficacy of radiofrequency ablation combined with transcatheter arterial chemoembolization. Cancer. 2010;116(23):5452–60.
46. Wu ZB, Si ZM, Qian S, Liu LX, Qu XD, Zhou B, et al. Percutaneous microwave ablation combined with synchronous transcatheter arterial chemoembo-

lization for the treatment of colorectal liver metastases: results from a follow-up cohort. Onco Targets Ther. 2016;9:3783–9.
47. Fong ZV, Palazzo F, Needleman L, Brown DB, Eschelman DJ, Chojnacki KA, et al. Combined hepatic arterial embolization and hepatic ablation for unresectable colorectal metastases to the liver. Am Surg. 2012;78(11):1243–8.
48. Alexander ES, Wolf FJ, Machan JT, Charpentier KP, Beland MD, Iannuccilli JD, et al. Microwave ablation of focal hepatic malignancies regardless of size: a 9-year retrospective study of 64 patients. Eur J Radiol. 2015;84(6):1083–90.
49. Wright AS, Lee FT Jr, Mahvi DM. Hepatic microwave ablation with multiple antennae results in synergistically larger zones of coagulation necrosis. Ann Surg Oncol. 2003;10(3):275–83.
50. McCarley JR, Soulen MC. Percutaneous ablation of hepatic tumors. Semin Intervent Radiol. 2010;27(3):255–60.
51. Elias D, Di Pietroantonio D, Gachot B, Menegon P, Hakime A, De Baere T. Liver abscess after radiofrequency ablation of tumors in patients with a biliary tract procedure. Gastroenterol Clin Biol. 2006;30(6–7):823–7.
52. Khan W, Sullivan KL, McCann JW, Gonsalves CF, Sato T, Eschelman DJ, et al. Moxifloxacin prophylaxis for chemoembolization or embolization in patients with previous biliary interventions: a pilot study. AJR Am J Roentgenol. 2011;197(2):W343–5.
53. Kim W, Clark TW, Baum RA, Soulen MC. Risk factors for liver abscess formation after hepatic chemoembolization. J Vasc Interv Radiol. 2001;12(8):965–8.
54. Berber E, Siperstein AE. Perioperative outcome after laparoscopic radiofrequency ablation of liver tumors: an analysis of 521 cases. Surg Endosc. 2007;21(4):613–8.
55. Wettstein M, Vogt C, Cohnen M, Brill N, Kurz AK, Modder U, et al. Serotonin release during percutaneous radiofrequency ablation in a patient with symptomatic liver metastases of a neuroendocrine tumor. Hepatogastroenterology. 2004;51(57):830–2.
56. Roy RC, Carter RF, Wright PD. Somatostatin, anaesthesia, and the carcinoid syndrome. Perioperative administration of a somatostatin analogue to suppress carcinoid tumour activity. Anaesthesia. 1987;42(6):627–32.
57. Oberg K, Kvols L, Caplin M, Delle Fave G, de Herder W, Rindi G, et al. Consensus report on the use of somatostatin analogs for the management of neuroendocrine tumors of the gastroenteropancreatic system. Ann Oncol. 2004;15(6):966–73.
58. Warner RR, Mani S, Profeta J, Grunstein E. Octreotide treatment of carcinoid hypertensive crisis. Mt Sinai J Med. 1994;61(4):349–55.
59. Hinshaw JL, Laeseke PF, Winter TC III, Kliewer MA, Fine JP, Lee FT Jr. Radiofrequency ablation of peripheral liver tumors: intraperitoneal 5% dextrose in water decreases postprocedural pain. AJR Am J Roentgenol. 2006;186(5 Suppl):S306–10.
60. Raman SS, Lu DS, Vodopich DJ, Sayre J, Lassman C. Minimizing diaphragmatic injury during radiofrequency ablation: efficacy of subphrenic peritoneal saline injection in a porcine model. Radiology. 2002;222(3):819–23.
61. Ahmed M, Liu Z, Humphries S, Goldberg SN. Computer modeling of the combined effects of perfusion, electrical conductivity, and thermal conductivity on tissue heating patterns in radiofrequency tumor ablation. Int J Hyperthermia. 2008;24(7):577–88.
62. Washburn WK, Dodd GD III, Kohlmeier RE, McCoy VA, Napier DH, Hubbard LG, et al. Radiofrequency tissue ablation: effect of hepatic blood flow occlusion on thermal injuries produced in cirrhotic livers. Ann Surg Oncol. 2003;10(7):773–7.
63. Bitsch RG, Dux M, Helmberger T, Lubienski A. Effects of vascular perfusion on coagulation size in radiofrequency ablation of ex vivo perfused bovine livers. Invest Radiol. 2006;41(4):422–7.
64. Park MH, Rhim H, Kim YS, Choi D, Lim HK, Lee WJ. Spectrum of CT findings after radiofrequency ablation of hepatic tumors. Radiographics. 2008;28(2):379–90; discussion 90–2.
65. Goldberg SN, Grassi CJ, Cardella JF, Charboneau JW, Dodd GD III, Dupuy DE, et al. Image-guided tumor ablation: standardization of terminology and reporting criteria. J Vasc Interv Radiol. 2009;20(7 Suppl):S377–90.
66. Goldberg SN, Gazelle GS, Compton CC, Mueller PR, Tanabe KK. Treatment of intrahepatic malignancy with radiofrequency ablation: radiologic-pathologic correlation. Cancer. 2000;88(11):2452–63.
67. Mazzaglia PJ, Berber E, Milas M, Siperstein AE. Laparoscopic radiofrequency ablation of neuroendocrine liver metastases: a 10-year experience evaluating predictors of survival. Surgery. 2007;142(1):10–9.
68. Choi H, Loyer EM, DuBrow RA, Kaur H, David CL, Huang S, et al. Radio-frequency ablation of liver tumors: assessment of therapeutic response and complications. Radiographics. 2001;21 Spec No:S41–54.
69. Sainani NI, Gervais DA, Mueller PR, Arellano RS. Imaging after percutaneous radiofrequency ablation of hepatic tumors: part 1, normal findings. AJR Am J Roentgenol. 2013;200(1):184–93.
70. Breedis C, Young G. The blood supply of neoplasms in the liver. Am J Pathol. 1954;30(5):969–77.
71. Madoff DC, Gupta S, Ahrar K, Murthy R, Yao JC. Update on the management of neuroendocrine hepatic metastases. J Vasc Interv Radiol. 2006;17(8):1235–49; quiz 50.
72. Mayo SC, de Jong MC, Bloomston M, Pulitano C, Clary BM, Reddy SK, et al. Surgery versus intra-arterial therapy for neuroendocrine liver metastasis: a multicenter international analysis. Ann Surg Oncol. 2011;18(13):3657–65.

73. Hoffmann RT, Paprottka P, Jakobs TF, Trumm CG, Reiser MF. Arterial therapies of non-colorectal cancer metastases to the liver (from chemoembolization to radioembolization). Abdom Imaging. 2011;36(6):671–6.
74. Gupta S, Yao JC, Ahrar K, Wallace MJ, Morello FA, Madoff DC, et al. Hepatic artery embolization and chemoembolization for treatment of patients with metastatic carcinoid tumors: the M.D. Anderson experience. Cancer J. 2003;9(4):261–7.
75. Ruszniewski P, Rougier P, Roche A, Legmann P, Sibert A, Hochlaf S, et al. Hepatic arterial chemoembolization in patients with liver metastases of endocrine tumors. A prospective phase II study in 24 patients. Cancer. 1993;71(8):2624–30.
76. Pitt SC, Knuth J, Keily JM, McDermott JC, Weber SM, Chen H, et al. Hepatic neuroendocrine metastases: chemo- or bland embolization? J Gastrointest Surg. 2008;12(11):1951–60.
77. Fiore F, Del Prete M, Franco R, Marotta V, Ramundo V, Marciello F, et al. Transarterial embolization (TAE) is equally effective and slightly safer than transarterial chemoembolization (TACE) to manage liver metastases in neuroendocrine tumors. Endocrine. 2014;47(1):177–82.
78. de Baere T, Arai Y, Lencioni R, Geschwind JF, Rilling W, Salem R, et al. Treatment of liver tumors with lipiodol TACE: technical recommendations from experts opinion. Cardiovasc Intervent Radiol. 2016;39(3):334–43.
79. Marrache F, Vullierme MP, Roy C, El Assoued Y, Couvelard A, O'Toole D, et al. Arterial phase enhancement and body mass index are predictors of response to chemoembolisation for liver metastases of endocrine tumours. Br J Cancer. 2007;96(1):49–55.
80. Dominguez S, Denys A, Madeira I, Hammel P, Vilgrain V, Menu Y, et al. Hepatic arterial chemoembolization with streptozotocin in patients with metastatic digestive endocrine tumours. Eur J Gastroenterol Hepatol. 2000;12(2):151–7.
81. Bhagat N, Reyes DK, Lin M, Kamel I, Pawlik TM, Frangakis C, et al. Phase II study of chemoembolization with drug-eluting beads in patients with hepatic neuroendocrine metastases: high incidence of biliary injury. Cardiovasc Intervent Radiol. 2013;36(2):449–59.
82. Joskin J, de Baere T, Auperin A, Tselikas L, Guiu B, Farouil G, et al. Predisposing factors of liver necrosis after transcatheter arterial chemoembolization in liver metastases from neuroendocrine tumor. Cardiovasc Intervent Radiol. 2015;38(2):372–80.
83. Guiu B, Deschamps F, Aho S, Munck F, Dromain C, Boige V, et al. Liver/biliary injuries following chemoembolisation of endocrine tumours and hepatocellular carcinoma: lipiodol vs. drug-eluting beads. J Hepatol. 2012;56(3):609–17.
84. Gee M, Soulen MC. Chemoembolization for hepatic metastases. Tech Vasc Interv Radiol. 2002;5(3):132–40.
85. Takayasu K, Shima Y, Muramatsu Y, Moriyama N, Yamada T, Makuuchi M, et al. Hepatocellular carcinoma: treatment with intraarterial iodized oil with and without chemotherapeutic agents. Radiology. 1987;163(2):345–51.
86. Carrasco CH, Charnsangavej C, Ajani J, Samaan NA, Richli W, Wallace S. The carcinoid syndrome: palliation by hepatic artery embolization. AJR Am J Roentgenol. 1986;147(1):149–54.
87. Gupta S, Johnson MM, Murthy R, Ahrar K, Wallace MJ, Madoff DC, et al. Hepatic arterial embolization and chemoembolization for the treatment of patients with metastatic neuroendocrine tumors: variables affecting response rates and survival. Cancer. 2005;104(8):1590–602.
88. Therasse E, Breittmayer F, Roche A, De Baere T, Indushekar S, Ducreux M, et al. Transcatheter chemoembolization of progressive carcinoid liver metastasis. Radiology. 1993;189(2):541–7.
89. Bloomston M, Al-Saif O, Klemanski D, Pinzone JJ, Martin EW, Palmer B, et al. Hepatic artery chemoembolization in 122 patients with metastatic carcinoid tumor: lessons learned. J Gastrointest Surg. 2007;11(3):264–71.
90. Roche A, Girish BV, de Baere T, Baudin E, Boige V, Elias D, et al. Trans-catheter arterial chemoembolization as first-line treatment for hepatic metastases from endocrine tumors. Eur Radiol. 2003;13(1):136–40.
91. Kennedy A, Nag S, Salem R, Murthy R, McEwan AJ, Nutting C, et al. Recommendations for radioembolization of hepatic malignancies using yttrium-90 microsphere brachytherapy: a consensus panel report from the radioembolization brachytherapy oncology consortium. Int J Radiat Oncol Biol Phys. 2007;68(1):13–23.
92. Salem R, Thurston KG. Radioembolization with yttrium-90 microspheres: a state-of-the-art brachytherapy treatment for primary and secondary liver malignancies: part 3: comprehensive literature review and future direction. J Vasc Interv Radiol. 2006;17(10):1571–93.
93. Murthy R, Kamat P, Nunez R, Madoff DC, Gupta S, Salem R, et al. Yttrium-90 microsphere radioembolotherapy of hepatic metastatic neuroendocrine carcinomas after hepatic arterial embolization. J Vasc Interv Radiol. 2008;19(1):145–51.
94. Saxena A, Chua TC, Sarkar A, Chu F, Liauw W, Zhao J, et al. Progression and survival results after radical hepatic metastasectomy of indolent advanced neuroendocrine neoplasms (NENs) supports an aggressive surgical approach. Surgery. 2011;149(2):209–20.
95. Kennedy AS, Dezarn WA, McNeillie P, Coldwell D, Nutting C, Carter D, et al. Radioembolization for unresectable neuroendocrine hepatic metastases using resin 90Y-microspheres: early results in 148 patients. Am J Clin Oncol. 2008;31(3):271–9.
96. Charnsangavej C, Carrasco CH, Wallace S, Richli W, Haynie TP. Hepatic arterial flow distribution with hepatic neoplasms: significance in infusion chemotherapy. Radiology. 1987;165(1):71–3.

97. Leung DA, Goin JE, Sickles C, Raskay BJ, Soulen MC. Determinants of postembolization syndrome after hepatic chemoembolization. J Vasc Interv Radiol. 2001;12(3):321–6.
98. Xing M, Lahti S, Kokabi N, Schuster DM, Camacho JC, Kim HS. 90Y radioembolization lung shunt fraction in primary and metastatic liver cancer as a biomarker for survival. Clin Nucl Med. 2016;41(1):21–7.
99. Ludwig JM, Ambinder EM, Ghodadra A, Xing M, Prajapati HJ, Kim HS. Lung shunt fraction prior to yttrium-90 radioembolization predicts survival in patients with neuroendocrine liver metastases: single-center prospective analysis. Cardiovasc Intervent Radiol. 2016;39(7):1007–14.
100. Strosberg JR, Cheema A, Kvols LK. A review of systemic and liver-directed therapies for metastatic neuroendocrine tumors of the gastroenteropancreatic tract. Cancer Control. 2011;18(2):127–37.
101. Lee E, Leon Pachter H, Sarpel U. Hepatic arterial embolization for the treatment of metastatic neuroendocrine tumors. Int J Hepatol. 2012;2012:471203.
102. Khan MS, Caplin ME. Therapeutic management of patients with gastroenteropancreatic neuroendocrine tumours. Endocr Relat Cancer. 2011;18(Suppl 1):S53–74.
103. Brown DB, Nikolic B, Covey AM, Nutting CW, Saad WE, Salem R, et al. Quality improvement guidelines for transhepatic arterial chemoembolization, embolization, and chemotherapeutic infusion for hepatic malignancy. J Vasc Interv Radiol. 2012;23(3):287–94.
104. Murthy R, Nunez R, Szklaruk J, Erwin W, Madoff DC, Gupta S, et al. Yttrium-90 microsphere therapy for hepatic malignancy: devices, indications, technical considerations, and potential complications. Radiographics. 2005;25(Suppl 1):S41–55.
105. Salem R, Thurston KG. Radioembolization with 90yttrium microspheres: a state-of-the-art brachytherapy treatment for primary and secondary liver malignancies. Part 2: special topics. J Vasc Interv Radiol. 2006;17(9):1425–39.
106. Jia Z, Paz-Fumagalli R, Frey G, Sella DM, McKinney JM, Wang W. Single-institution experience of radioembolization with yttrium-90 microspheres for unresectable metastatic neuroendocrine liver tumors. J Gastroenterol Hepatol. 2017;32(9):1617–23.
107. Peterson JL, Vallow LA, Johnson DW, Heckman MG, Diehl NN, Smith AA, et al. Complications after 90Y microsphere radioembolization for unresectable hepatic tumors: an evaluation of 112 patients. Brachytherapy. 2013;12(6):573–9.
108. Memon K, Lewandowski RJ, Mulcahy MF, Riaz A, Ryu RK, Sato KT, et al. Radioembolization for neuroendocrine liver metastases: safety, imaging, and long-term outcomes. Int J Radiat Oncol Biol Phys. 2012;83(3):887–94.
109. Kennedy AS, McNeillie P, Dezarn WA, Nutting C, Sangro B, Wertman D, et al. Treatment parameters and outcome in 680 treatments of internal radiation with resin 90Y-microspheres for unresectable hepatic tumors. Int J Radiat Oncol Biol Phys. 2009;74(5):1494–500.
110. Paprottka PM, Hoffmann RT, Haug A, Sommer WH, Raessler F, Trumm CG, et al. Radioembolization of symptomatic, unresectable neuroendocrine hepatic metastases using yttrium-90 microspheres. Cardiovasc Intervent Radiol. 2012;35(2):334–42.
111. Therasse P, Arbuck SG, Eisenhauer EA, Wanders J, Kaplan RS, Rubinstein L, et al. New guidelines to evaluate the response to treatment in solid tumors. European Organization for Research and Treatment of Cancer, National Cancer Institute of the United States, National Cancer Institute of Canada. J Natl Cancer Inst. 2000;92(3):205–16.
112. Bruix J, Sherman M, Llovet JM, Beaugrand M, Lencioni R, Burroughs AK, et al. Clinical management of hepatocellular carcinoma. Conclusions of the Barcelona-2000 EASL conference. European Association for the Study of the Liver. J Hepatol. 2001;35(3):421–30.
113. Salem R, Lewandowski RJ, Gates VL, Nutting CW, Murthy R, Rose SC, et al. Research reporting standards for radioembolization of hepatic malignancies. J Vasc Interv Radiol. 2011;22(3):265–78.
114. Ibrahim SM, Nikolaidis P, Miller FH, Lewandowski RJ, Ryu RK, Sato KT, et al. Radiologic findings following Y90 radioembolization for primary liver malignancies. Abdom Imaging. 2009;34(5):566–81.
115. Riaz A, Kulik L, Lewandowski RJ, Ryu RK, Giakoumis Spear G, Mulcahy MF, et al. Radiologic-pathologic correlation of hepatocellular carcinoma treated with internal radiation using yttrium-90 microspheres. Hepatology. 2009;49(4):1185–93.
116. Mosconi C, Cappelli A, Pettinato C, Golfieri R. Radioembolization with yttrium-90 microspheres in hepatocellular carcinoma: role and perspectives. World J Hepatol. 2015;7(5):738–52.

Systemic Therapy for the Management of Neuroendocrine Tumor Liver Metastases

Stephanie M. Kim and Jennifer R. Eads

Introduction

Gastroenteropancreatic neuroendocrine tumors (GEP-NETs) are a rare, heterogeneous group of cancers with increasing incidence. As expected, the prognosis for patients with metastatic disease is worse than for those with localized disease. The use of systemic therapy is only indicated in patients with metastatic disease, and treatment options depend on tumor grade and site of the primary tumor. Somatostatin analogues are the mainstay of treatment in grade 1 and grade 2 intestinal neuroendocrine tumors, and their combination with targeted therapies, liver-directed therapies, and peptide receptor radionuclide therapy has resulted in extended overall survival. Treatment options for grade 1 and grade 2 pancreatic NETs include somatostatin analogues, liver-directed therapy, targeted therapies, cytotoxic chemotherapy and peptide receptor radionuclide therapy. Grade 3 neuroendocrine carcinomas are aggressive and associated with poor survival. While systemic chemotherapy is the mainstay of therapy for patients with this disease, the data for effective therapies in this disease are very limited, and clinical trials assessing chemotherapy regimens are ongoing.

Epidemiology and Clinical Presentation

Gastroenteropancreatic neuroendocrine tumors are rare malignancies; however they have demonstrated increasing incidence over the last few decades. A retrospective study of the Surveillance, Epidemiology, and End Results (SEER) database reported that from 1973 to 2007, the incidence of GEP-NETs in the United States increased from 1.00 per 100,000 to 3.65 per 100,000 [1]. This phenomenon may be the result of increased awareness of the disease among physicians and improved diagnostic testing.

As diagnostic tools improve, it is increasingly evident that GEP-NETs represent a heterogeneous group of cancers, arising from neuroendocrine cells throughout the gastroenteropancreatic system and demonstrating a range of histopathologic features and clinical behavior. In an attempt to lessen ambiguity in defining neuroendocrine

S. M. Kim
Division of Hematology and Oncology,
University Hospitals Seidman Cancer Center,
Case Comprehensive Cancer Center,
Cleveland, OH, USA
e-mail: Stephanie.Kim@UHhospitals.org

J. R. Eads (✉)
Division of Hematology and Oncology,
Perelman Center for Advanced Medicine,
University of Pennsylvania, Philadelphia, PA, USA
e-mail: jennifer.eads@uhhospitals.org

Table 22.1 2010 WHO classification scheme

WHO class	Definition	Ki-67 index (%)	Mitotic count (per 10 hpf[a])	Grade
1	NET[b]	≤2	<2	G1
2	NET	3–20	2–20	G2
3	NEC[c]	>20	>20	G3
4	MANEC[d]	N/A[e]	N/A	N/A
5	Hyperplasia/dysplasia	N/A	N/A	N/A

[a]*hpf* high-powered field
[b]*NET* neuroendocrine tumor
[c]*NEC* neuroendocrine carcinoma
[d]*MANEC* mixed adeno-neuroendocrine carcinoma
[e]*N/A* not applicable

neoplasms, the World Health Organization (WHO) published a classification scheme in 2010, stratifying GEP-NETs based on their proliferation rate (Table 22.1) [2].

In addition, GEP-NETs demonstrate a range of clinical manifestations. Functional tumors can produce symptoms related to hormone secretion, whereas nonfunctional tumors do not secrete hormones but can be symptomatic due to tumor bulk [3]. Functional tumors arising from the midgut (jejunum, ileum, appendix, proximal colon), also called carcinoids, may result in carcinoid syndrome. These patients have symptoms related to increased serotonin production including flushing and diarrhea [4]. Symptoms often develop after the tumor is metastatic, and patients with bulky liver disease have an increased risk of developing cardiac carcinoid, a rare syndrome characterized by the right-sided endocardial deposition of fibrous plaques [4]. A small proportion, approximately 10%, of pancreatic NETs are also functional and can produce a variety of symptoms based on the type of cell involved and hormone produced [5]. Such tumors may include gastrinomas, VIPomas (vasoactive intestinal peptide), glucagonomas, insulinomas, and somatostatinomas [3]. Treatment strategies for these tumors are directed toward symptom control as well as antiproliferation.

Among all types and grades of tumor, the presence of metastatic disease is common, particularly involving the liver. At diagnosis, an estimated 40–50% of tumors are already metastatic, likely due to the indolent behavior of many GEP-NETs [6, 7]. As would be expected, the presence of metastasis is a poor prognostic factor, with primary tumor site and tumor grade also carrying prognostic significance [8, 9]. In a retrospective SEER database study of 35,618 patients, those with metastatic disease had a markedly worse median overall survival (OS) as compared with those with localized disease. Patients with metastatic well-differentiated tumors had a significantly worse median OS of 33 months as compared to 223 months in patients with localized disease. Among patients with poorly differentiated tumors, median OS was 5 months in patients with metastatic disease as compared to 34 months in patients with localized disease [9]. In addition, pancreatic neuroendocrine tumors (PNETs) carry a worse prognosis than intestinal primary tumors, with a median OS of 24 months in metastatic PNETs and 56 months in those with metastases from a small bowel primary [9].

Given that patients with metastatic disease do not have a curable condition, there is ongoing investigation for effective treatment strategies. While curative surgery is available for resectable tumors and may at times be used in patients with metastatic disease to debulk tumor burden and/or provide palliative benefit, multimodality therapy for unresectable or metastatic tumors is aimed at controlling symptoms and prolonging life. Treatment modalities for each group of tumors are discussed in detail below. Table 22.2 summarizes the major phase II/III studies, and Table 22.3 summarizes ongoing clinical trials.

Table 22.2 Major randomized phase II/III trials in G1/G2 neuroendocrine tumors

	N	Tumor type	Primary endpoint	Treatment arms	Result	Statistical benefit
PROMID Rinke et al. 2009 [11]	85	Well-differentiated midgut NETs	TTP[a]	• Octreotide LAR • Placebo	• 14.3 mos[b] • 6 mos	HR[c] 0.34, $p = 0.000072$
RADIANT-2 Pavel et al. 2011 [17]	429	G1/G2 NETs	PFS[d]	• Everolimus + octreotide LAR • Octreotide LAR	• 16.4 mos • 11.3 mos	HR 0.77, $p = 0.026$
RADIANT-3 Yao et al. 2011 [30]	410	G1/G2 NETs	PFS	• Everolimus • Placebo	• 11 mos • 4.6 mos	HR 0.35, $p < 0.001$
Raymond et al. 2011 [33]	171	Well-differentiated PNETs	PFS	• Sunitinib • Placebo	• 11.4 mos • 5.5 mos	HR 0.42, $p < 0.001$
CLARINET Caplin et al. 2014 [13]	204	Well- or moderately differentiated nonfunctioning NETs	PFS	• Lanreotide • Placebo	• Not reached • 18 mos	HR 0.47, $p < 0.001$
RADIANT-4 Yao et al. 2016 [18]	302	Well-differentiated nonfunctional NETs	PFS	• Everolimus • Placebo	• 11 mos • 3.9 mos	HR 0.48, $p < 0.00001$
Wolin et al. 2015 [53]	110	Carcinoids	% pts with symptom control	• Pasireotide LAR • Octreotide LAR	• 20.9% • 26.7%	OR[e] 0.73, $p = 0.53$
CALGB 80701 Kulke et al. 2015 [36]	150	Well- or moderately differentiated PNETs	PFS	• Everolimus + bevacizumab • Everolimus	• 16.7 mos • 14.0 mos	HR 0.80, $p = 0.12$ ($\alpha = 0.15$)
NETTER-1 Strosberg et al. 2017 [28]	229	Well-differentiated midgut NETs	PFS	• ^{177}Lu-Dotatate + best supportive care • Octreotide	• Rate of PFS at 20 mos was 65.2% • 10.8%	HR 0.21, $p < 0.0001$
SWOG S0158 Yao et al.	427	G1/G2 NETs	PFS	• Octreotide + bevacizumab • Octreotide + interferon-alpha	• 16.6 mos • 15.4 mos	HR 0.93, $p = 0.55$

[a]*TTP* time to progression
[b]*mos* months
[c]*HR* hazard ratio
[d]*PFS* progression-free survival
[e]*OR* odds ratio

Table 22.3 Ongoing clinical trials

	Type of study	Estimated completion date	Estimated enrollment	Patient population	Treatment arms	Primary endpoint
NCT01841736 (A021202)	Phase II	Dec 2016	165	G1/G2 GI NETs	• Pazopanib • Placebo	PFS[a]
NCT01824875 (E2211)	Phase II	Jul 2017	145	Advanced PNETs	• Temozolomide • Temozolomide + capecitabine	PFS
NCT02820857	Phase II	Jan 2020	124	G3 NEC, 2nd line setting	• FOLFIRI + bevacizumab • FOLFIRI	OS[b]
NCT02113800	Phase II	Feb 2018	40	G3 NEC, 2nd line setting	• Everolimus	AE[c]
NCT02595424 (EA2142)	Phase II	Jan 2018	126	G3 NEC, 1st line setting	• Temozolomide + capecitabine • Cisplatin + etoposide	PFS

[a]*PFS* progression-free survival
[b]*OS* overall survival
[c]*AE* adverse effects

Grade 1 and 2 Gastrointestinal Neuroendocrine Tumors

Somatostatin Analogues

Grade 1 and grade 2 gastrointestinal neuroendocrine tumors, also called carcinoids, are slow-growing cancers generally unresponsive to cytotoxic chemotherapy, and the mainstay of treatment is somatostatin receptor inhibition. Given their high levels of expression on intestinal NETs, somatostatin receptors are a natural target for somatostatin analogues and provide benefit in the form of both symptom relief for functional tumors and antiproliferative benefit [10]. The binding of somatostatin to its receptors on the tumor surface results in the inhibition of serotonin production by the tumor. While the body does produce somatostatin, the therapeutic use of endogenous somatostatin is limited by its half-life, as it is rapidly inactivated [10]. Octreotide was the first synthetic somatostatin analogue and was eventually developed into a long-acting repeatable (LAR) octreotide acetate. Octreotide and other somatostatin analogues are effective in controlling hormone secretion from functional NETs and thus were initially approved for symptomatic management of carcinoid syndrome.

In addition to symptom control, octreotide has an antitumor effect in well-differentiated midgut carcinoids. The PROMID phase III trial randomized 85 patients with treatment-naïve well-differentiated metastatic midgut NETs to receive either octreotide LAR or placebo [11]. This approach demonstrated a benefit in median progression-free survival (PFS) of 14 months in the octreotide group versus 6 months in the placebo group (HR 0.34, 95% CI 0.20–0.59, $p = 0.000072$). A subgroup analysis suggested no difference in time to progression between patients with a functional and a nonfunctional tumor (HR 1.38, 95% CI 0.81–2.37, $p = 0.24$). This study overall reported an antitumor benefit for octreotide in both functional and nonfunctional well-differentiated metastatic midgut NETs, and as a result, it is the current frontline standard of care therapy for treatment of this disease [12].

To further evaluate the antiproliferative benefit of somatostatin analogues in a broader group of well-differentiated NETs, lanreotide was tested in patients with nonfunctional tumors in the phase III CLARINET trial [13]. A total of 204 patients with an advanced grade 1 or 2 NET of the pancreas, midgut, hindgut, or unknown origin were randomized to receive lanreotide or placebo. A clear benefit in median PFS was shown in the lanreotide group (median PFS not reached) versus 18 months in the placebo group. Eighty-eight patients continued on an open-label extension study and ultimately showed a median

PFS in the lanreotide group of 32.8 months [14]. Of note, this study included more patients with a large hepatic tumor volume compared with the PROMID study. Positive results from this study confirmed that treatment with a somatostatin analogue could be initiated as treatment for patients with well-differentiated NETs arising in a primary site beyond just the midgut and also in patients with either a functional or nonfunctional tumor. Patients harboring a large tumor volume in the liver also derived survival benefit.

Targeted Therapies

The mammalian target of rapamycin (mTOR) pathway has been implicated in neuroendocrine tumor pathogenesis [15]. As such, everolimus, an oral inhibitor of mTOR, has been studied extensively as a treatment option in G1 and G2 NETs. An initial phase II study combining everolimus and octreotide showed a modest response rate of 20% in 60 patients with carcinoid and PNETS [16]. The combination was further evaluated in RADIANT-2, a phase III trial that randomized 429 patients with previously treated advanced carcinoid to everolimus plus octreotide or placebo plus octreotide [17]. The median PFS for the everolimus group compared with the placebo group was 16.4 months versus 11.3 months; however this did not achieve statistical significance (HR 0.77, 95% CI 0.59–1.00, $p = 0.026$). RADIANT-4 was subsequently designed to test everolimus as a monotherapy in patients specifically with nonfunctioning tumors. A total of 302 patients with previously treated G1 and G2 nonfunctional NETs of intestinal and lung origin were randomized to everolimus or placebo [18]. Median PFS was 11 months in the everolimus group compared with 3.9 months in the placebo group (HR 0.48, 95% CI 0.35–0.67, $p < 0.00001$), confirming a role for everolimus in nonfunctioning low- to intermediate-grade NETs of the lung and GI tract.

Interferon-Alpha

Interferon (IFN) was first studied as a therapeutic strategy in neuroendocrine tumors in the 1980s, when it was becoming clear that cytotoxic agents were largely ineffective. Interferon-alpha was felt to be a promising antiproliferative agent, but its use was limited by its toxicity. A phase II trial enrolling patients with progressive well-differentiated GI and pancreatic NETs showed that pegylated-interferon-alpha (PEG-IFN) produced a partial response or stable disease in 13 of 17 patients, with no grade 3 or 4 toxicities [19]. Interest in combining interferon with octreotide and comparing it to new anti-angiogenic targeted agents led to the SWOG 0158 study. In this phase III trial, 427 patients with an advanced G1 or G2 NET were randomized to octreotide plus IFN versus octreotide plus bevacizumab. Although there was a higher radiographic response rate in the bevacizumab group compared with the interferon-alpha group (12% versus 4%), there was no PFS difference between the two treatment arms (HR 0.93, 95% CI 0.73–1.18, $p = 0.55$). While one arm did not appear superior to the other, given that interferon-alpha and octreotide both have activity in this disease entity, this study suggested that bevacizumab and interferon-alpha likely have similar antitumor activity [20].

Peptide Receptor Radionuclide Therapy (PRRT)

With the many attractive features of somatostatin analogues—an effective antiproliferative agent, an effective therapy for reducing hormone-mediated symptoms, a tumor-specific targeted therapy, and the ability to use radiolabeled somatostatin analogues to visualize NETs radiographically—peptide receptor radionuclide therapy (PRRT) was developed as a treatment strategy in carcinoids. PRRT was initially studied using [^{111}In-DTPA^0]octreotide, the radiolabeled somatostatin analogue used for the octreotide scan. Unfortunately, tumor responses with this agent were uncommon [21]. However, interest in this modality continued as more radiolabeled somatostatin analogues were developed. [^{90}Y-DOTA^0,Tyr^3]octreotide showed promise in inducing partial and complete remissions

[22–24], and the newest radiolabeled somatostatin analogue, [^{177}Lu-DOTA^0,Tyr^3]octreotate, showed similar activity but less hematologic toxicity than [^{90}Y-DOTA^0,Tyr^3]octreotide in a phase I/II trial comparing the two [25–27]. PRRT utilizing [^{177}Lu-DOTA^0,Tyr^3]octreotate, or ^{177}Lu-Dotatate, ultimately showed a progression-free survival benefit over octreotide in the phase III NETTER-1 study [28]. In this trial, 229 patients with well-differentiated (Ki-67 < 20%) metastatic midgut NETs, with the presence of somatostatin receptors confirmed by octreotide scan and progression on previous octreotide LAR, were randomized to ^{177}Lu-Dotatate plus octreotide LAR 30 mg versus high-dose octreotide LAR 60 mg alone. At the time of initial analysis, the 20-month progression-free survival rate was 65.2% in the ^{177}Lu-Dotatate group (95% CI 50.0–76.8) versus 10.8% in the control group (95% CI 3.5–23.0), with the median PFS not yet reached in the ^{177}Lu-Dotatate group and 8.4 months in the control group (HR 0.21; 95% CI 0.13–0.33, $p < 0.0001$). The response rate, a secondary objective, was 18% in the PRRT group vs 3% in the octreotide alone group ($p < 0.001$). The most common adverse effects in the PRRT group were nausea (59%) and vomiting (47%), compared with the control group (12% and 10%, respectively). Grade 3 or 4 toxicities were uncommon in the PRRT group, including lymphopenia (9%), vomiting (7%), diarrhea (3%), fatigue (2%), and thrombocytopenia (2%), compared with no grade 3 or 4 hematologic toxicities in the control group. These results demonstrate that PRRT is strikingly efficacious in terms of its progression-free survival benefit without significant added toxicities as compared with previous therapies making it an exciting new treatment modality for the management of metastatic carcinoid. A great unknown at this time, however, is where this modality should be used in relation to other treatment options. This is of significant importance as there is some overlap in toxicity profiles, and it would be ideal to minimize toxicities experienced so as to allow patients to ultimately receive all forms of available treatment.

G1/G2 Pancreatic Neuroendocrine Tumors

Somatostatin Analogues

While somatostatin analogues are used for symptom control for carcinoids and functional G1 and G2 pancreatic neuroendocrine tumors (PNETs), the data is less clear on an antiproliferative tumor benefit in nonfunctional PNETs. While the PROMID study excluded PNETs, the phase III CLARINET study included 91 well- and moderately differentiated PNETs with a Ki-67 < 10% (out of a total $n = 204$). The progression-free survival in the overall study population of patients lanreotide as part of the open-label extension study was reported as 32.8 months [14], versus a median PFS of 18 months in the placebo arm from the core study [13]. As such, there is consensus that somatostatin analogues may be used as an antiproliferative agent in the management of PNETs, particularly in patients with a Ki-67 < 10%. Despite the Ki-67 cutoff identified in this study, this is generally not used to make treatment decisions for patients receiving PNETs, and a large majority of patients with a well- or moderately differentiated PNET will receive treatment with a somatostatin analogue. Further studies delineating a Ki-67 cutoff value are needed in order to stratify patients to receive somatostatin analogues versus initiation of more aggressive therapy [6].

Targeted Therapies

Prior to the advent of targeted therapies, cytotoxic chemotherapy was the only approved treatment option in this disease. The activity of everolimus in intestinal NETs as discussed previously prompted evaluation in advanced PNETs. A single-arm phase II study assessing daily everolimus in patients with PNETs who had developed disease progression while on cytotoxic therapy demonstrated a median PFS of 16 months [29]. The activity of everolimus was subsequently confirmed by comparing it to placebo in the phase III RADIANT-3 study, which randomized

410 patients with advanced G1 and G2 PNETs to receive either everolimus or placebo. Median PFS was 11 months in the everolimus group versus 4.6 months in the placebo group, establishing everolimus as a therapeutic standard for patients with advanced PNETs [30].

In addition to mTOR inhibitors, inhibition of angiogenesis has been investigated in G1 and G2 PNETs, which are highly vascular tumors and are known to express vascular endothelial growth factor (VEGF) and platelet-derived growth factor receptors (PDGFR) [31]. Sunitinib, a small molecule tyrosine kinase inhibitor with activity against VEGFR, PDGFR, as well as other growth factor receptors, was evaluated in a phase II study, demonstrating a response rate of 16.7% and maintaining stable disease in 68% of patients with PNETs ($n = 66$) [32]. Of note, there did not appear to be activity in carcinoids, with a response rate of only 2.4% in 41 carcinoid patients. A phase III study confirmed the efficacy of sunitinib in PNETs, randomizing 171 patients to receive either sunitinib or placebo [33]. The study was stopped early in favor of the sunitinib group, with a median PFS of 11.4 months compared to 5.5 months in the placebo group, establishing sunitinib as a treatment standard in PNET. Based on the success of sunitinib, another VEGF inhibitor, bevacizumab, was found in a single-arm phase II study to have a median PFS of 13.6 months in 22 patients with G1/G2 advanced PNETs [34], similar to the progression-free survival from the phase III sunitinib study.

As both mTOR and angiogenesis pathways had been implicated in the pathogenesis of this disease and agents targeting both of these pathways had shown treatment benefit, dual pathway inhibition has been investigated. Bevacizumab was studied in combination with temsirolimus in a single-arm, phase II study, showing a response rate of 41% and a median PFS of 13.2 months in 58 patients with advanced G1/G2 PNETs [35]. In PNETs, combination therapy with bevacizumab and everolimus was studied in CALGB 80701, a phase II trial that randomized 150 patients with advanced PNETs to everolimus plus bevacizumab or everolimus alone [36]. The authors demonstrated an improved progression-free survival in the combination arm as compared to everolimus alone with a PFS of 16.7 months versus 14 months, respectively ($\alpha = 0.15$; HR 0.80, 95% CI 0.55–1.17, $p = 0.12$). Also observed was an increased response rate in the combination arm, as compared to single-agent everolimus at 31% and 12%, respectively ($p = 0.005$). Despite these positive results, the overall rate of grade 3 or 4 adverse events was much higher in the combination arm compared with everolimus alone at 81% vs 49%. This degree of toxicity, along with a modest PFS benefit, is likely to limit the use of combination therapy with an mTOR inhibitor and an anti-angiogenic agent in clinical practice. However, aside from cytotoxic chemotherapy, this regimen does show one of the better response rates so may be used in particular cases where a reduction in tumor burden is desired.

Additional tyrosine kinase inhibitors have also been investigated in early clinical trials. In a phase II study of advanced PNETs and carcinoids, sorafenib, a multi-targeted kinase inhibitor, demonstrated a modest response rate of 10% [37]. A phase II study of pazopanib, a multitargeted agent against VEGF, PDGFR, and c-KIT, in 52 patients with advanced G1 and G2 NETs showed a 21.9% response rate in PNETs ($n = 32$); however no response was detected in the carcinoid group ($n = 20$) [38]. Median PFS, a secondary endpoint, was promising in both groups, 14.4 months in the PNET cohort (95% CI 5.9–22.9) and 12.2 months in the carcinoid cohort (95% CI 3–19.9). Finally, cabozantinib, a multi-targeted kinase inhibitor against VEGF, MET, AXL, and RET, has been studied in a single-arm phase II trial that enrolled 61 patients with advanced PNETs ($n = 20$) and carcinoids ($n = 41$) [39]. Response rate, the primary endpoint, was found to be 15% in the PNET cohort (95% CI 5–36) and 15% in the carcinoid cohort (95% CI 7–28). Median PFS, a secondary endpoint, was 21.8 months in the PNET cohort (95% CI 8.5–32) and 31.4 months in the carcinoid cohort (95% CI 8.5-not reached), suggesting an improvement in survival with cabozantinib compared with historical results. A randomized phase III study assessing pazopanib versus placebo in patients with advanced carcinoid has been conducted with results pending at this time (A021202, NCT01841736). A phase III study assessing cabozantinib in PNETs and carcinoids is currently in development.

Cytotoxic Chemotherapy

The main goal of cytotoxic therapy in PNETs is to reduce the tumor burden in bulky or progressive disease. This can be beneficial in regard to controlling tumor growth as well as decreasing the level of hormone production in patients with functional tumors. As such, response rate is an important endpoint in these clinical trials. Initially, streptozocin combinations were assessed for tumor response in PNETs. Moertel et al. randomized 105 patients with advanced PNETs to streptozocin plus 5FU versus streptozocin plus doxorubicin versus chlorozotocin alone [40]. The combination of streptozocin plus doxorubicin offered a PFS benefit of 20 months as compared with 6.9 months in the streptozocin plus 5FU group. In another single-arm phase II study, the triplet regimen of streptozocin, doxorubicin, and 5FU produced a response rate of 30% in 84 patients with advanced PNETs and a median PFS of 9.3 months [41]. Despite the favorable results observed in these studies, streptozocin-based regimens are not commonly used in clinical practice due to the unfavorable side effect profile including nausea, vomiting, myelosuppression, renal insufficiency, and fatigue.

Temozolomide-based regimens have demonstrated promising results in several early clinical studies. A combination of temozolomide and thalidomide was evaluated in a single-arm phase II study of 29 patients with advanced NETs. In this study, a response rate of 45% was observed in PNETs ($n = 11$), whereas 7% of carcinoid patients showed tumor response ($n = 14$) [42]. Temozolomide in combination with bevacizumab also showed promise in a single-arm phase II study of 33 patients with advanced NETs, with a response rate of 33% in PNETs ($n = 15$) and 0 carcinoid patients showing a response [43]. The combination of temozolomide and capecitabine was studied in a single-center retrospective study of 30 patients with PNETs. In this study a response rate of 70% was reported [44]. As this was the highest response rate observed among any treatment regimen for treatment of this disease, a large prospective study was conducted assessing temozolomide vs temozolomide plus capecitabine in patients with advanced PNETs (E2211). The results of this important trial are pending at this time.

G3 Neuroendocrine Carcinomas

Cytotoxic Chemotherapy

G3 neuroendocrine carcinomas (NECs) are aggressive cancers, and treatment is limited to cytotoxic chemotherapy. There is little data to guide therapy; however much of the guidelines for high-grade neuroendocrine carcinomas are extrapolated from clinical trials in small cell carcinoma [45, 46]. Furthermore, most of the data evaluating a NEC-specific population are retrospective or small phase II studies. In 1999, a retrospective study examined the response rates of 53 patients with well-differentiated NETs or poorly differentiated NECs after receiving cisplatin plus etoposide chemotherapy [47]. The poorly differentiated group had a much higher response rate of 41% as compared with 9% in the well-differentiated group. The three-drug combination of carboplatin, etoposide, and paclitaxel was evaluated in a phase II study of 78 patients with poorly differentiated NECs. The reported response rate in this study was 53%, with no obvious advantage in efficacy over standard doublet therapy [48]. As such, this three-drug combination is not commonly used; however taxane-based therapy is a common choice for second-line therapy.

Regimens other than platinum and etoposide have been investigated in small retrospective studies in the second-line setting. FOLFOX showed a partial response of 29% in a French single-center retrospective study of 20 patients [49]. Temozolomide, alone or in combination with capecitabine and with or without bevacizumab, showed a partial response of 33% in a retrospective study of 25 patients from two oncology centers in Norway and Sweden [50]. Based on the results of this study, a temozolomide-based regimen has been thought by many to be a potential alternative treatment strategy to platinum and etoposide chemotherapy. The efficacy of these regimens needs further evaluation; however prospective studies have historically been difficult due to the rarity of this disease. As platinum and etoposide have not ever been officially evaluated in G3 NECs previously, there is an ongoing randomized phase II clinical trial of cisplatin or carboplatin and etoposide versus temozolomide and capecitabine (EA2142, NCT02595424). The results of this study should finally provide some prospective data regarding the role of each of these treatment regimens in patients with advanced G3 NECs.

Whether this group of heterogeneous cancers can be further stratified is an ongoing question in G3 NEC. The NORDIC study in 2012 analyzed clinical data from 74 studies in G3 NEC for predictive and prognostic factors [51]. This study identified a possible subgroup of patients with an improved survival. Patients with a Ki-67 less than 55% had a median survival of 14 months compared with 10 months in patients with Ki-67 greater than 55%. The data also suggested that patients with a Ki-67 less than 55% are not as responsive to platinum-based chemotherapy compared to patients with a Ki-67 greater than 55% (RR 15% versus 42%). These results underscored the idea that NECs are a heterogeneous group of cancers that are not fully classified and with a wide range of clinical behavior and prognosis [52]. Further delineating tumor types in this group and offering treatment that best fits their clinical risk would greatly benefit this patient population, and this is an area of active investigation.

> **Conclusion**
>
> GEP-NETs are a diverse group of cancers, and systemic therapy for metastatic disease is an ongoing area of clinical investigation. In particular, PRRT in well-differentiated carcinoids and PNETs has made a dramatic improvement in extending progression-free and overall survival. Targeted small molecule therapies in combination with somatostatin analogues have proved to be effective in G1/G2 intestinal and pancreatic NETs. With the rapid evolution of treatment options for patients with both PNETs and carcinoids, one unknown question at this time is how to best sequence these agents so as to provide patients with the greatest longevity while keeping toxicity to a minimum. As patients with these diseases have relatively long periods of survival, this question will likely take many years to answer, but it is an active area of investigation. G3 NECs continue to be associated with poor survival and limited treatment options, and ongoing clinical trials may help to further risk stratify this group.

References

1. Lawrence B, Gustafsson BI, Chan A, Svejda B, Kidd M, Modlin IM. The epidemiology of gastroenteropancreatic neuroendocrine tumors. Endocrinol Metab Clin North Am. 2011;40(1):1–18.
2. Rindi G, Petrone G, Inzani F. The 2010 WHO classification of digestive neuroendocrine neoplasms: a critical appraisal four years after its introduction. Endocr Pathol. 2014;25(2):186–92.
3. Eads JR, Meropol NJ. A new era for the systemic therapy of neuroendocrine tumors. Oncologist. 2012;17(3):326–38.
4. Oberg KE. Gastrointestinal neuroendocrine tumors. Ann Oncol. 2010;21(Suppl 7):vii72–80.
5. Halfdanarson TR, Rabe KG, Rubin J, Petersen GM. Pancreatic neuroendocrine tumors (PNETs): incidence, prognosis and recent trend toward improved survival. Ann Oncol. 2008;19(10):1727–33.
6. Pavel M, O'Toole D, Costa F, Capdevila J, Gross D, Kianmanesh R, et al. ENETS Consensus Guidelines update for the management of distant metastatic disease of intestinal, pancreatic, bronchial neuroendocrine neoplasms (NEN) and NEN of unknown primary site. Neuroendocrinology. 2016;103(2):172–85.
7. Frilling A, Modlin IM, Kidd M, Russell C, Breitenstein S, Salem R, et al. Recommendations for management of patients with neuroendocrine liver metastases. Lancet Oncol. 2014;15(1):e8–21.
8. Pape UF, Berndt U, Muller-Nordhorn J, Bohmig M, Roll S, Koch M, et al. Prognostic factors of long-term outcome in gastroenteropancreatic neuroendocrine tumours. Endocr Relat Cancer. 2008;15(4):1083–97.

9. Yao JC, Hassan M, Phan A, Dagohoy C, Leary C, Mares JE, et al. One hundred years after "carcinoid": epidemiology of and prognostic factors for neuroendocrine tumors in 35,825 cases in the United States. J Clin Oncol. 2008;26(18):3063–72.
10. Lamberts SW, van der Lely AJ, de Herder WW, Hofland LJ. Octreotide. N Engl J Med. 1996;334(4):246–54.
11. Rinke A, Muller HH, Schade-Brittinger C, Klose KJ, Barth P, Wied M, et al. Placebo-controlled, double-blind, prospective, randomized study on the effect of octreotide LAR in the control of tumor growth in patients with metastatic neuroendocrine midgut tumors: a report from the PROMID Study Group. J Clin Oncol. 2009;27(28):4656–63.
12. National Comprehensive Cancer Network. Neuroendocrine tumors (Version 2.2017). 2017. https://www.nccn.org/professionals/physician_gls/pdf/neuroendocrine.pdf. Accessed 6 Apr 2017.
13. Caplin ME, Pavel M, Cwikla JB, Phan AT, Raderer M, Sedlackova E, et al. Lanreotide in metastatic enteropancreatic neuroendocrine tumors. N Engl J Med. 2014;371(3):224–33.
14. Caplin ME, Pavel M, Cwikla JB, Phan AT, Raderer M, Sedlackova E, et al. Anti-tumour effects of lanreotide for pancreatic and intestinal neuroendocrine tumours: the CLARINET open-label extension study. Endocr Relat Cancer. 2016;23(3):191–9.
15. Moreno A, Akcakanat A, Munsell MF, Soni A, Yao JC, Meric-Bernstam F. Antitumor activity of rapamycin and octreotide as single agents or in combination in neuroendocrine tumors. Endocr Relat Cancer. 2008;15(1):257–66.
16. Yao JC, Phan AT, Chang DZ, Wolff RA, Hess K, Gupta S, et al. Efficacy of RAD001 (everolimus) and octreotide LAR in advanced low- to intermediate-grade neuroendocrine tumors: results of a phase II study. J Clin Oncol. 2008;26(26):4311–8.
17. Pavel ME, Hainsworth JD, Baudin E, Peeters M, Horsch D, Winkler RE, et al. Everolimus plus octreotide long-acting repeatable for the treatment of advanced neuroendocrine tumours associated with carcinoid syndrome (RADIANT-2): a randomised, placebo-controlled, phase 3 study. Lancet. 2011;378(9808):2005–12.
18. Yao JC, Fazio N, Singh S, Buzzoni R, Carnaghi C, Wolin E, et al. Everolimus for the treatment of advanced, non-functional neuroendocrine tumours of the lung or gastrointestinal tract (RADIANT-4): a randomised, placebo-controlled, phase 3 study. Lancet. 2016;387(10022):968–77.
19. Pavel ME, Baum U, Hahn EG, Schuppan D, Lohmann T. Efficacy and tolerability of pegylated IFN-alpha in patients with neuroendocrine gastroenteropancreatic carcinomas. J Interf Cytokine Res. 2006;26(1):8–13.
20. Yao JC, Guthrie KA, Moran C, Strosberg JR, Kulke MH, Chan JA, et al. Phase III prospective randomized comparison trial of depot octreotide plus interferon alfa-2b versus depot octreotide plus bevacizumab in patients with advanced carcinoid tumors: SWOG S0518. J Clin Oncol. 2017;35(15):1695–703. https://doi.org/10.1200/JCO.2016.70.4072.
21. Kwekkeboom DJ, Mueller-Brand J, Paganelli G, Anthony LB, Pauwels S, Kvols LK, et al. Overview of results of peptide receptor radionuclide therapy with 3 radiolabeled somatostatin analogs. J Nucl Med. 2005;46(Suppl 1):62S–6S.
22. Waldherr C, Pless M, Maecke HR, Haldemann A, Mueller-Brand J. The clinical value of [90Y-DOTA]-D-Phe1-Tyr3-octreotide (90Y-DOTATOC) in the treatment of neuroendocrine tumours: a clinical phase II study. Ann Oncol. 2001;12(7):941–5.
23. Bushnell DL Jr, O'Dorisio TM, O'Dorisio MS, Menda Y, Hicks RJ, Van Cutsem E, et al. 90Y-edotreotide for metastatic carcinoid refractory to octreotide. J Clin Oncol. 2010;28(10):1652–9.
24. Imhof A, Brunner P, Marincek N, Briel M, Schindler C, Rasch H, et al. Response, survival, and long-term toxicity after therapy with the radiolabeled somatostatin analogue [90Y-DOTA]-TOC in metastasized neuroendocrine cancers. J Clin Oncol. 2011;29(17):2416–23.
25. Bodei L, Cremonesi M, Grana CM, Fazio N, Iodice S, Baio SM, et al. Peptide receptor radionuclide therapy with (1)(7)(7)Lu-DOTATATE: the IEO phase I-II study. Eur J Nucl Med Mol Imaging. 2011;38(12):2125–35.
26. Romer A, Seiler D, Marincek N, Brunner P, Koller MT, Ng QK, et al. Somatostatin-based radiopeptide therapy with [177Lu-DOTA]-TOC versus [90Y-DOTA]-TOC in neuroendocrine tumours. Eur J Nucl Med Mol Imaging. 2014;41(2):214–22.
27. Bodei L, Kidd M, Paganelli G, Grana CM, Drozdov I, Cremonesi M, et al. Long-term tolerability of PRRT in 807 patients with neuroendocrine tumours: the value and limitations of clinical factors. Eur J Nucl Med Mol Imaging. 2015;42(1):5–19.
28. Strosberg J, El-Haddad G, Wolin E, Hendifar A, Yao J, Chasen B, et al. Phase 3 trial of 177Lu-Dotatate for midgut neuroendocrine tumors. N Engl J Med. 2017;376(2):125–35.
29. Yao JC, Lombard-Bohas C, Baudin E, Kvols LK, Rougier P, Ruszniewski P, et al. Daily oral everolimus activity in patients with metastatic pancreatic neuroendocrine tumors after failure of cytotoxic chemotherapy: a phase II trial. J Clin Oncol. 2010;28(1):69–76.
30. Yao JC, Shah MH, Ito T, Bohas CL, Wolin EM, Van Cutsem E, et al. Everolimus for advanced pancreatic neuroendocrine tumors. N Engl J Med. 2011;364(6):514–23.
31. Fjallskog ML, Lejonklou MH, Oberg KE, Eriksson BK, Janson ET. Expression of molecular targets for tyrosine kinase receptor antagonists in malignant endocrine pancreatic tumors. Clin Cancer Res. 2003;9(4):1469–73.
32. Kulke MH, Lenz HJ, Meropol NJ, Posey J, Ryan DP, Picus J, et al. Activity of sunitinib in patients with advanced neuroendocrine tumors. J Clin Oncol. 2008;26(20):3403–10.
33. Raymond E, Dahan L, Raoul JL, Bang YJ, Borbath I, Lombard-Bohas C, et al. Sunitinib malate for the treatment of pancreatic neuroendocrine tumors. N Engl J Med. 2011;364(6):501–13.

34. Hobday TJ, Yin J, Pettinger A, Strosberg JR, Reidy DL, Chen HX, Erlichman C. Multicenter prospective phase II trial of bevacizumab (bev) for progressive pancreatic neuroendocrine tumor (PNET). J Clin Oncol. 2015;33(15 Suppl):4096.
35. Hobday TJ, Qin R, Reidy-Lagunes D, Moore MJ, Strosberg J, Kaubisch A, et al. Multicenter phase II trial of temsirolimus and bevacizumab in pancreatic neuroendocrine tumors. J Clin Oncol. 2015;33(14):1551–6.
36. Kulke MH, Niedzwiecki D, Foster NR, Fruth B, Kunz PL, Kennecke HF, et al. Randomized phase II study of everolimus versus everolimus plus bevacizumab in patients with locally advanced or metastatic pancreatic neuroendocrine tumors, CALGB 80701. J Clin Oncol. 2015;33(Suppl 15):4005.
37. Hobday TJ, Rubin J, Holen K, Picus J, Donehower R, Marschke R, Maples W, Lloyd R, Mahoney M, Erlichman C. MC044h, a phase II trial of sorafenib in patients with metastatic neuroendocrine tumors (NET): a Phase II Consortium study. J Clin Oncol. 2007;25(90180):4504.
38. Phan AT, Halperin DM, Chan JA, Fogelman DR, Hess KR, Malinowski P, et al. Pazopanib and depot octreotide in advanced, well-differentiated neuroendocrine tumours: a multicentre, single-group, phase 2 study. Lancet Oncol. 2015;16(6):695–703.
39. Chan JA, Abrams TA. Phase II trial of cabozantinib in patients with carcinoid and pancreatic neuroendocrine tumors. J Clin Oncol. 2017;35(4 Suppl):228.
40. Moertel CG, Lefkopoulo M, Lipsitz S, Hahn RG, Klaassen D. Streptozocin-doxorubicin, streptozocin-fluorouracil or chlorozotocin in the treatment of advanced islet-cell carcinoma. N Engl J Med. 1992;326(8):519–23.
41. Kouvaraki MA, Ajani JA, Hoff P, Wolff R, Evans DB, Lozano R, et al. Fluorouracil, doxorubicin, and streptozocin in the treatment of patients with locally advanced and metastatic pancreatic endocrine carcinomas. J Clin Oncol. 2004;22(23):4762–71.
42. Kulke MH, Stuart K, Enzinger PC, Ryan DP, Clark JW, Muzikansky A, et al. Phase II study of temozolomide and thalidomide in patients with metastatic neuroendocrine tumors. J Clin Oncol. 2006;24(3):401–6.
43. Chan JA, Stuart K, Earle CC, Clark JW, Bhargava P, Miksad R, et al. Prospective study of bevacizumab plus temozolomide in patients with advanced neuroendocrine tumors. J Clin Oncol. 2012;30(24):2963–8.
44. Strosberg JR, Fine RL, Choi J, Nasir A, Coppola D, Chen DT, et al. First-line chemotherapy with capecitabine and temozolomide in patients with metastatic pancreatic endocrine carcinomas. Cancer. 2011;117(2):268–75.
45. Sorbye H, Strosberg J, Baudin E, Klimstra DS, Yao JC. Gastroenteropancreatic high-grade neuroendocrine carcinoma. Cancer. 2014;120(18):2814–23.
46. Eads JR. Poorly differentiated neuroendocrine tumors. Hematol Oncol Clin North Am. 2016;30(1):151–62.
47. Mitry E, Baudin E, Ducreux M, Sabourin JC, Rufie P, Aparicio T, et al. Treatment of poorly differentiated neuroendocrine tumours with etoposide and cisplatin. Br J Cancer. 1999;81(8):1351–5.
48. Hainsworth JD, Spigel DR, Litchy S, Greco FA. Phase II trial of paclitaxel, carboplatin, and etoposide in advanced poorly differentiated neuroendocrine carcinoma: a Minnie Pearl Cancer Research Network Study. J Clin Oncol. 2006;24(22):3548–54.
49. Hadoux J, Malka D, Planchard D, Scoazec JY, Caramella C, Guigay J, et al. Post-first-line FOLFOX chemotherapy for grade 3 neuroendocrine carcinoma. Endocr Relat Cancer. 2015;22(3):289–98.
50. Welin S, Sorbye H, Sebjornsen S, Knappskog S, Busch C, Oberg K. Clinical effect of temozolomide-based chemotherapy in poorly differentiated endocrine carcinoma after progression on first-line chemotherapy. Cancer. 2011;117(20):4617–22.
51. Sorbye H, Welin S, Langer SW, Vestermark LW, Holt N, Osterlund P, et al. Predictive and prognostic factors for treatment and survival in 305 patients with advanced gastrointestinal neuroendocrine carcinoma (WHO G3): the NORDIC NEC study. Ann Oncol. 2013;24(1):152–60.
52. Kidd M, Modlin I, Oberg K. Towards a new classification of gastroenteropancreatic neuroendocrine neoplasms. Nat Rev Clin Oncol. 2016;13(11):691–705.
53. Wolin EM, Jarzab B, Eriksson B, Walter T, Toumpanakis C, Morse MA, et al. Phase III study of pasireotide longacting release in patients with metastatic neuroendocrine tumors and carcinoid symptoms refractory to available somatostatin analogues. Drug Des Devel Ther. 2015;9:5075–86.

Patient Selection and Guidelines for Resection and Liver-Directed Therapies: Non-colorectal, Non-neuroendocrine Liver Metastases

Zhi Ven Fong, George A. Poultsides, and Motaz Qadan

Introduction

The liver represents a common site of metastatic disease, particularly from gastrointestinal neoplasms, given its role in the portal circulation. Hepatic resection and liver-directed therapies have been associated with favorable survival for patients with colorectal cancer liver metastases, with most contemporary studies reporting a 5-year survival rate of 40% or higher [1–3]. Similarly, surgical treatment of hepatic metastases from well-differentiated neuroendocrine tumors has been shown to be beneficial, with 5-year survival rates reaching 70% [4, 5]. For both diseases, these improved outcomes have largely been a result of a multidisciplinary approach, including advances in systemic chemotherapy, patient selection, preoperative staging, and intraoperative and perioperative management.

With these encouraging results, surgeons have been exploring the indications of liver resections for metastatic disease from other primary tumors. However, little is known regarding the appropriateness of surgical treatment of non-colorectal, non-neuroendocrine (NCNN) liver metastases. This is largely due to the rarity of isolated liver metastases from such primaries and the fact that most studies have reported on outcomes of liver metastasectomy from a multitude of primary sites without a specific focus on individual histologic subtypes [6, 7]. In this chapter, we aim to review the current literature on the surgical treatment of NCNN liver metastases with emphasis on prognostic indicators and patient selection strategies for treatment.

Epidemiology of Non-colorectal, Non-neuroendocrine Liver Metastases

In a recent large systematic review of all NCNN liver metastasis cohort studies, Uggeri and colleagues identified 30 studies encompassing 3849 patients with NCNN liver metastases, of whom 83.4% underwent surgical treatment. In their review, the most common primary site for patients

Z. V. Fong
Codman Center for Clinical Effectiveness in Surgery, Massachusetts General Hospital and Harvard Medical School, Boston, MA, USA
e-mail: ZFONG@PARTNERS.ORG

G. A. Poultsides (✉)
Division of Surgical Oncology, Department of Surgery, Stanford University Medical Center, Stanford University School of Medicine, Stanford University Hospital, Stanford, CA, USA
e-mail: gpoultsides@stanford.edu

M. Qadan
Codman Center for Clinical Effectiveness in Surgery, Massachusetts General Hospital and Harvard Medical School, Boston, MA, USA

Division of Surgical Oncology, Department of Surgery, Massachusetts General Hospital, Boston, MA, USA
e-mail: mqadan@mgh.harvard.edu

with NCNN liver metastases was the breast (917 out of 3849 patients, 23.8%), followed by the genitourinary (840 out of 3849 patients, 21.8%) and gastrointestinal tract (763 out of 3849 patients, 19.8%). Genitourinary primaries included organ sites such as gonads, kidneys, and uterine. Gastrointestinal primary sites included esophagus, stomach, pancreas, small bowel, gallbladder, and the biliary tract. Melanoma primaries comprised 7.7% of the cohort, and lung primaries 2.2%. Other less commonly reported primary lesions included soft tissue sarcomas, as well as head and neck, and adrenal primary sites.

Survival Outcomes

Of all the categories of NCNN liver metastasis primary sites, the **genitourinary** group appears to be associated with the best overall survival outcomes, with studies demonstrating a median survival of more than 60 months (Table 23.1) [8–14]. Within this subgroup, resections of NCNN liver metastases of ovarian [8, 9, 11, 15] and renal [8, 13, 16–20] primary sites were associated with the best outcomes, demonstrating pooled median survivals of 67.8 and 67.9 months, respectively. This was followed by those of testicular origin, with a pooled median survival of 61.7 months [8, 11, 12, 14, 21]. Conversely, those of uterine origin were associated with poorer survival, with studies reporting a median survival of 32 months [8]. It should be noted, however, that these data were limited to results provided by a single retrospective study of 43 patients, and more data points are likely needed to better identify the role of surgical treatment of NCNN liver metastases from the uterus [8]. As expected, all stated outcomes appear favorable at face value when compared with patients who were not felt to be candidates for surgical resection, with expected survival rates for patients with ovarian, renal, and uterine cancer being in the 10- to 20-month range with chemotherapy alone [22, 23].

Table 23.1 Pooled survival outcomes after resection of non-colorectal, non-neuroendocrine liver metastases

Category	Tumor type	No. of studies	No. of patients	Survival (months)		
				Median	Minimum	Maximum
Breast	Breast	27	1281	44.3	8	75
Gastrointestinal		31	684	22.3	5	58
	Esophagus	2	23	16.3	16	18
	GE junction	1	25	14	14	14
	Gastric	18	481	20.6	8.8	58
	Pancreas	2	55	18.1	13	20
	Duodenum	3	38	32.4	23	38
	Cholangiocarcinoma	1	13	28	28	28
	Gallbladder	3	21	26.2	5	42
	Small bowel	1	28	58	58	58
Genitourinary		16	549	63.4	5.4	142
	Testicular	4	153	61.7	5.4	82
	Ovary	4	119	67.8	26.3	98
	Renal	7	234	67.9	16	142
	Uterine	1	43	32	32	32
Others		35	1082	23.7	10	72
	GIST	5	106	31.9	28.8	40
	Sarcoma	4	189	53.8	23	72
	Melanoma	19	646	21.8	10	41
	Lung	2	36	16.1	16	17
	Head and neck	1	15	18	18	18
	Adrenal	4	90	40.9	22.8	63

Adapted from *Fitzgerald TL, Brinkley J, Banks S, et al. The benefits of liver resection for non-colorectal, non-neuroendocrine liver metastases: a systematic review. Langenbecks Arch Surg 2014; 399:989–1000*

The category with the second longest survival outcomes was **breast** as the primary site of NCNN liver metastases. In the largest study of breast cancer liver metastases treated surgically, Adam and colleagues evaluated long-term outcomes in 460 patients, and reported 5- and 10-year survivals of 41% and 22%, respectively, with an impressive median survival of 45 months [8]. These findings have been fairly congruent with other smaller series [6, 24–27], with more than 20 other studies reporting on 1281 patients pooling a median survival of 44.3 months [28]. In a comparative study, Mariani and colleagues reported an 80.7% 3-year survival rate in patients undergoing liver resection for metastatic breast cancer, which was significantly higher than the 50.9% survival in a matched cohort of patients who underwent observation [29]. This translated to a threefold lower risk of death in a subsequent adjusted analysis. A recent Markov model cost-utility analysis by Spolverato and colleagues demonstrated that liver resection followed by postoperative conventional systemic therapy in patients with breast cancer liver metastases was more cost-effective when compared with systemic therapy alone, particularly in patients with estrogen receptor-positive tumors [30]. Similarly, Sadot and colleagues demonstrated improved recurrence-free survival for patients undergoing surgical treatment versus medical therapy alone, thereby providing patients with significant periods of time off of systemic chemotherapy [31].

In contrast to patients with genitourinary and breast-derived liver metastases, patients with liver metastases originating from the **noncolorectal gastrointestinal tract** have been associated with poorer survival, with reported median survivals of approximately 20 months. This is largely driven by the dismal prognosis after liver resection of metastases from esophageal and pancreatic cancer, with reported median survivals of 6–8 months [8, 32, 33]. These figures are similar to expected survivals of patients with metastatic esophageal and pancreatic cancer who do not undergo resection [34, 35]. In a rare case-controlled study by Slotta and colleagues, the authors demonstrated no difference in survival in patients with metastatic liver cancer of gastrointestinal origin when undergoing surgical resection versus observation [36]. There are, however, certain subsets of gastrointestinal primaries that are associated with more favorable survival outcomes. For example, resection of small bowel adenocarcinoma liver metastases can be associated with prolonged survival, with median survival ranging from 32 months to as high as 58 months in selected patients [8, 33]. Along the same lines, liver metastasectomy for intestinal-type peri-ampullary cancers (intestinal-type ampullary or duodenal) has been shown to be associated with longer survival (median 23 versus 13 months) compared with their pancreaticobiliary-type counterparts (pancreatic, distal cholangiocarcinoma or pancreaticobiliary-type ampullary) [33]. Last, resections of liver metastases from gastrointestinal stromal tumors (GIST) have been associated with a median survival ranging from 28 to 40 months in the pre-imatinib era [37–40]. However, since its discovery, this agent has drastically altered the natural history of this disease in both the localized and metastatic settings, and in a later study of patients who received adjuvant imatinib, the 5-year survival after liver metastasectomy was shown to exceed 50% (Fig. 23.1) [41].

Survival outcomes for **melanoma**-derived liver metastases reported in the literature have been largely incongruent. In a cohort study of 148 patients performed by Adam and colleagues, the authors reported a 5-year and median survival of 21% and 20 months, respectively, in resected patients [8]. However, in a separate multi-institutional study by Groeschl and colleagues, the 5-year and median survival was 36% and 39 months, respectively [6]. This difference may be explained by the site of the primary melanoma; ocular melanomas are more likely to metastasize to the liver as the sole site of metastases, whereas cutaneous melanomas are usually more widely disseminated by the time they are detected in the liver [42, 43]. In addition, it is important to understand that ocular melanoma is largely unresponsive to immunotherapy agents, which have recently been demonstrated to have significant efficacy for stage IV cutaneous malignant melanoma. As such, whereas the surgical

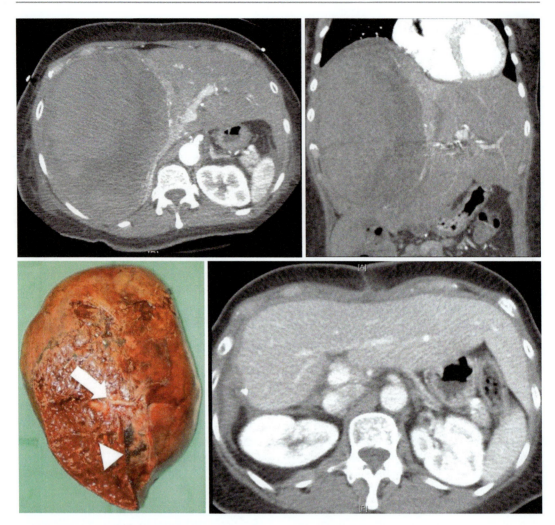

Fig. 23.1 Liver metastasectomy for GIST. A 65-year-old woman who presented with acute-onset right upper quadrant pain and anemia, 3 years s/p resection of a jejunal GIST. Computed tomography imaging (top row) revealed a large liver metastasis replacing the right hepatic lobe with intratumoral hemorrhage. The tumor was resected with a right hepatectomy via the anterior approach. The specimen is shown in the bottom left image. Note the stapled origin of the right hepatic vein (arrow) and the groove of the retrohepatic vena cava (triangle). Imaging 6 weeks postoperatively (bottom right) shows adequate hypertrophy of the liver remnant

treatment of cutaneous melanoma liver metastases may be considered the last resort, resection of liver ocular melanoma may generally be viewed as the first-line option. In an analysis of 255 patients with ocular melanoma liver metastases who underwent liver resection, the median survival reported was 27 months if microscopically complete (R0) resection is achieved [44]. However, the presence of miliary disease often precludes the performance of an R0 resection for this disease [43, 44].

Prognostic Factors of Survival

Perhaps the most comprehensive assessment of prognostic factors in patients with NCNN liver metastases treated surgically is the assessment of 1452 patients performed by Adam and colleagues [8]. As demonstrated above, among the most important prognostic factors is the **primary tumor site**, as evidenced by large differences in outcomes seen between patients with genitourinary primary cancers compared with gastrointestinal cancers such as pancreatic ductal adenocarcinoma. Patients with breast cancer were also associated with favorable outcomes, with a 1.3 times greater adjusted likelihood of 5-year survival when compared to other primary sites.

Next, and largely similar to colorectal and neuroendocrine liver metastases, a longer **disease-free interval** from the diagnosis of the primary tumor to the diagnosis of liver metastasis is typically suggestive of favorable tumor biology and improved survival after metastasectomy. Patients who develop hepatic metastases greater than 24 months after initial primary cancer diagnosis had a better prognosis compared to those diagnosed within 12 months, with a 1.8 times higher likelihood of improved survival compared with a disease-free interval of less than 12 months.

Additionally, the presence of **extrahepatic disease** at the time of surgical resection of NCNN liver metastases is also associated with a worse survival [8]. These factors, which reflect tumor biology, represent the strong independent prognostic factors, which are critical in the evaluation of patients for surgical resection. In addition, **chemoresponsiveness** and **growth rate** of metastases are additional alternative measures of tumor biology that possess independent prognostic capacity in the evaluation of patients for hepatic surgical resection.

Finally, **treatment-** and **tumor burden-related factors** are independent predictors of long-term survival as well. Patients who had a limited hepatectomy were 1.3 times more likely to achieve 5-year survival when compared to those requiring an extended hepatectomy. Similarly, patients who had an R0 resection were 1.9 times more likely to achieve long-term survival compared to patients with an R1 or R2 resection [8]. These factors are likely surrogates of disease extent and tumor biology rather than a reflection of the true impact of technical factors associated with liver resection. This is evident by other studies consistently demonstrating the association between **number** and **size of liver metastases**, and margin status, with overall survival [45–48]. Table 23.2 provides a comprehensive list of identified prognostic factors for patients undergoing resection of NCNN liver metastases, along with supporting studies for each factor.

Table 23.2 List of identified prognostic factors in patients with resected non-colorectal, non-neuroendocrine liver metastases and supporting citations for each factor

Prognostic factor	Citations demonstrating association with overall survival
Gender	[32]
Preoperative liver-directed therapy	[49]
Synchronous vs. metachronous	[45, 48, 50–52]
Primary site and histological subtype	[8, 12, 32, 36, 45–47, 49–57]
Symptomatic at the time of resection	[57]
Extent of hepatectomy	[8, 32, 45, 57]
Macroscopically incomplete resection (R2)	[45, 52, 55]
R1 margin status	[8, 45, 46, 51, 53]
Adjuvant treatment	[8, 12, 45, 47, 49, 54–56]
Extrahepatic disease	[8, 48, 49, 53, 55, 58]
Disease-free interval prior to metastatic presentation	[7, 46, 47]
Postoperative complications	[45, 59]
Number of metastases	[32, 45–48, 59]
Size of metastases	[6, 47, 57, 60, 61]
Presence of vascular invasion	[6]
Lymph node metastases	[6, 32, 60]
Disease-free survival	[8, 47, 52, 57]
Blood transfusion	[59]

Selecting Patients for Surgical Resection of NCNN Liver Metastases

It is critical to note that almost all of the cited studies above are small, descriptive, and retrospective. In addition, most lack a control group for comparison. As such, conclusions derived from such studies must be interpreted with extreme caution. For example, systemic therapies for stage IV cutaneous malignant melanoma have evolved dramatically in the last 5 years. In addition, these studies represent highly selected cohorts of patients in whom tumor biology has been determined to be favorable enough to suggest surgery, and arguably patients might have survived long even without surgical resection.

The decision to proceed with surgical treatment of patients with NCNN liver metastases should be based on very cautious evaluation in the multidisciplinary setting, taking into account the potential morbidity and mortality of the proposed liver resection, the alternative treatment strategies, and the aforementioned prognostic factors. Although there are no clearly defined guidelines to determine patient selection in patients with NCNN liver metastases, the decision to proceed with liver metastasectomy in this setting should be based on multiple factors, which can be summarized below:

1. Tumor biology (pace of disease, disease-free interval, and response to systemic therapies)
2. Site and histology of the primary tumor
3. Tumor burden (size of lesions, number of lesions, and presence of extrahepatic disease)
4. Patient-related factors, such as need for "chemotherapy holiday" or intolerance of nonsurgical therapies
5. The understanding that surgical resection may not represent cure, but could "set the clock back" and offer a period of time off of chemotherapy
6. A clear understanding of surgical morbidity and mortality during informed consent
7. Consensus agreement at multidisciplinary tumor board of tertiary academic referral center

Figure 23.2 depicts a suggested framework to select patients for surgical treatment of their NCNN liver metastases. The first level of decision-making considers assessment of the patient's tumor biology. This includes assessing the disease-free interval, which is defined by the time between the resection of the primary tumor and the development of the liver metastases. The longer the disease-free interval, the more indolent the tumor biology, and the more likely a patient is to benefit from surgical treatment of their liver disease. Additionally, tumor biology should incorporate patients' response to chemotherapy, with chemosensitivity representing a predictor of improved survival, in diseases where effective systemic therapies are available.

Next, the site of the primary tumor should be evaluated. Patients with tumors of genitourinary and breast primary are typically better suited for surgical resection for their metastatic liver dis-

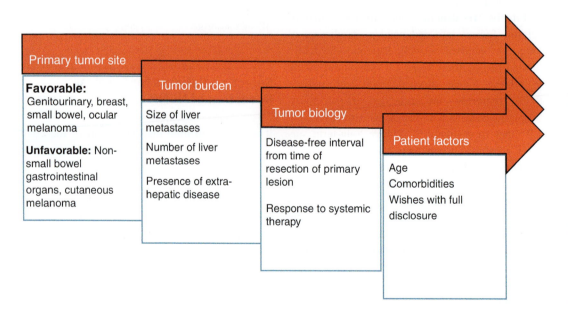

Fig. 23.2 Suggested framework for selecting patients for surgical resection of their non-colorectal, non-neuroendocrine liver metastases

ease. Considerations should be given to patients with small bowel or ocular melanoma primaries as well. Patients with gastrointestinal (aside from small bowel) origins will likely not benefit from hepatic resection for their metastatic disease, thus sparing them the unnecessary morbidity and mortality from an extensive operation.

The third level of decision-making centers around the extent of tumor burden. This includes the number and size of liver metastases, vessel involvement, and presence of extrahepatic disease. Patients with multifocal, extensive, bulky disease, with macroscopic vessel involvement, will likely not benefit from resection. In general, resection should be reserved for patients with solitary or limited NCNN hepatic metastatic disease.

The fourth and final stage includes patient-related factors. Patients' comorbidities and functional status are used to determine operative candidacy prior to embarking on a major abdominal operation. In addition, intolerance to chemotherapy and the desire to seek a break from chemotherapy ("chemotherapy holiday") are patient factors that must be compassionately considered in the evaluation for hepatic resection. Above all, it is important to ensure that patients and their families understand that liver resection in this setting is aimed at minimizing tumor burden and prolonging survival, but is not typically curative per se. A detailed discussion of morbidity and mortality, fully disclosing the expected outcomes in terms of survival and recurrence, should take place. As highlighted above, input from a multidisciplinary tumor board should routinely be obtained when considering liver resection for NCNN metastases.

Summary

Hepatic resection for NCNN liver metastases remains a controversial topic in surgical oncology, given the heterogeneity of histologies and the limited high-quality data on the best approach to patient selection. Liver resection appears to be beneficial in a highly selected group of such patients, with the greatest survival benefit demonstrated in patients with prolonged disease-free intervals between resection of primary disease and liver metastases, limited liver disease burden with no extrahepatic metastases, and those with tumors responsive to systemic therapy. Patients benefiting most from surgical treatment appear to be those with metastases arising from genitourinary and occasionally breast cancer, ocular melanoma, and small bowel primary cancers. The decision to proceed with surgical resection should be individualized and made in a center with expertise in hepatic resection and with consensus sought in the multidisciplinary setting.

References

1. Malik HZ, Prasad KR, Halazun KJ, et al. Preoperative prognostic score for predicting survival after hepatic resection for colorectal liver metastases. Ann Surg. 2007;246:806–14.
2. Quan D, Gallinger S, Nhan C, et al. The role of liver resection for colorectal cancer metastases in an era of multimodality treatment: a systematic review. Surgery. 2012;151:860–70.
3. Simmonds PC, Primrose JN, Colquitt JL, et al. Surgical resection of hepatic metastases from colorectal cancer: a systematic review of published studies. Br J Cancer. 2006;94:982–99.
4. Mayo SC, de Jong MC, Pulitano C, et al. Surgical management of hepatic neuroendocrine tumor metastasis: results from an international multi-institutional analysis. Ann Surg Oncol. 2010;17:3129–36.
5. Mayo SC, de Jong MC, Bloomston M, et al. Surgery versus intra-arterial therapy for neuroendocrine liver metastasis: a multicenter international analysis. Ann Surg Oncol. 2011;18:3657–65.
6. Groeschl RT, Nachmany I, Steel JL, et al. Hepatectomy for noncolorectal non-neuroendocrine metastatic cancer: a multi-institutional analysis. J Am Coll Surg. 2012;214:769–77.
7. Cordera F, Rea DJ, Rodriguez-Davalos M, et al. Hepatic resection for noncolorectal, nonneuroendocrine metastases. J Gastrointest Surg. 2005;9:1361–70.
8. Adam R, Chiche L, Aloia T, et al. Hepatic resection for noncolorectal nonendocrine liver metastases: analysis of 1,452 patients and development of a prognostic model. Ann Surg. 2006;244:524–35.
9. Abood G, Bowen M, Potkul R, et al. Hepatic resection for recurrent metastatic ovarian cancer. Am J Surg. 2008;195:370–3; discussion 373.
10. Bosquet JG, Merideth MA, Podratz KC, et al. Hepatic resection for metachronous metastases from ovarian carcinoma. HPB (Oxford). 2006;8:93–6.

11. Merideth MA, Cliby WA, Keeney GL, et al. Hepatic resection for metachronous metastases from ovarian carcinoma. Gynecol Oncol. 2003;89:16–21.
12. Elias D, Cavalcanti de Albuquerque A, Eggenspieler P, et al. Resection of liver metastases from a noncolorectal primary: indications and results based on 147 monocentric patients. J Am Coll Surg. 1998;187:487–93.
13. Ruys AT, Tanis PJ, Nagtegaal ID, et al. Surgical treatment of renal cell cancer liver metastases: a population-based study. Ann Surg Oncol. 2011;18:1932–8.
14. Goulet RJ Jr, Hardacre JM, Einhorn LH, et al. Hepatic resection for disseminated germ cell carcinoma. Ann Surg. 1990;212:290–3; discussion 293–4.
15. Roh HJ, Kim DY, Joo WD, et al. Hepatic resection as part of secondary cytoreductive surgery for recurrent ovarian cancer involving the liver. Arch Gynecol Obstet. 2011;284:1223–9.
16. Alves A, Adam R, Majno P, et al. Hepatic resection for metastatic renal tumors: is it worthwhile? Ann Surg Oncol. 2003;10:705–10.
17. Weitz J, Blumgart LH, Fong Y, et al. Partial hepatectomy for metastases from noncolorectal, nonneuroendocrine carcinoma. Ann Surg. 2005;241:269–76.
18. Stief CG, Jahne J, Hagemann JH, et al. Surgery for metachronous solitary liver metastases of renal cell carcinoma. J Urol. 1997;158:375–7.
19. Staehler MD, Kruse J, Haseke N, et al. Liver resection for metastatic disease prolongs survival in renal cell carcinoma: 12-year results from a retrospective comparative analysis. World J Urol. 2010;28:543–7.
20. Langan RC, Ripley RT, Davis JL, et al. Liver directed therapy for renal cell carcinoma. J Cancer. 2012;3:184–90.
21. You YN, Leibovitch BC, Que FG. Hepatic metastasectomy for testicular germ cell tumors: is it worth it? J Gastrointest Surg. 2009;13:595–601.
22. Motzer RJ, Mazumdar M, Bacik J, et al. Survival and prognostic stratification of 670 patients with advanced renal cell carcinoma. J Clin Oncol. 1999;17:2530–40.
23. Temkin SM, Fleming G. Current treatment of metastatic endometrial cancer. Cancer Control. 2009;16:38–45.
24. Adam R, Aloia T, Krissat J, et al. Is liver resection justified for patients with hepatic metastases from breast cancer? Ann Surg. 2006;244:897–907; discussion 907–8.
25. Pocard M, Pouillart P, Asselain B, et al. Hepatic resection in metastatic breast cancer: results and prognostic factors. Eur J Surg Oncol. 2000;26:155–9.
26. Abbott DE, Brouquet A, Mittendorf EA, et al. Resection of liver metastases from breast cancer: estrogen receptor status and response to chemotherapy before metastasectomy define outcome. Surgery. 2012;151:710–6.
27. Thelen A, Benckert C, Jonas S, et al. Liver resection for metastases from breast cancer. J Surg Oncol. 2008;97:25–9.
28. Fitzgerald TL, Brinkley J, Banks S, et al. The benefits of liver resection for non-colorectal, non-neuroendocrine liver metastases: a systematic review. Langenbecks Arch Surg. 2014;399:989–1000.
29. Mariani P, Servois V, De Rycke Y, et al. Liver metastases from breast cancer: surgical resection or not? A case-matched control study in highly selected patients. Eur J Surg Oncol. 2013;39:1377–83.
30. Spolverato G, Vitale A, Bagante F, et al. Liver resection for breast cancer liver metastases: a cost-utility analysis. Ann Surg. 2017;265:792–9.
31. Sadot E, Lee SY, Sofocleous CT, et al. Hepatic resection or ablation for isolated breast cancer liver metastasis: a case-control study with comparison to medically treated patients. Ann Surg. 2016;264:147–54.
32. Bresadola V, Rossetto A, Adani GL, et al. Liver resection for noncolorectal and nonneuroendocrine metastases: results of a study on 56 patients at a single institution. Tumori. 2011;97:316–22.
33. de Jong MC, Tsai S, Cameron JL, et al. Safety and efficacy of curative intent surgery for peri-ampullary liver metastasis. J Surg Oncol. 2010;102:256–63.
34. Polee MB, Hop WC, Kok TC, et al. Prognostic factors for survival in patients with advanced oesophageal cancer treated with cisplatin-based combination chemotherapy. Br J Cancer. 2003;89:2045–50.
35. Conroy T, Desseigne F, Ychou M, et al. FOLFIRINOX versus gemcitabine for metastatic pancreatic cancer. N Engl J Med. 2011;364:1817–25.
36. Slotta JE, Schuld J, Distler S, et al. Hepatic resection of non-colorectal and non-neuroendocrine liver metastases—survival benefit for patients with non-gastrointestinal primary cancers—a case-controlled study. Int J Surg. 2014;12:163–8.
37. Shima Y, Horimi T, Ishikawa T, et al. Aggressive surgery for liver metastases from gastrointestinal stromal tumors. J Hepatobiliary Pancreat Surg. 2003;10:77–80.
38. DeMatteo RP, Shah A, Fong Y, et al. Results of hepatic resection for sarcoma metastatic to liver. Ann Surg. 2001;234:540–7; discussion 547–8.
39. Nunobe S, Sano T, Shimada K, et al. Surgery including liver resection for metastatic gastrointestinal stromal tumors or gastrointestinal leiomyosarcomas. Jpn J Clin Oncol. 2005;35:338–41.
40. Xia L, Zhang MM, Ji L, et al. Resection combined with imatinib therapy for liver metastases of gastrointestinal stromal tumors. Surg Today. 2010;40:936–42.
41. Pawlik TM, Vauthey JN, Abdalla EK, et al. Results of a single-center experience with resection and ablation for sarcoma metastatic to the liver. Arch Surg. 2006;141:537–43; discussion 543–4.
42. Pawlik TM, Zorzi D, Abdalla EK, et al. Hepatic resection for metastatic melanoma: distinct patterns of recurrence and prognosis for ocular versus cutaneous disease. Ann Surg Oncol. 2006;13:712–20.
43. Rivoire M, Kodjikian L, Baldo S, et al. Treatment of liver metastases from uveal melanoma. Ann Surg Oncol. 2005;12:422–8.
44. Mariani P, Piperno-Neumann S, Servois V, et al. Surgical management of liver metastases from uveal

melanoma: 16 years' experience at the Institut Curie. Eur J Surg Oncol. 2009;35:1192–7.
45. Earle SA, Perez EA, Gutierrez JC, et al. Hepatectomy enables prolonged survival in select patients with isolated noncolorectal liver metastasis. J Am Coll Surg. 2006;203:436–46.
46. Berney T, Mentha G, Roth AD, et al. Results of surgical resection of liver metastases from non-colorectal primaries. Br J Surg. 1998;85:1423–7.
47. Duan XF, Dong NN, Zhang T, et al. Comparison of surgical outcomes in patients with colorectal liver metastases versus non-colorectal liver metastases: a Chinese experience. Hepatol Res. 2012;42:296–303.
48. Lindell G, Ohlsson B, Saarela A, et al. Liver resection of noncolorectal secondaries. J Surg Oncol. 1998;69:66–70.
49. Treska V, Liska V, Skalicky T, et al. Non-colorectal liver metastases: surgical treatment options. Hepatogastroenterology. 2012;59:245–8.
50. Takada Y, Otsuka M, Seino K, et al. Hepatic resection for metastatic tumors from noncolorectal carcinoma. Hepatogastroenterology. 2001;48:83–6.
51. Lendoire J, Moro M, Andriani O, et al. Liver resection for non-colorectal, non-neuroendocrine metastases: analysis of a multicenter study from Argentina. HPB (Oxford). 2007;9:435–9.
52. Harrison LE, Brennan MF, Newman E, et al. Hepatic resection for noncolorectal, nonneuroendocrine metastases: a fifteen-year experience with ninety-six patients. Surgery. 1997;121:625–32.
53. Yedibela S, Gohl J, Graz V, et al. Changes in indication and results after resection of hepatic metastases from noncolorectal primary tumors: a single-institutional review. Ann Surg Oncol. 2005;12:778–85.
54. van Ruth S, Mutsaerts E, Zoetmulder FA, et al. Metastasectomy for liver metastases of non-colorectal primaries. Eur J Surg Oncol. 2001;27:662–7.
55. Goering JD, Mahvi DM, Niederhuber JE, et al. Cryoablation and liver resection for noncolorectal liver metastases. Am J Surg. 2002;183:384–9.
56. Verhoef C, Kuiken BW, IJzermans JN, et al. Partial hepatic resection for liver metastases of non-colorectal origin, is it justified? Hepatogastroenterology. 2007;54:1517–21.
57. Ercolani G, Vetrone G, Grazi GL, et al. The role of liver surgery in the treatment of non-colorectal non-neuroendocrine metastases (NCRNNE). Analysis of 134 resected patients. Minerva Chir. 2009;64:551–8.
58. Karavias DD, Tepetes K, Karatzas T, et al. Liver resection for metastatic non-colorectal non-neuroendocrine hepatic neoplasms. Eur J Surg Oncol. 2002;28:135–9.
59. Takemura N, Saiura A, Koga R, et al. Long-term results of hepatic resection for non-colorectal, non-neuroendocrine liver metastasis. Hepatogastroenterology. 2013;60:1705–12.
60. O'Rourke TR, Tekkis P, Yeung S, et al. Long-term results of liver resection for non-colorectal, non-neuroendocrine metastases. Ann Surg Oncol. 2008;15:207–18.
61. Marudanayagam R, Sandhu B, Perera MT, et al. Hepatic resection for non-colorectal, non-neuroendocrine, non-sarcoma metastasis: a single-centre experience. HPB (Oxford). 2011;13:286–92.

Part IV

Evolving Therapies

Liver Transplantation for Other Cancers

24

Sandra Garcia-Aroz, Min Xu, and William C. Chapman

Liver Transplantation for Other Primary Liver Malignancies

Liver Transplantation for Cholangiocarcinoma

Introduction

Cholangiocarcinoma (CCA) arises from epithelial cells of the intrahepatic and extrahepatic bile ducts. These tumors are classified in three groups: perihilar, or Klatskin tumors accounting for 60% to 70% of all CCA; distal CCA, usually treated with Whipple resection when feasible, accounting for 20–30% of the cases; and intrahepatic CCA accounting for the remaining 5–10% of CCA [1]. Cholangiocarcinoma represents 3% of all gastrointestinal malignancies and is the second most common primary malignancy of the liver after hepatocellular carcinoma. The incidence and mortality of CCA has been increasing worldwide [2]. More than 3000 Americans are diagnosed with cholangiocarcinoma each year [3, 4]. Primary sclerosing cholangitis (PSC),

S. Garcia-Aroz · M. Xu · W. C. Chapman (✉)
Section of Transplantation, Division of General Surgery, Transplant Center, Department of Surgery, Washington University School of Medicine Saint Louis, Saint Louis, MO, USA
e-mail: garcia-arozs@wustl.edu; min.xu@wustl.edu; chapmanw@wustl.edu

polycystic liver disease, chronic intrahepatic stone disease (hepatolithiasis), and chronic liver disease are some of the predisposing risk factors for development of CCA. The association between PSC and cholangiocarcinoma, especially perihilar disease, is now well established. The strong association between chronic intrahepatic stone disease and intrahepatic CCA (ICCA) has also been observed in a large number of patients. Chronic liver disease such as cirrhosis and viral infection are also recognized as risk factors, especially for development of ICCA. CCA from any location has historically been considered a contraindication for liver transplantation (LT), but based on the promising results of several studies, today it is considered as an indication for liver transplantation in highly selected cases in some centers.

Clinical Presentation and Diagnosis

As mentioned above, CCA can arise from differing locations in the biliary tree, and this will influence clinical manifestations. Extrahepatic CCA (perihilar and distal CCA) usually become symptomatic when the biliary tract becomes obstructed. Symptoms for these tumors include jaundice, pruritus, dark urine, and/or cholangitis, although cholangitis is uncommon unless the biliary tree has been instrumented. On the other hand, ICCA often manifests differently; some patients can be asymptomatic with the tumor being detected incidentally, or they may present with a history of abdominal pain, malaise, and weight loss. On physical examination, patients with extrahepatic CCA may be jaundiced at presentation, sometimes with a palpable mass in the right upper quadrant, or present with fever, while right upper quadrant tenderness or weight loss are more commonly seen in patients with ICCA [5].

The first step in the diagnosis of CCA is suspecting it. Patients with a compatible clinical presentation, such as jaundice or other symptoms/signs of biliary obstruction, and patients with underlying diseases at high risk of CCA (e.g., PSC) should have liver biochemical tests and tumor markers (CA 19-9, CEA, and AFP) [5, 6]. Laboratory studies will show a cholestatic pattern with elevated bilirubin, as well as elevated alkaline phosphatase levels in patients with an extrahepatic CCA, while ICCA patients usually have a normal bilirubin level. The increase in gamma-glutamyl transpeptidase (GGT) levels will confirm the hepatic origin of elevated alkaline phosphatase. CA 19-9 is a consolidated tumor marker for CCA diagnosis, although its specificity is limited and it may be elevated in benign conditions such as cholangitis, or in other malignancies such as pancreatic cancer. CEA may be elevated in CCA but it's neither sufficiently sensitive nor specific to make the diagnosis of CCA. Serum levels of AFP may be checked to consider the presence of biphenotypic tumors (combined CCA with hepatocellular carcinoma) [7]. Once the diagnosis of CCA is suspected as a possibility based on laboratory testing and clinical features, imaging studies are used to confirm the diagnosis [8]. Ultrasound often represents the initial imaging test that is performed, especially when the treating physician is concerned about possible gallstone disease. Ultrasound may demonstrate the presence of a mass, with or without biliary tract dilatation, and can rule out gallstones as a possible cause or contributor to the biliary obstruction. An obstructing malignant lesion is suggested by ductal dilatation in the absence of stones. ICCA are often seen as a solitary solid mass within the hepatic parenchyma. Contrast-enhanced cross-sectional imaging is mandatory in all cases of suspected CCA [1, 5]. CT or MR/MRCP has similar utility, although MR/MRCP often provides slightly more information than CT and has less associated nephrotoxicity. CT has shown higher accuracy diagnosing ICCA than extrahepatic CCA [9]. MRCP provides a superior anatomical assessment of the bile ducts and tumor characteristics for hilar CCA. In patients with an extrahepatic lesion, ERCP is often performed (after cross-sectional imaging) to confirm diagnostic information (i.e., biliary obstruction), perform tissue sampling, and allow for therapeutic intervention (stent placement) when needed [8, 10].

Cholangiocarcinoma Resection

Surgical resection represents the best option for curative treatment of CCA. As a highly aggressive tumor, CCA is usually unresectable at the time of diagnosis in the majority of cases. Distal CCA have the highest resectability rate, while perihilar and intrahepatic tumors present lower rates [11].

Patients must meet certain requirements to be eligible for resection. Absence of disseminated disease, including absence of lymph node involvement beyond the usual boundaries of planned pancreatic resection (e.g., para-aortic nodal metastases) and distant hematogenous metastases, is required for resection [12, 13]. These criteria are necessary to consider the tumor suitable for resection but, sometimes, the presence of advanced liver disease (PSC) and/or insufficient hepatic functional reserve may result in resectable tumors but nonsurgical candidates.

Outcomes after resection vary based on tumor location. Distal CCA can reach survivals as high as 55–62% at 5-year post-resection in selected patients with complete resection (R0) and early-stage tumors (need reference). In patients with regional lymph node involvement survival rates are significantly worse. The usual procedure for these tumors is a Whipple resection. The procedure for ICCA usually involves liver resection in an attempt to obtain negative margins (complete resection, R0). Again, survival rates vary based on tumor stage [14, 15]. For localized tumors, with complete resection and absence of regional lymph nodes, survival rates reach 44–63% [12, 16–19]. Perihilar CCA present high early recurrence rates if the resection is limited to the bile duct. Outcomes after resection are improved when modifying the surgical technique and adding partial hepatectomy to the bile duct resection, which is required in almost all cases of hilar cholangiocarcinoma. With the practice of this more aggressive surgery, 5-year survival rates have become as high as 50%, but they are accompanied by an increase in surgical mortality and morbidity [20–23].

Liver Transplantation

Initially, liver transplantation for CCA was associated with low survival and high recurrence rates after LT (need reference). For this reason, CCA was considered an absolute contraindication for liver transplantation for many years. The Pittsburg group published their experience with LT for perihilar cholangiocarcinoma during 1980–1996 [24]. They reported 1-, 3-, and 5-year survival rates of 60%, 32%, and 25%, respectively, after LT compared to survival rates of 74%, 34%, and 9%, respectively, after liver resection. These survival rates significantly improved in early-stage tumors with R0 resection and uninvolved regional lymph nodes. After promising results in highly selected patients, the Mayo Clinic group developed a well-defined and highly specific protocol to select hilar CCA patients for LT, starting their protocol in 1993 [25].

Mayo Protocol for Perihilar Cholangiocarcinoma

In 2000, the Mayo Clinic group, published a study of LT in 11 CCA patients after neoadjuvant therapy with chemoirradiation [25]. Inclusion criteria for the study included patients with demonstrated CCA by cytology or biopsy or patients with a mass lesion suspicious of malignancy and CA 19-9 greater than 100 U/mL. The presence of a resectable tumor was not an exclusion criteria in patients with PSC. Patients without PSC were not included in the study if their tumor was resectable. Patients with tumors below the cystic duct were excluded, as well as patients with more advanced disease (i.e., any involved lymph nodes except for periductal nodes in the hilum which are not generally sampled, intrahepatic, or extrahepatic metastatic disease). Their protocol consisted of external beam radiation over 3 weeks plus chemotherapy with 5-FU for three consecutive days during the first week of radiation as the initial phase. Two to 3 weeks later, transcatheter irradiation (brachytherapy) was used as a local boost. Subsequently, oral 5-FU (Xeloda) is given as maintenance therapy until transplantation occurs or until the patient develops a contraindication (e.g., metastatic disease) with a pattern of 5 weeks with treatment, 1 week off (doses are shown in Fig. 24.1). Two to 6 weeks after brachytherapy, patients undergo staging laparotomy to evaluate for possible disease outside the bile ducts and liver. If there was no evidence of extrahepatic disease (i.e., peritoneal or nodal disease), patients continued with oral 5-FU until LT.

The results of this study significantly improved outcomes observed in patients undergoing LT with unresectable perihilar CCA, and were significantly better than outcomes described in other studies using adjuvant therapy after LT in CCA patients. This protocol was associated with a 92% disease-free survival with a median follow-up of 37 months, compared to 1-year survival of 53% showed by Baylor group using adjuvant therapy with radiation and 5-FU after LT [26]. After this successful experience with the Mayo protocol, patients with extrahepatic CCA could undergo LT when resective surgery is not an option because of underlying liver disease, including PSC, or due to unresectable but localized hilar tumors. The number of LT for CCA has increased since that time with reported 5-year survival rates >60% [27].

Current Organ Allocation and Patient Selection

In 2009, the United Network for Organ Sharing/Organ Procurement and Transplantation Network (UNOS/OPTN) approved the granting of routine exception MELD points for patients with perihilar CCA that meet general protocol requirements. The MELD score was set equal to the current standard assigned for HCC for approved patients. In 2017, OPTN policies determine that candidates

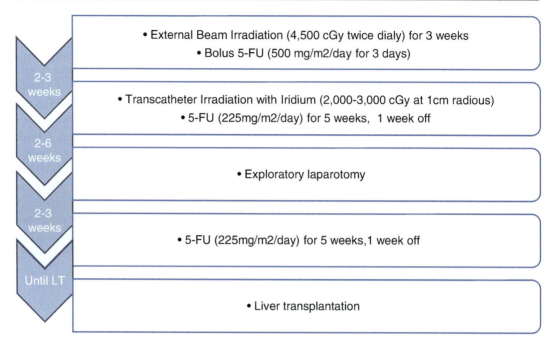

Fig. 24.1 Mayo Clinic protocol

for LT will receive 22 MELD exception points if they meet all the conditions described in Table 24.1, including the following: neoadjuvant therapy; absence of lymph node metastasis/extrahepatic disease/intrahepatic metastasis; a cholangiography study showing a stricture suspicious of malignancy plus CA 19.9 > 100 or cytology/biopsy of CCA; a CT study with no mass, or if a mass is present, it must be <3 cm; possible metastasis must be studied and excluded; and operative staging after neoadjuvant therapy must be done before LT [28].

Liver Transplantation for Perihilar Cholangiocarcinoma

As previously described, surgery represents the unique opportunity of cure for patients with perihilar CCA. Despite this fact, outcomes after standard surgical resection are not encouraging. Complete resection is an option in only 25–40% of patients presenting with hilar cholangiocarcinoma. And in those who do undergo curative surgical resection, overall survival rates after 5-year post-resection are around 50%, in the best reported series [20–23]. The benefit of adjuvant therapy after compete resection is uncertain. There are no prospective randomized clinical trials that determine the benefit of chemotherapy or chemoradiation after complete resection and retrospective studies that have been published describe conflicting results [29–32]. Regarding adjuvant chemoradiotherapy, several retrospective studies have shown better outcomes after complete and microscopically incomplete resection compared to cases that did not receive adjuvant chemoradiotherapy [33–35]. Similarly, there is no level one evidence that adjuvant chemotherapy alone improves survival after complete resection.

Tumors with invasion of major vessels, bilateral second order duct involvement, or low hepatic reserve that are unresectable, can be considered for LT. As previously indicated, initial experiences with LT for CCA were not satisfactory until the Mayo Clinic group published its experience, and neoadjuvant therapy with chemoradiation was established as mandatory before LT for CCA [25]. Following the establishment of this neoadjuvant protocol, several groups reported their experience with LT and outcomes were

Table 24.1 OPTN policies for MELD exception

1. Submit a written protocol for patient care to the Liver and Intestinal Organ Transplantation Committee that must include *all* of the following:
   (a) Candidate selection criteria
   (b) Administration of neoadjuvant therapy before transplantation
   (c) Operative staging to exclude any patient with regional hepatic lymph node metastases, intrahepatic metastases, or extrahepatic disease
   (d) Any data requested by the Liver and Intestinal Organ Transplantation Committee
2. Document that the candidate meets the diagnostic criteria for hilar CCA with a malignant appearing stricture on cholangiography and *one* of the following:
   (a) Biopsy or cytology results demonstrating malignancy
   (b) Carbohydrate antigen 19-9 greater than 100 U/mL in absence of cholangitis
   (c) Aneuploidy
   The tumor must be considered unresectable because of technical considerations or underlying liver disease
3. If cross-sectional imaging studies demonstrate a mass, the mass must be less than 3 cm
4. Intrahepatic and extrahepatic metastases must be excluded by cross-sectional imaging studies of the chest and abdomen at the time of the initial application for the MELD/PELD exception and every 3 months before the MELD/PELD score increases
5. Regional hepatic lymph node involvement and peritoneal metastases must be assessed by operative staging after completion of neoadjuvant therapy and before liver transplantation. Endoscopic ultrasound-guided aspiration of regional hepatic lymph nodes may be advisable to exclude patients with obvious metastases before neoadjuvant therapy is initiated
6. Transperitoneal aspiration or biopsy of the primary tumor (either by endoscopic ultrasound, operative, or percutaneous approaches) must be avoided because of the high risk of tumor seeding associated with these procedures

The candidate must meet all the qualifications

comparable to those obtained by the Mayo group. In 2005, the Mayo Clinic group reported the results of 71 patients with perihilar cholangiocarcinoma; 26 underwent resection and 38 underwent liver transplantation [36]. The neoadjuvant protocol was updated: patients initially received external-beam radiation (45 Gy in 30 fractions, 1.5 Gy twice daily) and continuous infusion of 5-flurouracil administered over 3 weeks. Brachytherapy (20 Gy at 1 cm in approximately 20–25 h) was administered 2 weeks following completion of external beam radiation therapy. After that, patients were treated with oral capecitabine, administered until the time of transplantation. Exploratory laparotomy was always performed to ascertain the absence of metastasis. One-, 3-, and 5-year survival rates in the transplant group were 92%, 82%, and 82%, respectively. They were significantly higher compared to 1-, 3-, and 5-year survivals found in the resection group (82%, 48%, and 21%, respectively). They also described a lower recurrence rate in the transplant group. They concluded that LT should be considered for patients with localized node-negative perihilar CCA as an alternative to resection. Predictors for tumor recurrence were analyzed; CA 19-9 > 100 units/mL at transplantation time, prior cholecystectomy, tumor grade, advanced age, the presence of a mass on imaging, perineural invasion, and residual tumor >2 cm were associated with higher risk of recurrence. A multicenter study for localized CCA with neoadjuvant chemoradiotherapy followed by LT was performed in 12 centers in the USA [27]. This study showed 2- and 5-year overall survival rates of 68% and 53%, respectively, whereas post-LT recurrence-free survival were 78% and 65%, respectively (Fig. 24.2) [27]. In conclusion, LT remains a controversial treatment, but it should be considered an alternative option in highly selected patients with unresectable perihilar CCA that are able to receive appropriate neoadjuvant treatment.

Liver Transplantation for Intrahepatic Cholangiocarcinoma

Similar to perihilar CCA cases, complete resection of the tumor with negative margins (R0) represents the only potential curative treatment for ICCA. Lymph node involvement has been demonstrated as an important prognostic factor. Outcomes after liver resection depend on tumor stage and achievement of complete resection. Five-year survival after resection varies among series, ranging between 11 and 40% [31, 37]. These percentages increase in a selected group of patients with no lymph node involvement and

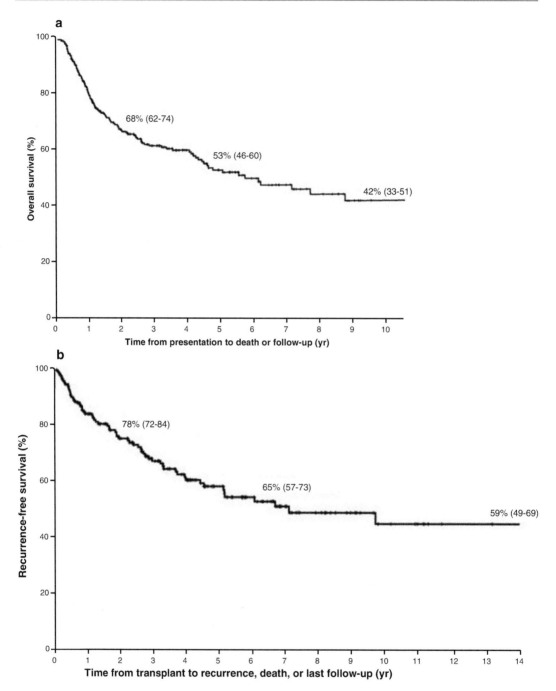

Fig. 24.2 Kaplan-Meier curves for intent-to-treat survival for the total population (left); recurrence-free survival for all transplanted patients (right)

complete resection with negative margins after surgery. For this group of patients, 5-year survival rates have been described between 44 and 63% [18, 38]. On the other hand, complete resection in these patients is achieved just in 30% of the cases, likely related to the advanced stage at presentation for most patients. A French group reported a study with 163 patients who underwent liver resection, and they analyzed the 5-year survival stratified by tumor stage. A significant drop-off in survival was showed between T1 and T2 tumors; 5-year survival for stage I (T1N0) tumors was 62%, while 5-year survival for stage II (T2N0) and stage III (T3N0, T1-3N1) tumors were 27% and 14%, respectively. The 5-year survival rate for the whole series was 32% [19]. In other studies, recurrence rates have been described as high as 60–65% [18].

Liver transplantation for ICCA demonstrated low survival rates and high recurrence rates in the 1990s. In several of the first series, the 5-year survival rates were below 20%, with recurrence rates of 60–84% [39, 40]. Based on these outcomes, liver transplantation for ICCA was considered a contraindication for LT. More recent studies have shown improved outcomes through in highly selected patients [41–43]. Most of these studies describe results of liver transplantation for ICCA and perihilar CCA in a combined fashion. Becker et al. reported, in a registry-based study, the outcomes in 280 patients who underwent LT for ICCA or perihilar CCA between 1987 and 2005, and 5-year survival rate was 68% for patients with diagnosed CCA [41]. Fu et al. showed a 3-year disease-free survival of 52% and recurrence rate of 45% in a retrospective study of 11 patients who underwent LT for ICCA [42]. Hong et al. presented a study in 2011, comparing results in patients with perihilar and ICCA who underwent LT or liver resection [43]. The study included 38 patients who underwent LT; 25 presented with ICCA and 13 patients presented with perihilar CCA and 19 patients who underwent liver resection; 12 of them presented with ICCA, and the other 7 had perihilar CCA. They reported a significantly higher 3- and 5-year recurrence-free rate in the LT group; 39% vs 6% and 33% vs 0%, respectively. Thirty-four patients of 38 (89%) who underwent LT presented with locally advanced tumors. They also reported better survival rates using neoadjuvant and adjuvant therapy compared with no therapy or adjuvant therapy alone. Regardless, LT for ICCA still remains controversial, and ICCA cannot be considered a standard indication for LT at this time. More studies are necessary to achieve suitable neoadjuvant/adjuvant protocols and an appropriate case selection to reach better outcomes.

Incidental Intrahepatic Cholangiocarcinoma and Biphenotypic Tumors

Cirrhosis and viral hepatitis B (HBV) and C (HCV) have been demonstrated to have a strong association with ICCA. This association is stronger for HCV than HBV. HCV also represents one of the main risk factors for the development of HCC. The incidence of HVC and cirrhosis is increasing, as well as its prevalence in patients diagnosed of ICCA. All these factors contribute to the occurrence of incidental ICCA and the diagnosis of biphenotypic tumors, intrahepatic cholangiocarcinoma + HCC (ICCA + HCC) in patients primarily diagnosed with HCC. These tumors, ICCA-HCC, are an uncommon type of primary liver malignancy, originating from the hepatocytes and cholangiocytes. Biphenotypic tumors account for 1–14% of all primary liver cancers, and they present histologic characteristics of both cholangiocarcinoma and hepatocellular carcinoma [44]. Most of these tumors are diagnosed and initially managed as either HCC or ICCA due to the lack of well-characterized radiologic properties, and they are correctly diagnosed after resection of the liver tumor or from liver explant specimens at the time of transplant. Improved cross-sectional imaging, especially with MR, has allowed more frequent suspicion of this variant compared with even 10 years ago.

Sapisochin et al. described recurrence rates of 60% after LT in a study that included ten patients with incidental biphenotypic tumors or incidental ICCA found in liver explants of patients initially diagnosed with HCC [45]. They compared this group of patients with a control group who underwent LT for HCC alone. One- and 5-year survival rates were lower in those with ICCA compared to the control group; 79% and 47% compared to 90% and 62%, respectively. Several studies have analyzed the outcomes after LT in cases of incidental ICCA or ICCA-HCC in patients initially thought to have HCC. Facciuto et al. presented a retrospective study with 32 patients that were found to have ICCA or biphenotypic tumor in liver explants [44]. Twenty-eight of them were originally incorrectly diagnosed as HCC. Tumor recurrence rate was 38%. They also analyzed 5-year recurrence rates based on tumor characteristics; tumors that met Milan size criteria (independently if there were ICCA or ICCA-HCC) had significantly lower recurrence rates than tumors that did not meet Milan criteria (10% vs 50%, respectively). Similarly, tumors within Milan criteria showed significantly higher survival rates than tumors beyond Milan criteria; 5-year survival rate for tumors within Milan was 78% compared to 32% in tumors beyond Milan. Again, these results showed that by improving patient selection criteria, LT could become a suitable therapeutic option for CCA patients achieving similar outcomes to those obtained with LT for HCC.

Liver Transplantation for Hepatoblastoma in Children

Hepatoblastoma is the most common primary hepatic malignancy in children. Its incidence is increasing in the USA with approximately 100 cases per year [46, 47]. Patients with hepatoblastoma are usually younger than 5 years old, and hepatoblastoma represents 1.2% of malignancies in patients younger than 15 years [48]. Diseases with an increased incidence of hepatoblastoma include Beckwith-Wiedemann syndrome, trisomy 21 and trisomy 18, Li-Fraumeni syndrome, von Gierke's disease, and familial adenomatous polyposis (FAP) [49]. Hepatoblastoma is also been associated with very low birthweight and maternal tobacco. There are several factors associated with treatment response and survival; if the tumor can be completely removed by resection, the presence of metastasis and histology of the tumor (pure fetal cell tumors are less aggressive than the ones with undifferentiated cells) are important predictors of outcome.

Staging

Previously utilized in the USA, the surgery-based Evans staging system required an exploratory laparotomy and an attempt to resection at diagnosis for all patients. Stage I included resected tumors with microscopically negative margins. Stage II classified resected tumors with microscopically positive margins. Stage III included unresectable tumors without metastasis, and stage IV was used to designate patients with unresectable tumors with metastasis.

Currently, the pretreatment extent of disease (PRETEXT) classification is used to determine the stage of the tumor. The PRETEXT classification is a radiology-based staging system and uses the number of hepatic sections free of disease to determine the stage of the tumor. It classifies hepatoblastomas in four groups (Table 24.2).

PRETEXT I and II are usually resectable at diagnosis or become resectable after neoadjuvant chemotherapy. PRETEXT III and IV may present vascular invasion, and chemotherapy is given to try to decrease the number of sections involved and/or eliminate vascular involvement.

Liver Resection

Liver resection aims to achieve a margin negative resection of the tumor (i.e., R0). This is achieved in less than half of the cases, as 60% of these tumors are unresectable at diagnosis. PRETEXT I and II tumors that present >1 cm of margin from major vessels usually undergo liver resection at diagnosis. Tumors that do not fit in

Table 24.2 Pretreatment extent of disease classification (PRETEX)

PRETEXT number	Definition
I	One section is affected; three adjacent sections are disease-free
II	One or two sections are involved, but two adjacent sections are free
III	Two or three sections are involved, and No 2 adjacent sections are free
IV	All for sections are involved
Plus (additional criteria)	C—caudate lobe involvement E—extrahepatic disease H—tumor rupture or intraperitoneal hemorrhage M—distant metastases N—lymph node metastases P—portal vein involvement V—vena cava and/or hepatic veins involvement

these categories undergo neoadjuvant chemotherapy, and after treatment, tumors that become PRETEXT (tumor stage after neoadjuvant chemotherapy) I, II, or III with no major vessels involvement are candidates for liver resection. When tumors remain unresectable after neoadjuvant therapy, LT represents an alternative treatment for these children [50].

Chemotherapy
Neoadjuvant treatment with chemotherapy in patients with unresectable hepatoblastomas at diagnosis has demonstrated a significantly improvement in resection rates. Cisplatin is the first-line agent used for these tumors since it is the most active in hepatoblastoma. Besides improvement in resection rates, cisplatin has shown better survival rates, in comparison with other agents that have been used in this disease. Doxorubicin is the second most commonly used agent, and it's usually combined with cisplatin when this is not administered alone [51]. Several studies have described the outcomes after treatment with different agents, but due to the presence of different risk stratification guidelines and surgical approaches, it's difficult to compare different chemotherapy lines directly. American groups show a greater predisposition for liver resection at diagnosis, whereas the European groups have favored delayed resection following neoadjuvant chemotherapy. The International Childhood Liver Tumors Strategy Group (SIOPEL) reported resection rates of 95% after chemotherapy among patients designated for neoadjuvant therapy before resection. There is no single chemotherapy regimen for patients with unresectable hepatoblastoma at diagnosis. In the USA, the chemotherapy regimen is based on cisplatin combined with 5-fluorouracil, vincristine, and doxorubicin [52], while European groups tend to favor cisplatin alone in patients with low risk and carboplatin combined with doxorubicin for patients with high risk (PRETEXT IV, metastatic tumor) [53, 54].

Liver Transplantation
In spite of the improvement obtained after the neoadjuvant treatment with chemotherapy, some tumors will remain unresectable after this treatment. These patients are the ones who will be considered for LT. The use of LT in pediatric patients for hepatoblastoma has increased over the last 30 years. Five LT were performed in 1990 in the USA for hepatoblastoma, while 43 LT were performed in 2013 [55]. The major criteria to consider LT in these cases are the presence of major vascular involvement and tumors that affect all four sections. Although initial studies described mixed outcomes for LT for hepatoblastoma, multiple studies have reported the efficacy of this treatment [30, 56, 57].

Patients with POSTEXT IV (PRETEXT IV after chemotherapy) with unifocal tumor and PRETEXT IV with multifocal tumors and absence of metastasis should be considered LT candidates. Patients with POSTEXT III with multifocal tumors and/or major vessels involvement should be also considered for LT. Some patients with POSTEXT III and major vessels involvement may be considered for nonconventional resection. Progression of metastatic disease or development of metastasis during neoadjuvant chemotherapy is usually considered a contraindication for liver transplantation. Despite these indications, all patients with PRETEXT III or IV should be referred to a center with liver transplantation to be able to consider that option if it's indicated.

Chemotherapy is continued while the patient is waiting for liver transplantation. Administration of prolonged chemotherapy should be avoided in patients with hepatoblastoma who are possible candidates for LT. The early referral to a specialized center with liver transplantation for consultation helps to avoid excessive toxicity due to prolonged chemotherapy. Four cycles of chemotherapy prior to transplantation are usually recommended [34], although this indication may be influenced by unpredictable factors such as organ availability or time between treatments.

The first cases of LT for hepatoblastoma were associated with poor outcomes mainly to the high rate of recurrence. In addition, most patients were not considered for adjuvant therapy during the initial series [58]. After neoadjuvant and adjuvant chemotherapy was introduced, these results improved showing higher survival and lower recurrence rates. Further studies have reported 5-year survival rates as high as 93% in patients who receive chemotherapy [30, 56, 57, 59]. In spite of this improvement, recurrence rates after LT for hepatoblastoma are still a concern. Poorer outcomes have been described once recurrence is developed after LT and recurrence rates have been reported up to 25% in some series.

Salvage liver transplantation has been also considered in children with previous attempt of resection. Several studies have compared LT in the setting of salvage treatment after surgery vs primary LT and poorer results have been shown in salvage LT [60–63]. Results in these studies are uniformly in favor of primary LT: all have described a lower survival rate and a higher recurrence rate in patients with salvage LT than patients receiving primary LT. A recent review of 292 patients from 29 centers report an overall survival rate of 76%. In this review, the authors compared survival rates between patients who underwent primary and salvage LT. At the time of publication 85% of patients who underwent primary LT were alive, compared to 41% of patients who underwent salvage liver transplantation [55].

Liver Transplantation to Treat Secondary Liver Cancers

Orthotopic liver transplantation (OLT) has been performed to treat secondary liver malignancies, such as neuroendocrine liver metastases, colorectal cancer liver metastases, and some other rare malignant liver metastases. However, the overall survival of patients with metastatic malignancies after OLT is substantially limited by tumor recurrence. OLT for liver metastases must achieve a comparable outcome as the patients without cancer to overcome the ethical dilemma posed by the mismatch of a relatively stable pool of deceased donors and the prolonging waitlist owing to the advanced surgical techniques and perioperative singe management. Unfortunately, there are no standard criteria of OLT for liver metastases, as for HCC with Milan criteria of OLT for hepatocellular carcinoma (HCC), although several guidelines have been proposed. In this section, we will briefly review the outcomes previous studies, current selection criteria for liver transplantation to treat metastases, and potential strategies to curb tumor recurrence in the future.

Liver Transplantation and Neuroendocrine Tumor Liver Metastases

The incidence of neuroendocrine tumor (NET) is less than 5 per 100,000, and the distribution of NET is highly variable with around 60% in the gastrointestinal tract, 30% in the pancreas, and 10% locating at other sites, for instance, the liver, endocrine organs, lungs, breasts, and skin [64]. The World Health Organization classified NET based on the mitotic index (MI) and Ki67 labeling index: low-grade G1 with an MI less than 2 per 10 high-power fields (HPF) and Ki67 positivity less than 3%, intermediate-grade G2 with and MI of 2–20 per 10 HPF and Ki67 positivity 3–20%, and high-grade G3 with an MI greater than 20 per 10 HPF, Ki67 positivity greater than 20% [65]. Multiple therapeutic modalities including cytotoxic chemotherapy, somatostatin analogs, interferon alpha therapy, molecular targeted therapy, locoregional therapies, and surgical strategies have been applied to treat NET [66].

Liver Transplantation to Treat Unresectable NET Liver Metastases

OLT has been performed to treated NET hepatic metastases for decades across North America and Europe, but it remains highly controversial. To date, liver transplantation is not routinely considered for NET liver metastases, and it is deemed as an investigational indication of unresectable NET liver metastases by the guideline of National Comprehensive Cancer Network, acknowledging the considerable tumor recurrence-associated risk (NCCN) [67].

Mazzaferro et al., famed for defining the Milan criteria of liver transplantation for patients with HCC, proposed the Milan criteria of liver transplantation for unresectable NET liver metastases; the 5-year overall survival (OS) and recurrence-free survival (RFS) were, respectively, 90% and 77% under this criteria after OLT for NET liver metastases [68]. In other studies, the 5-year OS and RFS ranged from 36% to 88% and 9% to 77%, respectively; one of the possible explanation of the excellent outcome in Mazzaferro et al.'s study is that only 10% patient in their cohort were symptomatic, while this proportion in all the other studies ranged from 32 to 100% [69–75], suggesting less hepatic involvement by NET in Mazzaferro et al.'s study. Unfortunately, some extensive studies using the UNOS database demonstrated the 5-year OS ranged from 47 to 58%, without complete RFS data [76–78]. Furthermore, a recent meta-analysis also suggested that the majority of patients undergoing liver transplantation ultimately developed NET recurrence although the 5-year survival rates were encouraging [79]. The overall and disease-free survival (DFS) rates of a representative study of OLT for NET liver metastases are shown in Fig. 24.3 [76]. These variable outcomes highlight the importance of patient selection for OLT to achieve better oncological outcome after liver transplantation to treat unresectable NET liver metastases.

Based on the best knowledge, the 2007 Milan criteria [68] and the 2012 European Neuroendocrine Tumor Society guidelines [80] recommended the following selection criteria for transplant candidates with unresectable NET: age less than 55 years, well-differentiated NET (Ki-67 less than 10%), absence of extrahepatic disease, primary tumor removed before transplantation, stable disease for at least 6 months before LT, and less than 50% liver involvement. Similarly, the OPTN/UNOS criteria for the consideration of exception is summarized as the following: recipient age less than 60 years; resection of primary malignancy and extrahepatic disease without any evidence of recurrence for at least 6 months; neuroendocrine metastasis limited to the liver, bilobar, not amenable to resection; tumors in the liver should meet the specified radiographic characteristics and negative metastatic workup, with metastatic surveillance every 3 months; tumor of origin gastroenteropancreatic with portal system drainage; well-differentiated and moderately differentiated (G1 and G2), mitotic rate less than 20/10 HPF with Ki-67-positive markers less than 20%; tumor metastases should not exceed 50% of the total liver volume; and presence of extrahepatic solid organ metastases should be an absolute contraindication [81].

In summary, unresectable NET liver metastases are ethically justifiable for OLT in some highly selected patients at present, and it is feasible to achieve comparable survival outcome as liver transplantation for noncancer patients. However, further studies are necessary to optimize the selection of transplant candidates and decrease the risk of long-term tumor recurrence. In addition many patients with hepatic neuroendocrine metastases have very long survival with regional therapy only, making it difficult to demonstrate the advantages of LT in this setting.

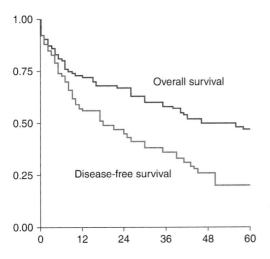

Fig. 24.3 The 5-year OS and DFS of patients underwent OLT for unresectable NET liver metastases

Strategies to Limit Tumor Recurrence After OLT for Unresectable NET Liver Metastases

OLT is investigationally indicated for candidates with unresectable NET liver metastases. Given the metastatic nature and late stage of most patients presenting for consideration of LT, tumor cells are very likely having been seeded into the systemic blood stream. Theoretically, only patients with tumors blood draining into the liver and tumors cells confined to the liver could have tumor-free survival after OLT. One of the possible techniques at this time but not yet included in the current guidelines is detecting the circulating tumor cell DNA and RNA. It has been shown that early changes in circulating tumor cells were associated with response and survival following treatment of metastatic neuroendocrine neoplasms [82, 83]. Moreover, enthusiasm also has been expressed in a consensus article of biomarkers for neuroendocrine tumor disease regarding the novel results of circulating DNAs and miRNAs from genomic technologies. The circulating multianalyte biomarkers were considered to be providing the highest sensitivity and specificity necessary for minimum disease detection [84], which may serve as a sufficient tool to select transplant candidates with minimized risk of tumor recurrence after OLT for unresectable NET liver metastases in the future.

Locoregional therapies such as radiofrequency ablation (RFA) and transarterial chemoembolization (TACE) as well systemic therapy including somatostatin analogs, interferon alpha therapy, cytotoxic chemotherapy, and targeted molecular therapies have been applied to relieve symptoms and reduce tumor burden [66]. However, it also remains unknown and to be investigated whether neoadjuvant therapies including neoadjuvant LRT could play an equal role in unresectable NET liver metastases as it does in HCC patients to downstage tumors or select transplant candidates with low risk of tumor recurrence.

Appropriate immunosuppressive therapy after liver transplantation is essential to maintain graft survival, and calcineurin inhibitors are the most used immunosuppressants. Studies have found that higher levels of immunosuppression were associated with higher tumor recurrence after liver transplantation for HCC [85–88], suggesting that a reduction in immunosuppression appears to be a reasonable approach to decrease the risk of HCC recurrence after transplantation. This method could apply to patients with unresectable NET liver metastasis after liver transplantation, although there is no clinical data available at this time [79]. Another promising approach is the application of antineoplastic immunosuppression as shown in a multicentric study with a high-level evidence; sirolimus improved the OS and RFS in the first 3–5 years especially in low-risk patients, but didn't improve long-term RFS after liver transplantation for HCC [89].

In summary, novel technologies and therapeutic modalities may be able to optimize the selection of transplant candidates with unresectable NET liver metastases and minimize the risk of tumor recurrence after liver transplantation in the future.

OLT and Colorectal Cancer Liver Metastases

Liver Transplantation and Unresectable CRC Liver Metastases

The primary metastatic site of patients diagnosed with colorectal cancer (CRC) is 60–70% in the liver, and up to 35% of metastatic CRC patients have metastases only in this organ [90]. Liver transplantation has been performed attempting to treat unresectable CRC liver metastases in the early stages of transplantation. However, the results in these cases discouraging, with very high recurrence rates and poor survival [91]. Before 1995, the 1- and 5-year survival rate after liver transplantation for unresectable CRC liver metastases according to the European Liver Transplant Registry was 62% and 18%, respectively [92]. Virtually, all the patients transplanted for unresectable CRC liver metastases suffered from tumor recurrence; thus liver transplantation was abandoned for unresectable CRC liver metastases at the majority of transplant centers [93]. In addition, there have been ethical concerns in light of the scarcity of liver donors and extremely high rate of tumor recurrence after transplantation [92, 94]. Currently, unresectable CRC liver metastases are still considered as an absolute contraindication for liver transplantation [95].

While many renowned experts of liver transplantation have called for extreme caution, efforts to utilize OLT for CRC liver metastases have not been entirely halted [93, 96–98]. In 2013, Hagness et al. from the Oslo University Hospital reported their experiences with liver transplantation in 21 patients performed over a 4.5-year time interval, and with 40% of patients evaluable at 3 years of follow-up and only 1 evaluable patient 5 years after transplantation. The estimate of the OS rates at 1, 3, and 5 years were 95%, 68%, and 60%, respectively. The disease-free survival was 35% at 1 year after liver transplant, and no patients had long-term disease-free survival [99]. This study was updated in 2015, and it was shown that the 5-year OS rate was 56% in patients treated by liver transplantation versus 9% in patients treated with first-line chemotherapy (Fig. 24.4a). However, no significant difference of DFS/PFS (progression-free survival) was found between transplantation and chemotherapy group (Fig. 24.4b). The authors explained the large difference in OS despite similar DFS/PFS was likely due to the recurrence or metastases in the liver transplantation group were often small, slowly growing lung lesions, whereas progression in the chemotherapy group was nonresectable liver metastases [100]. In this setting, liver transplantation is essentially a salvage surgery for debulking. Salvage liver resection for hepatocellular carcinoma has been shown to be able to provide disease control for a small number of unresectable HCC after downstaging [101], and perhaps in the setting of CRC liver metastases, LT may provide potential survival benefit [102].

Interestingly, the investigators from the same group from Oslo also initiated a phase III clinical trial to compare liver transplantation in selected patients with resectable CRC liver metastases to determine benefit compared to patients receiving liver resection, and it is estimated to be completed in 2027. Technically resectable patients would be randomized to arm A receiving either liver transplantation or resection; nonresectable patients with the metachronous or synchronous disease would be assigned to arm B or C, receiving either liver transplant or chemotherapy only, respectively (www.clinicaltrials.gov, NCT01479608). This ongoing trial remains highly controversial as it is difficult to be ethically justified at present. In an ideal setting, a patient with resectable CRC liver metastases could benefit more from liver transplantation oncologically over resection only if the radiologically visible and invisible metastatic tumors are limited to the native liver. Technically, it is currently almost impossible to select such a perfect candidate for liver transplantation. It is also highly unlikely that tumors cells are only limited in the liver given the metastatic nature and the often late stage of the disease.

Strategies to Limit Tumor Recurrence After OLT for Unresectable CRC Liver Metastases

To date, nearly all the patients with unresectable CRC liver metastases have suffered tumor recur-

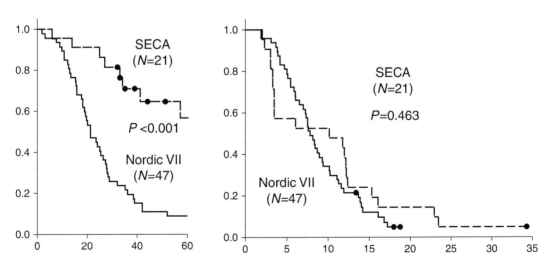

Fig. 24.4 The OS and PFS of CRC liver metastases after OLT (SECA study) or chemotherapy (Nordic VII study)

rence after liver transplantation, and there is insufficient selection criteria and treatment to decrease the tumor recurrence. However, ongoing studies of CRC and liver transplantation for other cancers such HCC and NET liver metastases could provide some clues.

Similar to NET, circulating CRC tumor cell [103], cell-free DNA [104, 105], and miRNA [106] have been reported as promising biomarkers for detection, monitoring, and survival prediction of patients with colorectal cancer. These emerging techniques might be helpful to select transplant candidates with unresectable CRC liver metastases in the future. It is also reported that 12.5% of patients with unresectable CRC liver metastases were downstaged to be resectable by chemotherapy; the 5-year survival was 33% overall despite a high rate of recurrence [101, 107, 108]. It remains unclear whether this strategy, the biomarkers cited above, would work in the setting of liver transplantation for unresectable CRC liver metastases. Avoidance of over-immunosuppression and consideration of immunosuppression with antineoplastic properties (e.g., m-TOR agents) might also be helpful to decrease the risk of tumor recurrence after liver transplantation for unresectable CRC liver metastases; these approaches will require further basic and clinical study. Studies have also been showing several promising novel treatment modalities for CRC, such as immune checkpoint therapies like PD-1 blockade [109], VEGF and/or EGFR antibody therapy, and genomic-driven treatments [110].

In summary, novel diagnostic methods and therapeutic agents may be able to optimize the selection of transplant candidates with unresectable CRC liver metastases and minimize the risk of tumor recurrence after liver transplantation.

Liver Transplantation and Other Liver Metastases

Liver transplantation cases also have been sporadically reported attempting to treat other unresectable malignant liver metastases from sarcoma ($n = 13$) [111], pancreatic pseudopapillary tumors ($n = 4$) [112–115], hemangiopericytoma ($n = 2$) [116, 117], breast cancer ($n = 1$) [118], and gastric cancer ($n = 1$) [119]. Essentially, almost all patients have developed tumor recurrence, and these liver metastases remain as contraindications for OLT.

Summary and Future

The scarcity of deceased-donor organs has led to strict allocation indications for liver transplantation for malignancies. Although liver transplantation may significantly increase the quality of life and overall survival, long-term tumor recurrence remains extremely high in the setting of metastatic disease to the liver. In the USA, the UNOS community has currently considered that transplantation for malignant liver diseases should receive exception points only when outcomes are substantially equivalent to results with standard indications, and only highly selected patient with liver malignancies can receive an exception MELD points at this time. Ongoing basic and clinical research of transplantation oncology may expand the indications of OLT for primary and secondary malignant liver diseases in the future.

References

1. Busuttil RW, Klintmalm G. Transplantation of the liver. 3rd ed. Philadelphia: Elsevier; 2015. p. 205–13.
2. Blechacz BR, Gores GJ. Cholangiocarcinoma. Clin Liver Dis. 2008;12(1):131–50, ix.
3. Shaib YH, Davila JA, McGlynn K, El-Serag HB. Rising incidence of intrahepatic cholangiocarcinoma in the United States: a true increase? J Hepatol. 2004;40(3):472–7.
4. Lazaridis KN, Gores GJ. Cholangiocarcinoma. Gastroenterology. 2005;128(6):1655–67.
5. Oliveira IS, Kilcoyne A, Everett JM, Mino-Kenudson M, Harisinghani MG, Ganesan K. Cholangiocarcinoma: classification, diagnosis, staging, imaging features, and management. Abdom Radiol (NY). 2017;42(6):1637–49.
6. Doherty B, Nambudiri VE, Palmer WC. Update on the diagnosis and treatment of cholangiocarcinoma. Curr Gastroenterol Rep. 2017;19(1):2.
7. Patel T. Cholangiocarcinoma—controversies and challenges. Nat Rev Gastroenterol Hepatol. 2011;8(4):189–200.

8. Mar WA, Shon AM, Lu Y, Yu JH, Berggruen SM, Guzman G, et al. Imaging spectrum of cholangiocarcinoma: role in diagnosis, staging, and posttreatment evaluation. Abdom Radiol (NY). 2016;41(3):553–67.
9. Petrowsky H, Wildbrett P, Husarik DB, Hany TF, Tam S, Jochum W, et al. Impact of integrated positron emission tomography and computed tomography on staging and management of gallbladder cancer and cholangiocarcinoma. J Hepatol. 2006;45(1):43–50.
10. Brandi G, Venturi M, Pantaleo MA, Ercolani G, GICO. Cholangiocarcinoma: current opinion on clinical practice diagnostic and therapeutic algorithms: a review of the literature and a long-standing experience of a referral center. Dig Liver Dis. 2016;48(3):231–41.
11. Jung DH, Hwang S, Song GW, Ahn CS, Moon DB, Kim KH, et al. Clinicopathological features and prognosis of intrahepatic cholangiocarcinoma after liver transplantation and resection. Ann Transplant. 2017;22:42–52.
12. DeOliveira ML, Cunningham SC, Cameron JL, Kamangar F, Winter JM, Lillemoe KD, et al. Cholangiocarcinoma: thirty-one-year experience with 564 patients at a single institution. Ann Surg. 2007;245(5):755–62.
13. Jonas S, Thelen A, Benckert C, Biskup W, Neumann U, Rudolph B, et al. Extended liver resection for intrahepatic cholangiocarcinoma: a comparison of the prognostic accuracy of the fifth and sixth editions of the TNM classification. Ann Surg. 2009;249(2):303–9.
14. Roayaie S, Guarrera JV, Ye MQ, Thung SN, Emre S, Fishbein TM, et al. Aggressive surgical treatment of intrahepatic cholangiocarcinoma: predictors of outcomes. J Am Coll Surg. 1998;187(4):365–72.
15. Puhalla H, Schuell B, Pokorny H, Kornek GV, Scheithauer W, Gruenberger T. Treatment and outcome of intrahepatic cholangiocellular carcinoma. Am J Surg. 2005;189(2):173–7.
16. Lang H, Sotiropoulos GC, Sgourakis G, Schmitz KJ, Paul A, Hilgard P, et al. Operations for intrahepatic cholangiocarcinoma: single-institution experience of 158 patients. J Am Coll Surg. 2009;208(2):218–28.
17. Choi SB, Kim KS, Choi JY, Park SW, Choi JS, Lee WJ, et al. The prognosis and survival outcome of intrahepatic cholangiocarcinoma following surgical resection: association of lymph node metastasis and lymph node dissection with survival. Ann Surg Oncol. 2009;16(11):3048–56.
18. Endo I, Gonen M, Yopp AC, Dalal KM, Zhou Q, Klimstra D, et al. Intrahepatic cholangiocarcinoma: rising frequency, improved survival, and determinants of outcome after resection. Ann Surg. 2008;248(1):84–96.
19. Farges O, Fuks D, Le Treut YP, Azoulay D, Laurent A, Bachellier P, et al. AJCC 7th edition of TNM staging accurately discriminates outcomes of patients with resectable intrahepatic cholangiocarcinoma: by the AFC-IHCC-2009 study group. Cancer. 2011;117(10):2170–7.
20. Burke EC, Jarnagin WR, Hochwald SN, Pisters PW, Fong Y, Blumgart LH. Hilar Cholangiocarcinoma: patterns of spread, the importance of hepatic resection for curative operation, and a presurgical clinical staging system. Ann Surg. 1998;228(3):385–94.
21. Tsao JI, Nimura Y, Kamiya J, Hayakawa N, Kondo S, Nagino M, et al. Management of hilar cholangiocarcinoma: comparison of an American and a Japanese experience. Ann Surg. 2000;232(2):166–74.
22. Nuzzo G, Giuliante F, Ardito F, Giovannini I, Aldrighetti L, Belli G, et al. Improvement in perioperative and long-term outcome after surgical treatment of hilar cholangiocarcinoma: results of an Italian multicenter analysis of 440 patients. Arch Surg (Chicago, IL: 1960). 2012;147(1):26–34.
23. Chamberlain RS, Blumgart LH. Hilar cholangiocarcinoma: a review and commentary. Ann Surg Oncol. 2000;7(1):55–66.
24. Iwatsuki S, Todo S, Marsh JW, Madariaga JR, Lee RG, Dvorchik I, et al. Treatment of hilar cholangiocarcinoma (Klatskin tumors) with hepatic resection or transplantation. J Am Coll Surg. 1998;187(4):358–64.
25. De Vreede I, Steers JL, Burch PA, Rosen CB, Gunderson LL, Haddock MG, et al. Prolonged disease-free survival after orthotopic liver transplantation plus adjuvant chemoirradiation for cholangiocarcinoma. Liver Transpl. 2000;6(3):309–16.
26. Goldstein RM, Stone M, Tillery GW, Senzer N, Levy M, Husberg BS, et al. Is liver transplantation indicated for cholangiocarcinoma? Am J Surg. 1993;166(6):768–71; discussion 71–2.
27. Darwish Murad S, Kim WR, Harnois DM, Douglas DD, Burton J, Kulik LM, et al. Efficacy of neoadjuvant chemoradiation, followed by liver transplantation, for perihilar cholangiocarcinoma at 12 US centers. Gastroenterology. 2012;143(1):88–98.e3; quiz e14.
28. OPTN. Allocation of Livers and Liver-Intestines 2017. https://optn.transplant.hrsa.gov/governance/policies/.
29. Kraybill WG, Lee H, Picus J, Ramachandran G, Lopez MJ, Kucik N, et al. Multidisciplinary treatment of biliary tract cancers. J Surg Oncol. 1994;55(4):239–45.
30. Pimpalwar AP, Sharif K, Ramani P, Stevens M, Grundy R, Morland B, et al. Strategy for hepatoblastoma management: transplant versus nontransplant surgery. J Pediatr Surg. 2002;37(2):240–5.
31. Mavros MN, Economopoulos KP, Alexiou VG, Pawlik TM. Treatment and prognosis for patients with intrahepatic cholangiocarcinoma: systematic review and meta-analysis. JAMA Surg. 2014;149(6):565–74.
32. Pitt HA, Nakeeb A, Abrams RA, Coleman J, Piantadosi S, Yeo CJ, et al. Perihilar cholangiocarcinoma. Postoperative radiotherapy does not improve

survival. Ann Surg. 1995;221(6):788–97; discussion 97–8.
33. Nakeeb A, Tran KQ, Black MJ, Erickson BA, Ritch PS, Quebbeman EJ, et al. Improved survival in resected biliary malignancies. Surgery. 2002;132(4):555–63; discission 63–4.
34. Ben-Josef E, Guthrie KA, El-Khoueiry AB, Corless CL, Zalupski MM, Lowy AM, et al. SWOG S0809: a phase II intergroup trial of adjuvant capecitabine and gemcitabine followed by radiotherapy and concurrent capecitabine in extrahepatic cholangiocarcinoma and gallbladder carcinoma. J Clin Oncol. 2015;33(24):2617–22.
35. Nelson JW, Ghafoori AP, Willett CG, Tyler DS, Pappas TN, Clary BM, et al. Concurrent chemoradiotherapy in resected extrahepatic cholangiocarcinoma. Int J Radiat Oncol Biol Phys. 2009;73(1):148–53.
36. Rea DJ, Heimbach JK, Rosen CB, Haddock MG, Alberts SR, Kremers WK, et al. Liver transplantation with neoadjuvant chemoradiation is more effective than resection for hilar cholangiocarcinoma. Ann Surg. 2005;242(3):451–8; discussion 8–61.
37. Spolverato G, Vitale A, Cucchetti A, Popescu I, Marques HP, Aldrighetti L, et al. Can hepatic resection provide a long-term cure for patients with intrahepatic cholangiocarcinoma? Cancer. 2015;121(22):3998–4006.
38. Tamandl D, Herberger B, Gruenberger B, Puhalla H, Klinger M, Gruenberger T. Influence of hepatic resection margin on recurrence and survival in intrahepatic cholangiocarcinoma. Ann Surg Oncol. 2008;15(10):2787–94.
39. Yokoyama I, Todo S, Iwatsuki S, Starzl TE. Liver transplantation in the treatment of primary liver cancer. Hepatogastroenterology. 1990;37(2):188–93.
40. Pichlmayr R, Weimann A, Oldhafer KJ, Schlitt HJ, Klempnauer J, Bornscheuer A, et al. Role of liver transplantation in the treatment of unresectable liver cancer. World J Surg. 1995;19(6):807–13.
41. Becker NS, Rodriguez JA, Barshes NR, O'Mahony CA, Goss JA, Aloia TA. Outcomes analysis for 280 patients with cholangiocarcinoma treated with liver transplantation over an 18-year period. J Gastrointest Surg. 2008;12(1):117–22.
42. Fu BS, Zhang T, Li H, Yi SH, Wang GS, Xu C, et al. The role of liver transplantation for intrahepatic cholangiocarcinoma: a single-center experience. Eur Surg Res. 2011;47(4):218–21.
43. Hong JC, Jones CM, Duffy JP, Petrowsky H, Farmer DG, French S, et al. Comparative analysis of resection and liver transplantation for intrahepatic and hilar cholangiocarcinoma: a 24-year experience in a single center. Arch Surg. 2011;146(6):683–9.
44. Facciuto ME, Singh MK, Lubezky N, Selim MA, Robinson D, Kim-Schluger L, et al. Tumors with intrahepatic bile duct differentiation in cirrhosis: implications on outcomes after liver transplantation. Transplantation. 2015;99(1):151–7.
45. Sapisochin G, Fidelman N, Roberts JP, Yao FY. Mixed hepatocellular cholangiocarcinoma and intrahepatic cholangiocarcinoma in patients undergoing transplantation for hepatocellular carcinoma. Liver Transpl. 2011;17(8):934–42.
46. Darbari A, Sabin KM, Shapiro CN, Schwarz KB. Epidemiology of primary hepatic malignancies in U.S. children. Hepatology (Baltimore, Md). 2003;38(3):560–6.
47. McLaughlin CC, Baptiste MS, Schymura MJ, Nasca PC, Zdeb MS. Maternal and infant birth characteristics and hepatoblastoma. Am J Epidemiol. 2006;163(9):818–28.
48. Pizzo PA, Poplack D. Principles and practice of pediatric oncology. 7th ed. Wolters Kluwer; 2016.
49. Suriawinata A. Pathology of malignant liver tumors [March 2017]. www.uptodate.com.
50. Powell CKH. AHEP0731: treatment of children with all stages of hepatoblastoma with temsirolimus added to high risk stratum treatment 2017 [March 2017]. www.chidrensoncologygroup.org.
51. Black CT, Cangir A, Choroszy M, Andrassy RJ. Marked response to preoperative high-dose cisplatinum in children with unresectable hepatoblastoma. J Pediatr Surg. 1991;26(9):1070–3.
52. Ortega JA, Douglass EC, Feusner JH, Reynolds M, Quinn JJ, Finegold MJ, et al. Randomized comparison of cisplatin/vincristine/fluorouracil and cisplatin/continuous infusion doxorubicin for treatment of pediatric hepatoblastoma: a report from the Children's Cancer Group and the Pediatric Oncology Group. J Clin Oncol. 2000;18(14):2665–75.
53. Perilongo G, Maibach R, Shafford E, Brugieres L, Brock P, Morland B, et al. Cisplatin versus cisplatin plus doxorubicin for standard-risk hepatoblastoma. N Engl J Med. 2009;361(17):1662–70.
54. Zsiros J, Brugieres L, Brock P, Roebuck D, Maibach R, Zimmermann A, et al. Dose-dense cisplatin-based chemotherapy and surgery for children with high-risk hepatoblastoma (SIOPEL-4): a prospective, single-arm, feasibility study. Lancet Oncol. 2013;14(9):834–42.
55. Trobaugh-Lotrario AD, Meyers RL, Tiao GM, Feusner JH. Pediatric liver transplantation for hepatoblastoma. Transl Gastroenterol Hepatol. 2016;1:44.
56. Srinivasan P, McCall J, Pritchard J, Dhawan A, Baker A, Vergani GM, et al. Orthotopic liver transplantation for unresectable hepatoblastoma. Transplantation. 2002;74(5):652–5.
57. Tiao GM, Bobey N, Allen S, Nieves N, Alonso M, Bucuvalas J, et al. The current management of hepatoblastoma: a combination of chemotherapy, conventional resection, and liver transplantation. J Pediatr. 2005;146(2):204–11.
58. Koneru B, Flye MW, Busuttil RW, Shaw BW, Lorber MI, Emond JC, et al. Liver transplantation for hepatoblastoma. The American experience. Ann Surg. 1991;213(2):118–21.

59. Zsiros J, Maibach R, Shafford E, Brugieres L, Brock P, Czauderna P, et al. Successful treatment of childhood high-risk hepatoblastoma with dose-intensive multiagent chemotherapy and surgery: final results of the SIOPEL-3HR study. J Clin Oncol. 2010;28(15):2584–90.
60. Hery G, Franchi-Abella S, Habes D, Brugieres L, Martelli H, Fabre M, et al. Initial liver transplantation for unresectable hepatoblastoma after chemotherapy. Pediatr Blood Cancer. 2011;57(7):1270–5.
61. Browne M, Sher D, Grant D, Deluca E, Alonso E, Whitington PF, et al. Survival after liver transplantation for hepatoblastoma: a 2-center experience. J Pediatr Surg. 2008;43(11):1973–81.
62. Otte JB. Paediatric liver transplantation—a review based on 20 years of personal experience. Transpl Int. 2004;17(10):562–73.
63. Kueht M, Thompson P, Rana A, Cotton R, O'Mahony C, Goss J. Effects of an early referral system on liver transplantation for hepatoblastoma at Texas Children's Hospital. Pediatr Transplant. 2016;20(4):515–22.
64. Hackl C, Schlitt HJ, Kirchner GI, Knoppke B, Loss M. Liver transplantation for malignancy: current treatment strategies and future perspectives. World J Gastroenterol. 2014;20(18):5331–44.
65. Oberg K, Castellano D. Current knowledge on diagnosis and staging of neuroendocrine tumors. Cancer Metastasis Rev. 2011;30(Suppl 1):3–7.
66. Grandhi MS, Lafaro KJ, Pawlik TM. Role of locoregional and systemic approaches for the treatment of patients with metastatic neuroendocrine tumors. J Gastrointest Surg. 2015;19(12):2273–82.
67. Kulke MH, Shah MH, Benson AB III, Bergsland E, Berlin JD, Blaszkowsky LS, et al. Neuroendocrine tumors, version 1.2015. J Natl Compr Canc Netw. 2015;13(1):78–108.
68. Mazzaferro V, Pulvirenti A, Coppa J. Neuroendocrine tumors metastatic to the liver: how to select patients for liver transplantation? J Hepatol. 2007;47(4):460–6.
69. van Vilsteren FG, Baskin-Bey ES, Nagorney DM, Sanderson SO, Kremers WK, Rosen CB, et al. Liver transplantation for gastroenteropancreatic neuroendocrine cancers: defining selection criteria to improve survival. Liver Transpl. 2006;12(3):448–56.
70. Lehnert T. Liver transplantation for metastatic neuroendocrine carcinoma: an analysis of 103 patients. Transplantation. 1998;66(10):1307–12.
71. Le Treut YP, Delpero JR, Dousset B, Cherqui D, Segol P, Mantion G, et al. Results of liver transplantation in the treatment of metastatic neuroendocrine tumors. A 31-case French multicentric report. Ann Surg. 1997;225(4):355–64.
72. Olausson M, Friman S, Cahlin C, Nilsson O, Jansson S, Wangberg B, et al. Indications and results of liver transplantation in patients with neuroendocrine tumors. World J Surg. 2002;26(8):998–1004.
73. Cahlin C, Friman S, Ahlman H, Backman L, Mjornstedt L, Lindner P, et al. Liver transplantation for metastatic neuroendocrine tumor disease. Transplant Proc. 2003;35(2):809–10.
74. Florman S, Toure B, Kim L, Gondolesi G, Roayaie S, Krieger N, et al. Liver transplantation for neuroendocrine tumors. J Gastrointest Surg. 2004;8(2):208–12.
75. Rosenau J, Bahr MJ, von Wasielewski R, Mengel M, Schmidt HH, Nashan B, et al. Ki67, E-cadherin, and p53 as prognostic indicators of long-term outcome after liver transplantation for metastatic neuroendocrine tumors. Transplantation. 2002;73(3):386–94.
76. Le Treut YP, Gregoire E, Belghiti J, Boillot O, Soubrane O, Mantion G, et al. Predictors of long-term survival after liver transplantation for metastatic endocrine tumors: an 85-case French multicentric report. Am J Transplant. 2008;8(6):1205–13.
77. Gedaly R, Daily MF, Davenport D, McHugh PP, Koch A, Angulo P, et al. Liver transplantation for the treatment of liver metastases from neuroendocrine tumors: an analysis of the UNOS database. Arch Surg (Chicago, IL: 1960). 2011;146(8):953–8.
78. Nguyen NT, Harring TR, Goss JA, O'Mahony CA. Neuroendocrine liver metastases and orthotopic liver transplantation: the US experience. Int J Hepatol. 2011;2011:742890.
79. Rossi RE, Burroughs AK, Caplin ME. Liver transplantation for unresectable neuroendocrine tumor liver metastases. Ann Surg Oncol. 2014;21(7):2398–405.
80. Pavel M, Baudin E, Couvelard A, Krenning E, Oberg K, Steinmuller T, et al. ENETS Consensus Guidelines for the management of patients with liver and other distant metastases from neuroendocrine neoplasms of foregut, midgut, hindgut, and unknown primary. Neuroendocrinology. 2012;95(2):157–76.
81. OPTN. Organ Procurement and Transplantation Network (OPTN): Guidelines for Neuroendocrine Tumors (NET). 2015. https://optn.transplant.hrsa.gov/resources/by-organ/liver-intestine/guidance-on-meld-peld-exception-review/#NET.
82. Khan MS, Kirkwood AA, Tsigani T, Lowe H, Goldstein R, Hartley JA, et al. Early changes in circulating tumor cells are associated with response and survival following treatment of metastatic neuroendocrine neoplasms. Clin Cancer Res. 2016;22(1):79–85.
83. Khan MS, Kirkwood A, Tsigani T, Garcia-Hernandez J, Hartley JA, Caplin ME, et al. Circulating tumor cells as prognostic markers in neuroendocrine tumors. J Clin Oncol. 2013;31(3):365–72.
84. Oberg K, Modlin IM, De Herder W, Pavel M, Klimstra D, Frilling A, et al. Consensus on biomarkers for neuroendocrine tumour disease. Lancet Oncol. 2015;16(9):e435–46.
85. Farkas SA, Schnitzbauer AA, Kirchner G, Obed A, Banas B, Schlitt HJ. Calcineurin inhibitor minimization protocols in liver transplantation. Transpl Int. 2009;22(1):49–60.
86. Schnitzbauer AA, Zuelke C, Graeb C, Rochon J, Bilbao I, Burra P, et al. A prospective randomised, open-labeled, trial comparing sirolimus-containing

versus mTOR-inhibitor-free immunosuppression in patients undergoing liver transplantation for hepatocellular carcinoma. BMC Cancer. 2010;10:190.
87. Zhu H, Sun Q, Tan C, Xu M, Dai Z, Wang Z, et al. Tacrolimus promotes hepatocellular carcinoma and enhances CXCR4/SDF-1α expression in vivo. Mol Med Rep. 2014;10(2):585–92.
88. Zhou S, Tan C, Dai Z, Zhu H, Xu M, Zhou Z, et al. Tacrolimus enhances the invasion potential of hepatocellular carcinoma cells and promotes lymphatic metastasis in a rat model of hepatocellular carcinoma: involvement of vascular endothelial growth factor-C. Transplant Proc. 2011;43(7):2747–54.
89. Geissler EK, Schnitzbauer AA, Zulke C, Lamby PE, Proneth A, Duvoux C, et al. Sirolimus use in liver transplant recipients with hepatocellular carcinoma: a randomized, multicenter, open-label phase 3 trial. Transplantation. 2016;100(1):116–25.
90. Hackl C, Gerken M, Loss M, Klinkhammer-Schalke M, Piso P, Schlitt HJ. A population-based analysis on the rate and surgical management of colorectal liver metastases in Southern Germany. Int J Color Dis. 2011;26(11):1475–81.
91. Hoti E, Adam R. Liver transplantation for primary and metastatic liver cancers. Transpl Int. 2008;21(12):1107–17.
92. Foss A, Adam R, Dueland S. Liver transplantation for colorectal liver metastases: revisiting the concept. Transpl Int. 2010;23(7):679–85.
93. Chapman WC. Liver transplantation for unresectable metastases to the liver: a new era in transplantation or a time for caution? Ann Surg. 2013;257(5):816–7.
94. Jones PD, Hayashi PH, Barritt AS IV. Liver transplantation in 2013: challenges and controversies. Minerva Gastroenterol Dietol. 2013;59(2):117–31.
95. Kim WR, Stock PG, Smith JM, Heimbach JK, Skeans MA, Edwards EB, et al. OPTN/SRTR 2011 Annual Data Report: liver. Am J Transplant. 2013;13(Suppl 1):73–102.
96. Martins PN, Movahedi B, Bozorgzadeh A. Liver transplantation for unresectable colorectal cancer liver metastases: a paradigm change? Ann Surg. 2015;262(1):e12.
97. Hernandez-Alejandro R, Wall WJ. The RAPID concept-novel idea or a bridge too far? Ann Surg. 2015;262(1):e10–1.
98. Eghtesad B, Aucejo F. Liver transplantation for malignancies. J Gastrointest Cancer. 2014;45(3):353–62.
99. Hagness M, Foss A, Line PD, Scholz T, Jorgensen PF, Fosby B, et al. Liver transplantation for nonresectable liver metastases from colorectal cancer. Ann Surg. 2013;257(5):800–6.
100. Dueland S, Guren TK, Hagness M, Glimelius B, Line PD, Pfeiffer P, et al. Chemotherapy or liver transplantation for nonresectable liver metastases from colorectal cancer? Ann Surg. 2015;261(5):956–60.
101. Adam R, Delvart V, Pascal G, Valeanu A, Castaing D, Azoulay D, et al. Rescue surgery for unresectable colorectal liver metastases downstaged by chemotherapy: a model to predict long-term survival. Ann Surg. 2004;240(4):644–57; discussion 57–8.
102. Tanaka K, Murakami T, Yabushita Y, Hiroshima Y, Matsuo K, Endo I, et al. Maximal debulking liver resection as a beneficial treatment strategy for advanced and aggressive colorectal liver metastases. Anticancer Res. 2014;34(10):5547–54.
103. Hardingham JE, Grover P, Winter M, Hewett PJ, Price TJ, Thierry B. Detection and clinical significance of circulating tumor cells in colorectal cancer—20 years of progress. Mol Med (Cambridge, Mass). 2015;21(Suppl 1):S25–31.
104. Basnet S, Zhang ZY, Liao WQ, Li SH, Li PS, Ge HY. The prognostic value of circulating cell-free DNA in colorectal cancer: a meta-analysis. J Cancer. 2016;7(9):1105–13.
105. Hao TB, Shi W, Shen XJ, Qi J, Wu XH, Wu Y, et al. Circulating cell-free DNA in serum as a biomarker for diagnosis and prognostic prediction of colorectal cancer. Br J Cancer. 2014;111(8):1482–9.
106. Zekri AR, Youssef AS, Lotfy MM, Gabr R, Ahmed OS, Nassar A, et al. Circulating serum miRNAs as diagnostic markers for colorectal cancer. PLoS One. 2016;11(5):e0154130.
107. Nuzzo G, Giuliante F, Ardito F, Vellone M, Pozzo C, Cassano A, et al. Liver resection for primarily unresectable colorectal metastases downsized by chemotherapy. J Gastrointest Surg. 2007;11(3):318–24.
108. Ivorra P, Sabater L, Calvete J, Camps B, Cervantes A, Bosch A, et al. [Effect of neoadjuvant chemotherapy on the results of resection of colorectal liver metastases]. Cir Esp. 2007;82(3):166–71.
109. Le DT, Uram JN, Wang H, Bartlett BR, Kemberling H, Eyring AD, et al. PD-1 blockade in tumors with mismatch-repair deficiency. N Engl J Med. 2015;372(26):2509–20.
110. Ciombor KK, Bekaii-Saab T. Emerging treatments in recurrent and metastatic colorectal cancer. J Natl Compr Canc Netw. 2013;11(Suppl 4):S18–27.
111. Husted TL, Neff G, Thomas MJ, Gross TG, Woodle ES, Buell JF. Liver transplantation for primary or metastatic sarcoma to the liver. Am J Transplant. 2006;6(2):392–7.
112. Kocman B, Jadrijevic S, Skopljanac A, Mikulic D, Gustin D, Buhin M, et al. Living donor liver transplantation for unresectable liver metastases from solid pseudo-papillary tumor of the pancreas: a case report. Transplant Proc. 2008;40(10):3787–90.
113. Dovigo AG, Diaz MB, Gutierrez MG, Selles CF, Grobas JP, Valladares M, et al. Liver transplantation as treatment in a massive metastasis from Gruber-Frantz pancreatic tumor: a case report. Transplant Proc. 2011;43(6):2272–3.
114. Lagiewska B, Pacholczyk M, Lisik W, Cichocki A, Nawrocki G, Trzebicki J, et al. Liver transplantation for nonresectable metastatic solid pseudopapillary pancreatic cancer. Ann Transplant. 2013;18:651–3.
115. Sumida W, Kaneko K, Tainaka T, Ono Y, Kiuchi T, Ando H. Liver transplantation for multiple liver

metastases from solid pseudopapillary tumor of the pancreas. J Pediatr Surg. 2007;42(12):e27–31.
116. Adams J, Lodge JP, Parker D. Liver transplantation for metastatic hemangiopericytoma associated with hypoglycemia. Transplantation. 1999;67(3):488–9.
117. Urata K, Ikegami T, Nakazawa Y, Ohno Y, Kobayashi A, Mita A, et al. Living-donor liver transplantation for hepatic metastasis from meningeal hemangiopericytoma: a case report. Transplant Proc. 2015;47(7):2274–7.
118. Wilson JM, Carder P, Downey S, Davies MH, Wyatt JI, Brennan TG. Treatment of metastatic breast cancer with liver transplantation. Breast J. 2003;9(2):126–8.
119. Song XM, Zhan WH, Wang JP, Lan P, He XS, Cai SR, et al. Radical resection of gastric or colorectal carcinoma combined with liver transplantation for gastric or colorectal carcinoma with multiple hepatic metastases. Chin J Gastrointes Surg. 2005;8(5):419–21.

Radiation Therapy for Liver Metastases

Arya Amini and Karyn A. Goodman

Introduction

Metastatic liver disease may originate from multiple primary malignancies, most commonly colorectal, lung, and breast cancers [1]. In colorectal cancer, up to 15–25% of patients present with synchronous metastases at diagnosis, and 50–70% will develop metastases to the liver at some point during their clinical course [2]. Cancers of the gastrointestinal tract commonly metastasize to the liver due to the draining blood supply via the portal circulation. Historically, metastatic disease to the liver was often treated with systemic therapy alone. Over time, however, oncologists have begun to recognize the broad continuum of metastatic disease ranging from single, solitary sites to diffuse disease. The term "oligometastases" [3, 4], which is now commonly used, refers to an intermediate stage of metastases where the number and site of metastatic disease is limited and potential local forms of treatment including surgery, radiation, and thermal ablation can be effectively used with curative intent. The rationale for adding local ablative therapies in certain metastatic patients who otherwise have well-controlled systemic disease is that many can progress at sites of increasing tumor burden including the liver.

With better combination of chemotherapy and targeted agents available today, median survival has more than tripled for patients with metastatic colorectal cancer from 10 to 30 months [5, 6]. Therefore, better control of systemic disease has led to the need for more ablative local therapy options, such as stereotactic body radiation therapy (SBRT), for unresectable hepatic tumors. Up to 40% of patients with metastatic colorectal cancer have been found to have disease confined to the liver and could therefore possibly benefit from liver-directed therapy. Even for patients with well-controlled extrahepatic disease, but liver-dominant metastases, the most likely cause of death is from local progression in the liver [7–9].

Prior to the introduction of intensity-modulated radiation therapy (IMRT) and SBRT, radiation oncologists were limited by the tolerance of the liver to radiation. In the past several decades, tremendous advances in the field of radiation oncology such as more sophisticated treatment planning software and improved imaging modalities that can be performed real time with treatment have led to the overall ability to more accurately deliver radiotherapy to the target lesion. With the emergence of these improved techniques, more focal treatments with higher doses of radiation can be delivered to metastatic liver lesions while sparing normal liver parenchyma.

A. Amini · K. A. Goodman (✉)
Department of Radiation Oncology,
University of Colorado Cancer Center,
Aurora, CO, USA
e-mail: aamini@coh.org;
karyn.goodman@ucdenver.edu

Unique Morphologic and Clinical Features of the Liver

The structure of the liver's functional subunits, or lobules, which are arranged in parallel makes it more sensitive to the volume effect of radiotherapy. Thus, historically, liver irradiation was limited due to toxicity concerns since liver radiotherapy was delivered using very large fields, often encompassing the entire organ. The primary dose-limiting toxicity from whole-liver radiation was radiation-induced liver disease (RILD). RILD is a clinical syndrome first described nearly 50 years ago in patients undergoing whole-liver radiation [10]. RILD is defined as a triad of anicteric hepatomegaly, ascites, and elevated liver enzymes, typically occurring 3 months after completing of radiation [11, 12]. Histologically, RILD involves veno-occlusive injury with fibrin deposition in the central veins [13]. Modern studies have demonstrated that transforming growth factor-β (TGF-β) leads to the stimulation of fibroblast migration and development of liver fibrosis in RILD [14]. This complication thus far has rarely been observed with modern techniques of radiation delivery, such as SBRT. Early reports demonstrated patients treated to doses exceeding 30 Gy had higher rates of RILD [15, 16]. The Radiation Therapy Oncology Group (RTOG) conducted a dose-escalation whole-liver radiation study (RTOG 8405) and reported rates of RILD for doses of 27–30 Gy and 33 Gy of 0% and 10%, respectively. However, these low doses of radiation were ineffective in controlling gross disease; thus palliative whole-liver RT was used infrequently in the management of liver metastases.

A unique aspect of the liver is its potential for regeneration after injury. Liver regeneration as a parallel organ has been well-established in surgical series after partial hepatectomy [17]. While there is limited data demonstrating liver regeneration following radiation, one can extrapolate that partial liver radiation could stimulate a similar mechanism of repair. With the introduction of computed tomography (CT)-based radiation planning, investigators began exploring partial liver radiation and found higher doses could be achieved while sparing normal liver parenchyma, potentially allowing for regeneration and repair. This leads to a series of trials evaluating higher-dose conformal radiation to the liver [18, 19]. Dawson and colleagues [18] reported partial liver irradiation to doses as high as 70–90 Gy (1.5 Gy twice daily fractions) could be tolerated. In a subsequent report of 203 patients [20], they found no cases of RILD when the mean liver doses were maintained below 31 Gy. While these studies demonstrated improvement in tumor control, sustained local response continued to be suboptimal [21].

Overview of Stereotactic Body Radiation Therapy

The introduction of SBRT allows for more intensive tumor dose escalation delivered over fewer treatments with high conformality. With these newer treatment planning techniques, the dose can be delivered to the tumor with steep dose gradients outside the target to limit the amount of normal liver parenchyma receiving radiation, thereby decreasing complication rates from the effect of the radiation dose to the uninvolved liver and adjacent normal structures. The integration of SBRT into the management of liver metastases can only be accomplished with sophisticated treatment planning systems, tumor motion control, and localization techniques to allow for accurate and consistent targeting of the tumor. These allow for ablative tumor doses while minimizing toxicity to critical organs at risk including uninvolved liver parenchyma, the chest wall, and the gastrointestinal tract.

There is also a theoretical benefit of delivering higher doses with each fraction of SBRT based on the direct effect of high-dose RT on tumor vasculature shown in preclinical models. For example, high-dose radiation with 10 Gy or higher in a single fraction has been shown to cause severe vascular damage in human tumor xenografts [22, 23]. Additionally, the vascular injury and ensuing chaotic intra-tumoral environment caused by high-dose fraction SBRT may significantly hinder the repair of radiation damage [24]. As the survival and proliferation of tumor cells are directly dependent on the blood supply, the vascular effects of SBRT may lead to the ablative effects seen clinically.

There are now several prospective trials (described later in this chapter) using single-fraction versus multifraction SBRT for liver metastasis (Table 25.1). The majority of these trials treated 1–5 liver metastases, with tumors measuring no greater than 6 cm in largest diameter. The trials included patients with both favorable and unfavorable prognoses and the majority of metastatic liver lesions were from colorectal cancer [25]. Results from these studies showed 1- and 2-year local control rates ranging from 70 to 100% and 60 to 90%, respectively.

There are several potential mechanisms accounting for the higher rate of local control in comparison with older radiation techniques. Fractionated SBRT allows for delivery of highly conformal treatment of targets that are in close proximity to critical structures, and this has been hypothesized to improve the therapeutic ratio, thereby reducing the risk of late complications potentially associated with a large single dose [26]. Lastly, from a radiobiologic standpoint, the higher dose per fraction with SBRT-based treatments has been shown to provide improved local control over standard fractionation [27].

Patient Selection for SBRT

Patients with liver metastases from colorectal cancer should be discussed in a multidisciplinary fashion to identify cases that may be resectable as well as to determine if patients have adequate hepatic function to be eligible for liver SBRT. Based on data from current prospective trials treating liver lesions with SBRT, patients considered for SBRT should typically have five or fewer lesions with a size of no more than 6 cm in maximum diameter [28]. All patients should have adequate baseline liver function tests and a sufficient uninvolved proportion of liver which can be spared. Tumors which are in close proximity to adjacent radiosensitive structures, such as those close to the hilum, can potentially be treated with SBRT, but the total dose and fractionation scheme may need to be adjusted to meet the dose constraints of the adjacent organs/structures. Outside of current published studies, SBRT to lesions that are large (>6 cm) or patients who present with multiple lesions need to be considered on a case by case basis and undergo therapy under the guidance of an established protocol/study.

Image-Guided Radiation Therapy (IGRT)

IGRT is the use of daily imaging prior to radiation to ensure proper treatment setup and is performed daily for patients undergoing SBRT. With the reliance on image guidance during delivery of radiotherapy, there is a greater need for accurate target localization. As opposed to lung lesions, visualization of tumors in the liver is limited based on non-contrast cone beam CT (CBCT) scan. Hence, radiation oncologists often recommend that fiducial markers be placed prior to the radiation planning session or simulation process (referred to as CT simulation) to allow for accurate identification of the target and to assess the motion of the target during respiration. Gold fiducials are often placed percutaneously into or around the liver lesion to assist in target identification; it is recommended that at least 2–3 markers be placed in order to triangulate where the tumor is located and for improved tumor tracking during treatment [29]. Occasionally, postoperative clips can also be used to localize the treatment target.

Most new linear accelerators can obtain higher-quality diagnostic X-rays and have onboard three-dimensional (3D) CT imaging, known as CBCT, which is the common modality used for IGRT during SBRT. This provides real-time assessment of tumor positioning, while the patient is lying on the treatment table. IGRT using imaging such as CBCT has significantly advanced the radiation oncology field, allowing for better target alignment, which is critical when treating with SBRT to organs such as the liver, as there is a substantial degree of inter- and intra-fraction variability.

Table 25.1 Select prospective studies of SBRT for liver metastases

Study	Inclusion	Number of patients	Type of metastasis	Total dose per fraction	Toxicity	Median follow-up (months)	Local control rate	Survival
Herfarth et al. (2001) [37]	1–3 lesions	37	Not reported	14–26 Gy/1	No significant toxicity reported	14.9 (mean)	18 mo: 67%	1 yr: 76% 2 yr: 55%
Hoyer et al. (2006) [39]	1–6 lesions, largest ≤6 cm	44	CRC (44)	45 Gy/3	1 liver failure 2 severe late GI	52	2 yr: 86%	1 yr: 67% 2 yr: 38%
Mendez-Romero et al. (2006) [40]	1–3 lesions, largest <7 cm	25	CRC (14), lung (1), breast (1), carcinoid (1)	37.5 Gy/3	Acute grade ≥ 3: 4 cases Late grade 3: 1 case	12.9	2 yr: 86%	1 yr: 85% 2 yr: 62%
Rusthoven et al. (2009) [42]	1–3 lesions, largest <6 cm	47	CRC (15), lung (10), breast (4), ovarian (3), esophageal (3), HCC (2), other (10)	60 Gy/3	Late grade 3/4: <2%	16	2 yr: 92% <3 cm: 100%	Median: 17.6 mo
Lee et al. (2009) [43]	No maximum number or size	68	CRC (40), breast (12), gallbladder (4), lung (2), anal (2), melanoma (2)	28–60 Gy/6 Median 42 Gy	Acute grade 3: 8 cases Grade 4: 1 case (thrombocytopenia)	10.8	1 yr: 71%	18 mo: 47%
Ambrosino et al. (2009) [44]	1–3 lesions, largest <6 cm	27	CRC (11), other (16)	25–60 Gy/3 Median 36 Gy	No significant toxicity reported	13	74%	Not reported
Goodman et al. (2010) [38]	1–5 lesions, largest <5 cm	26	CRC (6), pancreatic (3), gastric (2), ovarian (2), other (6)	18–30 Gy/1	Late grade 2: 4 cases (2 GI, 2 soft tissue/rib)	17.3	1 yr: 77%	1 yr: 62% 2 yr: 49%
Rule et al. (2011) [45]	1–5 lesions	27	CRC (12), carcinoid (3), melanoma (2), other (10)	30 Gy/3, 50 Gy/5, 60 Gy/5	No grade 2 or higher reported	20	30 Gy: 56% 50 Gy: 89% 60 Gy: 100%	30 Gy: 56% (2 yr) 50 Gy: 67% (2 yr) 60 Gy: 50% (2 yr)
Scorsetti et al. (2013) [46]	1–3 lesions, largest <6 cm	61	CRC (29), breast (11), gynecologic (7), other (14)	52.5–75 Gy/3	No grade 3 or higher reported	24	91%	1 yr: 80% 2 yr: 70%

Abbreviations: *SBRT* stereotactic body radiotherapy, *yr* year, *mo* months, *CRC* colorectal cancer, *HCC* hepatocellular carcinoma

Motion Management During Treatment

The small, focal radiation fields used for SBRT could potentially miss the liver target if tumor motion with respiration is unaccounted for as this motion can be quite significant. Studies have shown that the liver can move as much as 1–8 cm in the superior-inferior direction and to a lesser degree from the anterior-posterior direction with respiration [30]. Variations in hollow organ filling due to gastric contents may also contribute to both inter- and intra-fraction motion. Because of the possibility of substantial liver motion, simply aligning the treatment field to bony landmarks during radiation delivery is not optimal. IGRT in combination with motion management is therefore frequently used for liver SBRT. Motion management incorporated in the radiation oncology clinic today can broadly be categorized as motion compensating or motion restricting [29].

Respiratory gating is a motion compensating technique consisting of beam radiation delivery at specific phases of the breathing cycle, usually during the expiratory phase where motion is the smallest and reproducibility is better. Tumor tracking is another motion compensating technique. For instance, the CyberKnife® system utilizes fiducial markers to localize the tumor [31, 32] and can track tumors in real time.

Motion restricting includes techniques such as abdominal compression and active breathing control (ABC). Abdominal compression uses a belt that compresses the abdominal cavity, increasing intra-abdominal pressure and limiting diaphragmatic respiratory motion, which translates to decreased liver motion during respiration. This technique can reduce the superior-inferior tumor motion by as much as 50% [33]. ABC is a technique used to deliver treatment while a patient holds his or her breath during a specific phase of the breathing cycle. This requires patient instruction on proper respiration patterns in addition to video tracking to deliver radiation at indicated points of the breathing cycle.

Patient Setup and Treatment

The radiation planning session, also referred to as the simulation process, should be done at least 3–5 days after placement of the fiducial markers to minimize any potential changes due to local inflammation or migration of the fiducial marker after the planning process. The simulation is the basis for the treatment planning process and includes the preparation of appropriate immobilization devices to keep the patient in the exact same position for treatment. A diagnostic CT scan with intravenous (IV) contrast and oral contrast if the target lesion(s) is near bowel is performed in the radiation oncology department. The CT images are taken, which are used for radiation planning purposes. Many institutions now employ four-dimensional (4D) CT to better delineate the motion of the liver lesion. 4D CT is acquired using a modified CT scanning technique that is synchronized with the respiratory pattern of the patient. The respiratory cycle of a patient is divided into numerous breathing phases, with end inspiration, end expiration, and interval phases between inspiration and expiration. For each breathing phase, a 3D construction is created, and these imaging sets at different breathing phases are constructed and analyzed to determine organ positions at all phases of respiration.

Most patients will also have a diagnostic multiphasic contrast-enhanced helical CT scan to assist in target localization. For liver tumors in particular, CT scans alone may not clearly delineate disease. Therefore, incorporation of a fluorodeoxyglucose positron emission tomography (FDG-PET) scan and magnetic resonance imaging (MRI) during planning can be helpful in better identifying the target. These additional images are fused to the simulation CT in the radiation oncology planning software.

Clinical Studies for Stereotactic Body Radiation Therapy for Liver Metastases

One of the first reports of the use of SBRT in extracranial tumors including liver was published by Blomgren and colleagues in 1998 [34, 35]. The study included 17 primary tumors and 21 liver metastases. Total radiation dose delivered was 20–45 Gy (mean 34.1 Gy) in 2–4 fractions. Actuarial local control of liver metastasis at 1- and 2-year intervals was 76% and 61%, respectively. There were no reported grade 3 or higher toxicities. A subsequent study of 34 patients with 42 lesions (13 lung, 6 hepatocellular, 23 lung or liver metastases) treated to 45 Gy in three fractions demonstrated a 2-year tumor control probability of 83.6% [36]. Tumor size appeared to be the greatest predictor of response with 95% local control rate in tumors <3 cm and only 58.3% in tumors ≥3 cm.

A summary of select prospective trials using SBRT for liver metastases is presented in Table 25.1. The majority of these trials treated 1–5 liver metastases, with tumors measuring no greater than 6 cm in the largest diameter. The trials included patients with both favorable and unfavorable prognoses [25]. The majority of metastatic liver lesions were from colorectal cancer. Overall, 1- and 2-year local control rates ranged from 70 to 100% and 60 to 90%, respectively. Median survival ranged from 10 to 34 months, with 2-year overall survival rates of 30–83%. The majority of these patients on long-term follow-up would later develop out-of-field metastases. The studies vary in dose heterogeneity, primary histology included, tumor volumes, total radiation dose, dose per fraction, and dosimetric planning criteria. Total radiation doses typically ranged from 30 to 60 Gy in 1–6 fractions. The following are all phase I or II trials. To date, there are no published phase III data.

Single-Fraction Stereotactic Body Radiation Therapy

There was early interest in single-fraction treatment for liver SBRT, similar to the single-fraction approach used in stereotactic radiosurgery for the brain. Herfarth and colleagues [37] from the University of Heidelberg were the first to report prospective outcomes of SBRT for liver metastases. The study enrolled 37 patients, with 55 liver metastases treated with single-fraction SBRT at a dose of 14–26 Gy. Local control at 18 months was reported to be 67%. No significant toxicities were recorded. There was a statistically significant difference in local tumor control between tumors treated with 14–20 Gy vs. 22–26 Gy, though this may have been due to a learning phase as investigators had noted local control also improved in patients who were enrolled later in the study, as more proper margin expansions were performed; patients enrolled in later years had an actuarial local control rate of 81% at 18 months [28, 37].

Goodman and colleagues [38] at Stanford University performed a phase I single-fraction dose-escalation study for primary and metastatic liver tumors. Of the 26 patients included, 19 patients had hepatic metastases. Total radiation dose was escalated from 18 to 30 Gy at 4-Gy increments. At a median follow-up of 17 months, there were no dose-limiting toxicities reported. There were nine acute grade 1, one acute grade 2, and two late grade 2 gastrointestinal toxicities observed. Local control at 1 year was 77%. For liver metastases patients, the 1- and 2-year overall survival rates were 62% and 49%, respectively. Investigators concluded that single-fraction SBRT is feasible with promising local control rates and tolerable side effects from treatment.

Hypofractionated Stereotactic Body Radiation Therapy

While the results of single-fraction liver SBRT appeared promising, the potential toxicity of the ultrahigh-dose radiotherapy in the abdomen leads many groups to evaluate the use of hypofractionated SBRT [39, 40]. Hoyer and colleagues [39] reported outcomes of 44 hepatic lesions treated with SBRT to 45 Gy divided in three fractions, with a 2-year actuarial local control of 79%. One- and two-year overall survival was 67% and 38%, respectively. Treatment-related toxicity included one patient who died of hepatic failure, one patient with colonic perforation requiring surgical management, and two patients with duodenal ulceration treated conservatively. In the trial by Méndez-Romero and colleagues [40], 34 liver metastases were treated to 37.5 Gy in three fractions. They reported a 2-year local control rate of 86%. One- and 2-year overall survival was 85% and 62%, respectively. There were three grade 3 toxicities documented among the patients with liver metastases.

In a phase I/II trial, investigators at the University of Colorado prospectively evaluated patients with three or fewer liver metastases, measuring less than 6 cm [41]. In the phase I portion of the trial which included 18 patients, the dose of SBRT was escalated from 36 to 60 Gy in three fractions, and no dose-limiting toxicity was observed. In the subsequent combined phase I/II multi-institutional trial, 47 patients with 63 liver metastases were enrolled and treated at seven participating institutions to 60 Gy in three fractions; 13 patients received <60 Gy, and 36 patients received 60 Gy [42]. Of patients with at least 6 months of radiographic follow-up after SBRT, only 3 infield local failures among 47 lesions occurred. At 2 years, the actuarial local control of all SBRT-treated lesions was 92%; among lesions <3 cm, the 2-year actuarial local control was 100%. Two-year overall survival was 30%. One patient experienced late grade 3 soft tissue breakdown. There were no reported grade 4–5 toxicities or RILD.

Investigators from Princess Margaret Hospital [43] also published their phase I trial of SBRT delivered in six fractions (median prescription dose of 41.8 Gy) to 68 patients with metastatic liver disease. Individualized radiation doses were chosen based on normal tissue complication probability (NTCP)-calculated risk of RILD at three risk levels (5%, 10%, and 20%). Observed 1-year local control was 71%, and no dose-limiting toxicity was observed. Two patients experienced acute grade 3 liver enzyme changes, and six patients had additional acute grade 3 toxicities including gastritis (2), nausea (2), lethargy (1), and thrombocytopenia (1). There was one grade 4 thrombocytopenia reported.

Ambrosino and colleagues [44] prospectively evaluated 27 patients with liver metastases treated with 25 to 60 Gy (median 36 Gy) delivered in three fractions. Mean tumor volume was 81.6 ± 35.9 ml. At a median follow-up of 13 months, crude local control was 74%. Mild to moderate transient hepatic dysfunction was observed in nine patients, pleural effusions in two patients, and partial portal vein thrombosis, pulmonary embolism, and upper gastrointestinal tract bleed in one patient each. Rule and colleagues [45] from the University of Texas Southwestern reported results from their phase I SBRT dose-escalation trial, with three dose groups, 30 Gy/3 fractions, 50 Gy/5 fractions, and 60 Gy /5 fractions. At 2 years, local control was 56%, 89%, and 100%, respectively. Two-year overall survival was 56%, 67%, and 50% accordingly. Further, there appeared to be a significant dose-response relationship between 30 and 60 Gy ($p = 0.009$). There were no grade 4–5 toxicity and one grade 3 asymptomatic transaminitis occurring in the 50 Gy cohort.

Investigators from Milan [46] reported on their phase II trial of 61 patients with 76 liver metastases treated to 25 Gy in three fractions. At a median follow-up of 12 months, the overall local control rate was 95%. One- and two-year overall survival was 80% and 70%, respectively. There were no reported events of RILD; one patient experienced late grade 3 chest wall pain.

Additional Studies

Chang and colleagues [47] performed a multi-institutional analysis reporting on prognostic factors following SBRT for colorectal cancer liver metastases. The study included 65 patients treated at three institutions. All patients had 1–4 lesions and received 1–6 fractions of SBRT to a median total dose of 42 Gy (range 22–60 Gy). The median follow-up was 1.2 years. On multivariate analysis, total dose of radiation, dose per fraction, and the BED were significantly associated with local control. Local disease control also appeared to be a borderline significant factor associated with improved overall survival under multivariate analysis ($p = 0.06$), demonstrating the impact local ablative therapy can have on overall survival. Chang and colleagues [47] further examined the correlation between total radiation dose and local control in a tumor control probability (TCP) model. Results from the TCP curves demonstrated that a 1-year local control rate exceeding 90% could be achieved when doses of 46–52 Gy in three fractions were delivered, concluding doses of 48 Gy or higher in three fractions should be offered if feasible.

Several studies have also evaluated the role of hypofractionation using more than five fractions. In one of the earlier studies, Sato and colleagues [48] evaluated 18 patients with 23 primary or metastatic liver lesions treated to a total dose of 50–60 Gy in 5–10 fractions. At 10-month follow-up, the crude local control rate was 100% with a 5% grade 1–2 and 5% grade 3–4 toxicity rate. A subsequent study by Wurm and colleagues [49] with three patients treated to a total dose of 74.8–79.2 Gy in 8–11 fractions also noted a local control rate of 100% (unspecified follow-up time). More recently, Katz and colleagues [50] published results of 174 metastatic liver lesions treated to a median total dose of 48 Gy (range, 30–55 Gy), delivered in 2–6 Gy fractions. At a median follow-up of 14.5 months, actuarial local control rates were 76% and 57% at 10 and 20 months accordingly. For liver metastases, the median overall survival was 14.5 months, and progression-free survival at 6 and 12 months was 46% and 24%, respectively. There was no grade 3 or higher toxicities reported.

The RTOG 0438 was a phase I trial of dose-escalated hypofractionated radiotherapy for hepatic metastases and is currently presented in abstract form only [51]. There were 26 patients enrolled, and four dose levels were achieved: 35–50 Gy in 5 Gy increments delivered in ten fractions. No dose-limiting toxicities were reported, although four patients (two patients at 45 Gy, two patients at 50 Gy) developed grade 3 toxicity. Investigators concluded that a hypofractionated regimen of 50 Gy in ten fractions is a reasonable and safe approach to treat metastatic liver lesions. Local control and survival outcomes have not been reported to date.

Long-Term Sequelae from Radiation

Most published series of liver SBRT have relatively short follow-up due to the nature of treating metastatic disease. Thus, the question remains as to what the long-term effects of SBRT may be on the biliary tree as well as the impact on overall liver function. The late effects of SBRT may become more significant as patients live longer with better systemic therapies. Fortunately, several small retrospective studies have reported data on long-term follow-up and toxicity from SBRT to the liver. Gunvén and colleagues [52] reported long-term radiation sequelae in 11 patients with up to 13-year follow-up. Follow-up tests included regular blood chemistry panels in addition to clearance of indocyanine green, and a segmental function study by single-photon emission computed tomography (SPECT) using hepatic iminodiacetic acid (HIDA) derivatives, including mebrofenin, to evaluate uptake by normal functioning hepatocytes. Their findings demonstrated overall elevations in liver serum values including alanine aminotransferase were uncommon, transient, and typically occurring within 2 years after SBRT; these findings were more common in patients with preexisting liver damage. Late liver function did not appear to be affected by treatment, even in the presence of cirrhosis. Two patients received equivalent 2 Gy (EQD_2) doses of 40 and 161 Gy to hilar structures, and no long-term bile duct damage was found. In two cases, moderate late liver dysfunction occurred – one patient after three courses of radiation and a second patient with cirrhosis after two liver resections and radiation.

One of the largest analyses of oligometastatic patients treated with SBRT with long-term follow-up was recently published by Fode and colleagues [53]. Their study included 321 patients (68% with liver metastases) with 587 lesions treated with SBRT over a 13-year period. The median follow-up was 5 years. Reported overall survival at 1, 3, 5, and 7.5 years was 80%, 39%, 23%, and 12%, respectively. Prognostic factors for overall survival in this study included performance status, solitary metastasis, metastasis measuring 30 mm or less, metachronous metastases, and pre-SBRT chemotherapy. Severe acute grade 3–4 toxicity occurred in 11 patients (3%), and late grade 3–4 toxicity occurred in 3 patients (1%). Specific to liver SBRT, one patient developed grade 3 gastritis and chronic skin reactions, and a second patient developed grade 3 chronic skin reaction after SBRT for liver metastases. An additional ten patients receiving SBRT to lung or liver experienced rib fractures 6–18 months after SBRT and were managed with pain medications. There were three possible treatment-related deaths: patient no. 1 deteriorated and died 6 weeks after SBRT; patient no. 2 died of hepatic failure 7 weeks after SBRT; and patient no. 3 developed a fistula from the stomach to the skin and died 15 months after SBRT. All three patients received total radiation dose of 45 Gy in three fractions (Fig. 25.1).

In a recent published quality of life analysis, Klein and colleagues [54] evaluated 222 patients treated with SBRT for hepatocellular carcinoma, liver metastases, or intrahepatic cholangiocarcinoma. SBRT total dose ranged from 24 to 60 Gy in six fractions. Prospective quality of life forms based on the European Organization for Research and Treatment of Cancer Quality of Life Questionnaire Core 30 (QLQ-C30) and/or Functional Assessment of Cancer Therapy-Hepatobiliary (FACT-Hep, version 4) questionnaires were provided at baseline and up to 12 months after treatment. Appetite and fatigue were clinically and statistically worse by 1 month but appeared to recover by 3 months after treatment. At 12 months, quality of life had improved in 23%, worsened in 39%, and was stable in 38%.

Future Directions

There are currently no randomized studies comparing SBRT and surgery for metastatic liver lesions, and there will likely not be one for some time, due to limited patient numbers and difficulty in accruing. Extrapolating from recent data published in non-small cell lung cancer (NSCLC), there appears to be promising results with SBRT when compared to surgery [55]. These results in lung cancer demonstrate the need for prospective trials evaluating outcomes comparing surgery to SBRT, for metastatic liver lesions are very much needed to assess local control rates, overall survival, and quality of life metrics. Further, given the heterogeneity in the currently published trials evaluating SBRT for liver metastases, multi-institutional prospective studies to evaluate the appropriate dose, fractionation scheme, and appropriate margins are urgently needed.

Additional data will also be needed to assess which noninvasive or minimally invasive modality to perform in select patients with liver metastases. There is currently at least one ongoing phase III randomized trial (NCT01233544) comparing radiofrequency ablation (RFA) to SBRT in colorectal cancer liver metastases [56]. The primary endpoint of the study is local progression-free survival.

Novel radiation delivery techniques including charged particle-based therapy may also provide an avenue for highly conformal dose-escalated treatment in liver tumors. Currently, most studies evaluating proton beam and carbon ion beam therapy have been in primary hepatocellular carcinoma. In several small, nonrandomized studies, for example, high-dose radiation with protons has demonstrated similar local control and survival rates to photon-based treatment in hepatocellular carcinoma [57–59]. Hong and colleagues evaluated respiratory-gated proton beam therapy for liver tumors, including primary hepatocellular carcinoma, intrahepatic cholangiocarcinoma, and liver metastasis, and found comparable local control rates and toxicity outcomes [60].

Delivery of SBRT with systemic therapies is also an integral part of the management for patients with metastatic liver disease. In patients with oligometastatic disease, the goal of SBRT is to minimize macrometastases, while systemic treatment is used to control micrometastases. Future studies evaluating combined modality treatment with SBRT and systemic therapies are needed.

Fig. 25.1 Example of liver stereotactic body radiation therapy (SBRT) plan treating to 50 Gy in five fractions with isodose lines representing the 50 Gy dose deposition prescribed to the target (green), with quick dose falloff represented by the 45 Gy (magenta) and 35 Gy lines (blue)

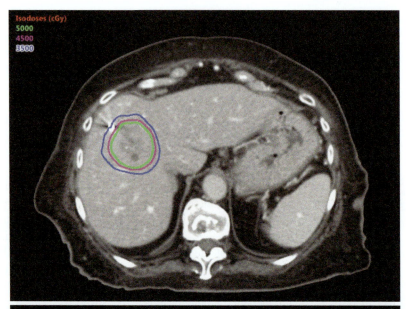

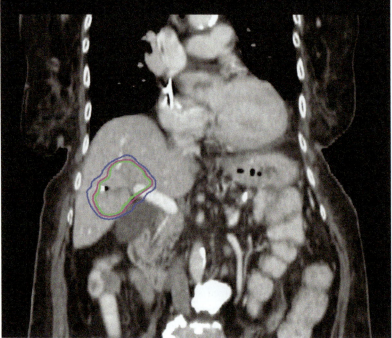

Conflicts of Interest The authors have no conflicts of interest to report.

References

1. Grover A, Alexander HR Jr. The past decade of experience with isolated hepatic perfusion. Oncologist. 2004;9:653–64.
2. Bozzetti F, Doci R, Bignami P, et al. Patterns of failure following surgical resection of colorectal cancer liver metastases: rationale for a multimodal approach. Recent Results Cancer Res. 1988;110:164–7.
3. Hellman S, Weichselbaum RR. Oligometastases. J Clin Oncol. 1995;13:8–10.
4. Weichselbaum RR, Hellman S. Oligometastases revisited. Nat Rev Clin Oncol. 2011;8:378–82.
5. Zuckerman DS, Clark JW. Systemic therapy for metastatic colorectal cancer. Cancer. 2008;112:1879–91.

6. Loupakis F, Cremolini C, Masi G, et al. Initial therapy with FOLFOXIRI and Bevacizumab for metastatic colorectal cancer. N Engl J Med. 2014;371:1609–18.
7. Crane CH, Koay EJ. Solutions that enable ablative radiotherapy for large liver tumors: fractionated dose painting, simultaneous integrated protection, motion management, and computed tomography image guidance. Cancer. 2016;122(13):1974–86.
8. Weiss L, Grundmann E, Torhorst J, et al. Haematogenous metastatic patterns in colonic carcinoma: an analysis of 1541 necropsies. J Pathol. 1986;150:195–203.
9. Wagner JS, Adson MA, Van Heerden JA, et al. The natural history of hepatic metastases from colorectal cancer. A comparison with resective treatment. Ann Surg. 1984;199:502–8.
10. Pan CC, Kavanagh BD, Dawson LA, et al. Radiation-associated liver injury. Int J Radiat Oncol Biol Phys. 2010;76:S94–100.
11. Lawrence TS, Robertson JM, Anscher MS, et al. Hepatic toxicity resulting from cancer treatment. Int J Radiat Oncol Biol Phys. 1995;31:1237–48.
12. Hawkins MA, Dawson LA. Radiation therapy for hepatocellular carcinoma: from palliation to cure. Cancer. 2006;106:1653–63.
13. Reed GB Jr, Cox AJ Jr. The human liver after radiation injury. A form of veno-occlusive disease. Am J Pathol. 1966;48:597–611.
14. Du SS, Qiang M, Zeng ZC, et al. Radiation-induced liver fibrosis is mitigated by gene therapy inhibiting transforming growth factor-beta signaling in the rat. Int J Radiat Oncol Biol Phys. 2010;78:1513–23.
15. Ingold JA, Reed GB, Kaplan HS, Bagshaw MA. Radiation hepatitis. Am J Roentgenol Radium Therapy, Nucl Med. 1965;93:200–8.
16. Austin-Seymour MM, Chen GT, Castro JR, et al. Dose volume histogram analysis of liver radiation tolerance. Int J Radiat Oncol Biol Phys. 1986;12:31–5.
17. Fausto N, Campbell JS, Riehle KJ. Liver regeneration. Hepatology. 2006;43:S45–53.
18. Dawson LA, McGinn CJ, Normolle D, et al. Escalated focal liver radiation and concurrent hepatic artery fluorodeoxyuridine for unresectable intrahepatic malignancies. J Clin Oncol. 2000;18:2210–8.
19. Robertson JM, Lawrence TS, Walker S, et al. The treatment of colorectal liver metastases with conformal radiation therapy and regional chemotherapy. Int J Radiat Oncol Biol Phys. 1995;32:445–50.
20. Dawson LA, Normolle D, Balter JM, et al. Analysis of radiation-induced liver disease using the Lyman NTCP model. Int J Radiat Oncol Biol Phys. 2002;53:810–21.
21. Mohiuddin M, Chen E, Ahmad N. Combined liver radiation and chemotherapy for palliation of hepatic metastases from colorectal cancer. J Clin Oncol. 1996;14:722–8.
22. Chen FH, Chiang CS, Wang CC, et al. Radiotherapy decreases vascular density and causes hypoxia with macrophage aggregation in TRAMP-C1 prostate tumors. Clin Cancer Res. 2009;15:1721–9.
23. Kioi M, Vogel H, Schultz G, et al. Inhibition of vasculogenesis, but not angiogenesis, prevents the recurrence of glioblastoma after irradiation in mice. J Clin Invest. 2010;120:694–705.
24. Song CW, Cho LC, Yuan J, et al. Radiobiology of stereotactic body radiation therapy/stereotactic radiosurgery and the linear-quadratic model. Int J Radiat Oncol Biol Phys. 2013;87:18–9.
25. Schefter TE, Kavanagh BD. Radiation therapy for liver metastases. Semin Radiat Oncol. 2011;21:264–70.
26. Gibbs IC, Levendag PC, Fariselli L, et al. Re: "The safety and efficacy of robotic image-guided radiosurgery system treatment for intra- and extracranial lesions: a systematic review of the literature" [Radiotherapy and Oncology 89 (2009) 245-253]. Radiother Oncol. 2009;93:656–7.
27. Timmerman RD, Kavanagh BD, Cho LC, et al. Stereotactic body radiation therapy in multiple organ sites. J Clin Oncol. 2007;25:947–52.
28. Dawood O, Mahadevan A, Goodman KA. Stereotactic body radiation therapy for liver metastases. Eur J Cancer. 2009;45:2947–59.
29. Hajj C, Goodman KA. Role of radiotherapy and newer techniques in the treatment of GI cancers. J Clin Oncol. 2015;33:1737–44.
30. Shirato H, Seppenwoolde Y, Kitamura K, et al. Intrafractional tumor motion: lung and liver. Semin Radiat Oncol. 2004;14:10–8.
31. Adler JR Jr, Chang SD, Murphy MJ, et al. The Cyberknife: a frameless robotic system for radiosurgery. Stereotact Funct Neurosurg. 1997;69:124–8.
32. Shirato H, Harada T, Harabayashi T, et al. Feasibility of insertion/implantation of 2.0-mm-diameter gold internal fiducial markers for precise setup and real-time tumor tracking in radiotherapy. Int J Radiat Oncol Biol Phys. 2003;56:240–7.
33. Heinzerling JH, Anderson JF, Papiez L, et al. Four-dimensional computed tomography scan analysis of tumor and organ motion at varying levels of abdominal compression during stereotactic treatment of lung and liver. Int J Radiat Oncol Biol Phys. 2008;70:1571–8.
34. Blomgren H, Lax I, Göranson H, et al. Radiosurgery for tumors in the body: clinical experience using a new method. J Radiosurg. 1998;1:63–74.
35. Blomgren H, Lax I, Naslund I, Svanstrom R. Stereotactic high dose fraction radiation therapy of extracranial tumors using an accelerator. Clinical experience of the first thirty-one patients. Acta Oncol. 1995;34:861–70.
36. Wada H, Takai Y, Nemoto K, Yamada S. Univariate analysis of factors correlated with tumor control probability of three-dimensional conformal hypofractionated high-dose radiotherapy for small pulmonary or hepatic tumors. Int J Radiat Oncol Biol Phys. 2004;58:1114–20.
37. Herfarth KK, Debus J, Lohr F, et al. Stereotactic single-dose radiation therapy of liver tumors: results of a phase I/II trial. J Clin Oncol. 2001;19:164–70.
38. Goodman KA, Wiegner EA, Maturen KE, et al. Dose-escalation study of single-fraction stereotactic

body radiotherapy for liver malignancies. Int J Radiat Oncol Biol Phys. 2010;78:486–93.
39. Hoyer M, Roed H, Traberg Hansen A, et al. Phase II study on stereotactic body radiotherapy of colorectal metastases. Acta Oncol. 2006;45:823–30.
40. Mendez Romero A, Wunderink W, Hussain SM, et al. Stereotactic body radiation therapy for primary and metastatic liver tumors: a single institution phase i-ii study. Acta Oncol. 2006;45:831–7.
41. Schefter TE, Kavanagh BD, Timmerman RD, et al. A phase I trial of stereotactic body radiation therapy (SBRT) for liver metastases. Int J Radiat Oncol Biol Phys. 2005;62:1371–8.
42. Rusthoven KE, Kavanagh BD, Cardenes H, et al. Multi-institutional phase I/II trial of stereotactic body radiation therapy for liver metastases. J Clin Oncol. 2009;27:1572–8.
43. Lee MT, Kim JJ, Dinniwell R, et al. Phase I study of individualized stereotactic body radiotherapy of liver metastases. J Clin Oncol. 2009;27:1585–91.
44. Ambrosino G, Polistina F, Costantin G, et al. Image-guided robotic stereotactic radiosurgery for unresectable liver metastases: preliminary results. Anticancer Res. 2009;29:3381–4.
45. Rule W, Timmerman R, Tong L, et al. Phase I dose-escalation study of stereotactic body radiotherapy in patients with hepatic metastases. Ann Surg Oncol. 2011;18:1081–7.
46. Scorsetti M, Arcangeli S, Tozzi A, et al. Is stereotactic body radiation therapy an attractive option for unresectable liver metastases? A preliminary report from a phase 2 trial. Int J Radiat Oncol Biol Phys. 2013;86:336–42.
47. Chang DT, Swaminath A, Kozak M, et al. Stereotactic body radiotherapy for colorectal liver metastases: a pooled analysis. Cancer. 2011;117:4060–9.
48. Sato M, Uematsu M, Yamamoto F, et al. Feasibility of frameless stereotactic high-dose radiation therapy for primary or metastatic liver cancer. J Radiosurg. 1998;1:233–8.
49. Wurm RE, Gum F, Erbel S, et al. Image guided respiratory gated hypofractionated Stereotactic Body Radiation Therapy (H-SBRT) for liver and lung tumors: initial experience. Acta Oncol. 2006;45:881–9.
50. Katz AW, Carey-Sampson M, Muhs AG, et al. Hypofractionated stereotactic body radiation therapy (SBRT) for limited hepatic metastases. Int J Radiat Oncol Biol Phys. 2007;67:793–8.
51. Katz AW, Winter KA, Dawson LA et al. RTOG 0438: a phase I trial of highly conformal radiation therapy for patients with liver metastases. J Clin Oncol. 30;2012 (suppl 4); abstr 257.
52. Gunven P, Jonas E, Blomgren H, et al. Undetectable late hepatic sequelae after hypofractionated stereotactic radiotherapy for liver tumors. Med Oncol. 2011;28:958–65.
53. Fode MM, Hoyer M. Survival and prognostic factors in 321 patients treated with stereotactic body radiotherapy for oligo-metastases. Radiother Oncol. 2015;114:155–60.
54. Klein J, Dawson LA, Jiang H, et al. Prospective longitudinal assessment of quality of life for liver cancer patients treated with stereotactic body radiation therapy. Int J Radiat Oncol Biol Phys. 2015;93:16–25.
55. Chang JY, Senan S, Paul MA, et al. Stereotactic ablative radiotherapy versus lobectomy for operable stage I non-small-cell lung cancer: a pooled analysis of two randomised trials. Lancet Oncol. 2015;16:630–7.
56. Radiofrequency ablation versus stereotactic radiotherapy in colorectal liver metastases (RAS01). https://clinicaltrials.gov/ct2/show/NCT01233544. Accessed 17 Mar 2016.
57. Chiba T, Tokuuye K, Matsuzaki Y, et al. Proton beam therapy for hepatocellular carcinoma: a retrospective review of 162 patients. Clin Cancer Res. 2005;11:3799–805.
58. Fukumitsu N, Sugahara S, Nakayama H, et al. A prospective study of hypofractionated proton beam therapy for patients with hepatocellular carcinoma. Int J Radiat Oncol Biol Phys. 2009;74:831–6.
59. Matsuzaki Y, Osuga T, Saito Y, et al. A new, effective, and safe therapeutic option using proton irradiation for hepatocellular carcinoma. Gastroenterology. 1994;106:1032–41.
60. Hong TS, DeLaney TF, Mamon HJ, et al. A prospective feasibility study of respiratory-gated proton beam therapy for liver tumors. Pract Radiat Oncol. 2014;4:316–22.

MRI-Guided Laser Ablation of Liver Tumors

Sherif G. Nour

Introduction

Ablative treatment, along with other forms of locoregional therapy, has become an integral part of the treatment paradigm for primary and secondary liver malignancies. Numerous reports [1–4] have demonstrated similar overall survival rates following ablative treatment and surgical resection for the management of small (≤3 cm) liver tumors.

Small hepatic tumors are being increasingly identified during metastatic work-ups and in the setting of evaluating patients with liver cirrhosis due to the vast improvements in diagnostic imaging capabilities. Advanced anatomic and functional abdominal MR imaging has become the primary imaging approach for evaluating liver disease at many institutions due to an established superiority over other imaging modalities [5].

Several options are currently available for ablative treatment of liver tumors, including tissue heating (e.g., radiofrequency (RFA) [6], laser [7], microwave [8], and focused ultrasound (HIFU)

S. G. Nour
Interventional MRI Program, Department of Radiology and Imaging Sciences, Emory University Hospitals and School of Medicine, Atlanta, GA, USA

Divisions of Abdominal Imaging, Interventional Radiology and Image-Guided Medicine, Department of Radiology and Imaging Sciences, Emory University Hospitals and School of Medicine, Atlanta, GA, USA
e-mail: sherif.nour@emoryhealthcare.org

[9]), tissue freezing (cryoablation [10]), and tissue damage by electric currents (irreversible electroporation (IRE) [11]). Most liver tumor ablations are currently performed with RFA or microwave ablation. In terms of efficacy in achieving tumor necrosis, no comparative series is available in the literature to support the use of one ablative technology versus the other. In our experience, the efficacy of ablation is not typically associated with the choice of ablative energy but is primarily related to the soundness of the technique and to the ability to identify the target, unequivocally clarify its margins, and adequately gauge the energy required to eradicate all the viable cells. Some inherent characteristics of the ablative energy may, however, favor its utilization in particular situations such as the use of microwave to achieve a larger ablation zone with a fewer probe punctures in a time-efficient manner [12] and the use of IRE to avoid heat sink while treating neoplasms in the vicinity of larger vascular structures [13].

Several reports of percutaneous laser ablation of hepatic tumors have surfaced more than a decade ago [7, 14, 15]. The technique has, however, subsequently fallen out of favor due to the complexity and invasive nature of introducers and the lack of advantage over simpler competing technologies when insertions were performed under CT guidance.

The approach for laser ablation discussed in this chapter represents a significant departure from those early practices and involves MRI identifica-

© Springer Nature Switzerland AG 2018
K. Cardona, S. K. Maithel (eds.), *Primary and Metastatic Liver Tumors*,
https://doi.org/10.1007/978-3-319-91977-5_26

tion of subtle, typically otherwise undetectable, liver tumors, followed by interactive MRI-guided insertion of smaller, minimally invasive, laser fibers and real-time monitoring of energy deployment, where the treatment endpoint is dictated by the individual tumor response rather than by predetermined vendor-recommended ablation parameters.

Principles of Laser Ablation

(Latin *ablat* "taken away," from *ab* "away" + *lat* "carried") [16].

Although the physical phenomenon producing tissue heating varies according to the source of thermal injury, the subsequent cascade of events leading to cell necrosis is quite similar regardless of the initial source of heating.

When using laser energy for deep tissue ablation, a laser applicator is inserted into the target tissue. When the laser system is operated, a flux of light photons is released in the tissues surrounding the laser applicator. The molecular elements in the tissues that absorb the light energy are called the "chromophores," which are the elements interacting with the laser photons deployed in the tissue during ablation. Numerous components of normal and abnormal tissues serve as naturally occurring chromophores, such as hemoglobin, myoglobin, bilirubin, melanin, and mitochondrial pigments [17, 18].

The absorbed energy excites orbital electrons from their original resting state. The difference in orbital energy levels inherent to each molecule dictates its affinity to absorb energy from a particular spectrum of light. The final three-dimensional distribution of laser power deposition in tissues is therefore the sum of photon absorption, scattering, and reflection and is primarily dependent on (a) laser wavelength, (b) tissue composition, and (c) applied energy level and duration.

Laser Wavelength

Laser lights come in a wide spectrum of wavelengths that serve different treatment goals when applied to human tissues. At one end of the spectrum are the short wavelength ultraviolet excimer lasers (wavelengths between 193 and 300 nm). These are highly absorbed by amino acids and have a limited power of tissue penetration (approximately 1 μm). The rapid water vaporization associated with the application of these short wavelength lasers does not allow sufficient time for heat radiation to create a meaningful ablative damage [19]. At the other end of the spectrum are the long wavelength lasers toward the infrared range and beyond. These are absorbed by a variety of natural tissue chromophores and are capable of deeper tissue penetration. As such, these are suitable lasers for controlled deep tissue ablation. Typically, several millimeters of depth penetration (up to 10–12 mm) are achievable with laser energies in the range of 600–1100 nm [19, 20]. Examples of lasers used for deep tissue ablation include diode lasers (wavelength 800–980 nm) and Neodymium: Yttirum Aluminum Garnet (Nd: YAG) lasers (wavelength 1064 nm) [17, 18, 21].

Tissue Composition

Laser-tissue interactions also depend on tissue composition, including the degree of tissue perfusion, proximity of target to large adjacent vessels, amount of pigment, fibrosis, necrosis, and the presence of distinct tissue interfaces (e.g., CSF space, diaphragm, etc.) adjoining the treated field. These variants should be considered when predicting the response of various tissues to deep laser ablative therapy. Tumor tissues have been shown to exhibit 33% more affinity to optical penetration compared to normal tissue at 1064 nm wavelength [17, 22]; however, the effects of many of the tissue composition factors have not been studied in a measured way and therefore require sufficient expertise of the treating physician with laser energy and familiarity with the treated organ(s) to ensure safe and efficacious treatment.

Applied Energy Level and Duration

The applied laser energy level and duration are other important factors in determining the ablative treatment effect. Interstitial tissue ablation is achieved by the continuous deposition of laser energy, usually in the range of 3–20 W over durations of 2–20 min [17], although higher energy levels have been also safely applied to achieve interstitial thermal tissue coagulation [23, 24]. The author's institution applies cycles of 12 W over 90–290 s for intracranial ablations [23] and 21–27 W over 120–180 s for extracranial applications [24]. Rapid heating delivered over a short duration of time results in tissue carbonization, steam buildup, and explosive ruptures at the laser fiber/tissue interface [19]. This impedes optical penetration in the tissues by up to 25% [17, 22] and leads to an ineffective ablation outcome, in the form of linear charring along the laser fiber rather than a sizeable zone of thermal damage. In order to avoid this effect, cool-tip technology is used, where the laser fiber's diffusing tip is housed within an applicator that contains circulating saline.

Role of MR Imaging Guidance

The ability to perform a focused percutaneous thermal treatment of liver tumors under image guidance has changed thermal ablation from an adjuvant surgical technique to a minimally invasive alternative to surgery that is more suited to a large sector of poor surgical candidates. Traditionally, image guidance during percutaneous thermal ablation is performed with CT or ultrasound to help a safe and precise placement of the ablative device into the targeted pathology. The ideal access trajectory during actual procedure execution is frequently different from that suggested on pre-procedure imaging data due to the shift of anatomical structures when using modified patient positions during treatment. Additionally, the guided approach provides updated information regarding the development of new pathological conditions that may alter treatment decision-making, such as the appearance of other tumor foci or the development of ascites.

A few institutions have added "interventional MRI" capabilities to their minimally invasive procedural armamentarium. At the author's institution, MRI-guided interventions have become an integral component of the routine procedural services and have contributed to a new refined approach to liver tumor ablation [25]. The new approach utilizes intra-procedural interventional MRI technology for (a) accurate mapping of hepatic tumor burden, (b) interactive navigation of the laser applicator into the target tumor(s), and (c) real-time monitoring of individual tumor response to the deposited ablative energy.

Accurate Mapping of Hepatic Tumor Burden

This is typically the initial step in MRI-guided laser ablation and is analogous to performing intraoperative high-resolution ultrasound on the exposed liver prior to surgical metastatectomy. This standard surgical step is performed intraoperatively, immediately before executing the surgical plan in order to detect any additional small liver tumors that were below the resolution of preoperative imaging work-up. Similarly, we use intra-procedural MRI to obtain high-resolution scans while inducing controlled apnea under general anesthesia and enhancing the visualization by using liver-specific contrast medium, gadoxetate disodium (Eovist®), to achieve accurate quantification of liver disease and confirm or modify the preexisting ablation plan. This approach has changed liver ablations from procedures geared toward identifying and treating known disease to a more comprehensive assessment that accounts for subtle previously unknown or newly developed disease.

Interactive Navigation of the Laser Applicator into the Target Tumor(s)

Percutaneous ablation procedures can be performed under ultrasound (US), computed tomography (CT), or magnetic resonance (MR) imaging guidance, all of which usually allow accurate placement of the ablative device into the targeted tumor. However, the additional specific features of MRI such as its excellent soft tissue contrast, high spatial resolution, multiplanar capabilities, and inherent sensitivity to temperature and blood flow [26–28] facilitate a greater suitability for accessing a wide variety of "difficult access" lesions in terms of tumor visibility, trajectory limitations, or proximity to vital structures.

MRI is being increasingly used for hepatic metastatic tumor work-up and for surveillance of patients with chronic liver disease. As such, it is not uncommon to identify sub-centimeter tumors that are too small to detect on CT or ultrasound scans. Some larger tumors also possess tissue characteristics that render them difficult to delineate except on MRI scans. MRI guidance becomes a necessity in these cases to ensure accurate tumor targeting during ablation. Without the availability of interventional MRI technology, the only alternative would be using surrounding tissue landmarks to access the approximate location of the tumor. This approach can result in either ineffective ablation due to missing part of or the entire targeted tumor or unnecessarily aggressive treatment due to the desire to eradicate all viable tissue of an originally unseen target. This latter scenario can be associated with a negative impact on liver reserve in patients who have already had prior surgical metastatectomies and/or multiple similarly aggressive ablative treatments.

In terms of trajectory limitations and proximity to vital structures, MRI guidance enables a safe and time-efficient navigation of the ablative device toward those "difficult-to-reach" targets. Examples include tumors at the extreme liver dome under the diaphragm. Access to these tumors under CT guidance requires expertise in triangulation techniques and is associated with a significant risk for the development of pneumothorax. Ultrasound is more suitable than CT for real-time ablative device guidance in oblique trajectories but can be hampered by air artifacts from the lung bases when targeting high subphrenic lesions. Other examples where MRI guidance is usually beneficial include tumors abutting the heart, gallbladder, colon, or liver hilum.

Real-Time Monitoring of Individual Tumor Response to the Deposited Ablative Energy

In addition to its role in accurate mapping of tumor burden and in interactive device navigation toward the target tumor, the major contribution of MR imaging to thermal ablation technology lies in its ability to monitor the zone of thermal tissue destruction during the procedure. This allows a real-time feedback on the status of energy deposition in the tissues and thereby facilitates direct control and adjustment of the thermal ablation zone size and configuration during the procedure. This technical refinement over the current standard of care practices translates to an added ability of the interventionist to compensate for deviations from preoperative predictions and to define the treatment endpoint without moving the patient from the interventional suite. As such, the treatment paradigm does not follow universal "vendor-recommended" ablation parameters but rather titrates the delivered treatment to the individual tumor response.

This ability to interactively monitor the zone of thermal tissue destruction may be achieved either by direct anatomical imaging of the zone of ablation or by creating a "thermal map" allowing real-time updates of temperature changes to be superimposed on the image of the ablation zone. This is achieved by computing and displaying phase changes during the deposition of heating energy in near real-time. These data are assigned color codes based on temperature thresholds and are displayed over the initial phase and/or magnitude (anatomical) image to reflect topographic updates in tissue temperature. The "total damage estimate map" is a modification of the "thermal map" that allows delineating tumor areas that have been exposed to lethal temperatures for a certain amount of time rather than highlighting the actual temperature distribution at the time of sampling. These features are exclusive to MR imaging and could not be reliably duplicated by any other currently used imaging modality.

With this elaborative and multifaceted role, the use of MRI to guide liver tumor ablation represents more than the utilization of a different imaging modality to guide the insertion of the ablative device. MRI guidance should rather be viewed as a comprehensive approach to percutaneous ablation technology that offers accurate pre-procedural quantification of tumor burden; allows a precise placement of the ablative device into the target tumor(s), with particular value in small, poorly visualized, and difficult-to-reach tumors; and facilitates a well-titrated energy deposition based on the actual response of the target tumor.

Rationale for Choosing Laser Ablative Energy

It has been our experience, as well as the experience of others, that effective treatment of liver tumors may be achieved with a variety of energy-based ablative technologies and that the treatment outcome is more dependent on the technique rather than on the actual source of utilized energy. In the previous section, we explained how the technique of thermal ablation can be markedly enhanced by incorporating modern interventional MRI technology into the various steps of the process.

As a relatively new mode of intervention that is being practiced exclusively in a limited number of institutions, interventional MRI is currently challenged by the lack of a dedicated MRI scanner design that offers a true procedural platform. As such, space restriction is always a complicating factor during MRI-guided interventions, even with the use of open-configuration scanners. The delivery system for deep tissue laser ablation consists of a thin flexible fiber optic, housed within a flexible cooling applicator. A short (14.5 cm), 14 gauge, introducing needle is typically used to carry this delivery system across the body wall into the target tumor within the liver. The laser fiber/applicator system exiting the body through the hub of the introducing needle can be easily bent to fit within the bore of the scanner. This arrangement requires only minimal additional space beyond the hub of the short introducing needle and circumvents the challenges of fitting the bulky handles and cables of other ablative devices (radiofrequency, microwave, etc.) within the magnet bore, particularly when attempting to treat larger patients.

In addition to simplifying the physical logistics of ablative treatment within the MRI environment, laser is also well-suited for MRI-guided ablation due to the lack of interference with imaging, allowing simultaneous treatment and scanning. This is the key feature in facilitating real-time ablation monitoring and constitutes the basis of offering a titrated, response-based, ablative treatment.

The sensitivity of MR imaging to the immediate changes occurring at the ablation zone and to the surrounding reactive tissue changes does, in fact, apply to all modes of thermal ablation. However, capturing these changes during some other treatments, such as radiofrequency (RF), is a complicated task due to RF interference with the scanner. This limitation can be circumvented during MRI-guided RF ablation by implementing intermittent MR scanning between the ablation cycles or by employing a special radiofrequency switching circuit to allow simultaneous RF ablation and MR imaging [29]. Microwave ablation may be monitored with simultaneous MRI scanning similar to laser ablation; however, there is no currently available commercial platform for real-time temperature mapping during microwave ablation. MRI has been reported to provide a reliable interactive visualization of the growing ice ball during cryoablation procedures. Early experiences with this phenomenon have been primarily based on monitoring of MRI-guided renal cryoablations [30–32]. MRI monitoring can provide the real-time feedback necessary to adjust the gas flow to individual cryoprobes in order to modify the size and shape of the forming ice ball. It is important, however, to note that the visualized leading edge of the ice ball during the procedure corresponds to 0 °C, which is a sublethal freezing point and results in incomplete treatment if used to indicate the treatment margin. Therefore, a 5–10 mm of ice ball, or more in the vicinity of large vessels, should be planned to extend beyond the margin of the target tumor to ensure proper coverage [33–35].

Interventional MRI Setup for Liver Laser Ablation

Performing liver laser ablation under MRI guidance and monitoring requires a dedicated *"interventional MRI suite"* that offers:

1. The ability to access the patient and perform the intervention within the bore of the scanner through an open biplanar or a wide-bore cylindrical magnet design
2. The ability to operate the scanner and review images at the patient's bedside
3. The ability to apply modern imaging techniques to achieve rapid near real-time interactive guidance of the introducing needle and laser applicator while maintaining sufficient image quality for continuous visualization of the typically small and/or difficult-to-reach target tumor
4. The ability to implement temperature mapping techniques for real-time monitoring of the intensity and distribution of deposited energy

In addition, the suite should be designed to accommodate general anesthesia and MRI-compatible versions of all instruments, and equipment should be readily available.

In their pioneering report on MRI-guided radiofrequency (RF) ablation, Lewin et al. [36] described the use of a biplanar low-field (0.2 T) magnet design that allows an abundant space for handling and navigating the RF probes. The low spatial and temporal resolutions of those low-field magnet designs have imposed a limitation on the level of complexity of supported interventions and on the practicality of subsequent larger-scale adoption. The trend in the field of interventional MRI have then favored a shift to higher-field interventions albeit at the expense of a relatively tighter room within the "wide-bore, open-configuration" 1.5 T interventional scanners.

The laser generator and saline pump are typically placed outside the MRI scanner room with the laser fibers and cooling tubes extended through the waveguide. As opposed to other ablative devices (e.g., radiofrequency or microwave), laser fibers do not contain any metallic components and do not require special attention to using an MRI-compatible version of the device. Additionally, bending the thin flexible laser fiber to fit within the magnet bore is not associated with the potentially damaging torque that occurs when attempting to bend the marketed flexible MRI-compatible RF probes. In the author's experience, this torque results in a significant shift of hepatic tissue and may cause inaccurate tip placement and potential tissue injury.

An adequate access trajectory can usually be planned while the patient is placed in the supine position on the MRI table. In some instances, a supine right anterior oblique or a prone position might be necessary to secure a safe trajectory. A flexible six-channel surface abdominal coil is used in conjunction with the built-in table coil to receive the MRI signal, which we typically accentuate by injecting gadoxetate disodium (Eovist®) at the beginning of the procedure as described above under *accurate mapping of hepatic tumor burden*. The surface coil we use (Siemens Healthcare, Erlangen, Germany) features four square-shaped openings, each measuring 4 × 4 in. It is important to realize that following the identification of the skin entry point (described below under *guidance phase*), the entire procedure field will be limited to the prepped and draped 4 × 4 in. square allowed through one of the coil openings. When placing the patient in the oblique position, it is advisable to place a second flexible coil between the patient and the lifting wedge to compensate for the lost signal at the relatively distant built-in table coil.

MRI-guided liver laser ablation can technically be performed under conscious IV sedation. Our practice at the Emory Interventional MRI Program has focused on offering this resource to patients who are otherwise not suitable candidates for conventional interventional radiologic procedures as a unique resource that maintains the minimally invasive treatment option for that subset of patients. This practice philosophy naturally filters referrals to the interventional MRI service to those medically and/or technically challenging cases. As such, the vast majority of procedures at our practice are performed under general anesthesia. In either case, the nurse administering conscious sedation and the general anesthesia team should be familiar with the requirements and limitations of working in the MRI environment. Performing interventional procedures within the MRI unit is associated with heightened traffic of personnel and hence an increased concern about MR safety issues, compared to the standard diagnostic MRI environment. All the staff involved in interventional procedures should receive formal MRI safety training and be issued card access to the scanner area (MRI Zone II). MRI-safe stretchers should be used to transport the patients from the pre-procedure care area (MRI Zone I) all the way to the interventional MRI suite (MRI Zone IV). Clipboards, pens, and paperclips are examples of small ferromagnetic items that are not infrequently overlooked even in the presence of experienced staff.

We perform our interventional MRI procedures on a 1.5 T cylindrical high-field, short-bore interventional MRI scanner (Magnetom Espree, Siemens Healthcare, Erlangen, Germany) while accessing the patient from the backside of the scanner. When using general anesthesia, the patient lays on the scanner in the "feet first" position allowing the anesthesia team to have access to the patient's head and to utilize the entire space around the front of the gantry.

Procedure Guidance and Treatment Monitoring

The procedure of MRI-guided liver laser ablation, similar to other MRI-guided ablation procedures, can generally be described under three distinct phases: the guidance phase, the confirmation phase, and the ablation/monitoring phase [37, 38].

The Guidance Phase

Following the initial gadoxetate disodium (Eovist®) scan, an updated map of the actual hepatic tumor burden is obtained, and the final decision on the number and location(s) of the tumor(s) to be targeted is made. The surface coil is placed over the patient's abdomen in such a way that one of the 4 × 4 in. coil openings resides over the approximate skin entry point and the margins of that coil opening are marked by fiducial markers. A rapid triorthogonal imaging sequence [39, 40] (usually a short repetition time (TR)/short echo time (TE) gradient echo sequence, such as fast low-angle shot (FLASH) or equivalent) is then planned in such a way that the three imaging planes intersect at the target tumor, while two of the planes are extended through safe trajectories to the same point at the skin surface. The next step is to test the entry point and the planned trajectory, usually with a syringe filled with dilute gadolinium. The coil opening is then fine-adjusted to bring the skin entry point to the center of the opening in order to allow room for subsequent angulations of the introducing needle during the guidance phase. When the procedure involves ablation of more than one tumor, the same process is then repeated for each target before prepping and draping the access site. In these cases, we typically try to converge all trajectories to the same entry point or to cluster them in close proximity to each other in order to fit within the small (4 × 4 in.) procedure field.

The introducing needle (14G, 14.5-cm-long) is then inserted through the skin and advanced into the targeted tumor under near-real-time interactive MR "fluoroscopic" guidance, applying repeated cycles of the same rapid triorthogonal imaging sequence used for the initial trajectory planning. This guidance phase consists of continuous imaging with automated sequential acquisition, reconstruction, and in-room display. The triorthogonal image plane MR guidance continuously acquires sets of adjustable sagittal, coronal, and axial scans that could be acquired relative to the needle axis, relative to the target tumor itself, or in any three arbitrary planes relative to each other and to the patient's body. In this method, the reconstruction and display program was modified to simultaneously project the three planes immediately as they were acquired.

Typically, the introducing needle is initially seen on only one or two of the three planes. The in-room monitor and controller are then utilized to co-localize the missing plane or planes on the planes where the electrode is already visualized. This process can be repeated whenever the needle is deflected out-of plane on any of the three planes.

The process of guiding an MR imaging-compatible introducing needle into a targeted tumor under MR fluoroscopy requires attention to the certain user-defined imaging parameters and needle trajectory decisions [41] because they can significantly affect needle visibility and thereby the accuracy and safety of the procedure. The guidance phase is typically performed using the freehand technique, although other modes of MR imaging guidance are technically applicable. Once the introducing needle has been placed into the target tumor, the stylet is removed and replaced by the laser applicator.

The Confirmation Phase

When the laser applicator is deemed in place within the target tumor on the rapid guidance scans, it is recommended that the applicator tip position be confirmed on various planes using higher spatial resolution, relatively lengthier turbo spin echo (TSE) scans prior to laser energy deployment. We typically use the Visualase™ (Medtronic, MN, USA) laser system for MRI-guided liver ablations. The 600-μm diode laser fiber used for liver ablations features a 15-mm-long diffusing tip and can generate up to a 2 × 3 cm oval-shaped ablation zone per application. For tumors smaller than 2 cm in diameter, the ideal placement of the laser applicator entails an applicator tip at the distal (furthest) margin of the tumor and an applicator shaft bisecting the width of the tumor. Larger tumors (2 or more cm in diameter) are expected to require more than one ablation cycle at different applicator positions, and the adequacy of initial placement should be assessed in light of the predetermined plan for the ablation procedure. Subsequent applicator placement(s) are typically based on feedback on the actual ablation progress as evaluated on intra-procedural temperature maps and intermittent magnitude (anatomical) MR imaging.

The Ablation/Monitoring Phase

When adequate placement of the laser applicator has been confirmed within the targeted tumor, the cooling pump is operated in order to provide a continuous flow of room-temperature saline around the laser fiber (housed within the cooled laser applicator). The purpose of this cooling is to prevent excessive heating and charring around the diffusing tip of the laser fiber. The building carbon at the laser/tumor interface would initially impede the transmission of light photons into the tumor, precluding an effective ablation and would eventually result in damage of the laser tip and its housing applicator.

The last safety check prior to embarking in the actual full ablation procedure consists of applying a small and brief test dose of laser (usually 9 W for 30 s) and simultaneously monitoring the location of the nidus of heating relative to the target tumor on real-time temperature maps. After confirming or adjusting the final location of the laser fiber to the ideal position, one or several laser ablation cycles are applied and monitored with real-time temperature maps and damage estimate maps, displayed over high-resolution anatomic images of the target tumor. This monitoring process can be performed and displayed on two perpendicular imaging planes simultaneously (typically axial and sagittal scans along the plane of the laser applicator) to ensure adequate coverage of all tumor margins, along with a surrounding rim of normal liver tissue. The laser ablation parameters can be adjusted for each cycle based on target size, adjacent vital structures, and user's experience and preference. We typically apply cycles of 21–27 W for 120–180 s and repeat/reposition as necessary based on the feedback from temperature/damage estimate monitoring. Electronic calipers can be placed over adjacent vital structures to trigger an automatic halt of laser energy deposition when a predetermined temperature threshold has been reached.

Once the induced thermal ablation zone is believed to encompass the entire tumor and a 5–10-mm cuff of normal adjacent tissue, we acquire a T1-weighted 3D imaging sequence (volumetric interpolated breath-hold examination (VIBE)) in axial, sagittal, and coronal planes and compare them to similar scans acquired immediately prior to ablation. This scan is sensitive to blood products, which is a constant finding within recently ablated tissues, and the identification of a bright signal encasing the circumference of the tumor on all three imaging planes has been, in our experience, a reliable indicator of the adequacy of ablation. Once this confirmation is achieved or additional repositioning and treatment of under-ablated margins is performed, the laser fiber/applicator system is withdrawn, and the final post-ablation/new baseline (TSE T2 and post-gadolinium VIBE) scans are acquired.

The patient is usually observed for 4–6 h before discharge unless admission is needed to manage complications.

References

1. Wang JH, et al. Survival comparison between surgical resection and radiofrequency ablation for patients in BCLC very early/early stage hepatocellular carcinoma. J Hepatol. 2012;56(2):412–8.
2. Ruzzenente A, et al. Surgical resection versus local ablation for HCC on cirrhosis: results from a propensity case-matched study. J Gastrointest Surg. 2012;16(2):301–11; discussion 311
3. Su TS, et al. Long-term survival analysis of stereotactic ablative radiotherapy versus liver resection for small hepatocellular carcinoma. Int J Radiat Oncol Biol Phys. 2017;98(3):639–46.
4. Pompili M, et al. Long-term effectiveness of resection and radiofrequency ablation for single hepatocellular carcinoma </=3 cm. Results of a multicenter Italian survey. J Hepatol. 2013;59(1):89–97.
5. Fowler KJ, Brown JJ, Narra VR. Magnetic resonance imaging of focal liver lesions: approach to imaging diagnosis. Hepatology. 2011;54(6):2227–37.
6. Aissou S, et al. Radiofrequency in the management of colorectal liver metastases: a 10-year experience at a single center. Surg Technol Int. 2016;Xxix:99–105.
7. Vogl TJ, et al. MR-controlled laser-induced thermotherapy (LITT) of liver metastases: clinical evaluation. Rontgenpraxis. 1996;49(7):161–8.
8. Ryu T, et al. Oncological outcomes after hepatic resection and/or surgical microwave ablation for liver metastasis from gastric cancer. Asian J Surg. 2017;
9. Diana M, et al. High intensity focused ultrasound (HIFU) applied to hepato-bilio-pancreatic and the digestive system-current state of the art and future perspectives. Hepatobiliary Surg Nutr. 2016;5(4):329–44.
10. Glazer DI, et al. Percutaneous image-guided cryoablation of hepatic tumors: single-center experience with intermediate to long-term outcomes. AJR Am J Roentgenol. 2017;209(6):1381–9.
11. Cohen EI, et al. Technology of irreversible electroporation and review of its clinical data on liver cancers. Expert Rev Med Devices. 2018;15(2):99–106.
12. Lubner MG, et al. Microwave ablation of hepatic malignancy. Semin Intervent Radiol. 2013;30(1):56–66.
13. Silk M, et al. The state of irreversible electroporation in interventional oncology. Semin Intervent Radiol. 2014;31(2):111–7.
14. Ishikawa T, et al. Laser induced thermotherapy for hepatocellular carcinoma. Nihon Rinsho. 2001;59 Suppl 6:601–5.
15. Albrecht D, et al. Laser-induced thermotherapy for palliative treatment of malignant liver tumors: results of a clinical study. Langenbecks Arch Chir Suppl Kongressbd. 1996;113:136–8.
16. http://www.oxforddictionaries.com/definition/english/ablation.
17. Izzo F. Other thermal ablation techniques: microwave and interstitial laser ablation of liver tumors. Ann Surg Oncol. 2003;10(5):491–7.
18. Germer CT, et al. Technology for in situ ablation by laparoscopic and image-guided interstitial laser hyperthermia. Semin Laparosc Surg. 1998;5(3):195–203.
19. Pearce J. Mathematical models of laser-induced tissue thermal damage. Int J Hyperth. 2011;27(8):741–50.
20. Jacques SL, Wang L. Monte Carlo modeling of light transport in tissues. In: Welch AJ, van MJC G, editors. Optical-thermal response of laser-irradiated tissue. New York: Plenum; 1995. p. 73–100.
21. Muralidharan V, Christophi C. Interstitial laser thermotherapy in the treatment of colorectal liver metastases. J Surg Oncol. 2001;76(1):73–81.
22. Germer CT, et al. Optical properties of native and coagulated human liver tissue and liver metastases in the near infrared range. Lasers Surg Med. 1998;23(4):194–203.
23. Willie JT, et al. Real-time magnetic resonance-guided stereotactic laser amygdalohippocampotomy for mesial temporal lobe epilepsy. Neurosurgery. 2014;74(6):569–84. discussion 584-5
24. Nour SG, Kooby DA, Maithel SK, Staley 3rd CA, Kitajima HD, Powell TE. Percutaneous laser ablation of hepatic metastases with realtime magnetic resonance thermometry monitoring. In: Proceedings of the American Society for Laser in Medicine and Surgery (ASLMS) 33rd annual meeting. 2013. Boston, MA, USA.
25. Nour SG, Kooby DA, Staley 3rd CA, Kitajima HD, Powell TE, Bowen MA, Gowda A, Burrow B, Small

WC, Torre WE. On percutaneous ablation of liver metastases: a method for mri-guided and monitored laser ablation of challenging lesions. In: Proceedings of the European Society for Magnetic Resonance in Medicine and Biology (ESMRMB) 29th annual scientific meeting. 2012. Lisbon, Portugal.
26. Schenck JF, et al. Superconducting open-configuration MR imaging system for image-guided therapy. Radiology. 1995;195(3):805–14.
27. Cline HE, et al. Magnetic resonance-guided thermal surgery. Magn Reson Med. 1993;30(1):98–106.
28. Cline HE, et al. Focused US system for MR imaging-guided tumor ablation. Radiology. 1995;194(3):731–7.
29. Hinshaw JL, Lee FT Jr. Image-guided ablation of renal cell carcinoma. Magn Reson Imaging Clin N Am. 2004;12(3):429–47. vi
30. Chin JL, et al. Magnetic resonance imaging-guided transurethral ultrasound ablation of prostate tissue in patients with localized prostate cancer: a prospective phase 1 clinical trial. Eur Urol. 2016;70(3):447–55.
31. Lindner U, et al. Image guided photothermal focal therapy for localized prostate cancer: phase I trial. J Urol. 2009;182(4):1371–7.
32. Raz O, et al. Real-time magnetic resonance imaging-guided focal laser therapy in patients with low-risk prostate cancer. Eur Urol. 2010;58(1):173–7.
33. Overduin CG, et al. Percutaneous MR-guided focal cryoablation for recurrent prostate cancer following radiation therapy: retrospective analysis of iceball margins and outcomes. Eur Radiol. 2017;27(11):4828–36.
34. Gage AA, Baust J. Mechanisms of tissue injury in cryosurgery. Cryobiology. 1998;37(3):171–86.
35. Baust JG, et al. Issues critical to the successful application of cryosurgical ablation of the prostate. Technol Cancer Res Treat. 2007;6(2):97–109.
36. Lewin JS, et al. Interactive MR imaging-guided biopsy and aspiration with a modified clinical C-arm system. AJR Am J Roentgenol. 1998;170(6):1593–601.
37. Nour SG. MRI-guided and monitored radiofrequency tumor ablation. Acad Radiol. 2005;12(9):1110–20.
38. Nour SG, Lewin JS. Radiofrequency thermal ablation: the role of MR imaging in guiding and monitoring tumor therapy. Magn Reson Imaging Clin N Am. 2005;13(3):561–81.
39. Nour SG, et al. A technique for MRI-guided transrectal deep pelvic abscess drainage. AJR Am J Roentgenol. 2008;191(4):1182–5.
40. Derakhshan JJ, et al. Characterization and reduction of saturation banding in multiplanar coherent and incoherent steady-state imaging. Magn Reson Med. 2010;63(5):1415–21.
41. Lewin JS, et al. Needle localization in MR-guided biopsy and aspiration: effects of field strength, sequence design, and magnetic field orientation. AJR Am J Roentgenol. 1996;166(6):1337–45.

Hepatic Artery Infusion Therapy for Primary Liver Tumors

Matthew S. Strand and Ryan C. Fields

Introduction

Liver cancer is the second most common cause of cancer death worldwide [1]. The two predominant types of primary liver tumors are hepatocellular carcinoma (HCC), accounting for 85% of primary liver cancers, and cholangiocarcinoma (CCA), which makes up most of the remaining 15% [2]. The incidence of both cancers is rising worldwide and in the United States [1, 3], yet while HCC is typically treated with resection for early, localized disease and transplant for advanced, non-resectable cases (generally in the setting of cirrhosis), fewer options exist for the treatment of locally advanced intrahepatic CCA (iCCA) or perihilar CCA.

The rationale for the use of HAI for liver tumors is that high doses of cytotoxic agents can be administered directly to tumors, while first-pass metabolism of many of these agents limits systemic toxicity. Additionally, tumors in the liver rely heavily on hepatic arterial inflow, while normal hepatocytes depend more on portal venous blood; thus arterial delivery of antineoplastic agents preferentially affects liver tumors [4]. Furthermore, both HCC and CCA have a propensity to spread or recur intrahepatically: since HAI therapy also treats the remaining liver, it also addresses a major site of disease progression [5, 6].

Sullivan and colleagues appear to be among the first to use arterial infusions of chemotherapy to treat tumors [7] beginning in the 1950s, including the treatment of liver metastasis from colorectal cancer [8]. Early experience with HAI in the United States in the 1970s included patients with both metastatic liver disease and primary liver tumors and was often combined with hepatic artery ligation [9]. These procedures appeared to induce responses but often incurred substantial morbidity [10]. Since then, a growing body of literature has validated HAI (without vascular ligation) for the treatment of advanced metastatic colorectal cancer [11] (see Section 3: Metastatic liver tumors; subsection E: Colorectal Cancer Liver Metastases; Chap. 17: Hepatic artery infusion therapy). This chapter will first review briefly the evidence for HAI therapy in HCC, predominantly from Asia, where it remains an important therapeutic modality. Attention will then be turned to the use of HAI therapy for cholangiocarcinoma.

M. S. Strand · R. C. Fields (✉)
Department of Surgery, Alvin J. Siteman Cancer Center, Barnes-Jewish Hospital, Washington University School of Medicine, St. Louis, MO, USA
e-mail: mstrand@wustl.edu; fieldsr@wustl.edu

Hepatic Artery Infusion Therapy for Hepatocellular Carcinoma

Mainstays of treatment for HCC include surgical resection, liver transplantation, transarterial chemoembolization (TACE), radioembolization or bland embolization, and microwave or radiofrequency ablation. Patients with HCC not amenable to resection or transplantation, with lesions too numerous or large for ablation and too widespread for TACE, or refractory to prior treatment have been considered candidates for hepatic arterial infusion (HAI) therapy. While early experience in HAI for HCC was reported in the United States, recent experience is described almost exclusively in Asia, where a much higher incidence of HCC and comparatively low rates of liver transplantation provide a larger candidate population.

The modern Asian experience with HAI for HCC appears to originate in 1995 with a report from Toyoda and colleagues [12]. They utilized a continuous infusion of 5-FU and cisplatin every other week in patients with advanced HCC, achieving a 1-year survival of 61.1%, compared to 8.2% in patients treated with a single arterial infusion of adriamycin and mitomycin C.

Subsequently, a multitude of studies have been conducted in Asia using HAI therapy for patients with unresectable HCC, advanced tumors (bilobar, diffuse, or vascular involvement), or recurrent disease (see Table 27.1). A variety of agents including 5-FU, cisplatin, epirubicin, etoposide, carboplatin, and IFN-α have been evaluated, either alone or in combination; for a summary of toxicities, see Table 27.2. While small (most studies involve fewer than 100 patients) and retrospective, nearly every study concluded that HAI therapy was effective, whether it was compared to systemic chemotherapy, best supportive care, or historical control cohorts. In general, HAI therapy with combinations of 5-FU, cisplatin, and either intramuscular or subcutaneous IFN-α appeared to confer the most benefit [12–28], while intra-arterial epirubicin did not appear effective [29, 30]. As a general rule of thumb, 5% of patients will have a complete response, and of the remaining patients, one third will have a partial response, one third will have stable disease, and one third will progress. Predictably, patients that demonstrated a radiographic response, whether complete or partial, had significantly better survival than those with stable or progressive disease on therapy. For this reason, efforts have been made to identify predictors of therapeutic response, and regular cross-sectional imaging to assess therapeutic response is indicated to inform prognosis and decide whether to continue, alter, or cease therapy. Multiple studies confirmed that patients with cirrhosis had a poorer overall survival [31], while those with hepatitis C had improved outcomes compared to those without hepatitis if concomitant ribavirin treatment was administered. For patients with portal vein tumor thrombus, HAI therapy remained effective [13, 32, 33]. While study populations and the treatments they received were heterogenous, median progression-free survival (PFS) ranged from 1.1 to 11.7 months, averaging 5.4 months across these studies. Median overall survival (OS) ranged from 3.5 to 19.7 months, averaging 11.2 months.

Hepatic Artery Infusion Therapy for Cholangiocarcinoma

For patients with CCA, locoregional therapy options are often fewer than in HCC, in part because of a historically limited candidacy for transplant but also because of the high incidence of perihilar CCA with invasion or abutment of hepatic vasculature, which are relative contraindications to ablative therapy. About 60% of all cases of CCA are intrahepatic or perihilar [34], but less than one third of these patients present with surgically resectable disease [35], with few eligible for transplant. With high recurrence rates of approximately 68–71% at about 2 years [36, 37], and a poor overall prognosis with 5-year survival rates of about 10–30% [38–45], transplant for CCA is less attractive compared to HCC, though improved 5-year survival rates of up to 82% can be obtained in a highly selected population [46] (see Section 4, Chap. 23: "Liver Transplantation for Other Cancers"). Thus a large

Table 27.1 Hepatic artery infusion therapy for hepatocellular carcinoma

Author Year	Title	Patients (treatment years)	Population	Agent/dose/frequency	Complications and toxicity	Results and conclusions
Fortner [9] 1973	Treatment of primary and secondary liver cancer by hepatic artery ligation and infusion chemotherapy	23	Unresectable HCC, carcinoid, and colorectal metastasis	FUDR (0.3 mg/kg) daily or methotrexate (2.5–5.0 mg) daily	4 patients died: one of liver failure, one of hepatorenal syndrome, one of methotrexate toxicity, one of liver necrosis, and one of pulmonary embolus	Response rate 78%, 50% remission Hepatic artery ligation and intra-arterial infusion is a safe and effective palliative operation
Ramming [58] 1976	Hepatic artery ligation and 5-fluorouracil infusion for metastatic colon carcinoma and primary hepatoma	16	Unresectable HCC and colorectal metastasis	5-FU (8 mg/kg) daily	Not reported	Six of seven patients with HCC had significant clinical improvement All six responding patients were alive at study conclusion (mean survival, 14 months)
Bern [10] 1978	Intra-arterial hepatic infusion and intravenous adriamycin for treatment of hepatocellular carcinoma: a clinical and pharmacology report	14	Unresectable HCC	Intra-arterial Adriamycin (4 patients) or intravenous Adriamycin (10 patients) every 3 weeks	6 patients died <14 days after IV therapy: 3 from liver failure, 1 from myocardial infarction, 1 from variceal hemorrhage, and 1 from pulmonary embolus 1 patient in the intra-arterial group died of duodenal necrosis	Average PR in the intra-arterial group: 5.6 months Average PR in the intravenous group: 6.8 months Adriamycin has activity in HCC; survival is improved compared to historical survival of 1–2 months

(continued)

Table 27.1 (continued)

Reed [59] 1981	The practicality of chronic hepatic artery infusion therapy of primary and metastatic hepatic malignancies: 10-year results of 124 patients in a prospective protocol	13	HCC	FUDR (0.3 mg/kg) continuous infusion	2 patients died of hepatic failure prior to evaluation	9 of 11 patients responded to treatment In responders, mean PFS was 12.7 months Median OS in responders: 11 months HAI with FUDR is practical and the therapy of choice for advanced HCC
Kajanti [60] 1986	Regional intra-arterial infusion of cisplatin in primary hepatocellular carcinoma. A phase II study	10 (1981–1984)	Unresectable HCC	Cisplatin (50 mg/m^2) for 24 h every 4 weeks	All patients had nausea and vomiting 4 patients had weight loss 1 patient had jaundice 1 patient died of uremia	Mean PFS: 11.7 months Mean OS: 19.7 months Intra-arterial cisplatin is useful in unresectable HCC
Tommasini [31] 1986	Intrahepatic doxorubicin in unresectable hepatocellular carcinoma. The unfavorable role of cirrhosis	16 (1978–1979)	Unresectable HCC, 8 with cirrhosis and 8 without	Doxorubicin (0.3 mg/kg/day) for 8 days	8 patients died prior to evaluation All patients had alopecia 14 patients had stomatitis 4 patients had abdominal pain, tachycardia, and diarrhea	PR 37.5% For 6 responders, median OS was 10 months Absence of cirrhosis is a prerequisite for use of intra-arterial doxorubicin in advanced HCC
Shepherd [61] 1987	Hepatic arterial infusion of mitoxantrone in the treatment of primary hepatocellular carcinoma	23	Unresectable HCC	Mitoxantrone (6 mg/m^2/day) for 3 days or 10 mg/m^2/day for 3 days	8 patients had granulocytopenia 6 patients had hepatic artery dissection, asymptomatic 4 patients had thrombocytopenia 2 patients had sepsis	PR 20%, SD 38%, PD 42% Median PFS among responders: 5 months Median OS: 5.5 months Mitoxantrone has activity against HCC and is well tolerated, but not clearly superior to systemic therapy

Doci [62] 1988	Intrahepatic chemotherapy for unresectable hepatocellular carcinoma	28 (1976–1983)	Unresectable HCC	Adriamycin (0.3 mg/kg/day) for 8 days every 4 weeks or 5-FU (15 mg/kg/day) for 15 days	16 patients had alopecia 3 patients had gastric bleeding 11 patients had liver failure 11 patients had ascites 11 patients had elevated transaminases 7 patients had catheter-related complications 2 patients had jaundice	Median OS was 3.5 months (6 months in non-cirrhotic patients, 2 months in cirrhotic patients) There is no clear benefit of HAI with adriamycin in advanced HCC
Patt [63] 1988	Hepatocellular carcinoma: A retrospective analysis of treatments to manage disease confined to the liver	10 (1976–1983)	Unresectable HCC	Adriamycin (10–40 mg/m^2) and mitomycin C (10 mg/m^2) on day 1 and then FUDR (75 mg/m^2) daily for 5 days	Not reported	73% response rate Median OS 9 months in HAI-treated patients compared to 2 months for patients receiving IV chemotherapy Arterial therapy may double survival rates in comparison with similar intravenous therapy
Toyoda [12] 1995	The efficacy of continuous local arterial infusion of 5-fluorouracil and cisplatin through an implanted reservoir for severe advanced hepatocellular carcinoma	21 (1991–1993)	Unresectable HCC	5-FU (500 mg) daily and cisplatin (5–10 mg) daily	Catheter malfunction in 6 patients, resolved in 5 Renal failure in 1 patient Stroke in 1 patient	PR 14.2%, SD 71.4%, PD 14.2% 61% 1-year survival (range 36–549 days) Continuous HAI with 5-FU and cisplatin is effective in controlling progression and maintaining QOL, with few side effects

(continued)

Table 27.1 (continued)

Author Year	Title	Patients (treatment years)	Population	Agent/dose/frequency	Complications and toxicity	Results and conclusions
Ando [64] 2002	Hepatic arterial infusion chemotherapy for advanced hepatocellular carcinoma with portal vein tumor thrombosis: analysis of 48 cases	48 (1990–2000)	Advanced HCC	Cisplatin (7 mg/m^2) for 5 days, 5-FU (170 mg/m^2) for 5 days Some patients went on to receive additional therapies, including additional intra-arterial therapy, systemic chemotherapy, and radical local therapies	Nausea 35% Peptic ulcer 13% Leukopenia or thrombocytopenia 13% Decline in hepatic function 13% Renal insufficiency 2% Hearing loss 2% Obstruction of catheter 10% Hematoma around injection port 8% Catheter infection 4% Dislodgement of catheter 2% Obstruction of hepatic artery 2%	CR 8%, PR 40%, SD 29%, PD 23% Median OS: 10.2 months HAI may be effective in patients with portal vein thrombosis. Hepatic function should be monitored during HAI therapy
Itamoto [65] 2002	Hepatic arterial infusion of 5-fluorouracil and cisplatin for unresectable or recurrent hepatocellular carcinoma with tumor thrombus of the portal vein	7 (1997–2000)	Unresectable or recurrent HCC with portal vein thrombosis	Intra-arterial CDDP (10 mg) for 5 days and 5-FU (250 mg) for 5 days, weekly for 3 or more weeks	3 patients had nausea or vomiting 2 patients had thrombocytopenia 2 patients had leukopenia 1 patient had liver dysfunction	PR 28.6%, SD 28.6%, PD 28.6%, unassessable 14.3% Median OS 7.5 months HAI with 5-FU and cisplatin can improve survival in patients with HCC and portal vein thrombus who are not candidates for surgery or TACE

Sakon [13] 2002	Combined intra-arterial 5-fluorouracil and subcutaneous interferon-alpha therapy for advanced hepatocellular carcinoma with tumor thrombi in the major portal branches	17 (1998–1999)	Unresectable HCC with portal vein involvement	Intra-arterial 5-FU (400–500 mg/day for 2 weeks) and interferon-α (5 million IU 3 times/week for 4 weeks) Some patients also received methotrexate, cisplatin, and leucovorin, but this was discontinued due to myelosuppression	Thrombocytopenia or leukopenia in 36% Depression in 18.2%	CR 27.3%, PR 45.5%, SD 9.1%, PD 18.2% Median OS—not reported Intra-arterial 5-FU and subcutaneous IFN-α is a promising therapy for advanced HCC with portal vein thrombus
Lai [32] 2003	Hepatic arterial infusion chemotherapy for hepatocellular carcinoma with portal vein tumor thrombosis	18 (2000–2003)	Unresectable HCC with portal vein tumor thrombus	CDDP (10 mg/day) and 5-FU (250 mg/day) for 5 days, for 4 weeks	Nausea and anorexia 28% Thrombocytopenia and leukopenia 11% Peptic ulcer 5.6% Elevated LFTs 11.2% Catheter obstruction 11.2% Catheter infection 11.2% Dislocation of catheter 5.6% Hematoma near injection port 5.6%	CR 0%, PR 33%, SD 39%, PD 28% Median OS: 9.5 months HAIC with cisplatin and 5-FU may be useful in the treatment of HCC complicated with portal vein tumor thrombus
Sumie [66] 2003	Interventional radiology for advanced hepatocellular carcinoma: comparison of hepatic artery infusion chemotherapy and transcatheter arterial lipiodol chemoembolization	37 (1996–1997)	Unresectable HCC	Cisplatin (10 mg), 5-FU (250 mg) for 5 days, 4 serial courses or TACE with lipiodol and epirubicin (20–30 mg) every 3–4 weeks	13 patients had anorexia 11 patients had fever 9 patients had abdominal pain 6 patients developed peptic ulcer 6 patients had a decline in liver function 3 patients had leukopenia and thrombocytopenia 2 patients had hepatic artery obstruction 1 patient each had infection and catheter obstruction	Median OS: 2.7 years for cisplatin/5-FU group Median OS: 1.7 years for TACE group HAI chemotherapy with cisplatin and 5-FU has a better antitumor effect than TACE

(continued)

Table 27.1 (continued)

Author Year	Title	Patients (treatment years)	Population	Agent/dose/frequency	Complications and toxicity	Results and conclusions
Hamada [14] 2004	Hepatic arterial infusion chemotherapy with the use of an implanted port system in patients with advanced hepatocellular carcinoma: prognostic factors	88 (1991–2002)	Unresectable or recurrent HCC	Cisplatin (10 mg/m^2) and 5-FU (1000 mg/m^2) every 1–4 weeks or doxorubicin or epirubicin (10–20 mg/m^2) every 2–4 weeks	8 patients had nausea, vomiting, and anorexia 6 patients had catheter occlusion 5 patients had hepatic arterial occlusion 3 patients had infection of the port 2 patients had leukopenia	CR 1%, PR 16%, MR 6%, SD 77% No progression Mean OS: 19.5 months Large tumor volume, high Okuda stage, high alkaline phosphatase, ascites, high AST, portal venous invasion, and lack of response to HAI therapy correlate with poor prognosis in HCC
Ota [15] 2005	Treatment of hepatocellular carcinoma with major portal vein thrombosis by combined therapy with subcutaneous interferon-alpha and intra-arterial 5-fluorouracil; role of type 1 interferon receptor expression	55 (1997–2003)	Unresectable HCC with portal venous tumor thrombi	Subcutaneous interferon-α (5 × 10^6 U, days 1, 3, 5 of each week) and intra-arterial 5-FU (300 mg/m^2/day) every 2 weeks for 2 sessions	Grade 3 or higher toxicity: Leukopenia 5.5% Anemia 1.8% Thrombocytopenia 9.1%	CR 14.5%, PR 29.1%, SD 7.3%, PD 49.1% Median PFS: 5.2 months Median OS: 11.8 months Subcutaneous interferon-α and intra-arterial 5-FU are effective in patients with advanced HCC with portal vein tumor thrombi. Clinical response correlates with IFNAR2 expression

Enjoji [67] 2005	Reevaluation of antitumor effects of combination chemotherapy with interferon-alpha and 5-fluorouracil for advanced hepatocellular carcinoma	28 (2003–2004)	Advanced HCC	Subcutaneous interferon-α (3×10^6 U, days 1, 3, 5 of each week) and intra-arterial 5-FU (500/day) for 5 days for 3 weeks, followed by 1-week rest. Patients received 1–4 cycles	NR	CR 3.6%, PR 17.9% PD 78.6% No survival data reported Discriminating between responders and nonresponders after HAI should be performed in order to triage nonresponders to other therapies
Yamasaki [16] 2005	Prognostic factors in patients with advanced hepatocellular carcinoma receiving hepatic arterial infusion chemotherapy	44 (1997–2002)	Unresectable HCC	Intra-arterial CDDP (10 mg) daily for 5 days with 5-FU (250 mg) daily for 5 days, with or without leucovorin or isovorin, for 4 weeks	NR	CR 11.4%, PR 27.3%, MR 4.5%, SD 27.3%, PD 29.5% 1-, 2-, 3-, and 5-year cumulative survival rates: 39%, 18%, 12% and 9% Addition of leucovorin or isovorin appears to improve response rate and survival compared to regimens without leucovorin or isovorin
Obi [17] 2006	Combination therapy of intra-arterial 5-fluorouracil and systemic interferon-alpha for advanced hepatocellular carcinoma with portal venous invasion	116 (2000–2004)	HCC with portal vein invasion	Intramuscular interferon-α (5 million U on days 1, 3, 5 of each treatment week) and intra-arterial 5-FU (500 mg days 1–5 of each week for the first 2 weeks of a 4-week cycle, for 3 cycles unless progressive disease on treatment	Fever 90% AST elevation 60% Leukopenia or thrombocytopenia 80% Nausea and vomiting 50% Stomatitis 1% Depression 1% There was only one grade 3 adverse event required cessation of treatment	CR 16%, PR 36%, SD 1.7%, PD 45.7% 1- and 2-year survival rates: 34% and 18% Combination of intramuscular IFN-α with intra-arterial 5-FU improved survival among complete responders; RCTs are needed

(continued)

Table 27.1 (continued)

Author Year	Title	Patients (treatment years)	Population	Agent/dose/frequency	Complications and toxicity	Results and conclusions
Ikeda [29] 2007	Hepatic arterial infusion chemotherapy with epirubicin in patients with advanced hepatocellular carcinoma and portal vein tumor thrombosis	45 (1999–2004)	Advanced HCC with tumor thrombosis	Intra-arterial epirubicin (60 mg/m^2) with dose reductions if needed, every 4–12 weeks	Grade 3 or greater toxicities: Leukopenia 27% Neutropenia 47% Anemia 4% Thrombocytopenia 9% Elevated AST 36% Elevated ALT 13%	PR 9%, SD 28.9%, SD 64% Median PFS: 1.1 months Median OS: 6.0 months HAI therapy with epirubicin alone appears to have little activity in patients with HCC and portal vein tumor thrombosis
Uka [19] 2007	Pretreatment predictor of response, time to progression, and survival to intra-arterial 5-fluorouracil/interferon combination therapy in patients with advanced hepatocellular carcinoma	55 (2003–2006)	Unresectable HCC	Intra-arterial 5-FU (500 mg/day, days 1–5 each week for 2 weeks) and intramuscular IFN-α (5 million U on days 1, 3, and 5 of each week) repeated monthly as tolerated or unless disease progression occurred	Grade 3 toxicities: Leukopenia 12.7% Thrombocytopenia 9.1% Catheter-associated infection: 9.1%	CR 2%, PR 27%, SD 29%, PD 22%, dropped out 20% Median PFS: 7.5 months Median OS: 9.0 months HCV antibody positivity may predict time to progression and survival in patients with advanced HCC receiving HAI with 5-FU and IFN-α
Ishikawa [33] 2007	Improved survival for hepatocellular carcinoma with portal vein tumor thrombosis treated by intra-arterial chemotherapy combining etoposide, carboplatin, epirubicin, and pharmacokinetic modulating chemotherapy by 5-FU and enteric-coated tegafur/uracil: a pilot study	10 (2002–2007)	Unresectable HCC with portal vein tumor thrombus	Etoposide (50 mg), carboplatin (300 mg), and epirubicin (60 mg) over 30 min and then 5-FU (500 mg/m^2) for 24 h, administered 3 out of every 4 weeks, or biweekly	No grade 3 or higher toxicities	CR or PR: 30%, SD or PD: 70% Median OS: 15.2 months 1-year survival: 70% (15% historical) 2-year survival: 20% (5% historical) HAI therapy for advanced HCC with portal vein tumor thrombus improves survival

Park [18] 2007	Repetitive short-course hepatic arterial infusion chemotherapy with high-dose 5-fluorouracil and cisplatin in patients with advanced hepatocellular carcinoma	41 (2001–2004)	Unresectable HCC	5-FU (500 mg/m^2) days 1–3, cisplatin (60 mg/m^2) on day 2, every 4 weeks	Grade 3 or greater toxicities 1 patient had leukopenia 2 patients had thrombocytopenia 2 patients had AST elevations 3 patients had ALT elevations 1 patient had alkaline phosphatase elevation 5 patients had bilirubin elevation 3 patients had nausea and vomiting 2 patients had infection 1 patients had catheter occlusion	PR 22%, SD 34.1%, 26.8% PD (17.1% unable to assess) Median DFS: 7 months Median OS: 12 months HAI with high dose 5-FU and cisplatin demonstrates clinical efficacy
Yoshikawa [68] 2008	Phase II study of hepatic arterial infusion of a fine-powder formulation of cisplatin for advanced hepatocellular carcinoma	80 (1999–2001)	Unresectable HCC	Cisplatin (65 mg/m^2) every 4–6 weeks	32.5% elevated AST 25% thrombocytopenia 22.5% anorexia 13% neutropenia 6.3% vomiting 3.8% elevated bilirubin 3.8% elevated GGT 2.5% elevated creatinine 1.3% leukopenia, anemia, abdominal pain, hypoalbuminemia, or elevated alkaline phosphatase	PR 33.7%, SD 46.3%, PD 13.8%, (unable to assess 6.2%) 1-year survival rate: 67.5% 2-year survival rate: 50.8% Intra-arterial cisplatin has substantial local and systemic toxicity, but high therapeutic efficacy suggests usefulness in the treatment of advanced HCC

(continued)

Table 27.1 (continued)

Author Year	Title	Patients (treatment years)	Population	Agent/dose/frequency	Complications and toxicity	Results and conclusions
Tanaka [30] 2008	A phase II trial of transcatheter arterial infusion chemotherapy with an epirubicin-lipiodol emulsion for advanced hepatocellular carcinoma refractory to transcatheter arterial embolization	20 (1998–2004)	TACE-refractory HCC	60 mg/m^2 epirubicin emulsified in lipiodol administered to feeding artery every 4–12 weeks	Leukocytopenia 35% Neutropenia 65% Thrombocytopenia 30% AST elevation 45% ALT elevation 35%	PR 5%, minor response 15%, SD 25%, PD 55% Median PFS: 1.1 months Median OS: 12.4 months HAI with epirubicin-lipiodol has only modest activity, and these findings do not support its use in practice
Ikushima [69] 2009	Transarterial infusion chemotherapy with epirubicin in water-in-oil-in-water emulsion for recurrent hepatocellular carcinoma in the residual liver after hepatectomy	18 (2002–2006)	Recurrent HCC after hepatectomy	Water-in-oil-in-water (W/O/W) emulsion containing epirubicin (60 mg), lipiodol (5 mL), and polyoxyethylene stearate	Grade II complications: Hypotension 77.8% Fever 11.1%	CR 33%, PR 45% 1-, 2-, and 3-year survival: 94%, 76%, and 76% HAI with W/O/W may be an effective treatment for patients with recurrent HCC after surgical resection
Kasai [20] 2009	Evaluation of newly developed combination therapy of intra-arterial 5-fluorouracil and systemic pegylated interferon alpha-2b for advanced hepatocellular carcinoma with portal venous invasion: preliminary results	9 (2006–2008)	HCC with portal vein thrombosis	Subcutaneous pegylated interferon-α (50–100 μg on day 1 of each week for 4 weeks) and intra-arterial 5-FU (250 mg/day, days 1–5 of each week for 4 weeks) for 2 to 3 cycles	Thrombocytopenia 22.2% Leukopenia/anorexia 22.2% General fatigue 22.2%	PR 77.8%, SD 11.1%, PD 11.1% 6- and 12-month survival: 88.9% and 77.8% Intra-arterial 5-FU and subcutaneous pegylated interferon-α may be useful as palliative treatment in HCC

Katamura [21] 2009	Intra-arterial 5-fluorouracil/ interferon combination therapy for advanced hepatocellular carcinoma with or without three-dimensional conformal radiotherapy for portal vein tumor thrombosis	16 (2003–2008)	HCC with portal vein thrombosis	Intramuscular IFN-α on days 1, 3, and 5 of each week and intra-arterial 5-FU (500 mg/body weight/day) on days 1–5 for 2 weeks, repeated as tolerated versus above regimen plus 3D conformal radiation therapy	Grade 3 or greater toxicities: Leukopenia 75.1% Thrombocytopenia 68.8% Anorexia 12.6%	Non-RT group: 6%, PR 13%, SD 50%, PD 31% RT-group: CR 6%, PR 19%, SD 50%, PD 25% Median PFS: 3.6 months in non-RT group, 3.8 months in RT group Median OS: non-RT group 7.9 months; RT group 7.5 months 5-FU/IFN with 3D-CRT for portal vein thrombosis improves the response rate of portal vein thrombosis
Ueshima [22] 2010	Hepatic arterial infusion chemotherapy using low-dose 5-fluorouracil and cisplatin for advanced hepatocellular carcinoma	52 (2004–2006)	Advanced HCC	5-FU (250–500 mg/day for days 1–5 for each week for the first 2 weeks) and CDDP (10 mg/day for 5 days/week for the first 2 weeks) After 2 weeks, the 5-U was increased to 1000 mg once a week, and CDDP changed to 10 mg a week	Grade 3 or greater toxicities: Leukocytopenia 19.2% Anemia 9.6% Thrombocytopenia 46.1% Neutropenia 23.1% Hyperbilirubinemia 13.5% Hepatic artery obstruction in 1 patient	CR 7.7%, PR 30.8%, SD 26.9%, PD 28.8% 1-, 2- and 3-year survival: 53.3%, 34.8%, and 26.1% HAI with 5-FU and CDDP is an effective treatment option for locally advanced HCC, but regular hematologic monitoring is necessary
Kim [70] 2010	A comparative study of high-dose hepatic arterial infusion chemotherapy and transarterial chemoembolization using doxorubicin for intractable, advanced hepatocellular carcinoma	36 (2006–2008)	Unresectable HCC	5-FU (500 mg/m²) days 1–3 and cisplatin (60 mg/m²) on day 2, repeated every 4 weeks or TACE with doxorubicin (10–60 mg) with lipiodol (5–10 mL) every 4–8 weeks	19 patients had hyperbilirubinemia 18 patients had elevated ALT 16 patients had GI toxicity 6 patients had thrombocytopenia 7 patients had neutropenia 3 patients had anemia	PR 16.7%, SD 33.3%, PD 44.4% for HAI PR 0%, SD 25.8%, PD 61.2% for TACE Median OS for HAI: 193 days Median OS for TACE: 119 days HAI might be safe and effective compared to TACE for advanced HCC

(continued)

Table 27.1 (continued)

Author Year	Title	Patients (treatment years)	Population	Agent/dose/frequency	Complications and toxicity	Results and conclusions
Woo [23] 2010	A randomized comparative study of high-dose and low-dose hepatic arterial infusion chemotherapy for intractable, advanced hepatocellular carcinoma	68 (2006–2008)	Unresectable HCC, most with portal vein tumor thrombi	High dose: 5-FU (500 mg/m^2) on days 1–3 and cisplatin (60 mg/m^2) on day 2 every 4 weeks or low dose: 5-FU (170 mg/m^2) days 1–5 and cisplatin (7 mg/m^2) on days 1–5 every 4 weeks	Grade 3 or greater toxicities: Anemia 2.9% Hyperbilirubinemia 2.9% Lung abscess 1.5% Port infection 1.5% Port occlusion 1.5%	High dose: PR 16.7%, SD 33.3%, PD 44.4% Low dose: PR 0%, SD 28.1%, PD 53.1% Median PFS high dose: 4.8 months Median OS high dose: 6.4 months Median PFS low dose: 3 months Median PFS high dose: 5.1 months Both HAI regimens are safe and effective in advanced HCC. High-dose HAI achieves a better tumor response compared to low-dose HAI

Kasai [24] 2011	Combination therapy of intra-arterial 5-fluorouracil and systemic pegylated interferon alpha-2b for advanced hepatocellular carcinoma	50 (2005–2008)	HCC with tumor thrombus	Intra-arterial 5-FU (250 mg/day, days 1–5 of each week for 2 weeks) and intramuscular IFN-α (3 million units on days 1, 3, and 5 of each week) or intra-arterial 5-FU and subcutaneous pegylated IFN-α or intra-arterial CDDP (50 or 100 mg) suspended in lipiodol (10 mL)	Overall toxicities: General fatigue 32% Anorexia 24% Nausea and vomiting 36% Fever 72% Leukopenia 22% Thrombocytopenia 13%	5-FU/PEG-IFN group ($n = 21$): PR 71.4%, SD 9.5%, PD 19.1% 5-FU/IFN group ($n = 12$): PR 8.3%, SD 41.7%, PD 50% CDDP group ($n = 17$): PR 17.6%, SD 11.7%, PD 70.7% Cumulative survival at 6, 12, 18, and 24 months by group: 5-FU/PEG-IFN group ($n = 21$): 5-FU/IFN group ($n = 12$): CDDP group ($n = 17$): Combination of intra-arterial 5-FU and subcutaneous pegylated IFN-α may be useful for patients with advanced HCC

(continued)

Table 27.1 (continued)

Author Year	Title	Patients (treatment years)	Population	Agent/dose/frequency	Complications and toxicity	Results and conclusions
Kim [71] 2011	Long-term clinical outcomes of hepatic arterial infusion chemotherapy with cisplatin with or without 5-fluorouracil in locally advanced hepatocellular carcinoma	138 (2002–2007)	Advanced HCC	Cisplatin (60 mg/m^2) alone every 4 weeks. Cisplatin (60 mg/m^2) on day 1 and 5-FU (500 mg/m^2) on days 1, 2, and 3 every 4 weeks	Grade 3 or higher toxicities: Leukopenia 13.8% Neutropenia 2.2% Anemia 0.7% Thrombocytopenia 2.9% AST elevation 7.2% ALT elevation 2.9% Bilirubin elevation 8.7% Mucositis 2.2% Nausea or vomiting 5.8% Diarrhea 0.7% Renal impairment 0.7% Port infection 2.2% Catheter occlusion 0.7%	Cisplatin only: CR 0%, PR 12.2%, SD 48.8%, PD 39.0% Cisplatin and 5-FU: CR 3.1%, PR 24.7%, SD 35.1%, PD 34.0%, unassessable 3.1% Median PFS cisplatin only: 4.6 months Median OS cisplatin only: 7.5 months Median PFS cisplatin and 5-FU: 7.0 months Median OS cisplatin and 5-FU: 12 months HAI is a promising approach for patients with advanced HCC; those treated with intra-arterial cisplatin and 5-FU derive the greatest benefit

Yamashita [25] 2011	Randomized, phase II study comparing interferon combined with hepatic arterial infusion of fluorouracil plus cisplatin and fluorouracil alone in patients with advanced hepatocellular carcinoma	114 (2003–2007)	Advanced primary and recurrent HCC	Group 1: 5-FU (300 mg/m^2/day) for 5 days × 2 weeks with interferon-α-2b (3 × 10^6 U, 3 times weekly) for 4 weeks Group 2: the same regimen plus cisplatin (20 mg/m^2) on days 1 and 8 of each 4 week cycle	Grade 3 or higher toxicity(Group 1/Group 2): Neutropenia 33.3/29.8% Leukopenia 31.6/21.1% Reduced Hgb 3.5/7.0% Thrombocytopenia 22.8/45.6% Prothrombin time elevation 1.8/5.3% Asthenia 5.3/1.8% Fever 0/1.8% Nausea 5.3/17.5% Vomiting 1.8/7.0% Mucositis 1.8/5.3% Liver function test elevation 17.5/7%	5-FU and IFN: CR 5.3%, PR 19.3%, SD 33.3%, PD 38.6%, unassessable 3.5% 5-FU, IFN, and cisplatin: CR 1.7%, PR 43.9%, SD 26.3%, PD 22.8%, unassessable 5.3% Median PFS 5-FU and IFN: 3.3 months Median PFS 5-FU, IFN, and CDDP: 6.5 months Median OS 5-FU and IFN: 10.5 months Median OS 5-FU, IFN, and CDDP: 17.6 months Adding CDDP increases the efficacy of HAI with 5-FU in conjunction with IFN-α
Nouso [26] 2013	Effect of hepatic arterial infusion chemotherapy of 5-fluorouracil and cisplatin for advanced hepatocellular carcinoma in the Nationwide Survey of Primary Liver Cancer in Japan	467 (2000–2005)	Advanced HCC	Intra-arterial 5-FU and CDDP (doses not specified)	NR	HAI group: CR 4%, PR 36.5%, SD 23.6%, PD 27.2%, undefined 8.7% HAI group: median OS 14 months No therapy group: median OS 5.2 months For advanced HCC, HAI is considered to be effective treatment

(continued)

Table 27.1 (continued)

Author Year	Title	Patients (treatment years)	Population	Agent/dose/frequency	Complications and toxicity	Results and conclusions
Song [27] 2015	A comparative study between sorafenib and hepatic arterial infusion chemotherapy for advanced hepatocellular carcinoma with portal vein tumor thrombosis	110 (2008–2013)	HCC with portal vein thrombosis	Intra-arterial 5-FU (500 mg/m^2) on days 1–3 and intra-arterial CDDP (60 mg/m^2) on day 2, with or without epirubicin (35 mg/m^2) on day 1, repeated every 3–4 weeks or sorafenib	Grade 3 or greater toxicities: HAI Group: Leukopenia 16% Neutropenia 64% Anemia 52% Thrombocytopenia 80% Hyperbilirubinemia 16% ALT elevation 36%	Sorafenib group: PR 13.3%, SD 31.7%, PD 55% HAI group: CR 2%, PR 22%, SD 66%, PD 10% Median PFS sorafenib: 2.1 months Median PFS HAI: 3.3 months Median OS sorafenib: 5.5 months Median OS HAI: 7.1 months HAI is comparable with sorafenib in terms of survival and time to progression but shows more favorable treatment responses for patients with HCC and portal vein tumor thrombus

Table 27.2 Reported toxicities of hepatic artery infusion therapy for hepatocellular carcinoma

Author Year	Therapy	Symptomatic		Hematologic		Clinical			Device-related			Other
		Nausea/ vomiting	Abdominal pain	Cytopenia	Elevated LFTs	Cholangitis	Death (unrelated to disease)		Device infection	Device malfunction or misperfusion	Device or artery thrombosis	
Fortner [9] 1973	FUDR (0.3 mg/kg) daily or methotrexate (2.5–5.0 mg) daily with hepatic artery ligation	NR	NR	NR	NR	NR	4/23 (liver failure; hepatorenal syndrome and methotrexate toxicity; liver necrosis; pulmonary embolus)		1/23	NR	NR	NR
Bern [10] 1978	Intra-arterial Adriamycin (4 patients) or intravenous Adriamycin (10 patients) every 3 weeks	6/11	NR	2/11 Thrombocytopenia 2/11 Neutropenia	3/11	NR	1/4 (duodenal necrosis)		1/11	NR	2/11	Alopecia 8/11 Stomatitis 2/11 Diarrhea 2/11 Sepsis 1/11
Reed [59] 1981	FUDR (0.3 mg/kg) continuous infusion	NR	NR	NR	NR	NR	2/13 (liver failure)		NR	NR	NR	NR
Kajanti [60] 1986	Cisplatin (50 mg/m²) for 24 h every 4 weeks	10/10	NR	NR	NR	NR	1/10 (cisplatin-induced renal failure)		NR	NR	NR	NR
Tommasini [31] 1986	Doxorubicin (0.3 mg/kg/day) for 8 days	NR	4/16	NR	NR	NR	8/16 (majority with liver failure, possibly related to disease progression)		NR	NR	NR	Alopecia 16/16 Stomatitis 14/16 Diarrhea 4/16

(continued)

Table 27.2 (continued)

Author Year	Therapy	Nausea/vomiting	Abdominal pain	Cytopenia	Elevated LFTs	Cholangitis	Death (unrelated to disease)	Device infection	Device malfunction or misperfusion	Device or artery thrombosis	
Shepherd [61] 1987	Mitoxantrone (6 mg/m^2/day) for 3 days or 10 mg/m^2/day for 3 days	2/28	NR	8/23 granulocytopenia 4/23 Thrombocytopenia 5/23 Neutropenia	NR	NR	NR	NR	NR	5/23 artery thrombosis (asymptomatic)	Sepsis 2/23 Alopecia 3/23
Doci [62] 1988	Adriamycin (0.3 mg/kg/day) for 8 days every 4 weeks or 5-FU (15 mg/kg/day) for 15 days	NR	NR	3/28	11/28	NR	1/28 (sepsis)	NR	2/28	4/28 artery thrombosis	16/28 alopecia 11/28 liver failure 3/28 gastric bleeding
Toyoda [12] 1995	5-FU (500 mg) daily and cisplatin (5–10 mg) daily	NR	NR	NR	NR	NR	NR	NR	6/21	NR	Stroke 1/21 Renal failure 1/21
Ando [64] 2002	Cisplatin (7 mg/m^2) for 5 days, 5-FU (170 mg/m^2) for 5 days Some patients went on to receive additional therapies, including additional intra-arterial therapy, systemic chemotherapy, and radical local therapies	17/48	NR	6/48	6/48	NR	2/48 (liver failure; sepsis)	2/48	6/48	1/48	Renal failure 1/48 Hearing loss 1/48 Peptic ulcer 6/48
Itamoto [65] 2002	Intra-arterial CDDP (10 mg) for 5 days and 5-FU (250 mg) for 5 days, weekly for 3 or more weeks	3/7	NR	2/7 Thrombocytopenia 2/7 Leukopenia	1/7	NR	NR	NR	NR	NR	NR

Sakon [13] 2002	Intra-arterial 5-FU (400–500 mg/day for 2 weeks) and interferon-α (5 million IU 3 times/week for 4 weeks) Some patients also received methotrexate, cisplatin, and leucovorin, but this was discontinued due to myelosuppression	NR	NR	6/17	NR	NR	NR	NR	Depression 2/17
Lai [32] 2003	CDDP (10 mg/day) and 5-FU (250 mg/day) for 5 days, for 4 weeks	5/18	NR	2/18	NR	6/18 (GI bleeding 3; sepsis 3)	2/18	3/18	NR	Peptic ulcer 1/18 Renal insufficiency 1/18
Sumie [66] 2003	Cisplatin (10 mg), 5-FU (250 mg) for 5 days, 4 serial courses or TACE with lipiodol and epirubicin (20–30 mg) every 3–4 weeks	NR	9/37	3/37	6/37	NR	NR	2/37	2/37	2/37	13/37 anorexia 11/37 fever
Hamada [14] 2004	Cisplatin (10 mg/m²) and 5-FU (1000 mg/m²) every 1–4 weeks or doxorubicin or epirubicin (10–20 mg/m²) every 2–4 weeks	8/88	NR	2/88	NR	NR	3/88	6/88	5/88	NR

(continued)

Table 27.2 (continued)

Author Year	Therapy	Nausea/vomiting	Abdominal pain	Cytopenia	Elevated LFTs	Cholangitis	Death (unrelated to disease)	Device infection	Device malfunction or misperfusion	Device or artery thrombosis
Ota [15] 2005	Subcutaneous interferon-α (5×10^6 U, days 1, 3, 5 of each week) and intra-arterial 5-FU ($300 \ mg/m^2/day$) every 2 weeks for 2 sessions	NR	NR	6/55 leukopenia 2/55 anemia 10/55 thrombocytopenia	NR	NR	NR	NR	NR	NR
Yamasaki [16] 2005	Intra-arterial CDDP (10 mg) daily for 5 days with 5-FU (250 mg) daily for 5 days, with or without leucovorin or isovorin, for 4 weeks	NR	NR	NR	NR	NR	9/44 (GI bleeding 4; liver failure 3; pneumonia 2)	NR	NR	NR
Ikeda [29] 2007	Intra-arterial epirubicin (60 mg/m^2) with dose reductions if needed, every 4–12 weeks	NR	NR	12/45 leukopenia 16/45 neutropenia 2/45 anemia 11/45 thrombocytopenia	6/45	NR	NR	NR	NR	NR
Uka [19] 2007	Intra-arterial 5-FU (500 mg/day days 1–5 each week for 2 weeks) and intramuscular IFN-α (5 million U on days 1, 3, and 5 of each week) repeated monthly as tolerated or unless disease progression occurred	NR	NR	7/55 leukopenia Thrombocytopenia 5/55	NR	NR	NR	5/55	NR	NR

Study	Regimen		Hematologic toxicity							Other
Park [18] 2007	5-FU (500 mg/m²) days 1–3, cisplatin (60 mg/m²) on day 2, every 4 weeks	3/41	NR	1/41 leukopenia 2/41 thrombocytopenia	9/41	NR	NR	2/41	1/41	NR	NR
Yoshikawa [68] 2008	Cisplatin (65 mg/m²) every 4–6 weeks	5/80	1/80	1/80 leukopenia 10/77 neutropenia 1/80 anemia 20/80 thrombocytopenia	15/80	NR	2 (1 myocardial infarction; 1 unknown)	NR	NR	NR	1/80 retroperitoneal hematoma and pancreatitis
Tanaka [30] 2008	60 mg/m² epirubicin emulsified in Lipiodol administered to feeding artery every 4–12 weeks	0/20	NR	Neutropenia 13/20 Leukopenia 7/20 Thrombocytopenia 6/20	7/20	NR	NR	NR	NR	NR	NR
Kasai [20] 2009	Subcutaneous pegylated interferon-α (50–100 μg on day 1 of each week for 4 weeks) and intra-arterial 5-FU (250 mg/day, days 1–5 of each week for 4 weeks) for 2–3 cycles	NR	NR	Thrombocytopenia 1/9	NR	NR	NR	NR	NR	NR	NR
Katamura [21] 2009	Intramuscular IFN-α on days 1, 3, and 5 of each week and intra-arterial 5-FU (500 mg/body weight/day) on days 1–5 for 2 weeks, repeated as tolerated versus above regimen plus 3D conformal radiation therapy	NR	NR	Leukopenia 3/16 Thrombocytopenia 5/16	NR	NR	NR	NR	NR	NR	Anorexia 1/16

(continued)

Table 27.2 (continued)

Author Year	Therapy	Nausea/ vomiting	Abdominal pain	Cytopenia	Elevated LFTs	Cholangitis	Death (unrelated to disease)	Device infection	Device malfunction or misperfusion	Device or artery thrombosis	
Ueshima [22] 2010	5-FU (250–500 mg/day for days 1–5 for each week for the first 2 weeks) and CDDP (10 mg/day for 5 days/week for the first 2 weeks) After 2 weeks, the 5-U was increased to 1000 mg once a week, and CDDP changed to 10 mg a week	NR	NR	Leukopenia 10/52 Anemia 5/52 Thrombocytopenia 22/52 Neutropenia 12/52	7/52	NR	NR	NR	NR	NR	NR
Kim [70] 2010	5-FU (500 mg/m^2) days 1–3 and cisplatin (60 mg/m^2) on day 2, repeated every 4 weeks or TACE with doxorubicin (10–60 mg) with lipiodol (5–10 mL) every 4–8 weeks	16/36	NR	Neutropenia 7/36 Thrombocytopenia 6/36 Anemia 3/36	Hyper-bilirubinemia 19/36 ALT elevation 18/36	NR	NR	NR	NR	NR	
Woo [23] 2010	High dose: 5-FU (500 mg/m^2) on days 1–3 and cisplatin (60 mg/m^2) on day 2 every 4 weeks Low dose: 5-FU (170 mg/m^2) days 1–5 and cisplatin (7 mg/m^2) on days 1–5 every 4 weeks	NR	NR	Neutropenia 2/68	Hyper-bilirubinemia 2/68	NR	NR	1/68	NR	1/68	Lung abscess 1/68

Kasai [24] 2011	Intra-arterial 5-FU (250 mg/day, days 1–5 of each week for 2 weeks) and intramuscular IFN-α (3 million units on days 1, 3, and 5 of each week) Intra-arterial 5-FU and subcutaneous pegylated IFN-α Intra-arterial CDDP (50 or 100 mg) suspended in lipiodol (10 mL)	18/50	NR	Leukopenia 11/50 Thrombocytopenia 13/50	NR	NR	NR	NR	Fatigue 16/50 Anorexia 12/50 Fever 36/50
Kim [71] 2011	Cisplatin (60 mg/m^2) alone every 4 weeks Cisplatin (60 mg/m^2) on day 1 and 5-FU (500 mg/m^2) on days 1, 2, and 3 every 4 weeks	9/36	NR	Anemia 2/36 Neutropenia 5/36 Thrombocytopenia 4/36	Hyper-bilirubinemia 7/36 ALT elevation 6/36	NR	NR	NR	NR
Yamashita [25] 2011	Group 1: 5-FU (300 mg/m^2/day) for 5 days × 2 weeks with interferon-α-2b (3 × 10^6 U, 3 times weekly) for 4 weeks Group 2: Same regimen plus cisplatin (20 mg/m^2) on days 1 and 8 of each 4 week cycle	13/114	NR	Neutropenia 36/114 Leukopenia 30/114 Anemia 6/114 Thrombocytopenia 39/114	14/114	NR	NR	NR	Fatigue 4/114 Mucositis 4/114

(continued)

Table 27.2 (continued)

Author Year	Therapy	Nausea/ vomiting	Abdominal pain	Cytopenia	Elevated LFTs	Cholangitis	Death (unrelated to disease)	Device infection	Device malfunction or misperfusion	Device or artery thrombosis
Song [27] 2015	Intra-arterial 5-FU (500 mg/m^2) on days 1–3 and intra-arterial CDDP (60 mg/m^2) on day 2, with or without epirubicin (35 mg/m^2) on day 1, repeated every 3–4 weeks or sorafenib	NR	NR	Leukopenia 8/50 Neutropenia 32/50 Anemia 26/50 Thrombocytopenia 40/50	Hyper-bilirubinemia 8/50 ALT elevation 18/50	NR	NR	NR	NR	NR

number of patients with intrahepatic or perihilar disease are not candidates for surgical resection or transplant. For this reason, alternative locoregional therapies have been sought to fill this treatment gap, including HAI therapy.

No randomized trials have compared systemic chemotherapy to HAI therapy for CCA to date. Therefore, as a benchmark for understanding the efficacy of HAI therapy for iCCA, we will first briefly review the natural history of patients receiving only systemic chemotherapy for this disease. One caveat is that most patients receiving chemotherapy alone have either unresectable or metastatic disease, whereas most centers consider metastasis to be a relative contraindication for HAI therapy. Studies of patients undergoing systemic chemotherapy therefore may have a higher overall stage compared to those undergoing HAI therapy.

Studies of systemic chemotherapy in CCA are limited to small series, often with inclusion of patients with other biliary, pancreatic, or ampullary cancers. Valle and colleagues established the superiority of cisplatin and gemcitabine over gemcitabine alone for patients with biliary tract cancer [47]. This randomized controlled trial allocated 410 patients with locally advanced or metastatic biliary tract cancer to receive either gemcitabine and cisplatin or gemcitabine alone. Patients receiving gemcitabine and cisplatin had a median survival of 11.7 months, compared to 8.1 months in the patients receiving gemcitabine alone. Among study enrollees, one quarter had locally advanced disease, while the remainder had metastases. A second study reported a median survival of 9.3 months for patients treated with chemotherapy for cholangiocarcinoma [48]. Thus the expected survival for a patient with unresectable or metastatic CCA treated with systemic chemotherapy is approximately 9–12 months.

Just as with studies of systemic chemotherapy, the results of HAI therapy in the treatment of CCA are difficult to interpret for several reasons. First, a relatively low incidence of disease means that most reports consist of small case series. Second, study populations are very heterogenous in terms of disease stage and overall tumor burden and prior systemic or local treatment. Last, treatment regimens vary widely in terms of agents used, dosage, frequency, and duration of treatment. Studies that employ HAI therapy for CCA are summarized in Table 27.3.

One of the first modern studies of HAI for CCA was reported by Tanaka and colleagues in 2002 [49]. HAI was administered to 11 patients with unresectable, liver-predominant stage II–IV intrahepatic CCA. Three drug regimens were used: one consisted of 5-fluorouracil (5-FU) adriamycin or epirubicin and mitomycin C and/or cisplatin, another contained 5-FU only, and a third consisted of 5-FU and cisplatin. Delayed complications were seen in three patients, including hearing deficit, pancytopenia, and cholangitis. Survival rates were 90.9% at 1 year, 50.5% at 2 years, 20.2% at 3 years, and 10.1% at 4 years, with a median survival of 26 months.

Mambrini and colleagues used oral capecitabine plus intra-arterial epirubicin and cisplatin in 20 patients with unresectable biliary cancer [50]. There were no complete responses (CR). Partial response (PR), stable disease (SD), and progressive disease (PD) were observed in 31.5%, 47.5%, and 21%, respectively. Despite a low response rate, median PFS and OS were 11.6 and 18 months, respectively.

Shitara and colleagues [51] treated 20 patients with unresectable iCCA with mitomycin C and degradable starch microspheres via intra-arterial infusion weekly until disease progression or unacceptable toxicity. There was one CR, nine PR, eight SD, and two PD for an overall response rate of 50%. Median PFS and OS were 8.3 and 14.1 months, respectively.

Jarnagin and colleagues treated 34 patients with unresectable iCCA or HCC with HAI consisting of FUDR and dexamethasone every 4 weeks until progression, excessive toxicity, or resectability occurred [52]. Of the 26 patients with iCCA, 14 had a PR, 11 had SD, and 1 had PD. There were no radiographic complete responses; however, one patient underwent resection which revealed complete tumor necrosis. Median PFS was 7.4 months, and disease-specific survival was 29.5 months, with patients with iCCA having a higher response rate (53.8%)

Table 27.3 Hepatic artery infusion therapy for cholangiocarcinoma

Author Year	Title	Patients (treatment years)	Population	Agent/dose/frequency	Grade 3 or higher complications and toxicity	Results and conclusions
Tanaka [49] 2002	Arterial chemoinfusion therapy through an implanted port system for patients with unresectable intrahepatic cholangiocarcinoma—initial experience	11 (1991–2000)	Unresectable iCCA	Intra-arterial: 5-FU only (1500 mg) every week or 5-FU (200–500 mg) and cisplatin (10 mg) for 5 days or 5-FU (250–500 mg every week) and adriamycin (30 mg q 4 weeks) or epirubicin (10 mg q week) and mitomycin C (4 mg q 2 weeks) or cisplatin (10 mg q week)	Hearing weakness and cholangitis in 1 patient improved with drug removal Pancytopenia in 1 patient, resolved after GMCSF administration Cholangitis and elevation of liver function tests in 3 patients, with 1 resulting in death 16 months after initiation of therapy, possibly also related to tumor progression	Survival rates: 90.9% at 1 year, 50.5% at 2 years, 20.2% at 3 years, and 10.1% at 4 years Median OS: 26 months HAI is relatively safe and appears to prolong survival
Mambrini [50] 2007	Capecitabine plus hepatic intra-arterial epirubicin and cisplatin in unresectable biliary cancer: a phase II study	20 (2004–2006)	Unresectable iCCA or eCCA	Intra-arterial epirubicin (50 mg/m^2), cisplatin (60 mg/m^2) every 3 weeks Oral capecitabine (1000 mg/m^2 twice a day	Severe gastroenteritis resulting in death in 1 patient, suspected to be related to dihydropyrimidine dehydrogenase gene polymorphism Leukopenia in 1 patient Nausea and emesis in 1 patient Mucositis in 2 patients Alopecia in 3 patients	PR 31.5%, SD 47.5%, PD 21%. Median PFS: 11.6 months Median OS: 18 months HAI therapy is feasible and active in CCA

Shitara [51] 2008	Hepatic arterial infusion of mitomycin C with degradable starch microspheres for unresectable intrahepatic cholangiocarcinoma	20 (2002–2006)	Unresectable iCCA	Intra-arterial mitomycin C (2 mg) and degradable starch micropsheres (300 mg) weekly	Anorexia in 1 patient Nausea and vomiting in 1 patient Gastroduodenal ulcer in 4 patients Abdominal pain in 2 patients	CR 5%, PR 45%, SD 40%, PD 10% Median PFS: 8.3 months Median OS: 14.1 months Intra-arterial mitomycin C and degradable starch microspheres are a feasible and effective treatment for unresectable iCCA
Jarnagin [52] 2009	Regional chemotherapy for unresectable primary liver cancer: results of a phase II clinical trial and assessment of DCE-MRI as a biomarker of survival	34 (2003–2007)	Unresectable iCCA or HCC	FUDR (0.16 mg/kg) and dexamethasone every 4 weeks	Abdominal pain in 1 patient Elevated bilirubin in 3 patients Diarrhea in 1 patient Pump misperfusion in 1 patient	PR 47.1%, SD 41.2%, PD 11.7% Median PFS: 7.4 months Median disease-specific survival: 29.5 months HAI therapy can be safe and effective HAI is more effective in iCCA than HCC Tumor perfusion characteristics as measured by MRI may predict treatment outcome
Inaba [72] 2011	Phase I/phase II study of hepatic arterial infusion chemotherapy with gemcitabine in patients with unresectable intrahepatic cholangiocarcinoma (JIVROSG-0301)	16 (2004–2006)	Unresectable iCCA	Intra-arterial gemcitabine (600 or 800 or 1000 mg/m^2)	Nausea in 1 patient Fatigue in 1 patient Elevated bilirubin in 1 patient Elevated GGT in 2 patients Elevated AST in 1 patient Elevated ALT in 1 patient Neutropenia in 5 patients	PR 7.7%, SD 61.5% PD 30.8% Median OS: 12.8 months Despite low toxicity of 1000 mg/m^2 intra-arterial gemcitabine, no clear efficacy was seen

(continued)

Table 27.3 (continued)

Author Year	Title	Patients (treatment years)	Population	Agent/dose/frequency	Grade 3 or higher complications and toxicity	Results and conclusions
Kemeny [53] 2011	Treating primary liver cancer with hepatic arterial infusion of floxuridine and dexamethasone: does the addition of systemic bevacizumab improve results?	22	Unresectable iCCA or HCC	Intra-arterial FUDR (0.16 mg/kg) and dexamethasone every 4 weeks Systemic bevacizumab (5 mg/kg) every other week	Alkaline phosphatase elevation in 7 patients Elevated SGOT in 5 patients Elevated bilirubin in 6 patients Need for biliary stent in 3 patients Thrombosis in 2 patients Myocardial infarction in 1 patient Hyperglycemia in 1 patient Syncope in 1 patient Hyponatremia in 1 patient Confusion in 2 patients Duodenal tear in 1 patient	PR 31.8%, SD 69.2% Median PFS: 8.45 months Median OS: 31.1 months The addition of bevacizumab increased biliary toxicity without a clear benefit in PFS or OS compared to FUDR alone
Ghiringhelli [56] 2013	Hepatic arterial infusion of gemcitabine plus oxaliplatin as second-line treatment for locally advanced intrahepatic cholangiocarcinoma: preliminary experience	12 (2008–2012)	Unresectable iCCA after failure of systemic chemotherapy	Intra-arterial gemcitabine (1000 mg/m^2) and oxaliplatin (100 mg/m^2) every 2 weeks	Neutropenia in 4 patients Thrombocytopenia in 3 patients Neuropathy in 2 patients Infection in 2 patients Oxaliplatin allergy in 2 patients Leukopenia in 1 patient	Overall response rate: 66% Tumor control rate: 91% Median PFS: 9.1 months Median OS: 20.3 months HAI is feasible and demonstrates a good efficacy in iCCA as second-line treatment

Sinn [54] 2013	Hepatic arterial infusion with oxaliplatin and 5-FU/folinic acid for advanced biliary tract cancer: a phase II study	37 (2004–2010)	Advanced biliary tract cancer	Intra-arterial oxaliplatin (85 mg/m²), folinate (170 mg/m²), and 5-FU (600 mg/m²)	Death in 2 patients, 1 from cholangitis and 1 from a rare immunological-mediated side effect from 5-FU Elevated bilirubin in 11 patients Elevated transaminases in 7 patients Abdominal pain in 3 patients Nausea in 1 patient Diarrhea in 1 patient Neurotoxicity in 1 patient Thrombocytopenia in 2 patients Leukocytosis in 4 patients Port thrombosis in 5 patients Port dislocation in 4 patients Port infection in 3 patients Defective port in 1 patient Vascular spasm in 1 patient	Median PFS: 6.5 months Median OS: 13.5 months HAI therapy is feasible and appears to be effective for advanced biliary tract cancer
Subbiah [55] 2013	Targeted therapy of advanced gallbladder cancer and cholangiocarcinoma with aggressive biology: eliciting early response signals from phase 1 trials	40 (2004–2012)	CCA and gallbladder cancer	Novel targeted inhibitors of MEK, VEGF, gamma-secretase, aurora kinase, and IGR-IR pathway 43% received HAI therapy	GI bleeding in 2 patients treated with angiogenesis inhibitors No other toxicities reported	Targeted therapies including HAI has comparable efficacy to first-, second-, and third-line FDA-approved therapies These therapies should be further explored in clinical trials
Massani [57] 2015	Intrahepatic chemotherapy for unresectable cholangiocarcinoma: review of literature and personal experience	11 (2008–2012)	Unresectable iCCA	Intra-arterial 5-FU (7 mg/kg) and oxaliplatin (100 mg/mq) and oral folinic acid (25 mg) every 15 days	Liver dysfunction and decompensation in 1 patient Hand-foot syndrome in 3 patients	PR 45.4%, SD 18.2%, PD 36.4% Mean OS: 17.6 months HAI chemotherapy is effective and may reduce tumors to the point of resectability

compared to patients with HCC (25%). They also showed that pretreatment and early posttreatment tumor perfusion characteristics using dynamic, contrast-enhanced MRI could be used to predict treatment outcome.

Inaba and colleagues conducted a phase I/phase II dose-finding study for the use of gemcitabine HAI therapy in patients with unresectable iCCA. Infusions were given every 4 weeks for a maximum of five infusions. Of 13 patients who received the recommended dose of 1000 mg/m^2, there were no CRs, only one PR, and three PDs. Although many included patients had prior treatment, median survival time was just 12.8 months. Given the lack of observed treatment response, the authors concluded that HAI therapy with gemcitabine could not be definitively recommended for iCCA and that it was unclear if it provided any benefit over standard chemotherapy in this heavily pretreated population.

Kemeny and colleagues [53] conducted a study in which they added systemic bevacizumab to HAI therapy with FUDR and dexamethasone in patients with primary liver cancer. Twenty-two patients were treated with HAI and bevacizumab, 18 with iCCA, and 4 with HCC. Seven patients (31.8%) had PR, while 15 (69.2%) had SD. No patients experienced CR or PD. Median PFS was 8.45 months, and median OS was 31.1 months. The addition of bevacizumab increased biliary toxicity without a clear benefit in PFS or OS.

Sinn and colleagues conducted a phase II clinical trial using HAI therapy with biweekly oxaliplatin, 5-FU, and folinic acid in patients with advanced biliary tract cancer (predominantly iCCA) [54]. Thirty-seven patients received a total of 432 cycles of therapy. Median PFS was 6.5 months and median OS was 13.5 months.

Subbiah and colleagues treated 40 patients with advanced cholangiocarcinoma or gallbladder cancer with a variety of targeted agents and locoregional therapies, including HAI therapy, anti-angiogenic, anti-HER-2/neu, and MAPK/ERK (MEK) inhibitors [55]. Of these patients, 17 received HAI therapy, of which 7 had either SD > 6 months or PR, the highest rate among any treatment group.

Ghiringhelli and colleagues evaluated the efficacy of HAI therapy with gemcitabine and oxaliplatin as second-line therapy in 12 patients with unresectable iCCA [56]. Patients received infusions every 2 weeks until disease progression, limiting toxicity, or technical problems were encountered. Median PFS and median OS were 9.1 months and 20.3 months, respectively. Despite all patients having previously received the same chemotherapy systemically, the overall response rate was 66%, and tumor control rate was 91%. Two patients had responses sufficient to undergo surgical resection with curative intent.

Massani and colleagues treated 11 patients from 2008 to 2012 with unresectable iCCA with HAI therapy consisting of fluorouracil and oxaliplatin and compared their results with published results of patients treated with systemic chemotherapy during the same time period [57]. After six cycles, five patients experienced PR, two had SD, and four had PD. Mean OS was 17.6 months for patients treated with HAI, which included two patients who responded sufficiently to undergo surgical resection.

With respect to adverse events, the most commonly reported toxicities involved nausea and vomiting, anorexia, leukopenia and thrombocytopenia, and derangements in liver function tests (see Table 27.4). Hepatic decompensation and cholangitis were rare but severe complications. Implant or implantation-related complications were reported as infrequent and generally resolvable and included port thrombosis, dislocation, and infection.

As for any chemotherapy, bone marrow toxicity and the resultant cytopenias may occur, so routine hematology studies are prudent. Hepatic decompensation and cholangiopathy are rare but potentially fatal complications, so routine liver function testing is warranted. In addition, regular assessment of treatment response by cross-sectional imaging may be useful for prognosis and triaging nonresponders to other therapies.

In summary, evidence supporting the use of HAI therapy for patients with unresectable iCCA is sparse. Because of the rarity of iCCA, many studies group patients with advanced biliary tract cancers (intra- and extrahepatic CCA, gallbladder

Table 27.4 Reported toxicities of hepatic artery infusion therapy for cholangiocarcinoma

Author Year	Therapy	Symptomatic		Hematologic		Clinical		Device-related			Other
		Nausea/vomiting	Abdominal pain	Cytopenia	Elevated LFTs	Cholangitis	Death	Device infection	Device malfunction or misperfusion	Device thrombosis	
Tanaka [49] 2002	Intra-arterial: 5-FU only (1500 mg) every week or 5-FU (200–500 mg) and cisplatin (10 mg) for 5 days or 5-FU (250–500 mg every week) and adriamycin (30 mg q 4 weeks) or epirubicin (10 mg q week) and mitomycin C (4 mg q 2 weeks) or cisplatin (10 mg q week)	NR	NR	1/11	3/11	3/11	1/11; due to cholangitis 16 months after starting therapy	NR	NR	NR	NR
Mambrini [50] 2007	Intra-arterial epirubicin (50 mg/m²), cisplatin (60 mg/m²) every 3 weeks Oral capecitabine (1000 mg/m² twice a day	1/20	NR	1/20	NR	NR	1/20; due to severe gastroenteritis attributed to dihydropyrimidine dehydrogenase gene polymorphism	NR	NR	NR	Mucositis 2/20 Alopecia 3/20

(continued)

Table 27.4 (continued)

Author Year	Therapy	Symptomatic		Hematologic		Clinical		Device-related			Other
		Nausea/ vomiting	Abdominal pain	Cytopenia	Elevated LFTs	Cholangitis	Death	Device infection	Device malfunction or misperfusion	Device thrombosis	
Shitara [51] 2008	Intra-arterial mitomycin C (2 mg) and degradable starch micropsheres (300 mg) weekly	1/20	2/20	NR	NR	NR	NR	NR	NR	NR	Anorexia 1/20 Diarrhea 1/20 Gastric ulcer 4/20
Jarnagin [52] 2009	FUDR (0.16 mg/kg) and dexamethasone every 4 weeks	NR	1/34	NR	3/34	NR	NR	3/34	2/34	NR	NR
Inaba [72] 2011	Intra-arterial gemcitabine (600 or 800 or 1000 mg/m^2)	1/16	NR	5/16	4/16	NR	NR	NR	5/16	NR	Fatigue 1/16 AST elevation 1/16
Kemeny [53] 2011	Intra-arterial FUDR (0.16 mg/kg) and dexamethasone every 4 weeks Systemic bevacizumab (5 mg/kg) every other week	NR	NR	NR	20/22	NR	NR	NR	NR	2/22	Elevated SGOT 5/16 Need for biliary stent 3/22 Myocardial infarction 1/22 Hyperglycemia 1/22 Syncope 1/22 Hyponatremia 1/22 Confusion 2/22 Duodenal tear 1/22

Ghiringhelli [56] 2013	Intra-arterial gemcitabine (1000 mg/m²) and oxaliplatin (100 mg/m²) every 2 weeks	4/12	NR	8/12	NR	NR	NR	2/12	1/12	NR	Neuropathy 4/12 Oxaliplatin allergy 2/12 Diarrhea 2/12
Sinn [54] 2013	Intra-arterial oxaliplatin (85 mg/m²), folinate (170 mg/m²), and 5-FU (600 mg/m²)	1/37	3/37	2/37	18/37	1/37	2/37; one from cholangitis, one from rare 5-FU side effect	3/37	5/37	5/37	Leukocytosis 4/37 Neuropathy 1/37 Diarrhea 1/37
Subbiah [55] 2013	Novel targeted inhibitors of MEK, VEGF, gamma-secretase, aurora kinase, and IGR-IR pathway 43% received HAI therapy	NR	NR	NR	NR	NR	0/40	NR	NR	NR	2 episodes of GI bleeding in patients treated with angiogenesis inhibitors; 1/40 with AV fistula
Massani [57] 2015	Intra-arterial 5-FU (7 mg/kg) and oxaliplatin (100 mg/mq) and oral folinic acid (25 mg) every 15 days	0/11	0/11	NR	NR	NR	NR	0/11	0/11	NR	Hepatic failure 1/11 Hand-foot syndrome 3/11

cancer, and ampullary cancer) together. Additionally, disease heterogeneity (with respect to prior treatment, tumor burden, and vascular involvement) and treatment heterogeneity (with respect to chemotherapeutic agents employed, doses, and frequency) also make conclusive interpretation difficult. Though selection bias and other potential confounders preclude a definitive conclusion, the range of median OS for patients with CCA treated with HAI is 12.8–31.1 months, which compares favorably with the median OS of 9.3–11.7 months reported in studies of systemic therapy.

References

1. Ryerson AB, Eheman CR, Altekruse SF, Ward JW, Jemal A, Sherman RL, et al. Annual Report to the Nation on the Status of Cancer, 1975-2012, featuring the increasing incidence of liver cancer. Cancer. 2016;122(9):1312–37.
2. Ananthakrishnan A, Gogineni V, Saeian K. Epidemiology of primary and secondary liver cancers. Semin Intervent Radiol. 2006;23(1):47–63.
3. Patel T. Increasing incidence and mortality of primary intrahepatic cholangiocarcinoma in the United States. Hepatology (Baltimore MD). 2001;33(6):1353–7.
4. Breedis C, Young G. The blood supply of neoplasms in the liver. Am J Pathol. 1954;30(5):969–77.
5. Nakajima T, Kondo Y, Miyazaki M, Okui K. A histopathologic study of 102 cases of intrahepatic cholangiocarcinoma: histologic classification and modes of spreading. Hum Pathol. 1988;19(10):1228–34.
6. Toyosaka A, Okamoto E, Mitsunobu M, Oriyama T, Nakao N, Miura K. Pathologic and radiographic studies of intrahepatic metastasis in hepatocellular carcinoma; the role of efferent vessels. HPB Surg. 1996;10(2):97–103; discussion -4.
7. Sullivan RD, Miller E, Sikes MP. Antimetabolite-metabolite combination cancer chemotherapy. Effects of intraarterial methotrexate-intramuscular Citrovorum factor therapy in human cancer. Cancer. 1959;12:1248–62.
8. Sullivan RD, Norcross JW, Watkins E Jr. Chemotherapy of metastatic liver cancer by prolonged hepatic-artery infusion. N Engl J Med. 1964;270:321–7.
9. Fortner JG, Mulcare RJ, Solis A, Watson RC, Golbey RB. Treatment of primary and secondary liver cancer by hepatic artery ligation and infusion chemotherapy. Ann Surg. 1973;178(2):162–72.
10. Bern MM, W MD Jr, Cady B, Oberfield RA, Trey C, Clouse ME, et al. Intraarterial hepatic infusion and intravenous adriamycin for treatment of hepatocellular carcinoma: a clinical and pharmacology report. Cancer. 1978;42(2):399–405.
11. Bhutiani N, Martin RC 2nd. Transarterial therapy for colorectal liver metastases. Surg Clin North Am. 2016;96(2):369–91.
12. Toyoda H, Nakano S, Kumada T, Takeda I, Sugiyama K, Osada T, et al. The efficacy of continuous local arterial infusion of 5-fluorouracil and cisplatin through an implanted reservoir for severe advanced hepatocellular carcinoma. Oncology. 1995;52(4):295–9.
13. Sakon M, Nagano H, Dono K, Nakamori S, Umeshita K, Yamada A, et al. Combined intraarterial 5-fluorouracil and subcutaneous interferon-alpha therapy for advanced hepatocellular carcinoma with tumor thrombi in the major portal branches. Cancer. 2002;94(2):435–42.
14. Hamada A, Yamakado K, Nakatsuka A, Takaki H, Akeboshi M, Takeda K. Hepatic arterial infusion chemotherapy with use of an implanted port system in patients with advanced hepatocellular carcinoma: prognostic factors. J Vasc Interv Radiol. 2004;15(8):835–41.
15. Ota H, Nagano H, Sakon M, Eguchi H, Kondo M, Yamamoto T, et al. Treatment of hepatocellular carcinoma with major portal vein thrombosis by combined therapy with subcutaneous interferon-alpha and intra-arterial 5-fluorouracil; role of type 1 interferon receptor expression. Br J Cancer. 2005;93(5):557–64.
16. Yamasaki T, Kimura T, Kurokawa F, Aoyama K, Ishikawa T, Tajima K, et al. Prognostic factors in patients with advanced hepatocellular carcinoma receiving hepatic arterial infusion chemotherapy. J Gastroenterol. 2005;40(1):70–8.
17. Obi S, Yoshida H, Toune R, Unuma T, Kanda M, Sato S, et al. Combination therapy of intraarterial 5-fluorouracil and systemic interferon-alpha for advanced hepatocellular carcinoma with portal venous invasion. Cancer. 2006;106(9):1990–7.
18. Park JY, Ahn SH, Yoon YJ, Kim JK, Lee HW, Lee DY, et al. Repetitive short-course hepatic arterial infusion chemotherapy with high-dose 5-fluorouracil and cisplatin in patients with advanced hepatocellular carcinoma. Cancer. 2007;110(1):129–37.
19. Uka K, Aikata H, Takaki S, Miki D, Kawaoka T, Jeong SC, et al. Pretreatment predictor of response, time to progression, and survival to intraarterial 5-fluorouracil/interferon combination therapy in patients with advanced hepatocellular carcinoma. J Gastroenterol. 2007;42(10):845–53.
20. Kasai K, Kuroda H, Ushio A, Sawara K, Takikawa Y, Suzuki K. Evaluation of newly developed combination therapy of intra-arterial 5-fluorouracil and systemic pegylated interferon alpha-2b for advanced hepatocellular carcinoma with portal venous invasion: preliminary results. Hepatol Res. 2009;39(2):117–25.
21. Katamura Y, Aikata H, Takaki S, Azakami T, Kawaoka T, Waki K, et al. Intra-arterial 5-fluorouracil/interferon combination therapy for advanced hepatocellular carcinoma with or without three-dimensional conformal radiotherapy for portal vein tumor thrombosis. J Gastroenterol. 2009;44(5):492–502.

22. Ueshima K, Kudo M, Takita M, Nagai T, Tatsumi C, Ueda T, et al. Hepatic arterial infusion chemotherapy using low-dose 5-fluorouracil and cisplatin for advanced hepatocellular carcinoma. Oncology. 2010;78 Suppl 1:148–53.
23. Woo HY, Bae SH, Park JY, Han KH, Chun HJ, Choi BG, et al. A randomized comparative study of high-dose and low-dose hepatic arterial infusion chemotherapy for intractable, advanced hepatocellular carcinoma. Cancer Chemother Pharmacol. 2010;65(2):373–82.
24. Kasai K, Ushio A, Kasai Y, Sawara K, Miyamoto Y, Oikawa K, et al. Combination therapy of intra-arterial 5-fluorouracil and systemic pegylated interferon alpha-2b for advanced hepatocellular carcinoma. Int J Clin Oncol. 2011;16(3):221–9.
25. Yamashita T, Arai K, Sunagozaka H, Ueda T, Terashima T, Yamashita T, et al. Randomized, phase II study comparing interferon combined with hepatic arterial infusion of fluorouracil plus cisplatin and fluorouracil alone in patients with advanced hepatocellular carcinoma. Oncology. 2011;81(5–6):281–90.
26. Nouso K, Miyahara K, Uchida D, Kuwaki K, Izumi N, Omata M, et al. Effect of hepatic arterial infusion chemotherapy of 5-fluorouracil and cisplatin for advanced hepatocellular carcinoma in the Nationwide Survey of Primary Liver Cancer in Japan. Br J Cancer. 2013;109(7):1904–7.
27. Song DS, Song MJ, Bae SH, Chung WJ, Jang JY, Kim YS, et al. A comparative study between sorafenib and hepatic arterial infusion chemotherapy for advanced hepatocellular carcinoma with portal vein tumor thrombosis. J Gastroenterol. 2015;50(4):445–54.
28. Enjoji M, Morizono S, Kotoh K, Kohjima M, Miyagi Y, Yoshimoto T, et al. Re-evaluation of antitumor effects of combination chemotherapy with interferon-alpha and 5-fluorouracil for advanced hepatocellular carcinoma. World J Gastroenterol: WJG. 2005;11(36):5685–7.
29. Ikeda M, Okusaka T, Ueno H, Morizane C, Iwasa S, Hagihara A, et al. Hepatic arterial infusion chemotherapy with epirubicin in patients with advanced hepatocellular carcinoma and portal vein tumor thrombosis. Oncology. 2007;72(3–4):188–93.
30. Tanaka T, Ikeda M, Okusaka T, Ueno H, Morizane C, Ogura T, et al. A phase II trial of transcatheter arterial infusion chemotherapy with an epirubicin-Lipiodol emulsion for advanced hepatocellular carcinoma refractory to transcatheter arterial embolization. Cancer Chemother Pharmacol. 2008;61(4):683–8.
31. Tommasini M, Colombo M, Sangiovanni A, Orefice S, Bignami P, Doci R, et al. Intrahepatic doxorubicin in unresectable hepatocellular carcinoma. The unfavorable role of cirrhosis. Am J Clin Oncol. 1986;9(1):8–11.
32. Lai YC, Shih CY, Jeng CM, Yang SS, Hu JT, Sung YC, et al. Hepatic arterial infusion chemotherapy for hepatocellular carcinoma with portal vein tumor thrombosis. World J Gastroenterol. 2003;9(12):2666–70.
33. Ishikawa T, Imai M, Kamimura H, Tsuchiya A, Togashi T, Watanabe K, et al. Improved survival for hepatocellular carcinoma with portal vein tumor thrombosis treated by intra-arterial chemotherapy combining etoposide, carboplatin, epirubicin and pharmacokinetic modulating chemotherapy by 5-FU and enteric-coated tegafur/uracil: a pilot study. World J Gastroenterol. 2007;13(41):5465–70.
34. DeOliveira ML, Cunningham SC, Cameron JL, Kamangar F, Winter JM, Lillemoe KD, et al. Cholangiocarcinoma: thirty-one-year experience with 564 patients at a single institution. Ann Surg. 2007;245(5):755–62.
35. Endo I, Gonen M, Yopp AC, Dalal KM, Zhou Q, Klimstra D, et al. Intrahepatic cholangiocarcinoma: rising frequency, improved survival, and determinants of outcome after resection. Ann Surg. 2008;248(1):84–96.
36. Jarnagin WR, Ruo L, Little SA, Klimstra D, D'Angelica M, DeMatteo RP, et al. Patterns of initial disease recurrence after resection of gallbladder carcinoma and hilar cholangiocarcinoma: implications for adjuvant therapeutic strategies. Cancer. 2003;98(8):1689–700.
37. Spolverato G, Kim Y, Alexandrescu S, Marques HP, Lamelas J, Aldrighetti L, et al. Management and outcomes of patients with recurrent intrahepatic cholangiocarcinoma following previous curative-intent surgical resection. Ann Surg Oncol. 2016;23(1):235–43.
38. Burke EC, Jarnagin WR, Hochwald SN, Pisters PW, Fong Y, Blumgart LH. Hilar Cholangiocarcinoma: patterns of spread, the importance of hepatic resection for curative operation, and a presurgical clinical staging system. Ann Surg. 1998;228(3):385–94.
39. Chamberlain RS, Blumgart LH. Hilar cholangiocarcinoma: a review and commentary. Ann Surg Oncol. 2000;7(1):55–66.
40. Launois B, Reding R, Lebeau G, Buard JL. Surgery for hilar cholangiocarcinoma: French experience in a collective survey of 552 extrahepatic bile duct cancers. J Hepato-Biliary-Pancreat Surg. 2000;7(2):128–34.
41. Nagino M, Nimura Y, Kamiya J, Kanai M, Uesaka K, Hayakawa N, et al. Segmental liver resections for hilar cholangiocarcinoma. Hepato-Gastroenterology. 1998;45(19):7–13.
42. Nakeeb A, Tran KQ, Black MJ, Erickson BA, Ritch PS, Quebbeman EJ, et al. Improved survival in resected biliary malignancies. Surgery. 2002;132(4):555–63; discussion 63-4.
43. Rea DJ, Munoz-Juarez M, Farnell MB, Donohue JH, Que FG, Crownhart B, et al. Major hepatic resection for hilar cholangiocarcinoma: analysis of 46 patients. Arch Surg (Chicago, IL: 1960). 2004, 139;(5):514. 23; discussion 23-5
44. Tsao JI, Nimura Y, Kamiya J, Hayakawa N, Kondo S, Nagino M, et al. Management of hilar cholangiocarcinoma: comparison of an American and a Japanese experience. Ann Surg. 2000;232(2):166–74.

45. Washburn WK, Lewis WD, Jenkins RL. Aggressive surgical resection for cholangiocarcinoma. Arch Surg (Chicago IL : 1960). 1995;130(3):270–6.
46. Rea DJ, Heimbach JK, Rosen CB, Haddock MG, Alberts SR, Kremers WK, et al. Liver transplantation with neoadjuvant chemoradiation is more effective than resection for hilar cholangiocarcinoma. Ann Surg. 2005;242(3):451–8. discussion 8-61
47. Valle J, Wasan H, Palmer DH, Cunningham D, Anthoney A, Maraveyas A, et al. Cisplatin plus gemcitabine versus gemcitabine for biliary tract cancer. N Engl J Med. 2010;362(14):1273–81.
48. Huitzil-Melendez FD, O'Reilly EM, Duffy A, Abou-Alfa GK. Indications for neoadjuvant, adjuvant, and palliative chemotherapy in the treatment of biliary tract cancers. Surg Oncol Clin N Am. 2009;18(2):361–79. x
49. Tanaka N, Yamakado K, Nakatsuka A, Fujii A, Matsumura K, Takeda K. Arterial chemoinfusion therapy through an implanted port system for patients with unresectable intrahepatic cholangiocarcinoma-initial experience. Eur J Radiol. 2002;41(1):42–8.
50. Mambrini A, Guglielmi A, Pacetti P, Iacono C, Torri T, Auci A, et al. Capecitabine plus hepatic intra-arterial epirubicin and cisplatin in unresectable biliary cancer: a phase II study. Anticancer Res. 2007;27(4c):3009–13.
51. Shitara K, Ikami I, Munakata M, Muto O, Sakata Y. Hepatic arterial infusion of mitomycin C with degradable starch microspheres for unresectable intrahepatic cholangiocarcinoma. Clin Oncol (R Coll Radiol). 2008;20(3):241–6.
52. Jarnagin WR, Schwartz LH, Gultekin DH, Gonen M, Haviland D, Shia J, et al. Regional chemotherapy for unresectable primary liver cancer: results of a phase II clinical trial and assessment of DCE-MRI as a biomarker of survival. Ann Oncol. 2009;20(9):1589–95.
53. Kemeny NE, Schwartz L, Gonen M, Yopp A, Gultekin D, D'Angelica MI, et al. Treating primary liver cancer with hepatic arterial infusion of floxuridine and dexamethasone: does the addition of systemic bevacizumab improve results? Oncology. 2011;80(3–4):153–9.
54. Sinn M, Nicolaou A, Gebauer B, Podrabsky P, Seehofer D, Ricke J, et al. Hepatic arterial infusion with oxaliplatin and 5-FU/folinic acid for advanced biliary tract cancer: a phase II study. Dig Dis Sci. 2013;58(8):2399–405.
55. Subbiah IM, Subbiah V, Tsimberidou AM, Naing A, Kaseb AO, Javle M, et al. Targeted therapy of advanced gallbladder cancer and cholangiocarcinoma with aggressive biology: eliciting early response signals from phase 1 trials. Oncotarget. 2013;4(1):156–65.
56. Ghiringhelli F, Lorgis V, Vincent J, Ladoire S, Guiu B. Hepatic arterial infusion of gemcitabine plus oxaliplatin as second-line treatment for locally advanced intrahepatic cholangiocarcinoma: preliminary experience. Chemotherapy. 2013;59(5):354–60.
57. Massani M, Nistri C, Ruffolo C, Bonariol R, Pauletti B, Bonariol L, et al. Intrahepatic chemotherapy for unresectable cholangiocarcinoma: review of literature and personal experience. Updat Surg. 2015;67(4):389–400.
58. Ramming KP, Sparks FC, Eilber FR, Holmes EC, Morton DL. Hepatic artery ligation and 5-fluorouracil infusion for metastatic colon carcinoma and primary hepatoma. Am J Surg. 1976;132(2):236–42.
59. Reed ML, Vaitkevicius VK, Al-Sarraf M, Vaughn CB, Singhakowinta A, Sexon-Porte M, et al. The practicality of chronic hepatic artery infusion therapy of primary and metastatic hepatic malignancies: ten-year results of 124 patients in a prospective protocol. Cancer. 1981;47(2):402–9.
60. Kajanti M, Rissanen P, Virkkunen P, Franssila K, Mantyla M. Regional intra-arterial infusion of cisplatin in primary hepatocellular carcinoma. A phase II study. Cancer. 1986;58(11):2386–8.
61. Shepherd FA, Evans WK, Blackstein ME, Fine S, Heathcote J, Langer B, et al. Hepatic arterial infusion of mitoxantrone in the treatment of primary hepatocellular carcinoma. J Clin Oncol. 1987;5(4):635–40.
62. Doci R, Bignami P, Bozzetti F, Bonfanti G, Audisio R, Colombo M, et al. Intrahepatic chemotherapy for unresectable hepatocellular carcinoma. Cancer. 1988;61(10):1983–7.
63. Patt YZ, Claghorn L, Charnsangavej C, Soski M, Cleary K, Mavligit GM. Hepatocellular carcinoma. A retrospective analysis of treatments to manage disease confined to the liver. Cancer. 1988;61(9):1884–8.
64. Ando E, Tanaka M, Yamashita F, Kuromatsu R, Yutani S, Fukumori K, et al. Hepatic arterial infusion chemotherapy for advanced hepatocellular carcinoma with portal vein tumor thrombosis: analysis of 48 cases. Cancer. 2002;95(3):588–95.
65. Itamoto T, Nakahara H, Tashiro H, Haruta N, Asahara T, Naito A, et al. Hepatic arterial infusion of 5-fluorouracil and cisplatin for unresectable or recurrent hepatocellular carcinoma with tumor thrombus of the portal vein. J Surg Oncol. 2002;80(3):143–8.
66. Sumie S, Yamashita F, Ando E, Tanaka M, Yano Y, Fukumori K, et al. Interventional radiology for advanced hepatocellular carcinoma: comparison of hepatic artery infusion chemotherapy and transcatheter arterial lipiodol chemoembolization. AJR Am J Roentgenol. 2003;181(5):1327–34.
67. Amieva M, Peek RM Jr. Pathobiology of helicobacter pylori-induced gastric cancer. Gastroenterology. 2016;150(1):64–78.
68. Yoshikawa M, Ono N, Yodono H, Ichida T, Nakamura H. Phase II study of hepatic arterial infusion of a fine-powder formulation of cisplatin for advanced hepatocellular carcinoma. Hepatol Res. 2008;38(5):474–83.
69. Ikushima I, Higashi S, Seguchi K, Ishii A, Ota Y, Shima M, et al. Transarterial infusion chemotherapy with epirubicin in water-in-oil-in-water emulsion for recurrent hepatocellular carcinoma in the residual liver after hepatectomy. Eur J Radiol. 2009;69(1):114–9.
70. Kim HY, Kim JD, Bae SH, Park JY, Han KH, Woo HY, et al. A comparative study of high-dose hepatic arterial infusion chemotherapy and transarterial chemoembolization using doxorubicin for intrac-

table, advanced hepatocellular carcinoma. Korean J Hepatol. 2010;16(4):355–61.
71. Kim BK, Park JY, Choi HJ, Kim DY, Ahn SH, Kim JK, et al. Long-term clinical outcomes of hepatic arterial infusion chemotherapy with cisplatin with or without 5-fluorouracil in locally advanced hepatocellular carcinoma. J Cancer Res Clin Oncol. 2011;137(4):659–67.
72. Inaba Y, Arai Y, Yamaura H, Sato Y, Najima M, Aramaki T, et al. Phase I/II study of hepatic arterial infusion chemotherapy with gemcitabine in patients with unresectable intrahepatic cholangiocarcinoma (JIVROSG-0301). Am J Clin Oncol. 2011;34(1):58–62.

Two-Stage Approach to Liver Resection

28

Kerollos Nashat Wanis
and Roberto Hernandez-Alejandro

Introduction

Surgery offers the greatest likelihood of cure for primary and secondary liver tumors. Both surgical resection and liver transplantation are utilized, but liver transplantation is typically reserved for patients with hepatocellular carcinoma in the context of cirrhosis. The main limitation of extensive surgical resection is the risk of postoperative liver failure due to a small future liver remnant (FLR). Systemic chemotherapy has contributed to treatment by controlling tumor growth and revealing cancer biology, but hepatotoxic agents raise further concerns in the context of major liver resection. Multiple techniques have emerged to address the problem of a small predicted FLR, and the development of two-stage hepatectomy represents the forefront of evolving therapeutic approaches.

In 1996, Bismuth and colleagues described a cohort of patients undergoing hepatectomy for primarily unresectable disease in which various techniques for achieving resectability were employed including what is now commonly known as two-stage hepatectomy [1]. Later, in 2000, Adam and colleagues elaborated on the technique in a paper dedicated to two-stage resection, describing 13 patients in whom the approach was feasible [2]. In Japan, Makuuchi had introduced portal vein embolization (PVE) in 1990 as a method for facilitating hypertrophy of the non-embolized liver segments prior to extended hepatectomy in order to minimize the risk of postoperative liver dysfunction [3]. In 2003, Jaeck and associates combined the two concepts, generating the classical description of two-stage hepatectomy with PVE [4]. This approach, as it was initially defined, involves resection of metastases in the FLR during the first stage, followed by right PVE and right or extended right hepatectomy (trisectionectomy) once adequate FLR hypertrophy is achieved. Over the subsequent decade, the indications and techniques for TSH continued to evolve.

The early and rapid development of this aggressive surgical approach arose from a need to innovate on the existing methods for achieving curative resection in patients with disseminated colorectal cancer. It was already well-recognized that liver resection is the only hope for cure in patients with colorectal cancer liver metastases (CRLM) and that patients with favorable tumor characteristics may achieve long-term survival [5–7]. In patients with ini-

K. N. Wanis
Department of Surgery, London Health Sciences Centre, Western University, London, ON, Canada
e-mail: Kerollos.Wanis@lhsc.on.ca

R. Hernandez-Alejandro (✉)
Division of Transplantation, HPB Surgery, Department of Surgery, University of Rochester, Rochester, NY, USA
e-mail: roberto_hernandez@urmc.rochester.edu

© Springer Nature Switzerland AG 2018
K. Cardona, S. K. Maithel (eds.), *Primary and Metastatic Liver Tumors*,
https://doi.org/10.1007/978-3-319-91977-5_28

tially unresectable CRLM, due to bilobar and multiple metastases or lesions located near major vascular or biliary structures, various surgical and nonsurgical techniques have emerged with the aim of achieving curative resection. In initial publications, a FLR size of 20% of the total liver volume was felt to be necessary, but, with more widespread usage of hepatotoxic chemotherapeutic agents and the rising prevalence of cholestasis, steatosis, and fibrosis, preserving a higher postoperative liver volume is essential. Consequently, a FLR of 30% is recommended based on the current evidence [8–10]. In order to achieve resectability in patients who initially have inadequate liver volumes, newer chemotherapeutic regimens have been applied with successful tumor response in a portion of patients initially deemed unresectable [11–13]. Furthermore, combining surgery with additional local techniques, including radiofrequency or microwave ablation in conjunction with chemotherapy, in order to allow complete treatment of the tumor load has also been performed, but outcome data remain limited [14]. The development of TSH, using PVE to exploit the potential of liver regeneration, has provided an alternate, and more convincing, option for feasible curative treatment in patients with extensive tumor volume [3].

Liver Regeneration

The liver's capacity for regeneration has been known and studied for many years. Although the clinical applications of this remarkable function are continuing to develop, interest in utilizing liver regeneration has existed for several decades. For patients requiring TSH, the success of surgical resection without postoperative hepatic dysfunction relies on the extraordinary ability of the liver to restore its mass and function, maintaining adequate metabolic function despite significant parenchymal loss or ischemic injury. The mechanisms underlying this unique and complex phenomenon are multifactorial and involve hemodynamic changes, release of growth factors, and cellular proliferation [15]. Liver regeneration, although commonly referred to as hypertrophy, actually occurs by hyperplasia, an increase in the number of liver cells by a precise and moderated process of cellular regeneration that responds to a proliferative stimulus and terminates once the original liver volume has been achieved [16]. Interestingly, this extraordinary potential for regeneration is restricted to a threshold of injury beyond which further resection or parenchymal insult results in limited restoration of hepatic mass and resultant liver dysfunction. This threshold has been explored in mouse models and may help to explain the etiology of small-for-size syndrome and post-hepatectomy liver failure in humans [17, 18].

The multiple mechanisms of hepatic regeneration have been most thoroughly studied in rodent models of two-thirds partial hepatectomy (PH). PH induces a profound hemodynamic shift toward the residual liver. While arterial flow relative to amount of liver tissue does not change, the portal vein must continue to drain the entire venous outflow of most of the gastrointestinal tract, spleen, and pancreas. This results in a tripling of the portal supply relative to liver volume. Subsequently, these hemodynamic shifts result in a dramatic increase in hepatocyte exposure to growth factors [19]. There are a myriad of growth factors involved in hepatic regeneration, but hepatocyte growth factor appears to be the most fundamental contributor in conjunction with epidermal growth factor rector ligands [19]. Interestingly, unlike in the skin, intestine, and blood, the main mediator of cellular hyperplasia in the liver is mature hepatocytes, and the role of liver progenitor cells is incompletely understood [16].

Portal vein occlusion (PVO) results in a similar hyperplastic response. Comparable hemodynamic changes occur; however, the hemodynamic shift is less pronounced following PVO. This is because, while PH results in complete redirection of arterial and portal flow to the residual liver, PVO causes a redistributive effect leading to complete portal vein flow to the non-embolized liver with increased arterial flow to the embolized segments due to the hepatic arterial buffer response [20, 21]. An overall increase in arterial flow in the common hepatic artery, mediated by the hepatic arterial buffer response, maintains constant flow to the non-embolized liver, resulting in an overall increase in blood flow to the FLR [22, 23]. The subsequent growth factor signaling, activation of proliferative quiescent hepatocytes, and self-limiting hyperplasia proceed in a similar fashion to PH.

Criteria for TSH

The criteria for feasibility of liver resection have undergone considerable evolution over the past decade. Aggressive resection for CRLM is a relatively new concept that challenges traditional resectability conditions that were based on number and size of hepatic tumors. More general criteria focusing on the remnant liver have previously been proposed: (1) preserving two contiguous hepatic segments; (2) preservation of adequate vascular inflow and outflow, as well as biliary drainage; and (3) preserving >30% FLR [24]. Adoption of PVO and TSH has further attenuated these principles, with technical feasibility relying on a careful appraisal of FLR volume and function. Consequently, in some cases, a single healthy liver segment may be sufficient to mitigate liver failure [25].

The decision to offer TSH should be based on an oncological and technical evaluation with multidisciplinary input. More specific criteria for TSH are based on the feasibility of complete tumor resection with pathologically cancer-free margins; the ability to preserve adequate FLR volume (usually ≥30% at completion of TSH); adequate inflow, outflow, and biliary drainage of the FLR; absence of extrahepatic disease, except for technically resectable lung metastases in selected patients; and satisfactory patient functional status. Lastly, the application of the TSH technique in patients with primary liver tumors (i.e., hepatocellular carcinoma and cholangiocarcinoma) is controversial due to the risk of post-hepatectomy liver failure in the context of underlying liver disease including cholestasis and/or fibrosis.

Assessment of FLR

Determining the need for two-stage hepatectomy requires accurate assessment of the FLR volume. The absolute volume of the FLR as well as the total liver volume can be measured using computed tomography (CT) volumetry [26]. Techniques for CT liver volumetry include semi-manual delineation of liver borders using traditional software or automated segmentation with more modern technology [27, 28]. Further validation of newer software is necessary, but automated segmentation and three-dimensional image reconstruction are likely to result in more efficient and specific measurement.

Since the volume of liver required to maintain homeostasis and prevent post-hepatectomy liver failure (PHLF) varies from patient to patient based on body size, FLR should be expressed as a proportion of the total liver volume (TLV). This proportion is defined as the standardized FLR (sFLR) and can be calculated by dividing the FLR by the TLV. In order to calculate the sFLR, an accurate estimation of the TLV must be obtained. CT volumetry can be applied to measure the total liver volume; however, the presence of tumors complicates this assessment since the total tumor volume must be subtracted from the liver volume in order to obtain the true TLV. This process has a number of important limitations. In addition to being tedious, the existence of multiple liver lesions or lesions with ill-defined borders can make the process error-prone and imprecise. In order to address this, a number of formulas have been proposed to estimate the TLV based on patient characteristics [29]. Most formulas rely on the relationship between TLV and the patient's body surface area (BSA) or body weight (BW). The most widely used is the Vauthey formula (TLV = 1267.28(BSA) − 794.41) [30], but the formula proposed by Johnson and colleagues (TLV = $1000(0.72\sqrt{BSA} + 0.171)^3$) has also been shown to have high accuracy [29, 31].

While assessment of future liver remnant volume is essential, it serves only as a surrogate for post-resection function and may be poorly correlated with function in compromised livers. Although improvements in preoperative assessment, perioperative care, and surgical technique have reduced the incidence of PHLF, it continues to be the main factor underlying mortality following liver resection [32]. To reduce liver failure-related morbidity, several tools have been proposed to quantify liver function independently of volume. These include biochemical classifications such as the Child-Pugh classification or Model for End-Stage Liver Disease (MELD score) [33]. In TSH, biochemical models which predict PHLF can be applied in the inter-stage period to identify patients at risk of liver failure following completion of stage two. These include 50–50 criteria, peak bilirubin >7 mg/dL, and the International Study Group of Liver Surgery (ISGLS) definition [34–37]. In addition to these biochemical tools, indocyanine green retention rate at 15 min (ICG R15) and ^{99m}Tc-mebrofenin hepatobiliary scintigraphy (HIDA) scan allow further stratification of liver function and have been more commonly utilized in Asian centers [38–40]. These technologies require further validation in North America and are being studied at several centers. At our institution, HIDA scan is routinely obtained prior to completion of TSH stage two. A hepatic uptake cutoff of 2.69%/min/m^2 has been validated, and patients with a FLR function greater than this value are unlikely to suffer PHLF-related mortality; however, further corroborating research is necessary [41].

Surgical Approach to TSH

First Stage

At the first stage, exploratory laparotomy is performed to exclude the possibility of peritoneal disease and to confirm the preoperative assessment of liver resectability. Ultrasound is used to confirm the preoperative imaging findings. If indicated, the FLR is then cleared of tumors with nonanatomical resection in order to preserve liver volume.

Portal Vein Occlusion

Portal vein ligation can be completed intraoperatively during the first stage. Alternatively, percutaneous portal vein embolization can be performed within a few days or weeks of stage one completion. The sFLR volume is then calculated 4–8 weeks after PVO using CT volumetry.

Inter-stage

In the initial description of TSH without PVE, chemotherapy was administered between stages [2], and administration of inter-stage chemotherapy does not appear to affect liver hypertrophy [42]. While some centers continue to advocate for this protocol in order to reduce the risk of disease progression between stages, its efficacy has not been proven [42–44]. The decision to offer inter-stage chemotherapy should be made with multidisciplinary input, and the potential advantages of additional systemic treatment should be weighed against the risk of delaying the second stage of TSH.

Second Stage

Once adequate FLR volume and function has been confirmed, the second laparotomy is completed. Typically, resection involves right hepatectomy or right trisectionectomy, depending on the tumor distribution (Fig. 28.1). Although less common, a left hepatectomy or left trisectionectomy can be performed using a right-sided FLR.

Techniques for Portal Vein Occlusion

Both PVL and PVE have been employed to induce hypertrophy of the FLR during TSH. Conflicting reports regarding the superiority of either technique have been published [45, 46]. Meta-analyses comparing PVE to PVL, without specifically limiting the analysis to TSH, suggest that FLR hypertrophy may be similar irrespective of the occlusion technique used [47, 48]. Nonetheless, it is generally believed that PVE is the superior technique for achieving reliable FLR hypertrophy. This is because PVE can more robustly occlude all portal vein branches, including occlusion of the segment IV portal vein branch, which is thought

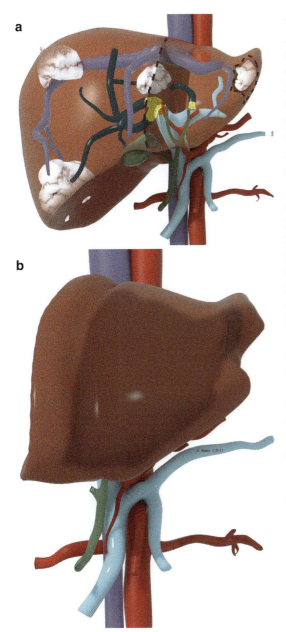

Fig. 28.1 (a) Illustration demonstrating extensive, challenging colorectal liver metastases. The dotted line demarcates the future liver remnant. Resection of metastases in the future liver remnant (left lateral section) is performed during the first stage of two-stage hepatectomy. Embolization of the right portal vein and segment IV portal vein branch is then performed, as illustrated. Extended right hepatectomy is performed during the second stage. (b) Illustration demonstrating the future liver remnant after two-stage hepatectomy with portal vein embolization (extended right hepatectomy)

to improve left lateral section regeneration [49]. As such, at centers with experienced interventional radiologists able to accomplish consistent embolization of all diseased segments, including segment IV, PVE should be preferred. Otherwise, PVL may offer adequate portal occlusion in most patients and has the advantage of reducing the total number of interventions required since it can be performed during the first stage of TSH.

PVE has been performed using various embolic materials [50, 51]. Excellent hypertrophic response has been obtained with the use of n-butyl 2-cyanoacrylate (NBCA), nonspherical polyvinyl alcohol particles (PVA), sodium tetradecyl sulfate foam (STS), and fibrin glue with iodized oil [52–55]. Distal tris-acryl microsphere embolization with proximal portal vein coiling has been shown to provide improved hypertrophy when compared with nonspherical PVA and may represent the best embolic material; however, no studies have compared microspheres with NBCA [56]. Overall, few studies have directly compared embolic agents, and the choice of agent is dependent on local availability and expertise.

Outcomes Following Classical TSH

While the two-stage approach to liver resection can be applied in a variety of primary and secondary liver tumors, the vast majority of published outcomes relate to its application for the treatment of CRLM. This reflects the most common and universally recommended indication for TSH. Several centers have published observational studies reporting the outcomes of TSH. Perioperative morbidity and mortality following TSH are acceptable, with poorer outcomes observed following the second stage during which the deportalized liver is removed. Pooled analysis of results has identified a first-stage morbidity of 17% and mortality of 0.5%, with a second-stage morbidity of 40% and mortality of 3%. Disease-free survival (DFS) tends to be poor following TSH, with a reported 3-year

DFS of 20%; however, 50% 3-year overall survival (OS) is excellent compared to historical controls treated with chemotherapy alone [12, 43, 57, 58]. Unfortunately, approximately one-third of patients do not reach the second stage due to disease progression and/or inadequate hypertrophy [59].

Associating Liver Partition and Portal Vein Ligation for Staged hepatectomy (ALPPS)

The conventional approach to two-stage hepatectomy is constrained by the major drawback of a prolonged waiting period between stages during which FLR hypertrophy occurs. While feasible in most patients, approximately 30% of the time the second stage cannot be completed [59]. The two main reasons for failure to complete two-stage hepatectomy are inadequate hypertrophy of the FLR or, more commonly, disease progression during the inter-stage hypertrophy period [57, 59]. Modifications of the original PVE technique, including embolization of segment IV provide an answer to the problem of inadequate hypertrophy [49]; however, short-interval disease progression continues to result in patient dropout between stages. The causes and implications of disease progression during conventional two-stage hepatectomy are topics of ongoing debate. It is unknown whether disease progression following portal vein occlusion is related to underlying tumor biology, or if tumor growth is stimulated by the prolonged period of liver ischemia and FLR hypertrophy. While the inter-stage period in conventional TSH has been hypothesized to act as a test of time for disease biology, this has not been proven, and some patients who may benefit oncologically from complete resection do not reach stage two with classical PVE or PVL.

Recently, ALPPS has emerged as an innovative technique to accelerate and intensify FLR hypertrophy, thereby reducing the time interval between stages and mitigating the risk of short-interval disease progression while avoiding postoperative liver failure. ALPPS was first reported in 2011 as a novel variation of two-stage hepatectomy [60, 61], and, since its introduction, it has generated considerable controversy and garnered mounting interest within the international hepatobiliary community. Enthusiasm for ALPPS has been moderated by concerns over elevated morbidity and mortality. Furthermore, due to its recent emergence, few long-term outcomes have been reported and many unanswered questions exist.

ALPPS was initially performed unintentionally in 2007 during a planned extended right hepatectomy for a perihilar cholangiocarcinoma [62]. An in situ division of the liver parenchyma along the falciform ligament combined with ligation of the right portal vein resulted in surprisingly accelerated and amplified growth of the left lateral section within 1 week. This facilitated subsequent right trisectionectomy, and the technique was later employed in planned approaches to patients with extensive, bilateral, or centrally located malignancies. The initial experience was published in 2012 [63], and, despite its infancy, the ALPPS approach has undergone considerable evolution since its introduction.

Technical Points

The initial description of ALPPS outlines the general approach, but many subsequent technical modifications have been suggested. The author's description of classical ALPPS is (Fig. 28.2):

- Stage one
  - Exploratory laparotomy with intraoperative assessment of resectability, including intraoperative liver ultrasonography
  - Cholecystectomy
  - Complete mobilization of the right lobe and caudate lobe including ligation and division of small venous branches draining directly into the inferior vena cava
  - Clearing of lesions from the FLR (if applicable)
  - Right portal vein ligation, approaching from behind the common hepatic duct, with preservation of the right hepatic artery and bile duct

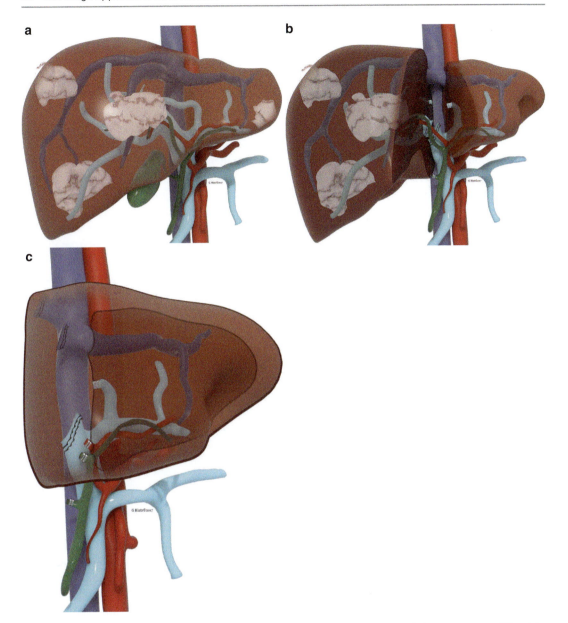

Fig. 28.2 (a) Illustration demonstrating extensive, challenging colorectal liver metastases, with a large central tumor and a small future liver remnant (FLR). Resection of the metastasis in the FLR (left lateral section) is required, with subsequent right trisectionectomy. ALPPS facilitates the necessary rapid hypertrophy of the FLR. (b) During ALPPS stage one, the metastasis in the left lateral section has been resected with a nonanatomic wedge resection, and an in situ parenchymal division has been performed starting anteriorly between segment IV and the left lateral section and targeting the right hilar plate. The right portal vein has been ligated along with the segment IV portal vein branch. (c) Hypertrophy of the future liver remnant is demonstrated. Right trisectionectomy has been completed during stage two of ALPPS. The middle hepatic vein, right hepatic vein, right bile duct, and right hepatic artery have been ligated

- Total parenchymal division at the right of the falciform ligament between segment IV and the left lateral section, targeting the right hilar plate
- Preservation of the right and middle hepatic veins, encircled with vessel loops
- Stage two
  - Division of the right hilar plate
  - Division of the right and middle hepatic veins
  - Completion of extended right hepatectomy (trisectionectomy)
  - Fixation of the left lateral section to the anterior abdominal wall

Variations

Numerous variations on the initial description have been reported [64]. Although limited data and no experimental studies exist comparing any of the modifications, several technical variants warrant mention. Firstly, portal vein ligation may be replaced with postoperative portal vein embolization in a modification termed hybrid ALPPS [65]. This approach may be applied in patients with tumors involving the right hilar plate in whom dissection around the right portal vein is not feasible. Secondly, the mechanism for achieving liver parenchymal splitting varies widely. While the initial technique of complete parenchymal transection continues to be commonly employed, partial transection of the parenchyma (typically, at least 50%), called partial ALPPS, has been proposed with the aim of improving the safety profile of stage one while inducing similar hypertrophy [66]. Other alternative methods, including radiofrequency ablation, microwave ablation, and tourniquet placement along the future line of liver transection, are practiced. The tourniquet modification has been termed associating liver tourniquet and portal ligation for staged hepatectomy (ALTPS) and offers an alternative technique for occluding vascular circulation during the first stage [67]. Lastly, due to the rapid hypertrophy induced by ALPPS, feasibility of TSH has been expanded to include patients with monosegment FLRs. Even some atypical FLRs, such as monosegment VI with venous drainage via an accessory right hepatic vein, have sufficed [68]. These resections are termed monosegment ALPPS, and individual cases may be named after the segment constituting the FLR [25].

In order to prevent segment IV ischemia and resultant infectious and biliary complications, specific attention should be paid to the blood supply and venous drainage of segment IV. During liver partition, the segment IV portal vein branch is transected; however, segment IV will have preserved blood supply through the segment IV arterial branch which usually arises from the left hepatic artery. Therefore, avoiding dissection of the hepatoduodenal ligament will minimize the risk of injury to the segment IV hepatic artery and prevent dearterialization. Moreover, preservation of the middle hepatic vein prevents postoperative venous congestion of segment IV and subsequent ischemia. If segment IV ischemia can be prevented, the hypothetical cascade of necrosis, biliary leak, severe sepsis, and death may be avoided in some patients. The author's preference is to preserve both the right and middle hepatic veins, in addition to the right hilar plate, placing vessel loops around all three structures during ALPPS stage one.

Laparoscopy has been used in one or both ALPPS stages and can be considered in the hands of surgeons highly experienced in both ALPPS and complex laparoscopic liver surgery [69]. Simultaneous ALPPS and colorectal resection for patients with synchronous colorectal liver metastases have also been performed at several high-volume ALPPS centers; however, the morbidity and mortality of this approach appear to be higher than after ALPPS alone [70].

Inter-stage Course

The principle advantage of ALPPS is extensive and accelerated FLR hypertrophy during the inter-stage interval. Compared to classical TSH, ALPPS achieves a FLR kinetic growth rate severalfold greater than conventional PVE and results in larger overall hypertrophy [71]. The two main explanations for accelerated growth are division of the microcirculation after liver partition and generation of circulatory growth factors. An experimental model in mice suggests that the later mechanism is the predominant driver of liver regeneration [72]. In this model, injection of plasma containing systemically released growth factors from ALPPS mice resulted in a comparable degree of liver hypertrophy in mice who were treated with PVL alone. The ensuing clinical significance is a truncated hypertrophy time of as little as 1 week with ALPPS, compared to several weeks with PVE.

The FLR size should be assessed before and after stage one with CT volumetry. However, it is important to recognize that volume alone is not necessarily an adequate indicator of function and that the majority of complications following ALPPS are related to sepsis associated with postoperative liver failure [37]. As such, assessment of FLR function prior to completion of stage two is important. For this purpose, the use of hepatobiliary scintigraphy (HIDA) or indocyanine green clearance may be considered. A mismatch between volume and function growth suggests a higher likelihood of liver failure, and, in these patients, stage two should be delayed or abandoned.

The inter-stage course is an important predictor of outcomes. Patients undergoing ALPPS who have an inter-stage course complicated by severe morbidity or signs of liver failure are at significantly higher risk of mortality if stage two is completed [73]. Specifically, those who meet International Study Group for Liver Surgery (ISGLS) criteria for postoperative liver failure or have a MELD score greater than 10 in the inter-stage period are at increased risk [37]. In those patients, as well as patients who have a complicated inter-stage course, consideration should be given to delaying or abandoning the second stage.

Indications for ALPPS

Since ALPPS has only recently been introduced, specific indications have yet to be defined. Typically, patients considered for ALPPS will

Table 28.1 Suggested criteria for ALPPS

Criteria
Oncological characteristics
Colorectal liver metastases
Absence of extrahepatic metastases (excluding resectable lung metastases)
Radiographical evidence of response to systemic chemotherapy after 4–6 cycles
Biochemical response to chemotherapy with reduction in serum carcinoembryonic antigen (CEA) level
Patient characteristics
Eastern Cooperative Oncology Group (ECOG) performance status 0 or 1
Absence of major medical comorbidities
Technical characteristics
Extensive bilobar metastases necessitating extended hepatectomy
Future liver remnant <30%
Technical feasibility of R0 resection

have bilateral, extensive hepatic tumor load that is initially unresectable. Furthermore, the FLR should be less than 30% and require rapid hypertrophy to facilitate two-stage resection. Regarding patient selection, the available evidence suggests that patients older than 60 and those with non-CRLM tumors have higher morbidity and mortality, perhaps due to cholestasis and/or parenchymal disease [37]. As such, until further evidence is available, ALPPS should generally be restricted to patients with CRLM. Nonetheless, some high-volume ALPPS centers may contemplate applying ALPPS in other tumors with caution and within a clinical trial setting. Lastly, in light of the higher perioperative risk associated with ALPPS, it should only be offered to patients without major comorbidities and good functional status. Based on the senior author's experience, specific criteria for ALPPS are suggested (Table 28.1).

Rescue ALPPS

In the subset of patients who fail to progress to stage two of conventional two-stage hepatectomy due to insufficient FLR hypertrophy during the 4–8-week growth period, few options exist. These options include repeated PVE with inclusion of the segment IV branches, embolization of the hepatic artery, and hepatic vein embolization. Hepatic vein embolization has been shown to be safe, while inducing additional hypertrophy in the setting of insufficient FLR growth following PVE, but there is limited evidence regarding the efficacy of these techniques and no comparative studies have been conducted [74, 75]. The rapid and reliable hypertrophy achieved by ALPPS has provided an alternative option [76]. In those patients with inadequate hypertrophy, but no evidence of inter-stage disease progression, laparotomy with liver partition results in accelerated FLR growth in a short period of time, facilitating reliable and expeditious completion of two-stage hepatectomy [77].

ALPPS Outcomes

Any discussion of ALPPS outcomes must be prefaced by acknowledging that ALPPS is in relative infancy and that a limited amount of high-quality evidence is available. Initial case series of ALPPS identified high morbidity and mortality [63, 78–82]. Subsequently, international registry-based studies have identified perioperative mortality of 9% and severe morbidity of 27% [37, 83]. These results are somewhat counterbalanced by other single center series demonstrating minimal perioperative morbidity and mortality with careful patient selection [84, 85]. Although no randomized controlled trial has been conducted, pooled analysis of observational studies suggests that ALPPS continues to have elevated perioperative risk compared to conventional TSH [86].

Evidence on long-term outcomes is even more limited. A case series on intermediate oncological outcomes reported 2-year overall survival of 59% [87]. Studies with longer follow-up examining both oncological outcomes and quality of life are eagerly anticipated.

Conclusion on ALPPS

Although some centers have adopted ALPPS as the primary approach to two-stage hepatectomy, the current paucity of data on long-term outcomes and the absence of experimental studies comparing conventional TSH with ALPPS do not support this decision. The good outcomes seen in some high-volume liver resection centers are encouraging and, if replicated in larger series, support the proliferation of ALPPS [84, 85, 88]. Perhaps the best current indication for ALPPS is in the setting of initially unresectable CRLM following failed PVE/PVL or in patients with monosegmental FLRs; however, ALPPS continues to be a topic of rich investigation and is currently in a phase of growing acceptance. While data from experimental, comparative studies are pending, TSH with PVE remains the gold standard for patients with extensive, bilobar or central liver tumors, and a very small predicted FLR.

> **Conclusion**
>
> TSH is an option for curative resection in patients with a very small predicted FLR. Careful patient selection and preoperative and inter-stage assessment of FLR function are essential. Conventional TSH with PVE remains the gold standard; however, ALPPS is adopting a growing role.

References

1. Bismuth H, Adam R, Lévi F, Farabos C, Waechter F, Castaing D, et al. Resection of nonresectable liver metastases from colorectal cancer after neoadjuvant chemotherapy. Ann Surg. 1996;224:509–20.
2. Adam R, Laurent A, Azoulay D, Castaing D, Bismuth H. Two-stage hepatectomy: a planned strategy to treat irresectable liver tumors. Ann Surg. 2000;232:777–85.
3. Makuuchi M, Thai BL, Takayasu K, Takayama T, Kosuge T, Gunvén P, et al. Preoperative portal embolization to increase safety of major hepatectomy for hilar bile duct carcinoma: a preliminary report. Surgery. 1990;107:521–7.
4. Jaeck D, Oussoultzoglou E, Rosso E, Greget M, Weber J-C, Bachellier P. A two-stage hepatectomy procedure combined with portal vein embolization to achieve curative resection for initially unresectable multiple and bilobar colorectal liver metastases. Ann Surg. 2004;240:1037–51.
5. Jaeck D, Bachellier P, Guiguet M, Boudjema K, Vaillant JC, Balladur P, et al. Long-term survival following resection of colorectal hepatic metastases. Br J Surg. 1997;84:977–80.

6. Fong Y, Fortner J, Sun RL, Brennan MF, Blumgart LH. Clinical score for predicting recurrence after hepatic resection for metastatic colorectal cancer: analysis of 1001 consecutive cases. Ann Surg. 1999;230:309–18.
7. Nordlinger B, Guiguet M, Vaillant JC, Balladur P, Boudjema K, Bachellier P, et al. Surgical resection of colorectal carcinoma metastases to the liver. A prognostic scoring system to improve case selection, based on 1568 patients. Cancer. 1996;77:1254–62.
8. Kishi Y, Abdalla EK, Chun YS, Zorzi D, Madoff DC, Wallace MJ, et al. Three hundred and one consecutive extended right hepatectomies: evaluation of outcome based on systematic liver volumetry. Ann Surg. 2009;127:171–9.
9. Shindoh J, Tzeng C-WD, Aloia TA, Curley SA, Zimmitti G, Wei SH, et al. Optimal future liver remnant in patients treated with extensive preoperative chemotherapy for colorectal liver metastases. Ann Surg Oncol. 2013;20:2493–500.
10. Shoup M, Gonen M, D'Angelica M, Jarnagin WR, DeMatteo RP, Schwartz LH, et al. Volumetric analysis predicts hepatic dysfunction in patients undergoing major liver resection. J Gastrointest Surg. 2003;7:325–30.
11. Pozzo C, Basso M, Cassano A, Quirino M, Schinzari G, Trigila N, et al. Neoadjuvant treatment of unresectable liver disease with irinotecan and 5-fluorouracil plus folinic acid in colorectal cancer patients. Ann Oncol. 2004;15:933–9.
12. Alberts SR. Oxaliplatin, fluorouracil, and leucovorin for patients with unresectable liver-only metastases from colorectal cancer: a North Central Cancer Treatment Group Phase II Study. J Clin Oncol. 2005;23:9243–9.
13. Ho WM, Ma B, Mok T, Yeo W, Lai P, Lim R, et al. Liver resection after irinotecan, 5-fluorouracil, and folinic acid for patients with unresectable colorectal liver metastases: a multicenter phase II study by the Cancer Therapeutic Research Group. Med Oncol. 2005;22:303–12.
14. Elias D, Baton O, Sideris L, Boige V, Malka D, Liberale G, et al. Hepatectomy plus intraoperative radiofrequency ablation and chemotherapy to treat technically unresectable multiple colorectal liver metastases. J Surg Oncol. 2005;90:36–42.
15. Michalopoulos GK, DeFrances MC. Liver regeneration. Science. 1997;276:60–6.
16. Riehle KJ, Dan YY, Campbell JS, Fausto N. New concepts in liver regeneration: new concepts in liver regeneration. J Gastroenterol Hepatol. 2011;26:203–12.
17. Lehmann K, Tschuor C, Rickenbacher A, Jang J, Oberkofler CE, Tschopp O, et al. Liver failure after extended hepatectomy in mice is mediated by a p21-dependent barrier to liver regeneration. Gastroenterology. 2012;143:1609–19.
18. Cataldegirmen G, Zeng S, Feirt N, Ippagunta N, Dun H, Qu W, et al. RAGE limits regeneration after massive liver injury by coordinated suppression of TNF-α and NF-κB. J Exp Med. 2005;201:473–84.
19. Michalopoulos GK. Liver regeneration. J Cell Physiol. 2007;213:286–300.
20. Kito Y, Nagino M, Nimura Y. Doppler sonography of hepatic arterial blood flow velocity after percutaneous transhepatic portal vein embolization. Am J Roentgenol. 2001;176:909–12.
21. Eipel C. Regulation of hepatic blood flow: the hepatic arterial buffer response revisited. World J Gastroenterol. 2010;16:6046.
22. Yokoyama Y, Nagino M, Nimura Y. Mechanisms of hepatic regeneration following portal vein embolization and partial hepatectomy: a review. World J Surg. 2007;31:367–74.
23. Lautt WW. Mechanism and role of intrinsic regulation of hepatic arterial blood flow: hepatic arterial buffer response. Am J Phys. 1985;249:G549–56.
24. Charnsangavej C, Clary B, Fong Y, Grothey A, Pawlik TM, Choti MA. Selection of patients for resection of hepatic colorectal metastases: expert consensus statement. Ann Surg Oncol. 2006;13:1261–8.
25. Schadde E, Malagó M, Hernandez-Alejandro R, Li J, Abdalla E, Ardiles V, et al. Monosegment ALPPS hepatectomy: extending resectability by rapid hypertrophy. Surgery. 2015;157:676–89.
26. Heymsfield SB, Fulenwider T, Nordlinger B, Barlow R, Sones P, Kutner M. Accurate measurement of liver, kidney, and spleen volume and mass by computerized axial tomography. Ann Intern Med. 1979;90:185–7.
27. Lodewick TM, Arnoldussen CWKP, Lahaye MJ, van Mierlo KMC, Neumann UP, Beets-Tan RG, et al. Fast and accurate liver volumetry prior to hepatectomy. HPB (Oxford). 2016;18:764–72.
28. Hermoye L, Laamari-Azjal I, Cao Z, Annet L, Lerut J, Dawant BM, et al. Liver segmentation in living liver transplant donors: comparison of semiautomatic and manual methods. Radiology. 2005;234:171–8.
29. Pomposelli JJ, Tongyoo A, Wald C, Pomfret EA. Variability of standard liver volume estimation versus software-assisted total liver volume measurement. Liver Transpl. 2012;18:1083–92.
30. Vauthey J-N, Abdalla EK, Doherty DA, Gertsch P, Fenstermacher MJ, Loyer EM, et al. Body surface area and body weight predict total liver volume in Western adults. Liver Transpl. 2002;8:233–40.
31. Johnson TN, Tucker GT, Tanner MS, Rostami-Hodjegan A. Changes in liver volume from birth to adulthood: a meta-analysis. Liver Transpl. 2005;11:1481–93.
32. Lafaro K, Buettner S, Maqsood H, Wagner D, Bagante F, Spolverato G, et al. Defining post hepatectomy liver insufficiency: where do we stand? J Gastrointest Surg. 2015;19:2079–92.
33. Hyder O, Pulitano C, Firoozmand A, Dodson R, Wolfgang CL, Choti MA, et al. A risk model to predict 90-day mortality among patients undergoing hepatic resection. J Am Coll Surg. 2013;216:1049–56.
34. Balzan S, Belghiti J, Farges O, Ogata S, Sauvanet A, Delefosse D, et al. The "50-50 Criteria" on postoperative day 5: an accurate predictor of liver failure and death after hepatectomy. Ann Surg. 2005;242:824–9.

35. Rahbari NN, Garden OJ, Padbury R, Brooke-Smith M, Crawford M, Adam R, et al. Posthepatectomy liver failure: a definition and grading by the International Study Group of Liver Surgery (ISGLS). Surgery. 2011;149:713–24.
36. Mullen JT, Ribero D, Reddy SK, Donadon M, Zorzi D, Gautam S, et al. Hepatic insufficiency and mortality in 1,059 noncirrhotic patients undergoing major hepatectomy. J Am Coll Surg. 2007;204:854–62.
37. Schadde E, Raptis DA, Schnitzbauer AA, Ardiles V, Tschuor C, Lesurtel M, et al. Prediction of mortality after ALPPS stage-1: an analysis of 320 patients from the International ALPPS Registry. Ann Surg. 2015;262:780–6.
38. Lam CM, Fan ST, Lo CM, Wong J. Major hepatectomy for hepatocellular carcinoma in patients with an unsatisfactory indocyanine green clearance test. Br J Surg. 1999;86:1012–7.
39. Cieslak KP, Bennink RJ, de Graaf W, van Lienden KP, Besselink MG, Busch ORC, et al. Measurement of liver function using hepatobiliary scintigraphy improves risk assessment in patients undergoing major liver resection. HPB (Oxford). 2016;18:773–80.
40. Chapelle T, Op De Beeck B, Huyghe I, Francque S, Driessen A, Roeyen G, et al. Future remnant liver function estimated by combining liver volumetry on magnetic resonance imaging with total liver function on 99mTc-mebrofenin hepatobiliary scintigraphy: can this tool predict post-hepatectomy liver failure? HPB (Oxford). 2016;18:494–503.
41. de Graaf W, van Lienden KP, Dinant S, Roelofs JJTH, Busch ORC, Gouma DJ, et al. Assessment of future remnant liver function using hepatobiliary scintigraphy in patients undergoing major liver resection. J Gastrointest Surg. 2010;14:369–78.
42. Muratore A, Zimmitti G, Ribero D, Mellano A, Viganò L, Capussotti L. Chemotherapy between the first and second stages of a two-stage hepatectomy for colorectal liver metastases: should we routinely recommend it? Ann Surg Oncol. 2012;19:1310–5.
43. Wicherts DA, Miller R, de Haas RJ, Bitsakou G, Vibert E, Veilhan L-A, et al. Long-term results of two-stage hepatectomy for irresectable colorectal cancer liver metastases. Ann Surg. 2008;248:994–1005.
44. Narita M, Oussoultzoglou E, Bachellier P, Rosso E, Pessaux P, Jaeck D. Two-stage hepatectomy procedure to treat initially unresectable multiple bilobar colorectal liver metastases: technical aspects. Dig Surg. 2011;28:121–6.
45. Robles R, Marín C, Lopez-Conesa A, Capel A, Perez-Flores D, Parrilla P. Comparative study of right portal vein ligation versus embolisation for induction of hypertrophy in two-stage hepatectomy for multiple bilateral colorectal liver metastases. Eur J Surg Oncol. 2012;38:586–93.
46. Homayounfar K, Liersch T, Schuetze G, Niessner M, Goralczyk A, Meller J, et al. Two-stage hepatectomy (R0) with portal vein ligation—towards curing patients with extended bilobular colorectal liver metastases. Int J Color Dis. 2009;24:409–18.
47. Pandanaboyana S, Bell R, Hidalgo E, Toogood G, Prasad KR, Bartlett A, et al. A systematic review and meta-analysis of portal vein ligation versus portal vein embolization for elective liver resection. Surgery. 2015;157:690–8.
48. Vyas S, Markar S, Partelli S, Fotheringham T, Low D, Imber C, et al. Portal vein embolization and ligation for extended hepatectomy. Indian J Surg Oncol. 2014;5:30–42.
49. Mise Y, Aloia TA, Conrad C, Huang SY, Wallace MJ, Vauthey J-N. Volume regeneration of segments 2 and 3 after right portal vein embolization in patients undergoing two-stage hepatectomy. J Gastrointest Surg. 2015;19:133–41.
50. Loffroy R, Favelier S, Chevallier O, Estivalet L, Genson P-Y, Pottecher P, et al. Preoperative portal vein embolization in liver cancer: indications, techniques and outcomes. Quant Imaging Med Surg. 2015;5:730–9.
51. Avritscher R, de Baere T, Murthy R, Deschamps F, Madoff DC. Percutaneous transhepatic portal vein embolization: rationale, technique, and outcomes. Semin Intervent Radiol. 2008;25:132–45.
52. de Baere T, Denys A, Paradis V. Comparison of four embolic materials for portal vein embolization: experimental study in pigs. Eur Radiol. 2009;19:1435–42.
53. de Baere T, Teriitehau C, Deschamps F, Catherine L, Rao P, Hakime A, et al. Predictive factors for hypertrophy of the future remnant liver after selective portal vein embolization. Ann Surg Oncol. 2010;17:2081–9.
54. Fischman AM, Ward TJ, Horn JC, Kim E, Patel RS, Nowakowski FS, et al. Portal vein embolization before right hepatectomy or extended right hepatectomy using sodium tetradecyl sulfate foam: technique and initial results. J Vasc Interv Radiol. 2014;25:1045–53.
55. Nagino M, Kamiya J, Nishio H, Ebata T, Arai T, Nimura Y. Two hundred forty consecutive portal vein embolizations before extended hepatectomy for biliary cancer: surgical outcome and long-term follow-up. Ann Surg. 2006;243:364–72.
56. Madoff DC, Abdalla EK, Gupta S, Wu T-T, Morris JS, Denys A, et al. Transhepatic ipsilateral right portal vein embolization extended to segment IV: improving hypertrophy and resection outcomes with spherical particles and coils. J Vasc Interv Radiol. 2005;16:215–25.
57. Lam VWT, Laurence JM, Johnston E, Hollands MJ, Pleass HCC, Richardson AJ. A systematic review of two-stage hepatectomy in patients with initially unresectable colorectal liver metastases. HPB (Oxford). 2013;15:483–91.
58. Koopman M, Antonini NF, Douma J, Wals J, Honkoop AH, Erdkamp FL, et al. Sequential versus combination chemotherapy with capecitabine, irinotecan, and oxaliplatin in advanced colorectal cancer (CAIRO): a phase III randomised controlled trial. Lancet. 2007;370:135–42.
59. Chua TC, Liauw W, Chu F, Morris DL. Summary outcomes of two-stage resection for advanced colorectal

liver metastases: two-stage resection of CLM. J Surg Oncol. 2013;107:211–6.
60. Baumgart J, Lang S, Lang H. A new method for induction of liver hypertrophy prior to right trisectionectomy: a report of three cases. HPB (Oxford). 2011;13(suppl 2):1–145.
61. de SE, Alvarez FA, Ardiles V. How to avoid postoperative liver failure: a novel method. World J Surg. 2011;36:125–8.
62. de Santibañes E, Clavien P-A. Playing Play-Doh to prevent postoperative liver failure: the "ALPPS" approach. Ann Surg. 2012;255:415–7.
63. Schnitzbauer AA, Lang SA, Goessmann H, Nadalin S, Baumgart J, Farkas SA, et al. Right portal vein ligation combined with in situ splitting induces rapid left lateral liver lobe hypertrophy enabling 2-staged extended right hepatic resection in small-for-size settings. Ann Surg. 2012;255:405–14.
64. Edmondson MJ, Sodergren MH, Pucher PH, Darzi A, Li J, Petrowsky H, et al. Variations and adaptations of associated liver partition and portal vein ligation for staged hepatectomy (ALPPS): many routes to the summit. Surgery. 2016;159:1058–72.
65. Li J, Kantas A, Ittrich H, Koops A, Achilles EG, Fischer L, et al. Avoid "All-Touch" by Hybrid ALPPS to achieve oncological efficacy. Ann Surg. 2016;263:e6–7.
66. Linecker M, Kambakamba P, Reiner CS, Linh Nguyen-Kim TD, Stavrou GA, Jenner RM, et al. How much liver needs to be transected in ALPPS? A translational study investigating the concept of less invasiveness. Surgery. 2017;161:453–64.
67. Robles R, Parrilla P, López-Conesa A, Brusadin R, de la Peña J, Fuster M, et al. Tourniquet modification of the associating liver partition and portal ligation for staged hepatectomy procedure. Br J Surg. 2014;101:1129–34.
68. Pineda-Solís K, Paskar D, Tun-Abraham M, Hernandez-Alejandro R. Expanding the limits of resectability: associating liver partition and portal vein ligation for staged hepatectomy (ALPPS) using monosegment 6, facilitated by an inferior right hepatic vein. J Surg Oncol. 2017;115(8):959–62.
69. Machado MAC, Makdissi FF, Surjan RC, Basseres T, Schadde E. Transition from open to laparoscopic ALPPS for patients with very small FLR: the initial experience. HPB (Oxford). 2017;19:59–66.
70. Wanis KN, Buac S, Linecker M, Ardiles V, Tun-Abraham ME, Robles-Campos R, et al. Patient survival after simultaneous ALPPS and colorectal resection. World J Surg. 2017;41:1119–25.
71. Croome KP, Hernandez-Alejandro R, Parker M, Heimbach J, Rosen C, Nagorney DM. Is the liver kinetic growth rate in ALPPS unprecedented when compared with PVE and living donor liver transplant? A multicentre analysis. HPB (Oxford). 2015;17:477–84.
72. Schlegel A, Lesurtel M, Melloul E, Limani P, Tschuor C, Graf R, et al. ALPPS: from human to mice highlighting accelerated and novel mechanisms of liver regeneration. Ann Surg. 2014;260:839–47.
73. Truant S, Scatton O, Dokmak S, Regimbeau J-M, Lucidi V, Laurent A, et al. Associating liver partition and portal vein ligation for staged hepatectomy (ALPPS): impact of the inter-stages course on morbi-mortality and implications for management. Eur J Surg Oncol. 2015;41:674–82.
74. Nagino M, Kanai M, Morioka A, Yamamoto H, Kawabata Y, Hayakawa N, et al. Portal and arterial embolization before extensive liver resection in patients with markedly poor functional reserve. J Vasc Interv Radiol. 2000;11(8):1063.
75. Hwang S, Lee S-G, Ko G-Y, Kim B-S, Sung K-B, Kim M-H, et al. Sequential preoperative ipsilateral hepatic vein embolization after portal vein embolization to induce further liver regeneration in patients with hepatobiliary malignancy. Ann Surg. 2009;249:608–16.
76. Tschuor C, Croome KP, Sergeant G, Cano V, Schadde E, Ardiles V, et al. Salvage parenchymal liver transection for patients with insufficient volume increase after portal vein occlusion – an extension of the ALPPS approach. Eur J Surg Oncol. 2013;39:1230–5.
77. Enne M, Shadde E, Björnsson B, Hernandez Alejandro R, Gayet B, Steinbruck K, et al. The ALPPS as salvage procedure after unsuccessful portal vein occlusion. "Give then another chance….". HPB (Oxford). 2016;e6:18.
78. Torres OJM, Fernandes E de SM, Oliveira CVC, Lima CX, Waechter FL, Moraes-Junior JMA, et al. Associating liver partition and portal vein ligation for staged hepatectomy (ALPPS): the Brazilian experience. Arq Bras Cir Dig. 2013;26:40–3.
79. Li J, Girotti P, Königsrainer I, Ladurner R, Königsrainer A, Nadalin S. ALPPS in right trisectionectomy: a safe procedure to avoid postoperative liver failure? J Gastrointest Surg. 2013;17:956–61.
80. Knoefel WT, Gabor I, Rehders A, Alexander A, Krausch M, Schulte am Esch J, et al. In situ liver transection with portal vein ligation for rapid growth of the future liver remnant in two-stage liver resection. Br J Surg. 2013;100:388–94.
81. Ratti F, Cipriani F, Gagliano A, Catena M, Paganelli M, Aldrighetti L. Defining indications to ALPPS procedure: technical aspects and open issues. Updat Surg. 2013;66:41–9.
82. Schadde E, Ardiles V, Slankamenac K, Tschuor C, Sergeant G, Amacker N, et al. ALPPS offers a better chance of complete resection in patients with primarily unresectable liver tumors compared with conventional-staged hepatectomies: results of a multicenter analysis. World J Surg. 2014;38:1510–9.
83. Schadde E, Ardiles V, Robles-Campos R, Malago M, Machado M, Hernandez-Alejandro R, et al. Early survival and safety of ALPPS: first report of the International ALPPS Registry. Ann Surg. 2014;260:829–38.
84. Hernandez-Alejandro R, Bertens KA, Pineda-Solis K, Croome KP. Can we improve the morbidity and mortality associated with the associating liver partition with portal vein ligation for staged hepatectomy

(ALPPS) procedure in the management of colorectal liver metastases? Surgery. 2015;157:194–201.
85. Alvarez FA, Ardiles V, de Santibañes M, Pekolj J, de Santibañes E. Associating liver partition and portal vein ligation for staged hepatectomy offers high oncological feasibility with adequate patient safety: a prospective study at a single center. Ann Surg. 2015;261:723–32.
86. Eshmuminov D, Raptis DA, Linecker M, Wirsching A, Lesurtel M, Clavien P-A. Meta-analysis of associating liver partition with portal vein ligation and portal vein occlusion for two-stage hepatectomy. Br J Surg. 2016;103:1768–82.
87. Björnsson B, Sparrelid E, Røsok B, Pomianowska E, Hasselgren K, Gasslander T, et al. Associating liver partition and portal vein ligation for staged hepatectomy in patients with colorectal liver metastases – intermediate oncological results. Eur J Surg Oncol. 2016;42:531–7.
88. Røsok BI, Björnsson B, Sparrelid E, Hasselgren K, Pomianowska E, Gasslander T, et al. Scandinavian multicenter study on the safety and feasibility of the associating liver partition and portal vein ligation for staged hepatectomy procedure. Surgery. 2016;159:1279–86.

Index

A
Abdominal compression, 84, 161, 315
Active breathing control (ABC), 315
Acute Physiology and Chronic Health Evaluation (APACHE) score, 4
Adjuvant chemotherapy, 294, 299
Adjuvant therapy, 294
Adriamycin, 334, 359
Alpha-fetoprotein (AFP) level, 45
American Society of Anesthesiologists (ASA) scale, 4
Angiogenesis, 218, 273
Antiemetics, 220
Anti-epidermal growth factor receptor (EGFR), 217
Anti-reflux microcatheters, 67
Anti-vascular endothelial growth factor (VEGF) antibodies, 217
Apoptosis-mediated cell death, 208
Associating liver partition and portal vein ligation for staged hepatectomy (ALPPS), 378
 criteria for, 381
 indications for, 381, 382
 inter-stage course, 380, 381
 outcomes, 382
 perihilar cholangiocarcinoma, 378
 rescue, 381, 382
 technical modification, 378, 380
 variation, 380
Associating liver tourniquet and portal ligation for staged hepatectomy (ALTPS), 380

B
Balloon occlusion microcatheters, 67
Barcelona Clinic Liver Cancer (BCLC) system, 46, 57, 58, 69
Benign hepatic tumors
 bile duct hamartomas, 21
 focal nodular hyperplasia, 18, 19
 hemangiomas, 15–18
 hepatic cyst, 15, 16
 hepatocellular adenomas, 19–21
 intrahepatic biliary cystadenoma, 21
Bevacizumab, 142, 218, 224, 226, 236, 240, 271, 273, 274
Bile duct hamartoma, 15, 21

Biliary intraepithelial neoplasia (BilIN)
 BilIN-3/CIS, 178
 definition, 177
 high-grade dysplasia, 178
 histopathologic diagnosis, 178, 179
 incidence, 178
 IPNBs, 179–181
 low-grade dysplasia, 178
 three-tiered grading scheme, 178
Biliary sclerosis (BS), 236
Biliary tract cancer, 137
 extrahepatic, 137
 intrahepatic (*see* Intrahepatic cholangiocarcinoma)
Bilobar disease, 243
Bilobar liver perfusion, 235
Biocompatible resin, 225
Biphenotypic tumors, 297, 298
Bland embolization, *see* Transarterial embolization (TAE)
Bleeding hepatocellular adenomas, 158, 160
Brachytherapy, 293
Brivanib, 92

C
Cabozantinib, 93, 144, 273, 274
Calcifications, 27
Cannulation, 235
Capecitabine, 118, 140, 274, 295, 359
Capillary hemangiomas, 16, 17
Carcinoembryonic antigen (CEA), 102, 225
Carcinoid syndrome, 270
Carcinoids, 268, 270, 274
CCA, *see* Cholangiocarcinoma (CCA)
Cetuximab, 218, 237, 240
Charged particle therapy, 130, 132
Charged particle-based therapy, 319
Charlson Comorbidity Index (CCI), 4
Chemoembolization, 57
Chemoresponsiveness, 283
Chemotherapy, 233, 299
Chemotherapy-associated liver injury (CALI), 218
Child-Pugh classification, 46, 47, 49, 64, 73–75, 78, 80, 83, 91, 94, 376

Child-Turcotte-Pugh (CTP) score, 6, 130
Chimeric antigen receptor (CAR) T cell therapy, 94
Chlorozotocin, 274
Cholangiocarcinoma (CCA), 99, 100
    classification, 291
    clinical presentation and diagnosis, 291, 292
    complications, 364
    current organ allocation and patient selection, 293, 294
    ICCA (*see* Intrahepatic cholangiocarcinoma (ICCA))
    incidence and mortality, 291 (*see also* Intrahepatic cholangiocarcinoma)
    locoregional therapy, 334
    perihilar cholangiocarcinoma
        adjuvant therapy, 294
        Kaplan-Meier curves, 295, 296
        Mayo protocol for, 293
        neoadjuvant therapy, 294, 295
        resection, 292, 293
    systemic chemotherapy in, 359
    toxicities of, 364–367
Cholangiocellular (biliary) cystadenocarcinoma, 27
Choledochal cysts, 190, 191
Chromogranin A levels, 259
Chromophores, 324
Chronic intrahepatic stone disease, 291
Ciliated hepatic foregut cysts, 191, 192
Cirrhosis, 7, 291, 297
Cisplatin, 274, 299, 359
CLOCC trial, 212
Coagulative necrosis, 207
Colorectal cancer (CRC), 233, 302–304, 311, 313, 316, 317, 319
Colorectal cancer liver metastases (CRLM), 6, 233, 373, 377
    ablative techniques, 199
        cryoablation, 210, 211
        image guidance, 208
        indications for, 207, 208
        irreversible electroporation, 213
        MWA, 209, 210
        percutaneous ablations, 208
        radiofrequency ablation, 208, 209
        thermal ablation, 211–213
    aggressive resection for, 375
    chemotherapy, 233
    external beam radiation therapy, 200
    FLR augmentation, 199
    HAI chemotherapy (*see* Hepatic artery infusion (HAI) therapy)
    margin status, 199
    minimally invasive approaches, 200
    multimodality therapy, 197
    non-resectional therapies, 200
    oncologic resectability, 198
    perioperative chemotherapy, 198, 199
    physiologic assessment, 197
    SIRT, 200
    surgical approach
        extent and distribution, 200, 201
        parenchymal-sparing hepatectomy, 201
        resection + ablation, 201
        two-stage hepatectomy, 202
    technical resectability, 198
    transarterial chemoembolization, 200
    treatment for, 217, 233
Colorectal cancer metastases, 28
Common bile duct (CBD), 234
Common hepatic artery (CHA), 234
Computerized tomography (CT) scan, 4, 15, 312, 315, 325, 326
    capillary hemangiomas, 17
    HCC, 23
    hepatic cyst, 15
    hepatocellular adenomas, 20
    mass-forming tumors, 25
    simulation, 313
Computerized tomography-guided high-dose brachytherapy (CT-HDRBT), 119
Conventional transarterial chemoembolization (cTACE), 63, 64, 68, 113–115, 218, 219, 221, 222
CRLM, *see* Colorectal cancer liver metastases (CRLM)
Cryoablation, 58, 59, 61, 210, 211, 256
Cryoablation-induced injury, 210
Cryoshock, 59, 61
cTACE, *see* Conventional transarterial chemoembolization (cTACE)
CyberKnife® system, 315
Cystic hamartomas, 187
Cystic liver metastases, 27
Cytoreduction, 243, 245, 246
Cytotoxic chemotherapy, 274, 275

D

DEBIRI, 116, 117, 222, 224
Degradable starch microsphere chemoembolization (DSM-TACE), 218
Dexamethasone, 220, 224, 236, 238, 260, 359, 364
Discontinue octreotide therapy, 256
Disease-free interval, 6, 283–285
Disease-free survival (DFS), 237, 301, 377
Disease-specific survival (DSS), 233
Dose-escalated radiotherapy, 129
Downstaging therapy, 41, 58, 70
Doxorubicin, 94, 274
Drug-eluting beads (DEBs), 258
Drug-eluting beads transarterial chemoembolization (DEB-TACE), 113, 115–117
Drug-eluting embolic transarterial chemoembolization (DEE-TACE), 63–65
    hepatitis C cirrhosis with TIPS, 65, 66
    TARE, 66–68
Drug-eluting embolics (DEEs), 64

E

Eastern Cooperative Oncology Group (ECOG) Performance Status, 4, 245
Embolotherapy, 260
Endoscopic retrograde cholangiopancreatography (ERCP), 103, 120, 292

Enucleation, 247–249
Eovist-enhanced magnetic resonance imaging (MRI), 7
Epirubicin, 334, 359
Etoposide, 274, 275
European Organization for Research and Treatment of Cancer Quality of Life Questionnaire Core 30 (QLQ-C30), 319
Everolimus, 145, 271–273
Exploratory laparotomy, 295
External beam radiation therapy (EBRT), 73
Extrahepatic disease, 4, 211, 249, 283
Extrahepatic perfusion, 235, 236

F

Fast low-angle shot (FLASH), 329
Fibrolamellar hepatocellular carcinoma, 23, 24
5-fluorouracil chemotherapy, 237, 240, 293, 364
5-fluorouracil, leucovorin, oxaliplatin (FOLFOX), 95, 139, 198, 224, 225, 237, 238, 274
Floxuridine (FUDR), 67, 233, 236, 238, 239
FLR, see Future liver remnant (FLR)
Fluorodeoxyglucose positron emission tomography (FDG-PET), 315
Focal Nodular Hyperplasia (FNH), 18, 19
FOLFIRI, 237, 238
Four-dimensional (4D) computerized tomography, 315
FUDR, see Floxuridine (FUDR)
Functional Assessment of Cancer Therapy-Hepatobiliary (FACT-Hep, version 4) questionnaires, 319
Future liver remnant (FLR), 3, 6, 373–375, 378, 381, 382
  assessment of, 7, 8, 375, 376
  atypical, 380
  augmentation, 199
  PVE, 376
  second laparotomy, 376

G

Gadoxetate disodium (Eovist®), 325, 328, 329
Gastroduodenal artery (GDA), 234, 235
Gastroenteropancreatic neuroendocrine tumors (GEP-NETs), 243, 245
  epidemiology and clinical presentation, 267–270
  grade 1 and 2, 272
    interferon-alpha, 271
    PNETs (see Pancreatic neuroendocrine tumors (PNETs))
    PRRT, 271, 272
    somatostatin analogues, 270, 271
    targeted therapies, 271
  G3 neuroendocrine carcinomas (NECs), cytotoxic chemotherapy, 274, 275
  somatostatin analogues, 267
Gastrointestinal stromal tumors (GIST), 281
Gemcitabine, 120, 218, 359
Gemcitabine-based combination chemotherapy, intrahepatic cholangiocarcinoma, 138
Genitourinary group, 280
Genitourinary primaries, 280

GEP-NETs, see Gastroenteropancreatic neuroendocrine tumors (GEP-NETs)
Giant hemangioma, 18
Gold fiducials, 313
Growth rate of metastases, 283
G3 neuroendocrine carcinomas (NECs), cytotoxic chemotherapy, 274, 275

H

Heat sink effect, 59, 62
Hemangiomas, 15–18
Hemihepatectomies, 246
Hepatectomy, 283
Hepatic adenomas (HAs)
  core needle biopsy, 169
  follow-up, 174
  hepatic artery embolization, 172, 173
  hypervascular HA, 173
  imaging, 169
  incidence rate, 170
  microwave ablation, 171
  prevalence, 169
  radiofrequency ablation, 170, 171, 173, 174
  risk factors, 170
  surgical management, 170
  surveillance, 174
Hepatic arterial drug-eluting bead (HAT-DEB) therapy, 218
  adverse effect, 221, 222
  oncologic outcomes, 222
  rationale, 220
  safety and efficacy, 223
  systemic therapy and surgery, 222, 224
  technical success and complications, 221, 222
  technique, 220, 221
Hepatic arterial infusion (HAI), 221
Hepatic arterial infusion pump (HAIP) placement, 234, 235
Hepatic arterial phase (HAP), 16
Hepatic arterial therapy (HAT)
  HAT-DEB therapy
    adverse effect, 221, 222
    oncologic outcomes, 222
    rationale, 220
    safety and efficacy, 223
    systemic therapy and surgery, 222, 224
    technical success and complications, 221, 222
    technique, 220, 221
  transarterial hepatic embolization
    rationale, 218
    reported technique, 218, 220
  Yttrium-90 (Y-90) radioembolization
    concomitant use with systemic chemotherapy, 225, 226
    efficacy and response evaluation, 225
    rationale and patient selection, 224
    safety and efficacy, 226
    surgery, 225, 226
    treatment and toxicity, 224, 225

Hepatic artery infusion (HAI) therapy, 202, 203
  in adjuvant setting, 236–239
  conversion to complete resection, 233
  disease-specific survival, 233
  FUDR, 233
  postoperative assessment, 236
  primary liver cancers
    CCA, 334, 359–368
    hepatocellular carcinoma, 334
    rationale for, 333
  randomized controlled trials, 237
  technical aspects
    complications, 235, 236
    continuous or bolus infusion, 234
    placement, 234, 235
    totally implantable infusion pumps, 234
  unresectable CRLM, 239, 240
Hepatic burden of disease (HBD), 225
Hepatic cysts, 15, 16
Hepatic focal nodular hyperplasia, 19
Hepatic hemangiomas, 17
Hepatic iminodiacetic acid (HIDA) derivatives, 318
Hepatic inflammatory adenoma, 21
Hepatic resection, 279
  oncologic appropriateness
    CRLM, 6
    HCC, 4–6
    ICC, 5
    preoperative evaluation, 4
  patient selection, surgical fitness of patient, 3, 4
  technical resectability
    assessment of liver function, 6, 7
    biliary anatomy, 7
    definition, 6
    FLR, 7, 8
    vascular inflow/outflow, 7
Hepatic venous balloon occlusion, 67
Hepatitis B (HBV), 297
Hepatitis C cirrhosis, 65, 66, 68
Hepatitis C virus (HCV), 45, 297
Hepatobiliary scintigraphy (HIDA), 381
Hepatoblastoma, in children
  chemotherapy, 299
  liver resection, 298, 299
  POSTEXT IV, 299
  PRETEXT III, 299
  staging, 298
Hepatocellular adenomas (HCAs), 19–21
  ablation, 161
  adenomatosis, 157
  β-catenin mutation, 155
  clinical presentation, 154
  complications, 158
  embolization, 160, 161
  follow-up, 162
  HNF1A, 154, 155
  IL6/JAK/STAT pathway, 155
  liver biopsy, 159, 160
  liver transplantation, 161
  macroscopic view, 154
  pregnancy, 161, 162
  radiological classification, 155–158
  risk factors, 153, 158, 159
  sonic hedgehog mutation, 155
  Wnt/β-catenin pathway, 155
Hepatocellular carcinoma (HCC), 23, 24, 52, 319, 333, 334
  CAR T cell therapy, 94
  checkpoint inhibitors, 93
  chemotherapy, 94, 95
  clinical prognostic indicators, 4
  DEEs, 64
  definition, 91
  EBRT, 73
  vs. ICC, 100, 102
  incidence of, 73
  Korean Practice guidelines, 73
  liver-directed radiotherapy, 73
  liver toxicity prevention
    absolute volume constraints, 83
    mean liver dose constraints, 80, 83
    relative volume constraints, 83
  liver transplantation for
    considerations for, 52
    disparities in access to transplantation, 39, 40
    downstaging therapy, 41
    exception policy, 38, 39
    history of, 38
    ITT, 50, 51
    LDLT, 41, 42
    MELD-based allocation, 38, 39
    Milan criteria, 40, 41, 48
    outcomes, 49
    overall survival and disease-free survival, 49–51
    patients with hepatocellular carcinoma, 52
    salvage transplantation, 51
    severe cirrhosis, 49
    UCSF criteria, 48
    UNOS modified TNM staging, 38
  local and systemic therapy, 95
  locoregional therapies (see Locoregional therapies)
  multifocality, 5
  National Comprehensive Cancer Network guidelines, 73
  patient-specific factors, 45
  PBR, 78–82
  preoperative assessment
    diagnosis, 45, 46
    surgical candidacy, 46
  radiation therapy, 73
  RTOG 1112 (NCT01730937) trial, 85
  SBRT, 75–78
  surgical resection (SR)
    considerations for, 52
    ITT, 50, 51
    nonanatomic resection, 48
    outcomes, 48
    overall survival and disease-free survival, 49–51
    patients selection, 46

in patient with Child-Pugh A cirrhosis, 46
patients with hepatocellular carcinoma, 52
salvage transplantation, 51
sFLR, 47
surgical resection in patient with Child-Pugh A cirrhosis, 47
TAE, 69, 70
treatment planning and delivery, 83–85
tumor size, 5
tyrosine kinase inhibitors, 91–93
vaccine therapy, 93, 94
vascular invasion, 5
Hepatoduodenal ligament, 234
HNF-1a-mutated hepatocellular adenoma, 22
Hypervascular hepatic lesion, 45
Hypervascular liver metastases, 28
Hypoattenuation, 27

I

Image-guided radiation therapy (IGRT), 313, 315
Imatinib, 281
Immunosuppressive therapy, 302
Indocyanine green (ICG), 7
Inflammatory hepatocellular adenoma (IHCA), 19, 155–159
Intensity-modulated radiation therapy (IMRT), 311
Intention-to-treat (ITT) analysis, 50
Interferon (IFN)-alpha, 271
Interleukin-2, 237
International Childhood Liver Tumors Strategy Group (SIOPEL), 299
International normalized ratio (INR), 38
International Study Group for Liver Surgery (ISGLS) criteria, 376, 381
Interstitial tissue ablation, 325
Interventional magnetic resonance imaging technology, 325, 326, 328, 329
Intestinal-type peri-ampullary cancers, 281
Intra-arterial chemotherapy, 236
Intraductal oncocytic papillary neoplasms, 181
Intraductal papillary neoplasms of the bile duct (IPNB), 179–181, 188, 189
Intraductal tubulopapillary neoplasm of the bile duct (ITPN), 181, 189, 190
Intraductal tumors, 25
Intrahepatic biliary cystadenoma, 15, 21
Intrahepatic cholangiocarcinoma (ICCA), 24, 26, 27, 113–119, 128–132, 142, 291, 292, 333, 359, 364
adjuvant therapy, 105, 106, 125, 126, 139–140
biliary drainage, 103
CA 19-9 biomarker, 100
CEA, 102
chemotherapy, 126
classification, 112
clinical presentation, 99–101
C-MET/hepatocyte growth factor (HGF), 144
CT-HDRBT, 119, 120
diagnosis, 100, 102, 111, 112
epidermal growth factor receptor (EGFR)/HER2 signaling pathways, 141, 142
ERCP, 120
fibroblast growth factor receptor (FGFR) 2 fusions, 142, 143
vs. HCC, 100, 102
hepatic tissue tolerance, 127
immunotherapy, 146
incidence, 99, 111, 125
incidental and biphenotypic tumors, 297, 298
intra-arterial therapies
cTACE, 113–115
DEB-TACE, 113, 115–118
RFA, 119
Y90-RE technique, 117–119
isocitrate dehydrogenase (IDH) 1/IDH2 mutations, 143, 144
locoregional therapy, 112, 113
low survival rates and high recurrence rates, 297
lymph node involvement, 295
mitogen-activated ERK kinase (MEK) pathway, 144, 145
molecular-targeted therapy, 140, 141
mortality, 99
multifocal, 6
neoadjuvant therapy, 105, 127, 128
pathology, 102
and perihilar CCA, 297
PI3K/AKT/mTOR pathway, 145
prognosis, 111
PTC, 120
radiotherapy
charged particle therapy, 130, 132
with chemotherapy, 132
dose-escalated radiotherapy, 129
liver-directed radiotherapy, 128
mandatory dose constraints for organs, 132
SBRT, 129–131
3D-CRT, 128, 129
whole-liver radiotherapy, 128
resectability assessment, 103–105
risk factors, 99, 111
routine staging laparoscopy, 105
SBRT, 120
staging of, 102, 103
surgical resection, 112, 137
survival rate, 137
systemic chemotherapy, 120, 137–139
TACE, 127
treatment, 104, 106, 107
tumor recurrence, 106
tumor size, 5
unresected tumors, 127
vascular endothelial growth factor (VEGF) agents, 142
Intrahepatic exophytic nodular tumors, 24
IRE, *see* Irreversible electroporation (IRE)
Irinotecan, 218, 238, 240
Irinotecan-based therapy, 221
Irreversible electroporation (IRE), 60, 61, 207, 208, 212, 213, 243, 249, 323

J
Joule-Thompson effect, 210

K
KRAS mutations, 141, 142, 144, 179, 199

L
LC Bead LUMI™ (BTG), 65
Lipiodol, 69, 114, 115, 258, 259
Liver metastasectomy, 284
Liver metastases, number and size of, 283
Liver regeneration, 374, 375
Liver transplantation (LT)
    ablation, 62
    CCA, 295
        classification, 291
        clinical presentation and diagnosis, 291, 292
        current organ allocation and patient selection, 293, 294
        ICCA (*see* Intrahepatic cholangiocarcinoma (ICCA))
        incidence and mortality, 291
        Mayo protocol for perihilar cholangiocarcinoma, 293
        perihilar cholangiocarcinoma, 294–296
        resection, 292, 293
    HCC
        considerations for, 52
        disparities in access to transplantation, 39, 40
        downstaging therapy, 41
        exception policy, 38, 39
        history of, 38
        ITT, 50, 51
        LDLT, 41, 42
        MELD-based allocation, 38, 39
        Milan criteria, 40, 41, 48
        outcomes, 49
        overall survival and disease-free survival, 49–51
        patients with hepatocellular carcinoma, 52
        salvage transplantation, 51
        severe cirrhosis, 49
        UCSF criteria, 48
        UNOS modified TNM staging, 38
    for hepatoblastoma in children
        chemotherapy, 299
        liver resection, 298, 299
        PERTEXT III, 299
        POSTEXT IV, 299
        staging, 298
    NERLMs, 251, 252
    NET (*see* Neuroendocrine tumor (NET))
    secondary liver cancer, 300
Liver, morphologic and clinical features of, 312
Liver-directed radiotherapy, 73
Liver-directed therapies, 41, 58, 279
    patient selection, 256, 257
    procedure, 257, 258
    treatment follow-up, 258
Living donor liver transplantation (LDLT), 37, 41, 42
Local recurrence-free survival (LRFS), 251
Locoregional therapies, 323, 334, 359, 364
    BCLC guidelines, 57, 58
    DEE-TACE, 64, 65
        hepatitis C cirrhosis with TIPS, 65
        TARE, 66–68
    ICC, 112, 113
    image-guided percutaneous ablation
        combination therapies, 62, 63
        cryoablation, 58, 59, 61
        IRE, 60–62
        liver transplantation, 62
        microwave ablation, 60
        MWA, 61
        vs. resection, 62
        RFA, 59–61
    image-guided transcatheter tumor therapies for, cTACE, 63, 64
    TAE, 68, 69
    transplant patient, approach to, 70
Long-acting repeatable (LAR) octreotide acetate, 270
Lymphadenectomy, 106, 112

M
Macroaggregated albumin (MAA), 224, 236
Magnetic resonance cholangiopancreatography(MRCP), 103, 111, 112, 191, 292
Magnetic resonance fluoroscopy, 330
Magnetic resonance imaging-guided laser ablation, 324, 325
    ablation/monitoring phase, 330, 331
    accurate mapping of hepatic tumor burden, 325
    confirmation phase, 330
    guidance phase, 329, 330
    interventional MRI setup, 328, 329
    IRE, 323
    laser ablative energy, choosing, 327
    microwave ablation, 323
    principles of, 324
        applied energy level and duration, 324, 325
        laser wavelength, 324
        tissue compositions, 324
    real-time monitoring of individual tumor response, 326, 327
    RFA, 323
    target tumor, laser applicator into, 325, 326
Magnetic resonance imaging (MRI), 4, 315
    FNH, 18
    HCC, 23
    hepatic cyst, 15
Mammalian target of rapamycin (mTOR) pathway, 271, 273
Mass-forming tumors, 25
Mebrofenin, 318
Melanoma, 280
Melanoma metastasis, 29
Melanoma-derived liver metastases, 281
MELD, *see* Model for end-stage liver disease (MELD)

Metroticket model, 40
Microcatheter, 260
Microwave ablation (MWA), 60, 61, 209, 210, 243, 248, 249, 251, 256, 323
Milan criteria, 5, 40–42, 46, 48, 49, 51, 62, 63, 251, 252
Milan size criteria, 298
Mitomycin C, 218, 237, 359
Mitotic index (MI), 300
Model for end-stage liver disease (MELD), 7, 38, 39, 46, 48, 293, 295, 304, 376, 381
Modified Response Evaluation Criteria in Solid Tumors (mRECIST), 41, 260
Molecular-targeted therapies, 217
Mucinous cystic neoplasms (MCNs), 181–183
Mucinous cystic neoplasms of liver (MCN-L), 187–189
Multicentric hepatocarcinogenesis, 5
MWA, *see* Microwave ablation (MWA)

N
National Cancer Database (NCDB) analysis, 106
National Comprehensive Cancer Network, 73, 300
Neoadjuvant protocol, 295
Neoadjuvant therapy, 299
Neuroendocrine Tumor Society guidelines, 301
Neuroendocrine tumors (NET), 243
    ablation modilities
        cryoablation, 256
        MWA, 256
        RFA, 256
    hepatic metastases, 255
    incidence of, 255
    liver-directed therapies
        patient selection, 256, 257
        procedure, 257–258
        treatment follow-up, 258
    strategies to limit tumor recurrence, 301, 302
    tumor ablation, 255–256
    unresectable, 300, 301
Neuroendocrine tumors liver metastases (NETLMs)
    anatomic liver resection, 246, 247
    categories, 243
    extent of resection, 245, 246
    liver transplantation, 251–252
    parenchymal-sparing procedures, 247
        ablative techniquess, 249, 251
        enucleation, 247–249
        wedge resections, 247
    patient selection, 244, 245
    SBNET metastases, 244
    surgical management of, 250–251
    survival rates, 243
Nivolumab, 93, 95, 146
Nonalcoholic steato-hepatitis (NASH), 218
Nonalcoholic steatohepatitis (NASH)-induced cirrhosis, 45
Non-colorectal gastrointestinal tract, 281
Non-colorectal metastases
    epidemiology of, 279, 280
    survival outcomes, 280–282

Non-neuroendocrine (NCNN) liver metastases, 279
    epidemiology of, 279, 280
    prognostic factors of survival, 282, 283
    selecting patients for surgical resection, 283–285
    survival outcomes, 280–282
Non-small cell lung cancer (NSCLC), 319
Nontargeted liver metastases, 222
Normal tissue complication probability (NTCP) model, 83, 317

O
Octreotide, 257, 270, 271
Ocular melanoma, 281, 285
Oligometastases, 311
Oligometastatic disease, 319
Oncocytic papillary cystadenocarcinomas, 181
Oral capecitabine plus intra-arterial epirubicin, 359
Organ Procurement and Transplantation Network (OPTN), 38
Orthotopic liver transplantation (OLT), 104
    CRC, 302–304
    NET, 300–302
Oxaliplatin, 238, 240, 364
OxMdG, 226

P
Pancreatic neuroendocrine tumors (PNETs), 268
    cytotoxic therapy, 274
    somatostatin analogues, 272
    targeted therapies, 272–274
Parenchymal-sparing hepatectomy (PSH), 201
Parenchymal-sparing procedures (PSP), 243, 244, 246, 247
    ablative technique, 249, 251
    enucleation, 247–249
    wedge resections, 247
Pazopanib, 143, 273
Pegylated-interferon-alpha (PEG-IFN), 271
Peptide receptor radionuclide therapy (PRRT), 271, 272
Percutaneous ablative technique, 251
Percutaneous transhepatic cholangiography (PTC), 120
Periductal infiltrating intrahepatic tumors, 24, 25
Periductal infiltrating tumors, 25
Perihilar cholangiocarcinoma, 293, 294, 297, 378
    adjuvant therapy, 294
    Kaplan-Meier curves, 295, 296
    Mayo protocol for, 293
    neoadjuvant therapy, 294, 295
Peripheral low-density area sign, 27
Peripheral washout sign, 27
Phase III CLARINET trial, 270
Platelet-derived growth factor receptors (PDGFR), 273
Portal hypertension, 7
Portal vein embolization (PVE), 47, 67, 373, 376, 377
Portal vein occlusion (PVO), 374, 376, 377
Portal vein tumor thrombus (PVT), 67
Portal venous phase (PVP), 16, 18, 20, 23
Post-hepatectomy liver failure (PHLF), 375
PRECISION V trial, 64

Preinvasive neoplastic cysts
   biliary intraepithelial neoplasia (BilIN)
      BilIN-3/CIS, 178
      definition, 177
      high-grade dysplasia, 178
      histopathologic diagnosis, 178, 179
      incidence, 178
      IPNBs, 179–181
      low-grade dysplasia, 178
      three-tiered grading scheme, 178
   choledochal cysts, 190, 191
   ciliated hepatic foregut cysts, 191, 192
   intraductal oncocytic papillary neoplasms, 181
   IPNB, 188, 189
   ITPN, 181, 189, 190
   MCN-L, 187–189
   MCNs, 181–183
PREMIERE trial, 69, 70
Pretreatment extent of disease (PRETEXT) classification, 298, 299
Primary liver cancers, HAI therapy
   CCA, 334, 359–364, 368
   hepatocellular carcinoma, 334
   rationale for, 333
Primary malignant hepatic tumors
   cholangiocellular (biliary) cystadenocarcinoma, 27
   HCC, 23, 24
   ICC, 24, 27
Primary sclerosing cholangitis (PSC), 127
Primary tumor site, 282
Progression-free survival (PFS), 238, 247, 270, 271, 334
PROMID phase III trial, 270
Proper hepatic artery (PHA), 234, 235
Proton beam and carbon ion beam therapy, 319
Proton beam radiation (PBR) therapy, 78–82
PSPs, see Parenchymal-sparing procedures (PSP)
PVE, see Portal vein embolization (PVE)

Q
Quantitative Analysis of Normal Tissue Effects in the Clinic (QUANTEC) organ-specific paper, 83

R
Radiation hepatitis, 80, 128
Radiation segmentectomy, 67
Radiation Therapy Oncology Group (RTOG), 312, 318
Radiation-induced liver disease (RILD), 312, 317
   clinical presentation, 80
   diagnosis, 80
   pathophysiology, 80
   treatment and prognosis, 80
Radioembolization, 66, 244
Radiofrequency (RF), 209, 327
Radiofrequency ablation (RFA), 59–63, 119, 208–213, 243, 247–249, 256, 302, 319, 323
Ramucirumab, 92
Rapidly filling hemangiomas, 18
Real-time temperature mapping, 327, 330
Regorafenib, 92, 143
Response Evaluation Criteria in Solid Tumors (RECIST), 224, 225, 260
Revised Cardiac Risk Index (RCRI), 4
RFA, see Radiofrequency ablation (RFA)
RILD, see Radiation-induced liver disease (RILD)

S
Salvage liver transplantation, 300
Salvage transplantation, 51
SARAH trial, 69
SBRT, see Stereotactic body radiation therapy (SBRT)
Sclerosed hemangiomas, 16, 18
Secondary (metastatic) malignant hepatic tumors, 27
Selective internal radiation therapy (SIRT), 66, 200, 259
Selective internal radiation, SIR-Spheres, 225
Simulation process, 315
Single-photon emission computed tomography (SPECT), 260, 318
Sinusoidal obstruction syndrome (SOS), 218
SIR-Spheres®, 67
SIRveNIB trial, 69
Small bowel adenocarcinoma liver metastases, 281
Small hepatic tumors, 323
Somatostatin analogues, 245, 267, 270–272
Sonography-guided microwave ablation, 119
Sorafenib, 69, 85, 91, 273
Standardized future liver remnant (sFLR) volume, 47
Steatotic hepatocellular adenomas, 156
Stereotactic body radiation therapy (SBRT), 311
   charged particle-based therapy, 319
   delivery of, 319
   in extracranial tumors, 315
   fractionated, 313
   HCC, 75–78
   high-dose RT, 312
   hypofractionation, 316–318
   ICC, 120, 129–131
   IGRT, 313
   local control, 313, 316
   long-term sequelae from radiation, 318, 319
   motion management, 315
   patient selection, 313
   patient setup and treatment, 315
   phase III randomized trial, 319
   prospective trials, 313, 314, 316, 319
   single-fraction treatment, 316
   TCP curves, 317
   vascular injury and ensuing chaotic intra-tumoral environment, 312
STOP-HCC trial, 69
Streptozocin, 274
Sunitinib, 91, 273
Surveillance, Epidemiology, and End Results (SEER) database, 267
Systemic chemotherapy, see Gastroenteropancreatic neuroendocrine tumors (GEP-NETs)
Systemic chemotherapy (CTx), 221

T

Targeted therapies, 141, 267, 271–274
Taxane-based therapy, 274
^{99m}Tc-mebrofenin hepatobiliary scintigraphy (HIDA) scan, 376
Temozolomide, 274, 275
Temperature mapping techniques, 328
Thalidomide, 274
TheraSpheres, 225
Thermal ablation, 211–213
Thermal map, 326
Three-dimensional (3D) computerized tomography imaging, 313
Three-dimensional conformal radiotherapy (3D-CRT), 74, 75, 128, 129
Tivantinib, 92, 144
Total damage estimate map, 326
Total liver volume (TLV), 8, 375
Transarterial and systemic therapies, 224
Transarterial chemoembolization (TACE), 62, 63, 95, 127, 200, 258–260, 302, 334
Transarterial chemoinfusion (TACI), 107
Transarterial drug-eluting beads, 218
Transarterial embolization (TAE), 63, 68–70, 258, 260
Transarterial hepatic embolization
  rationale, 218
  reported technique, 218, 220
Transarterial radioembolization (TARE), 63, 66–68, 106, 259–261
Transarterial therapies
  patient selection, 259, 260
  procedure, 260
  TAE therapy, 258
  TARE, 259
  transarterial chemoembolization (TACE), 258, 259
  treatment follow-up, 260, 261
Transcatheter irradiation, 293
Transjugular intrahepatic portosystemic shunt (TIPS), 38, 66
Transverse arteriotomy, 235
Treatment- and tumor burden-related factors, 283
Tremelimumab, 95
Transarterial chemoembolization (TACE), 302
Tumor ablation, 255, 256
Tumor control probability (TCP) model, 317
Tumor necrosis, 221
Turbo spin echo (TSE) scans, 330
T1-weighted images
  hemangiomas, 18
  hepatocellular adenomas, 20
T2-weighted images
  colorectal cancer metastases, 28
  FNH, 18
  hemangiomas, 18
  hepatic hemangiomas, 16
  hepatocellular adenomas, 20
  ICC, 27

Two-stage hepatectomy (TSH), 202, 375, 376, 378, 380–382
  ALPPS, 378
    criteria for, 381
    indications for, 381, 382
    inter-stage course, 380, 381
    outcomes, 382
    perihilar cholangiocarcinoma, 378
    rescue, 381, 382
    technical modification, 378, 380
    variation, 380
  criteria for, 375
  first stage, 376
  FLR, 374–376
  inter-stage chemotherapy, 376
  liver regeneration, 374, 375
  outcomes, 377, 378
  PVE, 373
  PVO, 376, 377
  second satge, 376
Two-thirds partial hepatectomy (PH), 374

U

Ultrasound, 257
  HCC, 23
  hemangiomas, 18
Un-enhanced computerized tomography, 20, 26
United Network for Organ Sharing (UNOS)/OPTN criteria, 38
Unresectable colorectal cancer liver metastases, 239, 240
Unresectable disease, 212, 233
University of California-San Francisco (UCSF) criteria, 41, 48

V

Vascular endothelial growth factor (VEGF), 92, 142, 144, 273
Vauthey formula, 375
Veno-occlusive injury, 312
Viral infection, 291
Visualase™ laser system, 330
Volumetric interpolated breath-hold examination (VIBE)), 331

Y

Yttrium-90 radioembolization (Y90-RE) technique, 117–119
concomitant use with systemic chemotherapy, 225, 226
efficacy and response evaluation, 225
rationale and patient selection, 224
safety and efficacy, 226
surgery, 225, 226
treatment and toxicity, 224, 225